Springhouse Review for NCLEX-PN

Fourth Edition

Springhouse Review for

NCLEX-PN

Fourth Edition

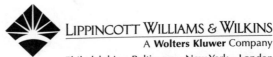

LIPPINCOTT WILLIAMS & WILKINS
A **Wolters Kluwer** Company

Philadelphia • Baltimore • New York • London
Buenos Aires • Hong Kong • Sydney • Tokyo

STAFF

Publisher
Judith A. Schilling McCann, RN, MSN

Editorial Director
David Moreau

Clinical Director
Joan M. Robinson, RN, MSN

Senior Art Director
Arlene Putterman

Clinical Editors
Kate McGovern, RN, MSN, CCRN (project manager);
Anita Lockhart, RN,C, MSN

Editors
Jaime L. Stockslager (senior associate editor), Kevin Haworth,
Brenna H. Mayer

Electronic Products Manager
John Macalino

Electronic Products Associate Editor
Liz Schaeffer

Copy Editors
Kimberly Bilotta, Scotti Cohn, Tom DeZego, Heather Ditch,
Amy Furman, Shana Harrington, Judy Orioli, Carolyn Peterson,
Marcia Ryan, Dorothy Terry, Patricia Turkington, Pamela Wingrod

Electronic Production Services
Diane Paluba (manager), Joyce Rossi Biletz (senior desktop assistant),
Donna S. Morris (project manager)

Manufacturing
Patricia Dorshaw (senior manager), Beth Janae Orr

Editorial Assistants
Danielle J. Barsky, Beverly Lane, Linda Ruhf

Indexer
Karen C. Comerford

The clinical procedures described and recommended in this publication are based on research and consultation with medical and nursing authorities. To the best of our knowledge, these procedures reflect currently accepted clinical practice; nevertheless, they can't be considered absolute and universal recommendations. For individual application, treatment recommendations must be considered in light of the patient's clinical condition and, before administration of new or infrequently used drugs, in light of the latest package-insert information. The authors and the publisher disclaim responsibility for any adverse effects resulting directly or indirectly from the suggested procedures, from any undetected errors, or from the reader's misunderstanding of the text.

NCLEXPN4 – D N O

04 03 02   10 9 8 7 6 5 4 3 2 1

Library of Congress Cataloging-in-Publication Data

Springhouse review for NCLEX-PN. — 4th ed.
    p. ; cm.
    Rev. ed. of: American nursing review for NCLEX PN / Leona A. Mourad. 3rd ed. c1998.
    Includes bibliographical references and index.
    1. Practical nursing — Examinations, questions, etc.
I. Mourad, Leona A. American nursing review for NCLEX PN.
II. Lippincott Williams & Wilkins.
    [DNLM: 1. Nursing, Practical — Examination Questions.
WY 18.2 S7696 2003]
RT62.M68 2003
610.73'076 — dc21
ISBN 1-58255-132-4 (pbk. : alk. paper)   2002011857

Contents

Contributors

Lula J. English, RN, MSN
Practical Nursing Instructor
Reid State Technical College
Evergreen, Ala.

Margaret M. Gingrich, RN, MSN
Associate Professor
Harrisburg (Pa.) Area Community College

Karla Jones, RN, MSN
Faculty, Nursing Department
Treasure Valley Community College
Ontario, Ore.

Carol Kohn-Keeth, RN, DNSc
Nurse Consultant and Complemental Faculty
Rush University College of Nursing
Chicago

Patricia B. Lisk, RN, BSN
Instructor
Augusta (Ga.) Technical College

Dawna Martich, RN, MSN
Clinical Trainer
American Healthways
Pittsburgh

Lourdes "Cindy" Reddy, MSN, MeD, CRNP, CPP, FAAPM
Nurse Practitioner Educator
Frankford Hospital School of Nursing
Philadelphia

Janet A. Rudolph, RN, MSN, CEN
Nursing Instructor
Brandywine School of Nursing
Coatesville, Pa.

Catherine Shields, RN, BSN
LPN Nurse Educator
Career and Technical Institute, School of Nursing
Lakehurst, N.J.

Willie B. Williams, RN, MS
Practical Nursing Instructor
Atlantic Technical Center
Coconut Creek, Fl.

Linda S. Wood, RN, MSN
Director of Practical Nursing
Massanutten Technical Center
Harrisonburg, Va.

You're ready to go out into the work force and show the world all that you've learned in the previous months, but you have one more step to take before you can practice with the title of "Licensed Practical Nurse"—you must first take the National Council Licensure Examination for Licensed Practical Nurses (NCLEX-PN). This test covers all areas of your nursing education, and you're worried that you won't remember everything that has been taught to you during the past several months. Don't fret; we have the tools you need to reach that final goal of becoming a licensed practical nurse. *Springhouse Review for NCLEX-PN* and its supplementary disc have been helping students pass the NCLEX-PN exam for years.

In this indispensable study tool, some of the most experienced nurses in the field have compiled their years of experience and expertise in order for you to have the knowledge, skills, guidance, and assurance you need to pass the comprehensive NCLEX exam with ease.

In addition to offering a wealth of coverage in all of the major clinical areas, *Springhouse Review for NCLEX-PN,* 4th Edition, shows you how to organize your review, highlights aspects of the testing procedure and, most important, helps you achieve NCLEX success. An 85-question pretest, including rationales for correct and incorrect answers, helps you identify areas in which you need the most review, allowing you to concentrate your study and save time. In addition, all of the questions have been updated to reflect the latest NCLEX-PN test plan.

Once you've identified the areas you need to concentrate on most, it's time to begin your review. Chapters 1 and 2 cover specifics about the NCLEX-PN exam, including test-taking strategies, preparation tips, and guidelines on how to organize your review. The indispensable tips found in this section help you manage your time and establish good study habits, resulting in the alleviation of your anxiety over taking the NCLEX-PN exam.

After this introduction to the test, chapters 3 and 4, an overview of the fundamentals of nursing, cover key topics and test points on nursing concepts and skills as well as maintaining homeostasis. The remaining chapters review the major nursing topics covered on the exam—perioperative, mental health, maternal-neonatal, pediatric, and adult nursing.

Each chapter presents diseases and disorders in an easy-to-use format that includes the nursing process. For example, the entry on heart failure includes a description of the disorder, its *possible causes; data collection findings; diagnostic findings;* associated *nursing diagnoses; treatment,* including *drug therapy options;* and *patient care goals.* Most important, the *nursing interventions* are broken down into bulleted lists with rationales for each intervention clearly identified. An *evaluation* of the patient goals finishes the nursing process coverage.

The review process is completed with a challenging 85-question posttest, which allows you to assess the effectiveness of your review. As if that weren't enough, the CD-ROM in the back of the book contains an additional 750 review questions to help build your confidence before you tackle the actual exam. On the disc, you can select review questions by subject or you can choose to answer questions in random order. After answering questions, you'll immediately receive feedback about your answers as well as rationales for correct and incorrect answer choices. The posttest and CD-ROM review questions are set in the same format as the pretest—a format identical to that of the NCLEX-PN exam—which will enhance your familiarity with the testing format as well as increase your knowledge and understanding of key information.

Study icons throughout the book help you organize your review sessions and enhance retention of information. These unique features include:

Fast fact—Key information is set off in shaded boxes throughout the text to help you repeat and recall important review material.

Spot check—Questions are randomly included throughout the text to verify that you understand the material.

Quick study — Limericks, mnemonics, and other creative strategies present easy ways to help you retain information.

Clinical situation — A variety of clinical situations that focus on the PN's role promote your understanding of nursing practice. Nursing principles are applied to advance your understanding, and questions are posed to promote further thought. You'll incorporate some of the valuable information you've learned in this book with the information you've learned in the classroom to solve these questions.

Nursing procedure — Commonly used nursing procedures are reviewed with detailed, step-by-step instructions.

To ensure NCLEX success, you not only need to carefully set up your review schedule but also need to make time to care for yourself. Get lots of rest, good nutrition, and adequate exercise so that you'll be in tip-top shape when you go to take the test. Preparing yourself physically, emotionally, and cognitively will surely lead to your success. You're almost through with your preparation to enter a rewarding and challenging career. As a new LPN, you'll become a part of the health care team during a time of renewal of patriotism, courage, and fortitude. I wish you the best of luck in your future.

Linda Sue Wood, RN, MSN
Director of Practical Nursing
Massanutten Technical Center
Harrisonburg, Va.

Instructions

The pretest has been designed to determine your knowledge base before you begin your study program for the NCLEX-PN. By analyzing the results, you can identify the areas in which you may wish to do more comprehensive study.

The pretest contains 85 questions, written in the format used in the computerized examination. Each question has four answer choices. Read each question and all possible answers carefully; then select the best answer.

Take no more than 85 minutes to complete the pretest. If you have difficulty understanding a question or you aren't sure of the answer, place a small mark next to the question number — but still select an answer, even if you have to guess. The mark will help you recall that you had trouble with that question. However, be aware that on the computerized examination, you will *not* be able to go back to a question or go on to the next question without selecting an answer choice.

In the pretest, possible answers are labeled A, B, C, and D to help identify the correct answer and the rationale. These letters don't appear in the actual computerized NCLEX-PN.

The pretest answer choices appear as:

A. Atonic
B. Dystonic
C. Hypotonic
D. Hypertonic

The NCLEX-PN answer choices appear as:

Atonic
Dystonic
Hypotonic
Hypertonic

Now, select a quiet room where you'll be undisturbed, set a timer for 85 minutes, and begin the first pretest.

After you've completed the pretest or the 85-minute time limit expires, check your responses against the correct answers provided on pages xx to xxx.

Questions

1. A client had an abdominal hysterectomy 10 hours ago. Which position should the nurse teach the client to avoid?
- ☐ **A.** High Fowler's
- ☐ **B.** Lateral recumbent
- ☐ **C.** Supine
- ☐ **D.** Side-lying

2. The physician orders an upper GI series for a client with GI complaints. The nurse teaches the client about the upper GI series. Which statement indicates that the client understands the instructions?
- ☐ **A.** "I'll have a special instrument passed through my mouth into my stomach."
- ☐ **B.** "I'll take several tablets the night before the test."
- ☐ **C.** "I'll drink a contrast medium while X-rays are taken."
- ☐ **D.** "I'll have a CT scan taken after I'm injected with a radioactive substance."

3. A client returns from surgery. Which nursing diagnosis takes priority at this time?
- ☐ **A.** Ineffective breathing pattern
- ☐ **B.** Deficient fluid volume
- ☐ **C.** Imbalanced nutrition: Less than body requirements
- ☐ **D.** Diarrhea

4. A client had abdominal surgery 2 days ago. Which data collection finding suggests that the client has developed a postoperative complication?
- ☐ **A.** Serous wound drainage
- ☐ **B.** Weakness when ambulating
- ☐ **C.** Abdominal distention
- ☐ **D.** Muscle soreness

5. Shortly after a multigravida client is admitted to the hospital in labor, her amniotic membranes rupture. Which action should the nurse take first?
- ☐ **A.** Check fetal heart tones.
- ☐ **B.** Turn the client onto her left side.
- ☐ **C.** Take the client's blood pressure.
- ☐ **D.** Change the pad under the client's buttocks.

6. A client is scheduled to receive a blood transfusion. During the transfusion, the nurse should observe for which sign or symptom of a transfusion reaction?
- ☐ **A.** Dizziness
- ☐ **B.** Chills
- ☐ **C.** Hypothermia
- ☐ **D.** Hyperreflexia

7. A 2-year-old child with cystic fibrosis is admitted to the hospital with pneumonia. The child receives aerosol treatments followed by percussion and postural drainage four times per day. Which nursing diagnosis takes priority for this client?
- ☐ **A.** Imbalanced nutrition: Less than body requirements related to appetite loss
- ☐ **B.** Anxiety (parental and child) related to acute illness
- ☐ **C.** Anticipatory grieving related to life-threatening illness
- ☐ **D.** Ineffective airway clearance related to tenacious tracheobronchial secretions

8. Which of the following reflexes should the nurse discuss and demonstrate to educate the parents about providing a safe environment for their neonate?
- ☐ **A.** Babinski's
- ☐ **B.** Stepping
- ☐ **C.** Tonic neck
- ☐ **D.** Prone crawl

9. A client with status asthmaticus is in severe respiratory distress. The nurse should maintain the client in which position?
- ☐ **A.** Upright sitting
- ☐ **B.** Side-lying
- ☐ **C.** Supine
- ☐ **D.** Prone

10. A client is admitted to the hospital with symptoms of left-sided heart failure. The physician prescribes digoxin (Lanoxin), 0.125 mg daily, and a low-sodium diet. When assessing this client, the nurse should expect to find which of the following signs?
- ☐ **A.** Tingling sensation in the fingers
- ☐ **B.** Dyspnea
- ☐ **C.** Abdominal distention
- ☐ **D.** Engorged neck veins

11. The physician informs a client that he'll need heart surgery. Later, the client tells the nurse angrily, "When you deal with a surgeon, you can only expect he'll want to cut you up." Which response by the nurse would be most appropriate?
- ☐ **A.** "I'm sure the surgeon knows what he's doing."
- ☐ **B.** "I think you're too upset to think clearly."
- ☐ **C.** "You're wondering if the surgery is necessary."
- ☐ **D.** "You're concerned about the skill of the surgeon."

12. A client has been placed on a low-sodium diet. The client would show an understanding of the dietary instructions by selecting which of the following foods as having the lowest sodium content?
- ☐ **A.** Canned tomato soup
- ☐ **B.** Broiled lobster
- ☐ **C.** Tapioca pudding
- ☐ **D.** Fresh string beans

13. A child undergoes a tonsillectomy and an adenoidectomy. During the early postoperative period, the nurse should observe the child closely for:
- ☐ **A.** frequent swallowing.
- ☐ **B.** intermittent moaning.
- ☐ **C.** incontinence.
- ☐ **D.** lethargy.

14. The husband of a client who is in labor asks the nurse what his role should be because his wife seems uncomfortable. The nurse explains that the coach's primary role is to be:
- ☐ **A.** an active support person throughout the labor.
- ☐ **B.** an observer who primarily participates during delivery.
- ☐ **C.** a witness to the labor and delivery experience.
- ☐ **D.** an information giver to all other family members not present at the birth.

15. A client is admitted to the hospital with signs and symptoms of a stroke. The client is unconscious on admission. The health care team starts an I.V. infusion and inserts a central venous pressure line. When the client is admitted to the nursing unit, the nurse should assign highest priority to which goal?
- ☐ **A.** Preventing skin breakdown
- ☐ **B.** Promoting urinary elimination
- ☐ **C.** Maintaining a patent airway
- ☐ **D.** Preserving muscle function

16. A child is scheduled for a tonsillectomy and an adenoidectomy. Preoperatively, which nursing assessment is essential?
- ☐ **A.** Examining for loose teeth
- ☐ **B.** Comparing the apical and radial pulse rates
- ☐ **C.** Checking the function of the facial nerve
- ☐ **D.** Determining the range of motion of the head and neck

17. A client begins to sob uncontrollably after learning that a tumor removed from the lung is cancerous. How should the nurse deal with this situation?
- ☐ **A.** Remain with the client and allow the client to cry.
- ☐ **B.** Leave the room and find out whether the client can have a sedative.
- ☐ **C.** Ask the client exactly what the physician said.
- ☐ **D.** Explain that it's important for the client not to cry now.

18. The physician prescribes an I.V. infusion of 1,000 ml of 5% dextrose in water every 12 hours for a client. The I.V. setup delivers 15 gtt/ml. Approximately how many drops should be administered each minute?
- ☐ **A.** 18
- ☐ **B.** 21
- ☐ **C.** 24
- ☐ **D.** 27

19. Two hours after a client delivers a neonate, the nurse assesses the client to determine whether she's ready for transfer to the postpartum unit. Which assessment finding warrants immediate nursing intervention?
- ☐ **A.** Temperature of 99.8° F (37.7° C); heart rate of 70 beats/minute
- ☐ **B.** Breasts soft and not tender; colostrum present
- ☐ **C.** Uterine fundus soft and located left of midline
- ☐ **D.** Moderate lochia rubra containing small clots

20. A client is receiving clonidine (Catapres). Which nursing action is appropriate for this client?
- ☐ **A.** Teach the client to change position slowly.
- ☐ **B.** Give the medication before meals.
- ☐ **C.** Instruct the client to take the medication with orange juice.
- ☐ **D.** Offer the client a cup of tea with meals.

21. While visiting a client who is recovering from a stroke, the client's husband asks the nurse, "Why does my wife have a splint on her hand?" The nurse explains that the splint is necessary to prevent:
- ☐ **A.** injury to the hand.
- ☐ **B.** deformity of the hand.
- ☐ **C.** muscle wasting in the hand.
- ☐ **D.** edema of the hand.

22. A client requires tracheal suctioning through the nose. Which nursing action would be incorrect?
- ☐ **A.** Lubricating the catheter with sterile water before beginning
- ☐ **B.** Applying suction when withdrawing the catheter from the nose
- ☐ **C.** Suctioning for 30 seconds
- ☐ **D.** Rotating the catheter when withdrawing it

23. A client with emphysema is scheduled to receive oxygen by nasal cannula. Which measure should the nurse take when caring for this client?
- ☐ **A.** Maintain the oxygen flow rate at no more than 3 L/minute.
- ☐ **B.** Increase the oxygen flow rate to 6 L/minute, if required.
- ☐ **C.** Teach the client to adjust the oxygen flow rate as needed.
- ☐ **D.** Change the oxygen tubing at each shift.

24. As the nurse assists a client with breathing exercises, the client says, "I don't feel any better. Why should I bother learning how to do these exercises?" How should the nurse respond?
- ☐ **A.** Tell the client that the physician ordered the exercises.
- ☐ **B.** Encourage the client to express his feelings.
- ☐ **C.** Ask the client whether he would like to do the exercises at another time.
- ☐ **D.** Inform the physician of the client's statements.

25. A client is admitted to the facility with a tentative diagnosis of acute pyelonephritis. To assess for risk factors for pyelonephritis, the nurse should ask the client which question?
- ☐ **A.** "Do you have pain in your back?"
- ☐ **B.** "Have you had a sore throat lately?"
- ☐ **C.** "Do you hold your urine for a long time before voiding?"
- ☐ **D.** "Have you taken any analgesics recently?"

26. A child is in skin traction. To help prevent a common complication of immobility, the nurse should include which measure in the child's care plan?
- ☐ **A.** Providing a high-fiber diet
- ☐ **B.** Keeping a soft light glowing in the corner of the room
- ☐ **C.** Measuring abdominal girth routinely
- ☐ **D.** Performing range-of-motion exercises to the legs at every shift

27. A law student who has been preparing for final exams comes to the student health center sobbing hysterically and hyperventilating. He says, "I haven't slept all night. I just can't go on." Which response by the nurse would be appropriate?
- ☐ **A.** "Relax, we all feel this way sometimes. You'll get through it."
- ☐ **B.** "Perhaps you need more time to study. Have you discussed this with your advisor?"
- ☐ **C.** "Studying for finals can be very stressful. Let's work on a plan that might be helpful."
- ☐ **D.** "You need to calm down. Lawyers have to learn to take a lot of stress."

28. A client has been in the manic phase of bipolar disorder for the past 8 days. During this time, the client has been hyperactive, hasn't sat down to eat meals, and has slept only 2 hours each night. Which strategy should the nurse use to help the client get adequate rest?
- ☐ **A.** Establish a bedtime routine.
- ☐ **B.** Place the client in seclusion during the night.
- ☐ **C.** Prevent the client from sleeping during the day.
- ☐ **D.** Encourage the client to nap throughout the day.

29. A client's son is 1 day old. She's upset because he sleeps most of the day and doesn't look at her often. Her interpretation is that her baby doesn't like her. The nurse's best response is:
- ☐ **A.** "Babies have no likes or dislikes; he'll like you later as his mother."
- ☐ **B.** "Babies sleep up to 20 hours per day. You'll notice him staying awake longer each week."
- ☐ **C.** "Babies sleep when they're getting sick; I'll take him to the nursery to be examined by the pediatrician."
- ☐ **D.** "Don't worry; he's just a baby."

30. A 2-year-old child is in Bryant's traction. Which measure should the nurse take to feed this child?
- ☐ **A.** Adjust the traction so the child can be turned to one side to eat.
- ☐ **B.** Temporarily stop the traction so the child can sit upright to eat.
- ☐ **C.** Ask the child's mother about the child's favorite eating position.
- ☐ **D.** Maintain the child in proper traction alignment during meals.

31. The nurse is caring for a postpartum client. To assess for thrombophlebitis, the nurse periodically should determine whether the client has:
- ☐ **A.** blood pressure discrepancy between the right and left legs.
- ☐ **B.** pain when the feet are dorsiflexed.
- ☐ **C.** limited range of motion in the legs.
- ☐ **D.** pitting edema in the lower extremities.

32. A client is admitted to the facility after falling at home. After X-rays confirm a fracture of the right hip, the client is placed in Buck's traction and scheduled for an open reduction and internal fixation. While the client is in Buck's traction, the nurse should:
- ☐ **A.** elevate the head of the bed 45 degrees.
- ☐ **B.** make sure the client's right heel touches the bed.
- ☐ **C.** remove the weights when bathing the client's legs.
- ☐ **D.** allow the weights to hang freely at the foot of the bed.

33. A client undergoes an open reduction and internal fixation to treat a fractured right hip. Five hours after surgery, the nurse should maintain the client's affected leg in which position?
- ☐ **A.** External rotation
- ☐ **B.** Abduction
- ☐ **C.** Flexion
- ☐ **D.** Hyperextension

34. The nurse on a psychiatric unit is assigned to stay with a severely depressed client. The nurse needs to go to the lavatory. How should the nurse manage this situation?
- ☐ **A.** The nurse should have another staff member inform the nurse-manager of the need for a replacement.
- ☐ **B.** The nurse should tell the client that she'll return in a few minutes.
- ☐ **C.** The nurse should ask another client to sit in for a while.
- ☐ **D.** The nurse should discontinue observation only when the client states that the depression has lifted.

35. A pregnant client is in the first stage of labor. The nurse should include which of the following measures in the client's care plan during this stage?
- ☐ **A.** Encouraging the client to lie on her left side
- ☐ **B.** Instructing the client to ambulate
- ☐ **C.** Urging the client to accept pain medication
- ☐ **D.** Advising the client to use learned breathing techniques

36. A child is receiving prednisone (Deltasone). The nurse knows that the mother understands the teaching about her child's prednisone therapy if she makes which statement?
- ☐ **A.** "I'll be sure to count my child's pulse every day."
- ☐ **B.** "I can't feed my child her favorite oatmeal for breakfast anymore."
- ☐ **C.** "I'll keep my child away from people with colds."
- ☐ **D.** "I'll make sure my child rests in bed every afternoon."

37. A 5-year-old child with leukemia has a platelet count of 20,000/mm³. Based on this information, the nurse should include which measure in the care plan?
- ☐ **A.** Provide a diet high in iron.
- ☐ **B.** Use hypoallergenic soap when bathing the child.
- ☐ **C.** Change the child's position every 2 hours.
- ☐ **D.** Inspect the child's skin for ecchymosis.

38. When measuring a client's blood pressure, the nurse sees that the client is having carpal spasms. Which action should the nurse take next?
- ☐ **A.** Assess for Babinski's reflex.
- ☐ **B.** Check for Chvostek's sign.
- ☐ **C.** Evaluate the client's apical pulse.
- ☐ **D.** Determine the client's level of consciousness.

39. A client who is scheduled for a frozen section biopsy and a possible mastectomy has difficulty understanding the surgeon's instructions. What's the most likely cause of her difficulty?
- ☐ **A.** She lacks knowledge of anatomy and physiology.
- ☐ **B.** She isn't interested in details.
- ☐ **C.** She has a high anxiety level.
- ☐ **D.** She has a limited mental ability.

40. At 38 weeks' gestation, a pregnant client comes to the clinic because her amniotic membranes have ruptured and she isn't having contractions. To confirm membrane rupture, the nurse should test the amniotic fluid for:
- ☐ **A.** glucose.
- ☐ **B.** pH
- ☐ **C.** color.
- ☐ **D.** albumin.

41. After a mastectomy, a client returns to her room with a wound drain attached to a Hemovac closed drainage system. The nurse caring for the client should take which measure?
- ☐ **A.** Clamp the wound catheter when emptying the Hemovac chamber.
- ☐ **B.** Flush the Hemovac chamber with sterile saline solution if it becomes clogged.
- ☐ **C.** Apply pressure around the wound catheter to promote drainage.
- ☐ **D.** Assess the client if the Hemovac chamber fills rapidly.

42. A client undergoes a mastectomy. Several days later, which finding by the nurse suggests that the client has accepted the alteration to her body?
- ☐ **A.** She's eager to be discharged.
- ☐ **B.** She asks when her sutures will be removed.
- ☐ **C.** She sits at the edge of the bed when the physician removes her dressing.
- ☐ **D.** She looks at the incision when the dressing is being changed.

43. After a cataract extraction, a client receives instructions on self-care. Which statement by the client indicates an understanding of the instructions?
- ☐ **A.** "I'll cover my mouth when I cough."
- ☐ **B.** "I'll get someone to pick up heavy objects from the floor."
- ☐ **C.** "I'll practice the Valsalva maneuver daily."
- ☐ **D.** "I'll sleep with two pillows under my head."

44. A client with Alzheimer's disease is at a group reality-orientation session. Several members of the group discuss the party they just attended. Which outcome suggests that the client is benefiting from this session?

☐ **A.** The client is quiet when others talk about the party.
☐ **B.** The client tells the group she wasn't at the party.
☐ **C.** The client says she wants to have a party now.
☐ **D.** The client talks about something that happened at the party.

45. A child is admitted to the facility with a tentative diagnosis of acute lymphocytic leukemia. Which of the following is a common sign of leukemia in children?

☐ **A.** Maculopapular rash
☐ **B.** Low-grade fever
☐ **C.** Photosensitivity
☐ **D.** Polydipsia

46. When obtaining a history from a client with cholelithiasis, the nurse should ask which question related to this disorder?

☐ **A.** "Are you more comfortable when you sleep in a sitting position?"
☐ **B.** "Do you get heartburn after a spicy meal?"
☐ **C.** "Do you have an intolerance to fatty foods?"
☐ **D.** "Do you have less flatus after taking an antacid?"

47. A client underwent abdominal surgery 6 hours ago. At 6 p.m., the client receives an order of meperidine (Demerol), 50 mg, as needed. Two hours later, the client complains of incisional pain. Which action should the nurse take?

☐ **A.** Place a heating pad against the client's abdomen.
☐ **B.** Repeat the meperidine dose.
☐ **C.** Turn the client onto the side and place a pillow behind the back.
☐ **D.** Give the client half the ordered dosage of meperidine.

48. After a cholecystectomy with a choledochostomy, a client returns to the medical-surgical unit with a T tube in place. The nurse should take which action related to the T tube?

☐ **A.** Irrigate it periodically.
☐ **B.** Connect it to a straight drainage system.
☐ **C.** Attach it to a low-suction apparatus.
☐ **D.** Aspirate it at least four times per day.

49. A client with a normal pregnancy visits the clinic. When teaching the client about nutrition, the nurse should provide which instruction?

☐ **A.** "Avoid salt whenever possible, and don't use salt when cooking."
☐ **B.** "Limit your intake of carbohydrates, such as bread, to improve your protein metabolism."
☐ **C.** "Peanut butter is a good source of protein to include in your diet."
☐ **D.** "Avoid eating fatty foods until after your baby is born."

50. A client with tuberculosis is to take isoniazid (INH) and rifampin (Rifadin). Which comment by the client indicates correct understanding of the medication regimen?

☐ **A.** "I'll take the medications until I regain my strength."
☐ **B.** "I'll take the medications as prescribed for over a year."
☐ **C.** "I'll take the medications with citrus juice."
☐ **D.** "I'll take the medications until my white blood cell count is normal."

51. A 76-year-old client is admitted to the hospital with a diagnosis of osteoarthritis. At a conference to discuss the client's progress, the nursing staff reports that the client looks at them intently when being questioned and answers inappropriately at times. Based on this information, the client should be evaluated for possible:

☐ **A.** hearing loss.
☐ **B.** perceptual defect.
☐ **C.** shortened attention span.
☐ **D.** cerebral oxygen deficit.

52. A client with heart failure is to be maintained on bed rest. For this client, the main purpose of bed rest is to:

☐ **A.** improve the heart's pumping action.
☐ **B.** enhance oxygenation of body tissues.
☐ **C.** decrease blood volume throughout the body.
☐ **D.** reduce the workload of the heart.

53. A schizophrenic client experiences auditory hallucinations. He tells the nurse that voices from another planet are commanding him to collect all metal cups. When responding, the nurse should tell the client that:

☐ **A.** it's all right for him to do what the voices tell him to do.
☐ **B.** she doesn't hear the voices.
☐ **C.** listening to music will obliterate the voices.
☐ **D.** he doesn't hear the voices.

54. The nurse encourages a postoperative client to move the legs. Contracting the leg muscles helps prevent which postoperative complication?
- [ ] **A.** Pleurisy
- [ ] **B.** Portal hypertension
- [ ] **C.** Hypostatic pneumonia
- [ ] **D.** Pulmonary embolism

55. When assessing a dehydrated infant, the nurse is most likely to detect which of the following signs?
- [ ] **A.** Heart rate of 100 beats/minute
- [ ] **B.** Absence of tears when crying
- [ ] **C.** Distended neck veins
- [ ] **D.** Bulging anterior fontanel

56. A client who suspects she's pregnant is given a pregnancy test. The presence of which hormone would confirm the pregnancy?
- [ ] **A.** Human chorionic gonadotropin
- [ ] **B.** Progesterone
- [ ] **C.** Follicle-stimulating hormone
- [ ] **D.** Luteinizing hormone

57. The nurse should instruct the client with Parkinson's disease to avoid which of the following activities?
- [ ] **A.** Walking in an indoor shopping mall
- [ ] **B.** Sitting on the deck on a cool summer evening
- [ ] **C.** Walking to the car on a cold winter day
- [ ] **D.** Sitting on the beach in the sun on a summer day

58. Shortly after a neonate is delivered, erythromycin (Ilotycin) is instilled into the neonate's eyes. This drug is given to prevent:
- [ ] **A.** ophthalmia neonatorum.
- [ ] **B.** retrolental fibroplasia.
- [ ] **C.** corneal keratitis.
- [ ] **D.** acute uveitis.

59. A client with insulin-dependent (type 1) diabetes mellitus is taking NPH insulin. The client sometimes engages in strenuous exercise. Which of these preexercise instructions should the nurse consider including in client teaching?
- [ ] **A.** "Take extra insulin."
- [ ] **B.** "Have a simple carbohydrate source available."
- [ ] **C.** "Rest for an hour."
- [ ] **D.** "Stretch and bend for 10 minutes."

60. A client with newly diagnosed adult-onset diabetes mellitus seems anxious when receiving instructions in self-care. The client tells the nurse, "What's the use? I can't be cured, so what's the sense in you telling me all this nonsense?" Which response by the nurse would be appropriate?
- [ ] **A.** "Getting tense and discouraged will only aggravate your condition."
- [ ] **B.** "Take one step at a time. None of us knows what will happen from day to day."
- [ ] **C.** "It's true, you'll have to modify your lifestyle, but your quality of life doesn't have to decline."
- [ ] **D.** "Don't feel so negative about the future. We're trying to help you better care for yourself."

61. A client receives instructions about high-calcium foods. The client shows an understanding of these instructions by selecting which food as having the most calcium?
- [ ] **A.** Liver
- [ ] **B.** Yogurt
- [ ] **C.** Bran muffin
- [ ] **D.** Carrots

62. A female client is diagnosed with gonorrhea. The nurse should assess her for which of the following signs?
- [ ] **A.** Lower abdominal pain
- [ ] **B.** Muscle rigidity
- [ ] **C.** Unsteady gait
- [ ] **D.** Reddish rash on the inner thighs

63. During labor, a client's amniotic membranes rupture. The nurse sees the umbilical cord protruding from the vagina. Which action should the nurse take?
- [ ] **A.** Encourage the client to breathe deeply.
- [ ] **B.** Turn the client onto her left side.
- [ ] **C.** Place the client in Trendelenburg's position.
- [ ] **D.** Place sterile pads under the client's buttocks.

64. A client is to receive 8 mg of morphine sulfate. The ampule contains 15 mg/ml. Approximately how much morphine should the nurse administer?
- [ ] **A.** 0.5 ml
- [ ] **B.** 0.7 ml
- [ ] **C.** 1.0 ml
- [ ] **D.** 1.5 ml

65. Tachycardia may result from:
- ☐ **A.** vagal stimulation.
- ☐ **B.** fear, anger, or pain.
- ☐ **C.** stress, pain, or vomiting.
- ☐ **D.** vomiting or suctioning.

66. A 63-year-old male is admitted to the medical-surgical unit before a left carotid endarterectomy. The nurse is completing an admission assessment. What pre-existing condition might the nurse expect to find with this client?
- ☐ **A.** Renal disease
- ☐ **B.** Atherosclerosis
- ☐ **C.** Crohn's disease
- ☐ **D.** Cervical dysplasia

67. A 5-year-old is admitted to the hospital for an elective tonsillectomy and adenoidectomy. During the admission assessment, which of the following observations calls for further evaluation?
- ☐ **A.** The child is chewing on his fingernails.
- ☐ **B.** The child is clutching a ragged teddy bear.
- ☐ **C.** The child is avoiding eye contact with the nurse.
- ☐ **D.** The child is sneezing frequently.

68. A client who has suffered a myocardial infarction (MI) is in the coronary care unit. The nurse suspects that the client is denying the seriousness of the medical condition. Which behavior supports this suspicion?
- ☐ **A.** The client refuses to eat solid food.
- ☐ **B.** The client says that tea made from heart-shaped leaves helps the heart.
- ☐ **C.** The client expects to return to work within 2 weeks.
- ☐ **D.** The client plans to do an oil painting for his daughter.

69. A client who was hospitalized for a myocardial infarction is being prepared for discharge. Which statement by the client indicates an understanding of the nurse's discharge instructions?
- ☐ **A.** "I'll stop walking when my pulse rate exceeds 80 beats/minute."
- ☐ **B.** "I'll wait about 1 hour after a meal before walking."
- ☐ **C.** "I'll use a ramp to walk the four steps into my house."
- ☐ **D.** "I'll walk for 10 minutes every 2 hours while awake."

70. A client is admitted to the hospital with a diagnosis of acute upper GI bleeding. Which nursing diagnosis takes highest priority for this client?
- ☐ **A.** Deficient fluid volume related to bleeding
- ☐ **B.** Impaired tissue integrity related to mucosal damage
- ☐ **C.** Impaired physical mobility related to weakness secondary to blood loss
- ☐ **D.** Anxiety related to critical illness

71. A client in an alcohol treatment center admits to drinking two to three cases of beer every weekend and reports experiencing several blackouts in the past few months. Which recommendation by the nurse would be appropriate?
- ☐ **A.** Monitor alcohol intake for the next 3 months.
- ☐ **B.** Reduce alcohol intake and attend Alcoholics Anonymous meetings.
- ☐ **C.** Limit drinking to special occasions only.
- ☐ **D.** Abstain from alcohol altogether.

72. The cervix of a client in labor is dilated 8 cm. Noting that the client bears down during contractions, the nurse teaches her to avoid doing this. Which observation during the client's next contraction indicates that the teaching was effective?
- ☐ **A.** The client pants when breathing.
- ☐ **B.** The client holds her breath.
- ☐ **C.** The client holds on to the side rails firmly.
- ☐ **D.** The client maintains a back-lying position.

73. To help prevent an infant from contracting infectious diarrhea, the nurse should instruct the mother in which topic?
- ☐ **A.** Introducing solid foods into the infant's diet
- ☐ **B.** Preparing, handling, and storing infant formula
- ☐ **C.** Having the child immunized
- ☐ **D.** Bringing the infant to the clinic for routine check-ups

74. A female college student is admitted to the hospital with toxic shock syndrome. She's confused, has a fever of 101° F (38.3° C), and has slow, shallow respirations. Which nursing diagnosis takes highest priority for this client?
- ☐ **A.** Deficient knowledge related to correct use of tampons
- ☐ **B.** Ineffective tissue perfusion (cerebral) related to low cardiac output

☐ **C.** Risk for infection related to streptococcal organisms

☐ **D.** Impaired gas exchange related to depressed respirations

75. A client complains of extreme fatigue and weakness after the 1st week of radiation therapy. Which of the following responses by the nurse would best reassure the client?

☐ **A.** "These symptoms result from radiation therapy. We'll monitor the laboratory and X-ray studies carefully."

☐ **B.** "These symptoms are part of your disease and can't be helped."

☐ **C.** "Don't be worried about these symptoms. Everyone feels this way after having radiation therapy."

☐ **D.** "This is a good sign. It means that only the cancer cells are dying."

76. A client with type 1 diabetes mellitus is admitted to the hospital with a diagnosis of ketoacidosis. Which client behavior is most likely to contribute to the development of ketoacidosis?

☐ **A.** Increasing the length of daily walks

☐ **B.** Neglecting to take insulin regularly

☐ **C.** Failing to adhere to the prescribed diet

☐ **D.** Working 8 hours per day

77. A client tells the nurse, "My husband and I have been married for 60 years. I don't understand why I always get cystitis and he doesn't." The nurse's explanation should include which information?

☐ **A.** The female urethra is shorter and closer to the rectum than the male urethra.

☐ **B.** Males have a greater resistance to bacterial organisms than females.

☐ **C.** The sphincter of the female meatus doesn't contract as tightly as that of the male.

☐ **D.** Toilet tissue is more likely to irritate the female meatus than the male meatus.

78. When preparing to administer NPH insulin to a client, the nurse should take which action?

☐ **A.** Rotate the vial between the hands.

☐ **B.** Warm the vial to body temperature by running hot water over it.

☐ **C.** Invert the vial for a few minutes.

☐ **D.** Aspirate the insulin without injecting air into the vial.

79. Which medication should the nurse have on hand to counteract adverse effects of heparin?

☐ **A.** Calcium gluconate

☐ **B.** Protamine sulfate

☐ **C.** Chlorambucil

☐ **D.** Lithium carbonate

80. After a transurethral prostatic resection, a client returns to the unit with an indwelling urethral catheter attached to a continuous bladder irrigating system. Within several hours, the client complains of bladder spasms. Which action should the nurse take initially?

☐ **A.** Determine whether clots are obstructing the catheter.

☐ **B.** Support the client in a side-lying position.

☐ **C.** Assess the client's vital signs.

☐ **D.** Administer prescribed pain medication.

81. On the 3rd day after a partial thyroidectomy, a client exhibits muscle twitching and hyperirritability of the nervous system. When questioned, the client reports numbness and tingling of the mouth and fingertips. Suspecting a life-threatening electrolyte disturbance, the nurse notifies the surgeon immediately. Which electrolyte disturbance most commonly follows thyroid surgery?

☐ **A.** Hypocalcemia

☐ **B.** Hyponatremia

☐ **C.** Hyperkalemia

☐ **D.** Hypermagnesemia

82. The nurse teaches a client about warfarin (Coumadin). Which statement by the client indicates the need for further instruction?

☐ **A.** "I'll use an electric razor when shaving."

☐ **B.** "I'll need to have periodic blood coagulation tests."

☐ **C.** "I'll expect my urine to be dark brown."

☐ **D.** "I'll check my skin to see whether I'm bruising more easily."

83. A client with a displaced fracture of the left femur is placed in balanced-suspension skeletal traction. The client complains of a sharp pain when the nurse dorsiflexes the affected foot. How should the nurse interpret this complaint?

☐ **A.** The client has thrombophlebitis.

☐ **B.** Osteomyelitis has set in.

☐ **C.** The client has developed compartment syndrome.

☐ **D.** Fragments of the fracture are displaced.

84. Which nursing measure is most likely to prevent further excoriation of an infant's bright red buttocks?
- ☐ **A.** Exposing the affected area to air
- ☐ **B.** Applying baby lotion to the affected area
- ☐ **C.** Using only disposable diapers
- ☐ **D.** Washing the affected area with warm water only

85. The nurse is obtaining a history from a client with suspected peptic ulcer disease. Which history finding is most likely to contribute to ulcer development?
- ☐ **A.** The client takes ibuprofen (Advil) daily for arthritis pain.
- ☐ **B.** The client operates a photocopy machine 8 hours per day, 5 days per week.
- ☐ **C.** The client has been on a strict vegetarian diet.
- ☐ **D.** The client has a family history of severe psoriasis.

Answers and rationales

In the pretest answers below, the question number appears in boldface type, followed by the letter of the correct answer. Rationales for correct answers and, where appropriate, for incorrect options follow. To help you evaluate your knowledge base and application of nursing behaviors, each rationale is classified as follows:
- nursing process step
- client needs category
- client needs subcategory
- cognitive level.

1. CORRECT ANSWER: A
High Fowler's position may cause pelvic congestion. The other options don't contribute to pelvic congestion and are desirable positions for this client.
Nursing process step: Planning
Client needs category: Physiological integrity
Client needs subcategory: Reduction of risk potential
Cognitive level: Analysis

2. CORRECT ANSWER: C
In an upper GI series, the client swallows barium and has X-rays of the stomach taken. Options A, B, and D don't apply to an upper GI series. A gastroscope is passed through the mouth into the stomach to observe the gastric mucosa to perform gastroscopy. The night before a gallbladder series, a client takes radiopaque tablets. A computed tomography (CT) scan isn't a component of an upper GI series.

Nursing process step: Evaluation
Client needs category: Safe, effective care environment
Client needs subcategory: Coordinated care
Cognitive level: Application

3. CORRECT ANSWER: A
An ineffective breathing pattern is a dangerous complication that can occur in a client recovering from general anesthesia. Option B may cause a problem but doesn't take priority over an ineffective breathing pattern. Options C and D aren't immediate postoperative problems.
Nursing process step: Evaluation
Client needs category: Safe, effective care environment
Client needs subcategory: Safety and infection control
Cognitive level: Application

4. CORRECT ANSWER: C
Postoperatively, persistent abdominal distention may indicate paralytic ileus. The other options are expected during the postoperative period.
Nursing process step: Data collection
Client needs category: Physiological integrity
Client needs subcategory: Reduction of risk potential
Cognitive level: Application

5. CORRECT ANSWER: A
When the amniotic membranes rupture, fluid is expelled through the vaginal canal and the cord may prolapse, possibly impeding fetal blood supply. The nurse should check fetal heart tones to assess fetal status. A position change isn't required unless the fetal heart rate is abnormal. Recording the client's blood pressure would be necessary only with signs of maternal distress. Changing the pad under the client would be done after checking the fetal heart tones.
Nursing process step: Implementation
Client needs category: Health promotion and maintenance
Client needs subcategory: Growth and development through the life span
Cognitive level: Comprehension

6. CORRECT ANSWER: B
Chills are a classic symptom of a transfusion reaction. The other options aren't associated with transfusion reactions.
Nursing process step: Data collection
Client needs category: Physiological integrity
Client needs subcategory: Pharmacological therapies
Cognitive level: Comprehension

7. CORRECT ANSWER: D

In cystic fibrosis, thick, tenacious tracheobronchial secretions may obstruct the airway. Ensuring a patent airway is the highest priority. Cystic fibrosis and pneumonia may cause fatigue and loss of energy. This results in loss of appetite, resulting in decreased food intake; however, option A isn't the highest priority. Options B and C also are appropriate nursing concerns and should be addressed in the care plan; however, they're secondary to ineffective airway clearance.

Nursing process step: Evaluation
Client needs category: Physiological integrity
Client needs subcategory: Physiological adaptation
Cognitive level: Analysis

8. CORRECT ANSWER: D

The neonate is capable of making crawling-forward movements. Discussion and demonstration of this neonate capability are important so that parents realize the danger of placing the neonate on a bed or changing table without sides. Babinski's, stepping, and tonic neck reflexes aren't specifically related to a safety concern that should be taught to the parents.

Nursing process step: Implementation
Client needs category: Safe, effective care environment
Client needs subcategory: Safety and infection control
Cognitive level: Application

9. CORRECT ANSWER: A

A client in status asthmaticus should be placed in the position that best promotes air exchange. Sitting upright eases the motion of the diaphragm and promotes a patent airway. The other positions don't promote air exchange.

Nursing process step: Implementation
Client needs category: Physiological integrity
Client needs subcategory: Basic care and comfort
Cognitive level: Analysis

10. CORRECT ANSWER: B

When the left side of the heart fails, fluid accumulates in the lungs, causing dyspnea. The other options are signs and symptoms of right-sided — not left-sided — heart failure.

Nursing process step: Data collection
Client needs category: Physiological integrity
Client needs subcategory: Pharmacological therapies
Cognitive level: Comprehension

11. CORRECT ANSWER: C

This response encourages the client to express his feelings. Option A denies the client's feelings. Option B is judgmental. Option D is inappropriate because the client hasn't expressed concern about the skill of the surgeon.

Nursing process step: Implementation
Client needs category: Psychosocial integrity
Client needs subcategory: Coping and adaptation
Cognitive level: Application

12. CORRECT ANSWER: D

Fresh vegetables, such as string beans, have the lowest sodium content (approximately 70 mg per cup) of the foods listed. The other options have more than 150 mg of sodium in an average portion and should be avoided by a client on a low-sodium diet.

Nursing process step: Evaluation
Client needs category: Physiological integrity
Client needs subcategory: Basic care and comfort
Cognitive level: Comprehension

13. CORRECT ANSWER: A

Frequent swallowing may indicate that the child is swallowing blood, a sign of excessive bleeding (hemorrhage). The other options may be expected during the early postoperative period.

Nursing process step: Data collection
Client needs category: Physiological integrity
Client needs subcategory: Reduction of risk potential
Cognitive level: Comprehension

14. CORRECT ANSWER: A

The primary role of the labor coach is to be actively involved in the birth process by providing emotional and physical support during the labor and delivery. Although the coach witnesses the events of the labor and birth and frequently is the one who shares this information with other family members, neither of these is the primary role.

Nursing process step: Implementation
Client needs category: Psychosocial integrity
Client needs subcategory: Psychosocial adaptation
Cognitive level: Application

15. CORRECT ANSWER: C
Maintaining a patent airway is a priority for any client who is unconscious. Although the other options are appropriate goals for an unconscious client, they aren't priorities.
Nursing process step: Planning
Client needs category: Physiological integrity
Client needs subcategory: Physiological adaptation
Cognitive level: Application

16. CORRECT ANSWER: A
Examining for loose teeth is essential because during the anesthetic phase of surgery, a loose tooth is likely to become completely dislodged and may be aspirated. The other options aren't essential preoperative assessments for this client.
Nursing process step: Data collection
Client needs category: Safe, effective care environment
Client needs subcategory: Safety and infection control
Cognitive level: Analysis

17. CORRECT ANSWER: A
Crying is an appropriate reaction to hearing distressing news; the nurse should remain with the client to provide comfort as needed. The nurse shouldn't leave the room; giving a sedative at this time would be premature. When a client is obviously distressed, it's the wrong time to try to obtain information. The client is venting feelings by crying and should be allowed to do so.
Nursing process step: Implementation
Client needs category: Psychosocial integrity
Client needs subcategory: Coping and adaptation
Cognitive level: Application

18. CORRECT ANSWER: B
About 21 drops/minute should be administered, based on the following calculation:

$$\frac{\text{Volume of infusion in ml} \times \text{Drip factor (gtt/ml)}}{\text{Time of infusion in minutes}} = \text{Drops/minute}$$

Therefore:
1,000 × 15/720 = 20.8, or 21 drops/minute.
Nursing process step: Implementation
Client needs category: Physiological integrity
Client needs subcategory: Pharmacological therapies
Cognitive level: Application

19. CORRECT ANSWER: C
A soft (relaxed) uterine fundus may lead to excessive bleeding, and uterine displacement may result from a distended bladder. The other options are within normal limits for a client 2 hours postpartum.
Nursing process step: Data collection
Client needs category: Health promotion and maintenance
Client needs subcategory: Growth and development through the life span
Cognitive level: Comprehension

20. CORRECT ANSWER: A
A client receiving clonidine or another antihypertensive medication should change position slowly to prevent postural hypotension. Clonidine can be taken either before or after meals. No therapeutic justification exists for taking it with orange juice. Overconsumption of tea and other stimulants should be discouraged in hypertensive clients.
Nursing process step: Implementation
Client needs category: Physiological integrity
Client needs subcategory: Pharmacological therapies
Cognitive level: Application

21. CORRECT ANSWER: B
After a stroke affecting the arm, fingers of the affected hand should be extended and the hand and wrist placed in a functional position to prevent deformity. (Be aware that in some instances hand splints may increase spasticity.)
Nursing process step: Implementation
Client needs category: Physiological integrity
Client needs subcategory: Basic care and comfort
Cognitive level: Comprehension

22. CORRECT ANSWER: C
Suctioning shouldn't continue for more than 12 seconds; suctioning for 30 seconds causes hypoxia. The other options describe correct actions to take before, during, or after suctioning.
Nursing process step: Implementation
Client needs category: Safe, effective care environment
Client needs subcategory: Safety and infection control
Cognitive level: Application

23. CORRECT ANSWER: A
A client with emphysema who requires oxygen should receive a maximum of 3 L/minute. A flow rate of 6 L/minute would be excessive. The client shouldn't adjust the oxygen flow rate. Changing the tubing at each shift is unnecessary.

Nursing process step: Implementation
Client needs category: Safe, effective care environment
Client needs subcategory: Safety and infection control
Cognitive level: Application

24. CORRECT ANSWER: B
A client who is upset with the treatment regimen should be given the opportunity to express his feelings. The other responses don't provide this opportunity.
Nursing process step: Implementation
Client needs category: Psychosocial integrity
Client needs subcategory: Coping and adaptation
Cognitive level: Application

25. CORRECT ANSWER: A
Back pain is a common symptom of pyelonephritis, which is a complication of lower urinary tract infections, such as cystitis and urethritis. The other options might elicit information about other renal problems but not about pyelonephritis.
Nursing process step: Data collection
Client needs category: Physiological integrity
Client needs subcategory: Reduction of risk potential
Cognitive level: Application

26. CORRECT ANSWER: A
A high-fiber diet helps prevent constipation, a common complication of immobility. Keeping a soft light glowing in the corner of the room and routinely measuring abdominal girth wouldn't prevent complications of immobility. Performing range-of motion exercises is impossible without interrupting traction, which is undesirable.
Nursing process step: Planning
Client needs category: Physiological integrity
Client needs subcategory: Reduction of risk potential
Cognitive level: Application

27. CORRECT ANSWER: C
The nurse's response should provide support and reassurance as well as open communication about forming a concrete plan for dealing with the client's issues. Option A invalidates the client's feelings and gives false reassurance. Option B is unrealistic; a client in severe anxiety can't think coherently enough to respond to such a suggestion. Option D negates the client's feelings and may cause further anxiety.

Nursing process step: Implementation
Client needs category: Psychosocial integrity
Client needs subcategory: Coping and adaptation
Cognitive level: Application

28. CORRECT ANSWER: D
The client's energy level is so high that a complete night's sleep probably is impossible; the nurse should use any "down" time to promote rest. The client's sleep pattern, including a bedtime routine, can be repatterned when the client comes "down" from the manic phase of the disorder (option A). During the manic phase, the client's energy level is so high that enforcing seclusion during the night isn't likely to promote sleep (option B). The nurse should encourage the client to sleep or rest at any time to prevent physical exhaustion (option D).
Nursing process step: Planning
Client needs category: Safe, effective care environment
Client needs subcategory: Coordinated care
Cognitive level: Analysis

29. CORRECT ANSWER: B
The nurse should tell the mother that neonates sleep up to 20 hours per day. This neonate is exhibiting normal behavior. The mother needs to be reassured that her baby is acting appropriately. Likes and dislikes are learned as children have experiences with people. These occur later as children develop. Because the neonate's behavior is normal, discussion of illness is inappropriate in response to this mother's comments. Mothers need reassurance. Telling a mother not to worry leads to more concern.
Nursing process step: Implementation
Client needs category: Psychosocial integrity
Client needs subcategory: Psychosocial adaptation
Cognitive level: Application

30. CORRECT ANSWER: D
For Bryant's traction to be effective, it must be continuous, with the child in proper traction alignment at all times. Options A and B interfere with proper traction. Option C is inappropriate because the child must remain in proper traction alignment when eating, regardless of the favorite eating position.
Nursing process step: Implementation
Client needs category: Safe, effective care environment
Client needs subcategory: Coordinated care
Cognitive level: Application

31. CORRECT ANSWER: B
Pain elicited by dorsiflexing the foot (positive Homans' sign) indicates thrombophlebitis. A blood pressure discrepancy between the right and left legs, limited range of motion in the legs, and dependent edema aren't signs of thrombophlebitis.
Nursing process step: Data collection
Client needs category: Health promotion and maintenance
Client needs subcategory: Growth and development through the life span
Cognitive level: Comprehension

32. CORRECT ANSWER: D
Weights on a traction apparatus should hang freely and unobstructed. The head of the bed should be elevated no more than 30 degrees. The affected heel should be raised off the bed. The weights shouldn't be removed from the traction apparatus.
Nursing process step: Planning
Client needs category: Physiological integrity
Client needs subcategory: Basic care and comfort
Cognitive level: Application

33. CORRECT ANSWER: B
After surgery for a fractured hip, the affected leg should be placed in abduction, using an abduction splint or pillows placed between the legs to separate them. The other positions may cause dislocation.
Nursing process step: Implementation
Client needs category: Physiological integrity
Client needs subcategory: Basic care and comfort
Cognitive level: Application

34. CORRECT ANSWER: A
A depressed client is at great risk for committing suicide and needs continuous observation. This client must not be left alone (options B and D). The nurse must not relinquish responsibilities to another client (option C).
Nursing process step: Implementation
Client needs category: Safe, effective care environment
Client needs subcategory: Coordinated care
Cognitive level: Application

35. CORRECT ANSWER: B
During the first stage of labor, ambulation helps to stimulate labor. Lying down (option A) and taking pain medication (option C) may slow early labor. The client should use learned breathing techniques only when she can no longer talk during contractions (option D).
Nursing process step: Planning
Client needs category: Health promotion and maintenance
Client needs subcategory: Growth and development through the life span
Cognitive level: Application

36. CORRECT ANSWER: C
Because prednisone increases susceptibility to infections, the child should be kept away from persons with infections. The other options describe limitations or activities that aren't necessary during prednisone therapy.
Nursing process step: Evaluation
Client needs category: Physiological integrity
Client needs subcategory: Pharmacological therapies
Cognitive level: Analysis

37. CORRECT ANSWER: D
A normal platelet count for a 5-year-old child ranges from 150,000 to 400,000/mm^3. Leukemia typically causes an extremely low platelet count, predisposing the child to hemorrhage. The nurse should check the child frequently for ecchymosis and other signs and symptoms of hemorrhage. The other options aren't relevant for a client with a below-normal platelet count.
Nursing process step: Data collection
Client needs category: Physiological integrity
Client needs subcategory: Reduction of risk potential
Cognitive level: Analysis

38. CORRECT ANSWER: B
Hypocalcemia is a possible cause of carpal spasm. To determine whether the client has hypocalcemia, the nurse should check for Chvostek's sign by tapping the facial nerve; in a positive response, indicating hypocalcemia, the facial muscles twitch. Babinski's reflex indicates damage to the central nervous system, not hypocalcemia. Neither the apical pulse nor the level of consciousness provides information relevant to carpal spasms.
Nursing process step: Implementation
Client needs category: Physiological integrity
Client needs subcategory: Reduction of risk potential
Cognitive level: Comprehension

39. CORRECT ANSWER: C

The client who faces a possible mastectomy obviously is apprehensive and anxious about the possibility of having cancer and losing a breast. A high anxiety level limits concentration and learning ability. No data suggest that the client lacks knowledge of anatomy and physiology, isn't interested in details, or has a limited mental ability.

Nursing process step: Evaluation
Client needs category: Psychosocial integrity
Client needs subcategory: Coping and adaptation
Cognitive level: Application

40. CORRECT ANSWER: B

To confirm rupture of the amniotic membranes, the nurse tests vaginal fluid with Nitrazine paper. With amniotic fluid, which is alkaline, the paper turns blue. Testing amniotic fluid for glucose, color, or albumin doesn't confirm membrane rupture.

Nursing process step: Data collection
Client needs category: Health promotion and maintenance
Client needs subcategory: Growth and development through the life span
Cognitive level: Application

41. CORRECT ANSWER: D

If the Hemovac chamber fills rapidly, it typically is filling with blood, indicating hemorrhage. To empty the chamber, the nurse simply opens it; clamping the catheter isn't necessary. Because patency of the Hemovac is maintained by suction, a saline solution flush isn't needed. Suction from the Hemovac, rather than pressure applied around the catheter, is used to promote drainage.

Nursing process step: Implementation
Client needs category: Physiological integrity
Client needs subcategory: Physiological adaptation
Cognitive level: Application

42. CORRECT ANSWER: A

A client who is eager to be discharged typically has accepted the alteration to her body and is willing to deal with the reaction of family and friends to the removal of her breast. The findings described in options B and C don't necessarily indicate such willingness. Option D isn't conclusive because it doesn't indicate the client's reaction when looking at the incision.

Nursing process step: Evaluation
Client needs category: Psychosocial integrity
Client needs subcategory: Coping and adaptation
Cognitive level: Comprehension

43. CORRECT ANSWER: B

After cataract surgery, the client must not stoop, bend, cough, or strain because these activities increase intraocular pressure and may damage the surgical site. The other options describe activities that increase intraocular pressure.

Nursing process step: Evaluation
Client needs category: Physiological integrity
Client needs subcategory: Reduction of risk potential
Cognitive level: Application

44. CORRECT ANSWER: D

The purpose of the reality-orientation session is to focus on the topic at hand. Talking about a specific event suggests that the client is following the discussion. Option A doesn't indicate whether the client is following the discussion. Option B doesn't reveal whether she's oriented to the present. Option C doesn't indicate whether she's aware of the discussion or is merely responding to the word "party."

Nursing process step: Evaluation
Client needs category: Psychosocial integrity
Client needs subcategory: Psychosocial adaptation
Cognitive level: Analysis

45. CORRECT ANSWER: B

Most children with acute lymphocytic leukemia have a low-grade fever. Maculopapular rash, photosensitivity, and polydipsia aren't common signs of leukemia.

Nursing process step: Data collection
Client needs category: Physiological integrity
Client needs subcategory: Physiological adaptation
Cognitive level: Knowledge

46. CORRECT ANSWER: C

Bile is necessary for fat digestion. Gallstones may block the common bile duct, leaving no bile available for digesting fat; this leads to an intolerance to fatty foods. Options A and B don't relate to fat digestion. Stools are accompanied by flatus (from lack of bile product), which is unrelated to antacids (option D).

Nursing process step: Data collection
Client needs category: Physiological integrity
Client needs subcategory: Physiological adaptation
Cognitive level: Application

47. CORRECT ANSWER: C

Changing the client's position is the most appropriate action because the pain may result from pressure on the incision. A position change also may promote drainage. Placing a heating pad on the abdomen is unlikely to ease incisional pain. Repeating the meperidine dose and giving the client half the ordered dosage of meperidine might be appropriate if a change in position isn't effective, but each of these actions requires a physician's order.

Nursing process step: Implementation
Client needs category: Physiological integrity
Client needs subcategory: Basic care and comfort
Cognitive level: Application

48. CORRECT ANSWER: B

The nurse should connect the T tube to a collection bag, which collects drainage by gravity (straight drainage system). There's no need to irrigate the tube (option A), attach it to suction (option C), or aspirate it (option D) after surgery. The physician may perform sterile saline irrigation if the client has thick bile or inadequate drainage.

Nursing process step: Implementation
Client needs category: Safe, effective care environment
Client needs subcategory: Safety and infection control
Cognitive level: Application

49. CORRECT ANSWER: C

Peanuts and other nuts are good sources of protein. The other options are incorrect because salt, carbohydrates, and fats are important to the diet of a pregnant woman and should not be avoided.

Nursing process step: Implementation
Client needs category: Physiological integrity
Client needs subcategory: Basic care and comfort
Cognitive level: Application

50. CORRECT ANSWER: B

Most clients must take antituberculosis medications for 18 to 24 months. Typically, they must continue to take these medications even if they no longer have symptoms (options A and D). Isoniazid is best taken on an empty stomach; vitamin C, such as from citrus juice, doesn't affect absorption of rifampin or isoniazid (option C).

Nursing process step: Evaluation
Client needs category: Physiological integrity
Client needs subcategory: Pharmacological therapies
Cognitive level: Application

51. CORRECT ANSWER: A

Many older persons have degenerative hearing loss. They may try to read lips and then misinterpret what has been said. No data suggest that the client has a perceptual defect, shortened attention span, or cerebral oxygen deficit.

Nursing process step: Data collection
Client needs category: Physiological integrity
Client needs subcategory: Reduction of risk potential
Cognitive level: Application

52. CORRECT ANSWER: D

Bed rest reduces the workload of the heart by decreasing tissue demands for oxygen. Cardiac glycosides, not bed rest, are used to improve the heart's pumping action (option A). Oxygen therapy is used to enhance oxygenation of body tissues (option B). Diuretics are prescribed to decrease the blood volume (option C).

Nursing process step: Planning
Client needs category: Physiological integrity
Client needs subcategory: Reduction of risk potential
Cognitive level: Application

53. CORRECT ANSWER: B

The nurse must not reinforce the client's hallucinations. Telling the client to listen to the voices would reinforce the hallucinations (option A). The nurse shouldn't say things that may not be true (option C). The voices are real to the client; telling him that he doesn't hear them isn't therapeutic (option D).

Nursing process step: Implementation
Client needs category: Psychosocial integrity
Client needs subcategory: Psychosocial adaptation
Cognitive level: Application

54. CORRECT ANSWER: D

Contracting the leg muscles helps to prevent pulmonary embolism, which occurs when a piece of a thrombus breaks off and enters the lung. Bed rest and inactivity promote such thrombus formation. Pleurisy, an inflammation of the lung pleura, typically results from spread of an infection from the lung. Portal hypertension usually is caused by liver damage. Hypostatic pneumonia results from inhibition of normal lung clearing mechanisms such as coughing.

Nursing process step: Planning
Client needs category: Physiological integrity
Client needs subcategory: Reduction of risk potential
Cognitive level: Application

55. CORRECT ANSWER: B
Absence of tears in a crying infant indicates dehydration, which causes a rapid heart rate (above 160 beats/minute in an infant). A heart rate of 100 beats/minute is within normal limits. Distended neck veins and bulging fontanels are signs of overhydration.
Nursing process step: Data collection
Client needs category: Physiological integrity
Client needs subcategory: Physiological adaptation
Cognitive level: Analysis

56. CORRECT ANSWER: A
Human chorionic gonadotropin is produced by the placenta and appears in maternal blood or urine 10 to 12 days after conception. Progesterone, follicle-stimulating hormone, and luteinizing hormone are hormones of the menstrual cycle.
Nursing process step: Data collection
Client needs category: Health promotion and maintenance
Client needs subcategory: Growth and development through the life span
Cognitive level: Knowledge

57. CORRECT ANSWER: D
The client with Parkinson's disease may be hypersensitive to heat, which increases the risk of hyperthermia, and he should be instructed to avoid sun exposure during hot weather.
Nursing process step: Planning
Client needs category: Health promotion and maintenance
Client needs subcategory: Prevention and early detection of disease
Cognitive level: Analysis

58. CORRECT ANSWER: A
Erythromycin is an antibiotic used to prevent ophthalmia neonatorum (ocular gonorrheal infection). It doesn't prevent other eye disorders, such as retrolental fibroplasia, corneal keratitis, or acute uveitis.
Nursing process step: Implementation
Client needs category: Physiological integrity
Client needs subcategory: Pharmacological therapies
Cognitive level: Application

59. CORRECT ANSWER: B
During exercise, the body uses more circulating glucose and calories, increasing the risk of a hypoglycemic reaction. Therefore, the client should make sure to have a simple carbohydrate source available to consume during exercise. Taking extra insulin before exercising would lower the blood glucose level further. Resting, stretching, and bending before exercising wouldn't alter the client's need for glucose during exercise.
Nursing process step: Planning
Client needs category: Health promotion and maintenance
Client needs subcategory: Prevention and early detection of disease
Cognitive level: Application

60. CORRECT ANSWER: C
Adult-onset insulin-dependent diabetes mellitus is compatible with a good quality of life as long as the client modifies the diet and uses insulin properly. A client who follows the prescribed regimen has few limitations. The other options don't convey this information and therefore are inappropriate responses.
Nursing process step: Implementation
Client needs category: Psychosocial integrity
Client needs subcategory: Coping and adaptation
Cognitive level: Application

61. CORRECT ANSWER: B
Milk, milk products (such as yogurt), and some green vegetables are good sources of calcium. The other options are lower in calcium.
Nursing process step: Evaluation
Client needs category: Health promotion and maintenance
Client needs subcategory: Prevention and early detection of disease
Cognitive level: Application

62. CORRECT ANSWER: A
Signs and symptoms of gonorrhea in females include lower abdominal pain, pain on urination, and vaginal discharge.
Nursing process step: Data collection
Client needs category: Physiological integrity
Client needs subcategory: Physiological adaptation
Cognitive level: Knowledge

63. CORRECT ANSWER: C

When the umbilical cord prolapses, pressure placed on the cord by the fetus may impede fetal oxygen supply. The nurse should take measures to help prevent pressure on the cord, such as placing the client's head lower than her legs (Trendelenburg's position). The other options wouldn't relieve pressure on the cord.

Nursing process step: Implementation
Client needs category: Physiological integrity
Client needs subcategory: Physiological adaptation
Cognitive level: Analysis

64. CORRECT ANSWER: A

The nurse should administer about 0.5 ml of morphine, as indicated by the following formula:

$$\frac{\text{Amount desired}}{\text{Amount on hand}} \times \text{Quantity} = \text{Amount to administer}$$

Therefore:
8 mg/15 mg x 1 ml = 0.53, or 0.5 ml.
Nursing process step: Implementation
Client needs category: Physiological integrity
Client needs subcategory: Pharmacological therapies
Cognitive level: Comprehension

65. CORRECT ANSWER: B

Tachycardia — overly rapid heart rate — may occur as a result of fear, anger, or pain. Bradycardia — slowed heart rate — can result from suctioning (causing vagal nerve stimulation), vomiting, and certain medications.
Nursing process step: Data collection
Client needs category: Health promotion and maintenance
Client needs subcategory: Prevention and early detection of disease
Cognitive level: Comprehension

66. CORRECT ANSWER: B

Arterial occlusive disease, which narrows the carotid artery, is a common complication of atherosclerosis. Predisposing factors include smoking, hypertension, hyperlipidemia, and diabetes. Renal disease, Crohn's disease, and cervical dysplasia aren't directly related to arterial occlusive disease.
Nursing process step: Data collection
Client needs category: Physiological integrity
Client needs subcategory: Reduction of risk potential
Cognitive level: Knowledge

67. CORRECT ANSWER: D

Frequent sneezing may indicate an allergy or infection such as a cold. If an infection is present, surgery usually is postponed. The other options suggest mild anxiety — not uncommon in a 5-year-old who is in a new situation.
Nursing process step: Data collection
Client needs category: Physiological integrity
Client needs subcategory: Reduction of risk potential
Cognitive level: Analysis

68. CORRECT ANSWER: C

A client who has had an MI must return to a modified routine slowly, with the physician determining how well the heart is tolerating increasing demands. Expecting to return to work within 2 weeks is unrealistic.
Nursing process step: Evaluation
Client needs category: Psychosocial integrity
Client needs subcategory: Coping and adaptation
Cognitive level: Analysis

69. CORRECT ANSWER: B

After a meal, the circulatory system (including the heart) must carry more blood to the stomach for digestion. Exercise, such as walking, also increases demands on the heart. To prevent both demands from occurring at once, the client should wait about 1 hour after a meal before exercising. The client need not measure the pulse rate when walking (option A). The client should be able to walk the four steps to the house without a ramp, although the pace may be slow (option C). Although the client should be encouraged to exercise, a rigid exercise schedule isn't desirable (option D).
Nursing process step: Evaluation
Client needs category: Health promotion and maintenance
Client needs subcategory: Prevention and early detection of disease
Cognitive level: Application

70. CORRECT ANSWER: A

Deficient fluid volume reflects a physiological need that's critical for life; using Maslow's hierarchy of needs, this need takes highest priority. The other options are less essential and therefore take lower priority.
Nursing process step: Evaluation
Client needs category: Physiological integrity
Client needs subcategory: Physiological adaptation
Cognitive level: Comprehension

71. CORRECT ANSWER: D
This client is addicted to alcohol and can't control what happens once consumption begins. Therefore, the client must abstain altogether.
Nursing process step: Planning
Client needs category: Safe, effective care environment
Client needs subcategory: Coordinated care
Cognitive level: Analysis

72. CORRECT ANSWER: A
It isn't possible to bear down and pant at the same time. Holding the breath may help the client to bear down rather than preventing it (option B). The client can hold on to the side rails (option C) or maintain a back-lying position (option D) while bearing down.
Nursing process step: Evaluation
Client needs category: Health promotion and maintenance
Client needs subcategory: Growth and development through the life span
Cognitive level: Application

73. CORRECT ANSWER: B
Infants most commonly contract infectious diarrhea through improper preparation, handling, or storage of formula. The other options are important topics to discuss with mothers of infants but don't relate directly to preventing infectious diarrhea.
Nursing process step: Implementation
Client needs category: Health promotion and maintenance
Client needs subcategory: Prevention and early detection of disease
Cognitive level: Application

74. CORRECT ANSWER: D
Ensuring airway patency and respirations is the highest priority. Option A takes lowest priority; option B is the second highest priority; option C, the third highest priority.
Nursing process step: Evaluation
Client needs category: Physiological integrity
Client needs subcategory: Physiological adaptation
Cognitive level: Comprehension

75. CORRECT ANSWER: A
Fatigue and weakness result from radiation treatment and usually don't represent disease progression. Option B is incorrect because the symptoms result from the treatment, not from the disease; they usually decrease after therapy ends. Option C belittles the client, who is obviously concerned about the symptoms. Option D is incorrect because radiation destroys normal cells as well as cancerous ones.
Nursing process step: Implementation
Client needs category: Physiological integrity
Client needs subcategory: Physiological adaptation
Cognitive level: Application

76. CORRECT ANSWER: B
Ketoacidosis (accumulation of ketones in the body) results from insufficient endogenous insulin and an elevated blood glucose level, such as from neglecting to take insulin regularly. Increasing the length of daily walks is more likely to cause hypoglycemia. Failing to adhere to the prescribed diet may cause hypoglycemia or hyperglycemia. Working 8 hours per day isn't a potential cause of ketoacidosis.
Nursing process step: Evaluation
Client needs category: Physiological integrity
Client needs subcategory: Reduction of risk potential
Cognitive level: Analysis

77. CORRECT ANSWER: A
Women are more susceptible than men to lower urinary tract infections, such as cystitis, because the female urethra is shorter and closer to the rectum, making it more vulnerable to bacteria.
Nursing process step: Implementation
Client needs category: Health promotion and maintenance
Client needs subcategory: Prevention and early detection of disease
Cognitive level: Application

78. CORRECT ANSWER: A
The active principle in NPH insulin is in the milky white precipitate. To ensure complete dispersion of the precipitate, the nurse must rotate the vial gently between the hands. Insulin should be administered at room temperature, not warmed. The nurse shouldn't invert the vial for a few minutes because this would allow the precipitate to settle. Inserting air into the vial is the correct procedure for insulin administration.
Nursing process step: Implementation
Client needs category: Physiological integrity
Client needs subcategory: Pharmacological therapies
Cognitive level: Application

79. CORRECT ANSWER: B

Protamine sulfate is the antidote for heparin sodium. When given I.V., it binds with heparin, rendering it ineffective within 5 minutes. The other options aren't heparin antidotes or antagonists.

Nursing process step: Planning
Client needs category: Physiological integrity
Client needs subcategory: Pharmacological therapies
Cognitive level: Comprehension

80. CORRECT ANSWER: A

The presence of clots in the urethral catheter may obstruct urine flow and cause bladder distension resulting in bladder spasms.

Nursing process step: Implementation
Client needs category: Physiological integrity
Client needs subcategory: Reduction of risk potential
Cognitive level: Analysis

81. CORRECT ANSWER: A

Hypocalcemia may follow thyroid surgery if the parathyroid glands were accidentally removed. Signs and symptoms of hypocalcemia may be delayed for up to 7 days after surgery. Thyroid surgery doesn't directly cause serum sodium, potassium, or magnesium abnormalities. Hyponatremia may occur if the client inadvertently received too much fluid; however, this can happen to any surgical client receiving I.V. fluid therapy, not just one recovering from thyroid surgery. Hyperkalemia and hypermagnesemia usually are associated with reduced renal excretion of potassium and magnesium.

Nursing process step: Evaluation
Client needs category: Safe, effective care environment
Client needs subcategory: Coordinated care
Cognitive level: Analysis

82. CORRECT ANSWER: C

Dark brown urine (hematuria) indicates bleeding of the urinary tract, which may signal an overdose of warfarin, an anticoagulant. During warfarin therapy, the client should use an electric razor to reduce the risk of injury (option A). The client must have periodic coagulation tests to determine whether clotting time is satisfactory (option B). Bruising may be a sign of bleeding into the skin, another potential sign of warfarin overdose (option D).

Nursing process step: Evaluation
Client needs category: Physiological integrity
Client needs subcategory: Reduction of risk potential
Cognitive level: Analysis

83. CORRECT ANSWER: C

Increasing pain on passive movement signals compartment syndrome, which results from increased venous pressure and decreased arterial perfusion in a confined space, leading to anoxia. Dorsiflexing the affected foot increases muscle stretching, worsening anoxia and pain. Unlike compartment syndrome, which causes sharp pain, thrombophlebitis causes dull, constant pain. Osteomyelitis usually causes continuous pain. No assessment data suggest that the traction apparatus is functioning improperly; therefore, the nurse has no reason to suspect that fragments of the fracture are displaced.

Nursing process step: Evaluation
Client needs category: Physiological integrity
Client needs subcategory: Reduction of risk potential
Cognitive level: Comprehension

84. CORRECT ANSWER: A

Exposure to air allows the skin to dry and heal. Bacteria grow best in a warm, moist environment, which is encouraged by applying baby lotion and using only occlusive disposable diapers. Washing the affected area with warm water only doesn't remove the offending bacteria.

Nursing process step: Implementation
Client needs category: Physiological integrity
Client needs subcategory: Basic care and comfort
Cognitive level: Application

85. CORRECT ANSWER: A

Ibuprofen is a nonsteroidal anti-inflammatory drug that can erode through the gastric mucosal barrier, predisposing the client to ulcer formation.

Nursing process step: Data collection
Client needs category: Physiological integrity
Client needs subcategory: Reduction of risk potential
Cognitive level: Analysis

Analyzing the pretest

Total the number of questions you answered incorrectly on the pretest. A score of 1 to 10 indicates that you have an excellent knowledge base; 11 to 15, good; 16 to 20, fair. If your incorrect responses total 21 or more, you'll need intensive study; a review course is recommended.

Taking the NCLEX-PN   Part 1

1 Understanding the NCLEX-PN

Introduction

Anyone who wants to practice as a licensed practical nurse (LPN) in the United States must be licensed by the nursing licensure authority in the state or territory in which she intends to practice. To obtain this license, you must pass the National Council Licensure Examination for Practical Nurses (NCLEX-PN). The NCLEX-PN is designed for one purpose: to determine whether it's appropriate for you to receive a license to practice as a nurse. By passing the NCLEX-PN, you demonstrate that you possess the minimum level of knowledge necessary to practice nursing safely.

Your success on the NCLEX-PN depends on three key elements:
- your nursing knowledge base
- your study program for the test
- your confidence level.

You also must understand the test administration method — the computerized adaptive testing (CAT) method.

Understandably, you may feel anxious about taking the examination on a computer, especially if you haven't had much practice with one. This chapter provides helpful information about applying for your license, registering for the NCLEX-PN, following the test plan, and using the computerized format.

To become more acquainted with taking a computerized examination and to obtain additional experience with NCLEX-PN questions, be sure to practice with the 750 review questions on the CD-ROM included with this book. You can select review or practice test modes or focus on a specific subject matter, nursing process step, or client needs category and subcategory. The questions are presented in a format similar to the actual examination and aren't included in this review book.

Application for licensure and registration

Obtaining a PN license is actually a two-step process. You must:
- complete a state board of nursing application
- complete the registration form in the NCLEX-PN Candidate Bulletin.

These key steps can help make the road to taking the NCLEX-PN smoother:
- **Make sure you're in good standing with your school financially.** Then you won't have any trouble having your transcript released. After graduation, your school will send your transcript to your state board of nursing.
- Contact your state board of nursing for an application for licensure. Your school may also provide you with an application. Make sure you're aware of the licensure requirements of the state where you plan to practice. Ask your school's nursing department or check with the appropriate state board of nursing.
- Fill out an application for a limited permit if you plan to start working before you take the NCLEX-PN.
- Read the application instructions carefully. Be aware that individual states have differences regarding what materials are required at the time of application. These may include:
  - 2″ × 2″ photograph
  - completed fingerprint card
  - an additional form if you're requesting verification of receipt of your application
  - proof that you have completed a course or have been trained in the identification and reporting of child abuse and in infection control and barrier precautions
  - your notarized signature.
- Submit your application or a certificate of nursing education, if required, to your nursing school for completion of the appropriate sections.

Viewing questions on the computer screen

These illustrations show the two types of questions you'll see on the computer screen when taking the computerized NCLEX-PN examination. The left screen shows a stand-alone question (one with no case study). The right screen shows a question that includes a case study.

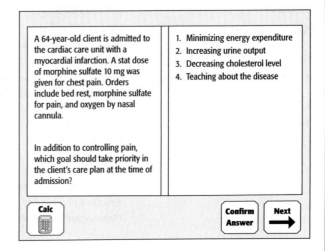

● Register with the appropriate educational testing service. Use the registration form within the NCLEX-PN Candidate Bulletin. Be sure to include a certified check, cashier's check, or money order for the fee. Call the educational testing group if you need more information or if you want to register by phone. Be aware that registering by phone using your credit card is quicker but it costs more.
● Consider sending your application by certified mail so you have confirmation of its delivery and receipt.
● Await receipt of your Authorization to Test form before making your appointment to take the test. You'll receive it from the educational testing group after your state board of nursing has notified them that you're eligible.
● Schedule your examination appointment by calling the candidate services center of your choice within the United States or its territories. Schedule your test for the time of day that you feel is your peak performance time.

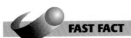

FAST FACT

Beginning in October 2002, the National Computer Systems, Inc., will manage the development and delivery of the NCLEX-PN at their sites across the United States. However, no major change in the testing process is anticipated.

● Keep the Authorization to Test form for the day of testing. It's required at the testing center on the day of the test. You'll also need two forms of current identification with your signature, including one with a recent photograph of yourself.

Computerized adaptive testing

Since 1994, the NCLEX-PN has been a computerized test in which a candidate must answer enough questions of various levels of difficulty to demonstrate minimum competence as an entry-level LPN. The CAT differs from the standard paper-and-pencil test in other ways as well. The most obvious difference is that, instead of sitting at a table with a test book and a pencil, you'll sit in front of a computer terminal, interacting with it as you take the examination.

The CAT chooses each test item based on your response to the previous question; the computer will "adapt" to your answers, correct or incorrect, by selecting harder or easier items for the next question. For example, at the start of the examination, a question of low-level difficulty may appear on the screen. If you answer this question correctly, the computer will then ask a more difficult question; if you answer incorrectly, the computer will ask an easier question. (See *Viewing questions on the computer screen.*)

Client needs categories

The NCLEX-PN assigns each question a certain category based on client needs. This chart lists client needs categories and subcategories and the approximate percentages of each type of question on the NCLEX-PN.

CATEGORY	SUBCATEGORIES	PERCENTAGE OF NCLEX-PN QUESTIONS
Safe, effective care environment	Coordinated care	6% to 12%
	Safety and infection control	7% to 13%
Health promotion and maintenance	Growth and development through the life span	4% to 10%
	Prevention and early detection of disease	4% to 10%
Psychosocial integrity	Coping and adaptation	6% to 12%
	Psychosocial adaptation	4% to 10%
Physiological integrity	Basic care and comfort	10% to 16%
	Pharmacological therapies	5% to 11%
	Reduction of risk potential	11% to 17%
	Physiological adaptation	13% to 19%

The database contains thousands of questions, each categorized according to the NCLEX-PN test plan and assigned a level of difficulty using a complex statistical formula. Every time you answer a question, the computer will search the database for the next appropriate question based on the difficulty level of the previous question and the accuracy of your response. This process continues until the computer can determine your competence in all areas of the test plan. Because each test is individualized, the number of questions can range from 85 to 205.

Mechanics of taking the CAT

The CAT begins with brief instructions and an opportunity to answer a few practice questions. Keep in mind:

● Computer experience isn't necessary. You'll only be using the button on the mouse to answer questions. This allows you to focus on the questions and not on the keyboard.

● Three small boxes are located at the bottom of the screen of each question. They include a CALCULATOR button, a NEXT button, and a CONFIRM ANSWER button. A tutorial will precede the examination to review how to use these buttons.

● Questions will appear on the screen one at a time. After you have confirmed your answer, the question will disappear; you can't return to the question.

● Answer every question, you can't skip questions and you aren't penalized for wrong answers.

● The number of questions can range from 85 to 205.

● The test will end when the computer has determined your competence level.

● Your state board of nursing will notify you of your results approximately 2 weeks to 1 month after testing. No test results are given over the phone.

NCLEX-PN test plan

All questions on the CAT NCLEX-PN adhere to a test plan, or blueprint. The NCLEX-PN draws questions from four categories of client needs that were developed by the National Council of State Boards of Nursing, the organization that sponsors and manages the NCLEX-PN. Client needs categories ensure that a wide variety of topics appear on every NCLEX-PN examination.

The National Council of State Boards of Nursing developed the client needs categories after conducting a work-study analysis of new PNs. All aspects of nursing care observed in the study were broken down into categories.

(See *Client needs categories.*) These categories were broken down further into subcategories. The four main client needs categories for the NCLEX-PN are:

- safe, effective care environment
- health promotion and maintenance
- psychosocial integrity
- physiological integrity.

Client needs categories and subcategories

Client needs categories and subcategories are used to develop the NCLEX-PN test plan, the content guidelines for the distribution of test questions. The people who write the questions and put the NCLEX-PN examination together use the test plan and client needs categories to make sure that a full spectrum of nursing activities are covered in the NCLEX-PN examination. Client needs categories appear in most NCLEX-PN review and question-and-answer review books, including this one. The truth is, however, that as a test-taker you don't have to concern yourself with client needs categories. You'll see those categories for each question and answer in this book and on the CD-ROM but they aren't identified on the actual NCLEX-PN.

An integrated examination

In nursing school, you may have had courses organized by the medical model. Courses were separated into such subjects as medical-surgical, pediatric, and psychiatric nursing. By contrast, the NCLEX-PN is integrated, meaning that different subjects are mixed together. As you answer the NCLEX-PN questions, you may encounter questions about clients (the NCLEX-PN term for patients) in any stage of life, from neonatal to geriatric. These clients may be of any background and may be completely healthy or extremely ill and have a variety of disorders.

The National Council of State Boards of Nursing has integrated these fundamental concepts throughout the NCLEX-PN:

- nursing process
- caring
- communication and documentation
- cultural awareness
- self-care
- teaching and learning.

2 Planning for success

Preparing for the examination

To prepare for the NCLEX-PN examination, you must study thoroughly, plan carefully, and master test-taking strategies. These tips can help ensure your success.

Create a good study plan

Here are some points to consider to ensure the effectiveness of your study plan:

● You may know more about some topics than others. Identify topics you feel less secure about. Become well versed in all topics the examination is likely to cover. When you're done studying, you should feel well prepared in every topic area.

● Study when you're alert. Study the difficult topics when you're most alert and energized, and study for topics that only require some refreshing during times when you're less alert. (See *Finding the right study space.*)

● Set up a basic schedule for studying. Using a calendar or organizer, determine how much time remains before you'll take the NCLEX-PN and set up a schedule. Set realistic goals. However, make sure you set aside time for normal activities.

● Become familiar with all parts of a test question.

● Take a review course or organize a study group with others planning to take the examination.

● Ask a nursing instructor or colleague for help or clarification if you encounter material that's unfamiliar to you or difficult to understand.

Keep focused

When you're faced with reviewing the amount of information covered by the NCLEX-PN, it's easy to become distracted and lose your concentration. When you lose concentration, you make less effective use of valuable study time. To help stay focused, keep these tips in mind:

● Alternate the order of the subjects you study during the day to add variety. Try alternating between topics you find most interesting and those you find least interesting.

● Approach studying with enthusiasm, sincerity, and determination.

● Once you have decided to study, begin immediately. Don't let anything interfere with your thought processes after you have begun.

● Concentrate on accomplishing one task at a time.

● Don't watch television or converse with friends while studying.

● Work continuously without interruption for a while, but don't study for such a long time that the whole experience becomes grueling or boring.

● Allow time for periodic breaks to give yourself a change of pace. Use these breaks to ease your transition into studying a new topic.

● When studying in the evening, wind down from your studies slowly. Don't move directly from studying to sleeping.

Finding the right study space

Having the right study space can be conducive to effective learning. Find a quiet, inviting study space that:

● is located in a convenient place, away from normal traffic patterns

● uses comfortable, soft lighting with which you can see clearly without eye strain

● has a temperature between 65° and 70° F

● contains flowers or green plants, familiar photographs or paintings, and easy access to soft instrumental background music

● doesn't have a television

● contains a solid chair that encourages good posture (avoid studying in bed – you'll be more likely to fall asleep and not accomplish your goals).

Take care of yourself

Don't neglect your physical and mental well-being in favor of studying longer hours. Maintaining your physical and mental health is critical for success in taking the NCLEX-PN. (See *Keeping yourself healthy.*)

Be prepared the day of testing

In order to properly prepare for the NCLEX-PN examination, follow these suggestions:

● Get a good night's sleep before the test.

● Eat a nutritious breakfast.

● Know your testing site location, and arrive at least 20 minutes early.

● Wear comfortable clothing, and bring a sweater or jacket because the room may be cool.

● Bring bottled water to drink, if desired.

● Make hotel arrangements in advance if you must travel and stay overnight.

● Bring your admission ticket and identification with you. You *must* present your Authorization to Test form as well as two forms of identification with your signature, including one with a recent photograph.

● Try to relax as much as you can but know that mild anxiety is normal.

● Be aware that a proctor will help you begin and will monitor security during the test.

● Know that the maximum time for the examination is 5 hours.

● Remember that the number of questions can range from 85 to 205.

Answering NCLEX-PN questions

Many of the questions you encounter on the NCLEX-PN will be long. As a result, it's easy to become overloaded with information. To focus on each question and to avoid becoming overwhelmed, use the following techniques to help answer NCLEX-PN questions:

● Determine what the question is asking.

● Identify relevant facts about the client described.

● Rephrase the question.

● Choose the best option.

Determine what the question is asking

Read the question twice. If the answer isn't apparent, break it down into easier, less intimidating terms to help you focus more accurately on the correct answer.

Identify the relevant facts

Sort out the relevant client information. Start by asking whether any of the information provided about the client isn't relevant.

Rephrase the question

After you have determined what the question is asking and identified the relevant facts about the client, consider rephrasing the question to make it clearer. Eliminate jargon and put the question in simpler, more personal terms.

Choose the best option

After you develop a strategy by applying the above steps, choose the best option for the question being asked.

Using key strategies

Regardless of the types of questions, there are four key strategies that will help you determine the correct answer for each question: Consider the nursing process, apply Maslow's hierarchy, consider patient safety, and consider verbal and nonverbal therapeutic communication.

Consider the nursing process

The nursing process steps include data collection, planning, implementation, and evaluation:

● Remember that data collection comes before planning, which comes before implementation, which comes before evaluation.

● If your question asks you to collect data or assess, you can immediately eliminate options that aren't assessment options.

The nursing process

The nursing process is a scientific method of applying nursing principles to client care. Understanding the different steps in the nursing process can help you determine which answer takes priority. Here's a list of common activities in nursing practice for each step of the nursing process.

Data collection or assessment: Gathering subjective and objective information about a client
- Collect information by reading hospital records and by observing verbal and nonverbal interactions among the client, family, friends, hospital staff, and other reliable sources.
- Examine common data sources for information.
- Recognize symptoms and findings.
- Assess the client's ability to perform activities of daily living (ADLs).
- Assess the client's environment.
- Assess the client's knowledge of his health problem.
- Assess the nurse's reaction to the client.
- Confirm all observations and perceptions by gathering additional data.
- Monitor the client personally rather than relying solely on machines.
- Communicate gathered information to other team members.

Planning: Establishing goals to meet client needs
- Include the client, family, friends, and other health team members in setting goals.
- Mutually establish goal priorities.
- Prepare a teaching plan appropriate for the client's ability.
- Anticipate the client's needs.
- Involve the client, family, friends, and other health care team members in developing care strategies.
- Document all information needed to manage the client's needs.

- Plan for the client's comfort and the maintenance of optimum functioning.
- Select the best nursing measures to deliver effective care.
- Coordinate the client's care with other providers.
- Formulate outcomes of nursing interventions.

Implementation: Carrying out actions that accomplish established goals
- Organize and manage the client's care.
- Perform or help the client perform ADLs.
- Provide comfort to the client.
- Help the client maintain optimum functioning.
- Teach the client and family about the client's condition, treatment, and care, and provide other instruction as appropriate.
- Apply proper technique in giving client care.
- Initiate lifesaving measures in life-threatening emergencies.
- Provide care that enables the client to achieve self-care and optimum independence.
- Supervise and validate the activities of other health care team members.
- Document all appropriate information.

Evaluation: Measuring the success of goal achievement
- Compare actual outcomes with expected outcomes.
- Evaluate client compliance with the prescribed therapy.
- Record the client's response to care.
- Change the care plan and reorder priorities as needed.

- Clearly understand what the question is asking. Are you assessing? Implementing? Remember you must assess before you can plan. (See *The nursing process*.)

Apply Maslow's hierarchy
Following Maslow's hierarchy of needs will help establish priorities:
- Physiologic needs are the most basic and the first needs to be met.
- The second needs to be met are safety and security, followed by loving and belonging, then self-esteem and, finally, self-actualization.

- Always satisfy the lowest-level needs first.
- Always ask yourself, "Does this choice make sense for this client?" Eliminate choices, even those that might normally take priority, if they don't make sense for a particular client's situation. (See *Maslow's hierarchy of needs*.)

Consider patient safety
- Use patient safety criteria for situations involving laboratory values, drug administration, or nursing care procedures.

Maslow's hierarchy of needs

Maslow's hierarchy of needs is a vital tool for establishing priorities on the NCLEX-PN. The list here provides a description of what constitutes each stage. The stages are arranged from the most basic to the most complex.

NEED	DESCRIPTION
Physiologic needs	<ul><li>Oxygen</li><li>Food</li><li>Elimination</li><li>Temperature control</li><li>Sex</li><li>Movement</li><li>Rest and comfort</li></ul>
Safety and security	<ul><li>Safety from physiologic and psychological threats</li><li>Protection</li><li>Continuity</li><li>Stability</li><li>Lack of danger</li></ul>
Love and belonging	<ul><li>Affiliation</li><li>Affection</li><li>Intimacy</li><li>Support</li><li>Reassurance</li></ul>
Self-esteem	<ul><li>Sense of self-worth</li><li>Self-respect</li><li>Independence</li><li>Dignity</li><li>Privacy</li><li>Self-reliance</li></ul>
Self-actualization	<ul><li>Recognition and realization of one's potential growth, health, and autonomy</li></ul>

Consider verbal and nonverbal therapeutic communication

- Listen to the client.
- Try to understand the client's needs.
- Promote clarification and insight about the client's condition.

More test-taking hints

- Read case studies carefully. They contain information you'll need to correctly answer the question.
- Pay special attention to such words as *best, most, first,* and *not* when reading the question (stem). These words, which may be italicized, capitalized, or otherwise highlighted, usually provide clues to the correct response. For example, consider the question, "What should the nurse do *first?*" All of the listed options may be appropriate nursing actions for the given circumstances, but only *one* action can take top priority.
- Try to predict the correct answer as you read the stem. If your predicted answer is among the four options, it's probably the correct response.
- Read each question and all options carefully before making your selection.
- If two options seem equally correct, reread them; they must differ in some way. Also reread the stem. You may

notice something you missed before that will aid your selection. If you're still unsure, make an educated guess. The computer won't let you skip a question.

● Choices that involve notifying the physician are usually incorrect. Remember the NCLEX-PN wants to see you, the nurse, at work.

● Remember some questions can get tricky, such as asking that something is "*no...*" or something is "*except...*". Be sure to read the question carefully before answering.

● Remain calm if a question focuses on an unfamiliar topic. Try to recall clients who have had problems similar to those in the question. Determine the nursing principles involved in your client's care and how they may apply to the test question. This may help you eliminate some options and may increase your chances of choosing the right answer.

● Take the necessary time for each question without spending excessive time on any one item. You'll have up to 5 hours to take the test. Pace yourself accordingly.

● Pay no attention to other candidates or the time they take to complete their tests. Because each test is individualized, some tests contain more questions than others.

● Take advantage of breaks during the test to give your mind and body a needed rest. The first mandatory break is given after 2 hours of testing and lasts 10 minutes. Candidates may take an optional break 90 minutes after testing resumes. If you tend to get hungry, bring a small snack with you to eat during the breaks. Do some stretching exercises during breaks to help you relax.

A final note

Developing and following an organized study plan will provide the best assurance that you're fully prepared to succeed on the NCLEX-PN. Approach the test with confidence. Good luck, and congratulations on choosing nursing as a career!

Introduction to fundamentals of nursing

Part II

5 Perioperative nursing 85

3 Nursing concepts and skills

Fundamentals: An overview

This chapter is divided into two main sections — nursing concepts and nursing skills — both of which are important in preparing for the NCLEX-PN. Drawing on your understanding of the structure of the NCLEX-PN and the discussion of study strategies previously presented, use this chapter as the basis for your review of the patient care problems that will be covered in the remainder of this book. The basic nursing concepts and skills contained in this chapter are essential for your understanding and application of the information contained in subsequent chapters.

Within chapter 3, and in subsequent chapters, you'll find strategies to help you understand and remember pertinent information. Watch for important logos, such as *Fast fact, Spot check,* and *Quick study,* which will help you understand, synthesize, and recall necessary information. There will also be short reviews of procedures found throughout the book.

Taking the NCLEX-PN is a daunting challenge, so some degree of apprehension is normal. However, organizing your efforts into a well-planned review will decrease your anxiety and improve your preparation for this critical examination. Remember that every practical nurse (PN) has gone through this experience and survived, and you can, too!

NURSING CONCEPTS

This section of the chapter reviews critical nursing concepts that are essential to effective nursing practice. Areas covered within this section include the nursing process, legal principles and nursing practice, therapeutic communication, growth and development, the family as the primary unit of health care, rehabilitation, grieving, geronto-logic nursing, home health care, infection control, and cultural and spiritual dimensions of care.

The nursing process

The nursing process — a scientific, systematic method of problem solving — forms the organizing framework for effective nursing practice. Using the nursing process in an ongoing, dynamic, and interactive manner with the client assures a scientific approach to, and continuous monitoring of, the nursing care received. (See *Steps of the nursing process,* page 14.)

Four steps make up the nursing process: data collection, planning and goal setting, implementation, and evaluation.

Data collection
● Involves collecting data and establishing a comprehensive database
● Entails recording subjective and objective data, including diagnostic test results

Planning and goal setting
● Involves identifying specific client needs and establishing nursing diagnoses according to a prescribed format and nomenclature

For a more detailed review of nursing diagnoses, see "Nursing diagnosis: A critical part of the nursing process," page 14. Additionally, refer to appendix B, NANDA Taxonomy II codes, which contains the most current list of nursing diagnoses approved by the North American Nursing Diagnosis Association (NANDA).
● Involves planning for how to:
– solve client problems according to priority

Steps of the nursing process

The nurse should proceed through the four steps of the nursing process, moving from data collection to evaluation. Depending on the evaluation findings, the nurse may update or change any of the previous steps.

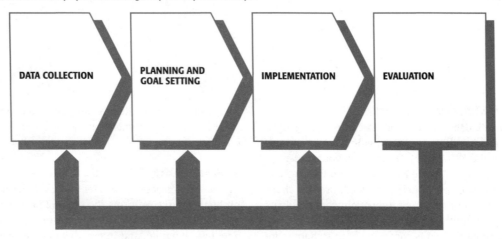

– identify goals or client outcomes to measure the effectiveness of nursing actions (goal setting is a mutual activity performed by the nurse and the client)

Implementation
● Involves nursing actions based on the plans that have been established to achieve the desired client outcomes
● Includes everything a nurse does to meet client needs, such as:
– teaching the client how to maintain his health
– administering treatments and medications
– providing support and comfort to the client and his family
– documenting all client care
– compensating for the client's inability to perform certain activities, as necessary
● Implies that the nurse understands the rationales for all nursing actions

Evaluation
● Focuses on the effectiveness of care the client receives
● Includes a review of the extent to which the nursing process has met its goals
– For goals achieved, no further action is necessary.
– For goals not achieved, the nurse retraces the nursing process steps to reassess the goals.

 SPOT CHECK

Why is it important to follow the steps of the nursing process? What might happen if you performed an action, even one that appeared critical, without the preliminary steps of data collection, planning and goal setting?
Even in critical situations, it's essential that the nurse assess the client before intervening. Although the need for rapid action may be critical, deciding on the correct action requires the nurse to accurately assess what's happening with the client. In emergency situations, data collection and planning must be done quickly – keeping the focus on the most important factors. Following the proper order of the steps of the nursing process will avoid making a serious situation even worse.

Nursing diagnosis: A critical part of the nursing process
The nursing diagnoses derived from the physical assessment and history data collected during the data collection step of the nursing process provide the basis for all subsequent nursing care.

Definition
A nursing diagnosis includes a clinical judgment about an individual, family, or community that has been reached through a deliberate, systematic process of data collection

and analysis of that data. The diagnosis provides the basis for prescribed, definitive therapy (for which the nurse is accountable) and concisely states the cause of the client's condition, if the cause is known.

The nursing diagnoses categories consider the physical, social, emotional, cognitive, spiritual, cultural, and environmental sources of disequilibrium experienced by each client. A nursing diagnosis focuses on the client's health care needs, whereas a medical diagnosis focuses on the client's disease.

The nursing process offers a way of thinking that's related to nursing care. The nursing diagnosis forms a vital and integral part of that process to make each client's care specific and individualized.

Components

A nursing diagnosis has these components:
● word or phrase about the degree or amount of change noted, indicated by words such as *imbalanced, impaired, ineffective, intolerance,* or *dysfunction*
● immediacy of the problem, commonly indicated by *actual* or *high risk*
● tissue or system involved, such as skin, bowel, bladder, or pulmonary or cardiac system
● type of problem, such as injury, fracture, or rape
● activity affected, such as mobility, coping, interaction, or home maintenance
● cause or etiology, which is indicated by the *related to* statement.

A well-constructed nursing diagnosis, therefore, sets the direction for the client's care plans and goals:
● The words *actual* and *high risk* help the nurse and client prioritize goals. For example, "actual impairment of skin integrity related to open sacral pressure ulcer" indicates the need to set as an immediate goal "The pressure ulcer will heal." or "The client will regain skin integrity with a healed pressure ulcer."
● The initial nursing diagnosis should refer to the tissue or system that's most in need of corrective care. Thus, a client with a myocardial infarction warrants an initial nursing diagnosis related to the cardiovascular system.
● Another high-priority nursing diagnosis concerns the client's deficient knowledge related to the diagnosis, treatment regimen (including its benefits and risks), and self-care needs. Teaching related to these factors is an initial and ongoing nursing activity as the client's treatment regimen proceeds, the condition changes, and the client regains independence.

Development

The efforts of many individuals created the current nursing diagnoses. Some of the first articles using "nursing diagnosis" were written by Chambers and Komorita and appeared in the early 1960s in the *American Journal of Nursing.* Other people associated with nursing diagnoses include Ackley, Carpenito, Kim, McFarland, Sparks, Taylor, and Gordon, each of whom has published books on the subject.

NANDA

The leading force in reviewing and developing new nursing diagnoses is NANDA, whose membership includes nursing experts from the various nursing disciplines.

Process

● Members meet yearly to review and refine established nursing diagnoses and to develop new ones.
● NANDA bases its diagnoses on human response patterns of exchanging, communicating, relating, valuing, choosing, moving, perceiving, knowing, and feeling. Other nursing diagnoses are derived from functional health patterns, such as activity and exercise, elimination, nutrition and metabolism, sleep and rest, cognition, perception, and coping and stress tolerance.

Legal principles and nursing practice

Law is a set of rules and principles derived from several sources and enforceable by legal processes. Laws provide a means of settling disputes, compensating for injuries caused by another, and disciplining and isolating individuals for wrongdoing as defined by society. Essential to any society's progress and survival, laws form an important basis for nursing practice.

Sources of law

Four sources of law — constitutions, judicial opinions, legislation, and regulations — form the legal basis of nursing practice.

Constitutions

Constitutions are documents that incorporate the basic principles by which an organization governs itself. The federal government and each state have written constitutions. The U.S. Constitution contains the fundamental laws of the nation, including:
● definition of the branches of government: legislative, executive, and judicial

● specification of a division of powers between federal and state governments

● establishing each citizen's basic rights; for example, the right to privacy, guaranteed to all citizens by the Fourteenth Amendment, supports a client's right to consent to or refuse treatment, even life-sustaining treatment.

Judicial opinions

A judicial opinion is the court's official position on a legal dispute, written by the judge who presides over the court case. Typically, judicial opinions emanate from appeals or higher courts in the state or federal court system as a result of disputes brought before lower courts by the litigants (those who bring the lawsuit or are otherwise involved in it). These opinions, which are published in what's called the *legal reporter system*, are also referred to as *case law* or *case decisions*.

Judicial opinions form precedent — a body of law that's commonly the basis for future decisions. Judicial opinions also address nursing practice in such areas as employment, licensure, malpractice and negligence, and crimes.

Legislation

Legislation is the set of rules created by the legislative branch of government at the federal, state, or local (city or county) level. The legislative branch of government, which meets periodically, is elected by the people. Also called *statutes* or *statutory law,* legislation is published and made available to the public; some states publish legislation in a book called a *code* or an *annotated code.* Nursing practice is shaped by many pieces of legislation, particularly the state nurse practice act and state and federal public health laws.

Legislation results from the legislative process, which involves studying issues; drafting a bill; discussing, compromising, redrafting the bill; and then voting for or against the bill's passage. A bill — the proposed law — usually becomes law when more votes are for passage than against it and after the governor (in state legislation) or the president (in federal legislation) signs the bill (in some circumstances, legislation can become law without this approval).

Regulations

Regulations are the rules created by the executive branch of government. The executive branch is headed by the governor of a state or the president of the United States. The legislative branch enacts laws granting the executive branch the authority to write regulations.

Regulations are created through the regulatory process, which involves the study of issues, the publication of the proposed rule, a period of public input (through written opinions or testimony at hearings), possible redrafting, and publication of the final regulation. Federal regulations are found in the Code of Federal Regulations, and state regulations are usually found in the state's Code of Regulations.

The government agency created by the state nurse practice act, usually called the *state board of nursing,* has the power to write specific rules that govern and control nursing practice within its jurisdiction.

Types of law

The three types of law are civil, administrative, and criminal law.

Civil law

Civil law refers to a wide range of legal issues that are unrelated to criminal acts. Usually, civil law involves disputes between two or more individuals or entities. Civil disputes related to safe nursing practice may involve an employment contract, a tort, or a violation of a client's rights. (See "Administrative disputes and nursing practice," page 22.)

Administrative law

Administrative law deals with the enforcement of government agencies' rules and regulations. Licensure and the state's power to discipline nurses are the ways states implement administrative law. A state can make rules that govern nursing based on its "police power," the power to act to protect public health, safety, and welfare; for instance, a state can prohibit a nurse from practicing nursing if the nurse is found guilty of unprofessional conduct.

Criminal law

Criminal law refers to a set of laws that define offenses against society. Crimes involve public wrongs (wrongs against society). The criminal justice and law enforcement systems exist to investigate, prosecute and, if the accused is found guilty, punish the offender.

Civil disputes and nursing practice

The law of the nurse's workplace is derived from federal and state statutes, judicial opinions, employer personnel handbooks, civil service rules, employer practice, collective bargaining agreements, and employment contracts.

A CONTRACT is a written or oral agreement between two or more individuals that includes several elements regarding formation, interpretation, and enforcement. A contract can be individual or collective (such as a union contract). It can specify the period within which the conditions of the agreement must be met. A contract may also include the elements *offer, acceptance,* and *consideration* (usually monetary compensation).

In nursing practice, civil disputes can arise that may involve torts and client rights.

Torts

A TORT is a private wrong or a breach of legal duty to the rights and interests of others. An injured litigant (usually called a PLAINTIFF) can receive remedy for a tort, commonly in the form of damages, if the litigant presents adequate evidence that an injury occurred. Courts recognize three types of torts: unintentional, intentional, and quasi-intentional.

Unintentional tort

An UNINTENTIONAL TORT is an act that fails to meet a duty owed to another person (the plaintiff) and leads to the person's injury. In nursing, the two most common types of unintentional tort are negligence and malpractice.

Negligence. NEGLIGENCE is an unintentional tort that involves four elements:
● duty — DUTY refers to the nurse's legal obligation to provide nursing care to a client. The nurse has the duty to meet a reasonable and prudent standard of care under the circumstances. The nurse must also deliver care as any other reasonable and prudent nurse would under similar circumstances. Standards of care are derived from policy and procedure manuals, nursing education, experience, and publications of professional associations and accreditation groups.
● breach of duty — BREACH OF DUTY is failure to provide the expected reasonable standard of care under the circumstances; it can take two forms. The nurse may fail to provide care (breach by *omission* of the duty), or the nurse may provide care in an unreasonable manner (breach by *commission* of the duty).
● proximate cause — PROXIMATE CAUSE refers to the causal connection between the breach of duty and the resulting injury. Proximate cause doesn't necessarily involve a direct cause-and-effect relationship, but the plaintiff must produce evidence that the nurse's action or inaction led to the plaintiff's injury. State laws vary in the language used to define proximate cause:
– If the definition uses the phrase *but for,* the plaintiff must prove that the injury wouldn't have occurred without (*but for*) the nurse's breach of duty.

– If the definition uses the phrase *substantial factor,* the plaintiff must prove that the nurse's breach of duty was a substantial factor in the injury.
– If the definition uses the term *foreseeability,* the plaintiff must prove that the nurse's breach of duty foreseeably led to the plaintiff's injury; that is, that the nurse should have known what would happen.
● damages — DAMAGES refers to physical and psychological injuries and to monetary compensation awarded to the plaintiff for incurring the injuries. The plaintiff must prove that an injury occurred and present evidence showing its monetary value. The plaintiff can request:
– COMPENSATORY DAMAGES, which are awarded to reimburse the plaintiff for the expenses, rehabilitation, and pain and suffering related to the injury
– NOMINAL DAMAGES, which are awarded to indicate a defendant's wrongdoing when little, if any, injury occurred
– PUNITIVE DAMAGES, which are awarded to the plaintiff in special circumstances (usually to punish the defendant for an especially egregious or outrageous act).

Malpractice. MALPRACTICE is negligence by a member of a profession (such as nursing); it differs from negligence only in that the standard or duty owed is a professional one based on special knowledge and skills.

The plaintiff in a malpractice action must prove all the elements of negligence, usually with expert witness testimony about the professional duty owed and how this duty was breached. However, not all states automatically apply a professional standard to nurses; some states apply a nonprofessional one and other states apply a professional standard only when the nurse's act requires special knowledge and skill.

Liability. Negligence and malpractice lawsuits also involve legal principles about who bears LIABILITY (responsibility) for resultant injuries. Two types of liability include:
● PERSONAL LIABILITY — responsibility for one's acts
● VICARIOUS LIABILITY — responsibility for another person's acts; such liability can take one of two forms:
– RESPONDEAT SUPERIOR addresses an employer's responsibility for injuries caused by an employee's negligent acts, if those acts were performed within the scope of employment and when an employment relationship existed. For example, if a hospital-employed nurse fails to detect a hematoma under the blood pressure cuff of a heavily heparinized client in the intensive care unit, the hospital *and* the nurse are liable.
– *Corporate liability* refers to an employer's responsibility for injury caused by an employee who acted according to

the employer's decisions (for example, because a hospital determines its budget, staff, and client population, the hospital — not the nurse — is liable for injury that results from understaffing).

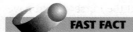

FAST FACT

If a client sustains injuries because a staff nurse administers the wrong drug or fails to monitor the client properly, the nurse can be found liable for those acts.

Nurses can avoid or defend negligence and malpractice lawsuits by following these principles:
● Know the standard of care — the duty owed the client — before delivering care.
● Deliver care that meets the standard of care.
● Document care accurately and concisely, following the health care facility's policies and procedures (documentation reflecting that a standard of care was met can serve as a nurse's best defense; the adage "If it wasn't charted, it wasn't done" receives credence in most jurisdictions).

Other defenses may apply to a nursing negligence case depending on the facts presented. For example, federally employed nurses hold personal immunity from liability (under federal legislation known as the *Federal Tort Claims Act*); all nurses hold immunity from liability for making a good faith report of child abuse, which all states require of nurses; and a case can be dismissed if the plaintiff doesn't file the lawsuit within a legislature-specified time, known as a *statute of limitation*.

Intentional tort

An INTENTIONAL TORT is a willful act that injures another person or the person's property. These acts include:
● ASSAULT — threat of imminent harmful or offensive bodily contact
● BATTERY — bodily contact with another person without the person's permission or consent
● FALSE IMPRISONMENT — unlawful restraint of a person against the person's will
● INTENTIONAL INFLICTION OF EMOTIONAL DISTRESS — extreme, outrageous, or intolerable conduct toward a person, causing emotional harm.

Quasi-intentional tort

A QUASI-INTENTIONAL TORT is an act that interferes with a person's intangible interests, such as privacy or reputation. A nurse may be charged with INVASION OF PRIVACY

and BREACH OF CONFIDENTIALITY for revealing personal information about a client to an unauthorized person. Or, a nurse may be charged with DEFAMATION for injuring the plaintiff's reputation in the community as the result of a false statement, either spoken (slander) or written (libel). False statements about another person's professional competence can lead to a defamation lawsuit. However, truth is a viable defense against a defamation charge.

Client rights

A PATIENT'S BILL OF RIGHTS, written by the American Hospital Association, contains a sample list of patient (client) rights. Although not law, this code lists many rights of clients legally recognized through sources of law previously mentioned. (See *A Patient's Bill of Rights*.)
Client rights include:
● informed consent
● freedom from unreasonable restraint
● right to refuse treatment
● right to privacy and confidentiality.

QUICK STUDY

Want an easy way to remember client rights as listed in A Patient's Bill of Rights? Remember this sentence: **I**ngrid **F**ries **R**ed **P**eppers.
    Informed consent
    Freedom from unreasonable restraint
    Right to refuse treatment
    Privacy and confidentiality right

Informed consent

INFORMED CONSENT refers to the client's involvement in and agreement with treatment decisions based on careful consideration of all information pertinent to his condition.
For informed consent to be recognized by the court, several conditions must be met:
● The consent must be voluntary.
● The information given to the client must include the nature of the proposed treatment, its foreseeable risks and benefits, alternatives to the proposed treatment, and the consequences of choosing to do nothing.
● The consent must be given by a person who is legally competent to do so.

The physician has the legal obligation to obtain a client's informed consent to medical treatment.

Nurses are commonly assigned the task of obtaining a signed consent form and witnessing the client's signature; doing so legally obligates the nurse, if called later, to testify

A Patient's Bill of Rights

Introduction

Effective health care requires collaboration between patients and physicians and other health care professionals. Open and honest communication, respect for personal and professional values, and sensitivity to differences are integral to optimal patient care. As the setting for the provision of health services, hospitals must provide a foundation for understanding and respecting the rights and responsibilities of patients, their families, physicians, and other caregivers. Hospitals must ensure a health care ethic that respects the role of patients in decision making about treatment choices and other aspects of their care. Hospitals must be sensitive to cultural, racial, linguistic, religious, age, gender, and other differences as well as the needs of people with disabilities.

The American Hospital Association presents A Patient's Bill of Rights with the expectation that it will contribute to more effective patient care and will be supported by the hospital on behalf of the institution and its medical staff, employees, and patients. The American Hospital Association encourages health care institutions to tailor this bill of rights to their patient community by translating or simplifying the language of this bill of rights as may be necessary to ensure that patients and their families understand their rights and responsibilities.

1. The patient has the right to considerate and respectful care.

2. The patient has the right to and is encouraged to obtain from physicians and other direct caregivers relevant, current, and understandable information concerning diagnosis, treatment, and prognosis.

Except in emergencies when the patient lacks decision-making capacity and the need for treatment is urgent, the patient is entitled to the opportunity to discuss and request information related to the specific procedures and/or treatments, the risks involved, the possible length of recuperation, and the medically reasonable alternatives and their accompanying risks and benefits.

Patients have the right to know the identity of physicians, nurses, and others involved in their care as well as when those involved are students, residents, or other trainees. The patient also has the right to know the immediate and long-term financial implications of treatment choices, insofar as they're known.

3. The patient has the right to make decisions about the plan of care prior to and during the course of treatment and to refuse a recommended treatment or plan of care to the extent permitted by law and hospital policy and to be informed of the medical consequences of this action. In case of such refusal, the patient is entitled to other appropriate care and services that the hospital provides or transfer to another hospital. The hospital should notify patients of any policy that might affect patient choice within the institution.

4. The patient has the right to have an advance directive (such as a living will, health care proxy, or durable power of attorney for health care) concerning treatment or designating a surrogate decision maker with the expectation that the hospital will honor the intent of that directive to the extent permitted by law and hospital policy.

Health care institutions must advise patients of their rights under state law and hospital policy to make informed medical choices, ask if the patient has an advance directive, and include that information in patient records. The patient has the right to timely information about hospital policy that may limit its ability to implement fully a legally valid advance directive.

5. The patient has the right to every consideration of privacy. Case discussion, consultation, examination, and treatment should be conducted so as to protect each patient's privacy.

6. The patient has the right to expect that all communications and records pertaining to his/her care will be treated as confidential by the hospital, except in cases such as suspected abuse and public health hazards when reporting is permitted or required by law. The patient has the right to expect that the hospital will emphasize the confidentiality of this information when it releases it to any other parties entitled to review information in these records.

7. The patient has the right to review the records pertaining to his/her medical care and to have the information explained or interpreted as necessary, except when restricted by law.

8. The patient has the right to expect that, within its capacity and policies, a hospital will make reasonable response to the request of a patient for appropriate and medically indicated care and services. The hospital must provide evaluation, service, and/or referral as indicated by the urgency of the case. When medically appropriate and legally permissible, or when a patient has so requested, a patient may be transferred to another facility. The institution to which the patient is to be transferred must first have accepted the patient for transfer. The patient must also have the benefit of complete information and explanation concerning the need for, risks, benefits, and alternatives to such a transfer.

9. The patient has the right to ask and be informed of the existence of business relationships among the hospital, educational institutions, other health care providers, or payers that may influence the patient's treatment and care.

(continued)

A Patient's Bill of Rights *(continued)*

10. The patient has the right to consent to or decline to participate in proposed research studies or human experimentation affecting care and treatment or requiring direct patient involvement, and to have those studies fully explained prior to consent. A patient who declines to participate in research or experimentation is entitled to the most effective care that the hospital can otherwise provide.

11. The patient has the right to expect reasonable continuity of care when appropriate and to be informed by physicians and other caregivers of available and realistic patient care options when hospital care is no longer appropriate.

12. The patient has the right to be informed of hospital policies and practices that relate to patient care, treatment, and responsibilities. The patient has the right to be informed of available resources for resolving disputes, grievances, and conflicts, such as ethics committees, patient representatives, or other mechanisms available in the institution. The patient has the right to be informed of the hospital's charges for services and available payment methods.

The collaborative nature of health care requires that patients, or their families/surrogates, participate in their care. The effectiveness of care and patient satisfaction with the course of treatment depend, in part, on the patient fulfilling certain responsibilities. Patients are responsible for providing information about past illnesses, hospitalizations, medications, and other matters related to health status. To participate effectively in decision making, patients must be encouraged to take responsibility for requesting additional information or clarification about their health status or treatment when they do not fully understand information and instructions. Patients are also responsible for ensuring that the health care institution has a copy of their written advance directive if they have one. Patients are responsible for informing their physicians and other caregivers if they anticipate problems in following prescribed treatment.

Patients should also be aware of the hospital's obligation to be reasonably efficient and equitable in providing care to other patients and the community. The hospital's rules and regulations are designed to help the hospital meet this obligation. Patients and their families are responsible for making reasonable accommodations to the needs of the hospital, other patients, medical staff, and hospital employees. Patients are responsible for providing necessary information for insurance claims and for working with the hospital to make payment arrangements, when necessary.

A person's health depends on much more than health care services. Patients are responsible for recognizing the impact of their lifestyle on their personal health.

Conclusion

Hospitals have many functions to perform, including the enhancement of health status; health promotion; prevention and treatment of injury and disease; the immediate and ongoing care and rehabilitation of patients; the education of health professionals, patients, and the community; and research. All these activities must be conducted with an overriding concern for the values and dignity of patients.

---

* These rights can be exercised on the patient's behalf by a designated surrogate or proxy decision maker if the patient lacks decision-making capacity, is legally incompetent, or is a minor.

---

about anything relating to what the nurse saw, heard, or knew about the consent.

A nurse who is concerned about the validity of an informed consent has a legal obligation to tell the physician and the nursing supervisor about the concerns and to document that she has done so.

Before a nurse obtains informed consent, the client's legal competence must be determined. Be aware that legal competence differs from medical or mental competence. It's a presumption established by the state legislatures (usually a chronological age such as 18 years); thus, everyone over age 18 is presumed legally competent, and everyone under age 18 is presumed legally incompetent.

For those under age 18 (known as *minors*), legislatures have established exceptions to the rule of presumed incompetency; unless one of these exceptions applies, informed consent for treatment of a minor must be obtained from the minor's parent or legal guardian.

Consent from a parent or guardian usually isn't required if the minor is married, has a child, lives independently, or seeks certain types of health care services (such as those for pregnancy, substance abuse, or a mental health problem).

After reaching the legal age, one can lose the legal capacity to consent only through a formal judicial process. In this proceeding, a court determines, usually on the basis of medical and psychiatric testimony, whether the person is incompetent; if the court finds the person incompetent, the court appoints a guardian (who becomes the person authorized to give informed consent).

In some situations, the court not only must rule on incompetency but also must determine whether the individual needs involuntary commitment to an institution for treatment. Before the court orders involuntary commitment, it must receive clear and convincing evidence that the individual poses a danger to himself or others with no other less restrictive treatment available. The rules to make these determinations vary among the states.

Under certain circumstances, informed consent may not be required, such as:
● In life-threatening emergencies, client consent is implied.
● A client may tell the physician that he doesn't want to know the appropriate information (known as *waiver*).
● The physician's professional judgment may dictate that fully informing a client would act as a substantial detriment to the client and cause harm (known as the physician's *therapeutic privilege*).

Freedom from unreasonable restraint
Freedom from unreasonable restraint recognizes the client's autonomy and freedom of movement. The client must receive care in a safe, prudent manner.

Health care providers can legally restrain a client under certain conditions previously defined by law and by the health care facility's policies and procedures. Conditions include:
● The restraints must be necessary to meet the client's therapeutic needs or to ensure the safety of the client or others.
● The least restrictive type of restraint must be used first.
● Use of restraints must be accompanied by a physician's order except in an emergency.
● Health care providers must closely monitor the client, periodically release the restraints, and remove them when the client's condition no longer warrants their use.
● Accurate and thorough documentation must reveal all pertinent details of the care given to the client, including how and why restraints were applied and removed.

Right to refuse treatment
The right to refuse treatment provides that every competent adult may refuse treatment, even life-sustaining treatment. Also known as the *right to withhold consent*, this right and all the requirements of informed consent apply to a client's decision to refuse treatment.

Similar to other client rights, the right to refuse treatment isn't absolute and must be considered by the court in relation to the interests of society. Thus, the client's right to refuse treatment may be outweighed by the court's responsibility to preserve human life, protect innocent third parties, prevent suicide, or maintain the ethical integrity of the medical profession.

Many states have enacted legislation that permits a client to make health care decisions in advance, such as:
● ADVANCE DIRECTIVE — a document written and signed by a patient before disabling illness occurs that includes information about the patient's decisions regarding future medical treatment; may also name someone to make choices for the patient if he's unable to do so (should become part of the client's medical record)
● LIVING WILL — a document in which a client instructs family and health care professionals about medical care that should or shouldn't be provided if the client becomes incapacitated (should become part of the client's medical record)
● DURABLE POWER OF ATTORNEY — a legal document in which a client identifies a proxy, or surrogate, decision maker in case he becomes incapacitated (should also be included in the client's medical record).

State laws vary on the issue of substituted consent; if the client lacks the capacity to make informed decisions, health care professionals usually turn to the client's family members and close friends, and the court may formally appoint them surrogate decision makers.

Right to privacy and confidentiality
The right to privacy and confidentiality recognizes a client's autonomy and right to be left alone. Because the client and the health care provider have a relationship based on trust, the client may reveal private information that will enhance treatment; in return, the health care provider must keep the information confidential.

The client has the right to access personal health records and to obtain a copy of the records. Health care providers have the responsibility to maintain health records in a secure, controlled manner.

Information can be revealed only with the client's permission or when required by law; for instance, physicians must report acquired immunodeficiency syndrome and other communicable diseases to the federal and state governments, but they must still keep such reports confidential.

Administrative disputes and nursing practice

State governments regulate nursing practice through an executive branch office, usually called a *state board of nursing*. Legislation known as the *state nurse practice act* creates the state board. Each state typically regulates several areas of nursing practice:
● the nursing profession's licensure examination (by determining the rules and requirements for admission or entry into nursing practice)
● in most states, the nurse practice act that defines the legal scope of nursing practice; the state can discipline, fine, censure, or take other appropriate steps against one who practices nursing without meeting the state requirements
● the professional conduct of licensed nurses (by defining unprofessional conduct); if a nurse is charged with unprofessional conduct, she has the right to due process, including notice of the specific charges, an opportunity to present evidence to counter the charge, and representation by an attorney hired by the nurse
● initiation of investigations, bringing charges of misconduct, and levying of disciplinary measures (investigations consider chemical impairment, including drug or alcohol abuse, which is the most common reason for disciplinary action against a nurse)
● nursing education by establishing the requirements of and approving the educational programs for nurse preparation.

Criminal disputes and nursing practice

In nursing practice, criminal disputes can arise that result in the conviction of nurses for such crimes as murder, fraud, patient abuse, and illegal use of controlled substances.

Most states recognize two types of crime: FELONIES and MISDEMEANORS (some states use the generic term *offenses*, categorizing these as crimes [felonies and misdemeanors] or violations). The primary difference between the types lies in the severity of the crime and thus in the length and type of sentence or penalty imposed on the convicted criminal.

Felonies entail more serious offenses and warrant lengthy prison sentences. Misdemeanors, which are less serious, usually result in a short prison sentence, a fine, or both. Keep in mind that, although the defendant in a criminal case may have committed a crime, he has constitutionally provided rights such as the right to legal counsel.

Criminal codes or statutes define the elements of each crime; the prosecutor must prove the existence of these elements beyond a reasonable doubt. For an act to be considered criminal, the prosecutor must prove the defendant's culpability — that is, that the defendant committed the act intentionally, knowingly, recklessly, or in a criminally negligent manner. However, mental impairment precludes the possibility of culpability; thus, the law doesn't support convicting a person who was affected by mental disease or a mental defect when committing the act. A person who is found not guilty by reason of insanity is committed to a treatment facility and is released after recovery. Definitions of mental impairment differ among jurisdictions.

Therapeutic communication

Therapeutic communication has a purpose and is goal-directed. It enhances the client's self-esteem, self-worth, and ability to function. Both nonverbal and verbal therapeutic communications exist. Aspects of verbal communication the nurse should be aware of include speech patterns, word selection, and honest presentation. Aspects of nonverbal communication the nurse should be aware of include touch, eye contact, facial expression, appearance, and gait.

The goals of therapeutic communication are directed toward the client's needs. The nurse should clarify the client's thoughts, feelings, and actions as well as explore new coping skills or behavior patterns. By utilizing the phases of therapeutic communication and focusing on nursing interventions and actions, the nurse can achieve the client's goal of self-discovery.

Phases of therapeutic communication

There are three phases of therapeutic communication: orientation and initiation, working and continuation, and termination and separation.

Orientation and initiation phase

The orientation and initiation phase is the initial introduction of client and nurse. Guidelines of this relationship are established, roles are clarified, and the setting, frequency, and duration of the relationship are established. (See *Characteristics of social and therapeutic relationships.*)

Working and continuation phase

The working and continuation phase of therapeutic communication involves dynamic interaction between the

Characteristics of therapeutic and social relationships

In an effective nurse-client relationship, the nurse uses therapeutic communication to shed light on and promote healthy changes in the client's behavior. The following chart contrasts important differences between a therapeutic relationship and a purely social one.

SOCIAL RELATIONSHIP	THERAPEUTIC RELATIONSHIP
● Focuses on mutual sharing, with each participant giving and receiving. ● Promotes mutual pleasure. ● Has no time constraints. ● Doesn't involve a contract. ● Doesn't require the participants to examine their behavior or possess a specialized knowledge base.	● Focuses on the client, with the nurse giving and the client receiving. ● Promotes client healing. ● Is time-limited. ● Involves a contract between nurse and client. ● Requires the nurse to have a sound understanding of human behavior and to examine the nurse's and the client's behaviors from a theoretical perspective.

nurse and the client. The nurse assists the client to reach certain goals.

Termination and separation phase

The termination and separation phase involves the evaluation of the goals as met or unmet. The client is able to express his emotional state at this stage.

Focus of nursing interventions

Nursing interventions focus on the individual, group, and family.

Individual

Nursing interventions should focus on the individual by emphasizing the client. This intervention is particularly helpful when the client is highly anxious or disorganized. It also affords the nurse greater control than a group or family setting.

Group

Nursing interventions should emphasize group work and the group processes. This intervention provides a supportive environment for group members to interact, share feelings and information, make decisions, develop socializing skills, and learn to do likewise in all interpersonal relationships.

Family

Nursing interventions should emphasize the client's family or significant other. Based on the concept that the client's identified psychological or physical problems affect the family or express family dysfunction, this intervention provides opportunities for the client's family members or significant other to alter and improve communication patterns, define desired relationships, and clarify roles. (See *The communication continuum.*)

The communication continuum

Words can help the nurse create a healing atmosphere. However, when poorly chosen, they can jeopardize nurse-client rapport and even harm the client's emotional well-being. Think of verbal communication as a continuum from destructive to constructive. Destructive communication can damage a client's self-esteem; constructive communication builds and preserves it.

DESTRUCTIVE COMMUNICATION	CONSTRUCTIVE COMMUNICATION
● Erodes self-esteem ● Conveys disrespect	● Promotes self-esteem ● Aids self-discovery ● Conveys respect

Techniques that facilitate communication

TECHNIQUE	DESCRIPTION	EXAMPLE
Silence	Refraining from speech to give the client (and the nurse) time to sort out thoughts and feelings	*Client:* "I hate you and everyone else." The nurse remains silent, with her body in an open position, and observes the client.
Self-disclosure	Sharing personal information at an opportune moment to convey understanding	*Client:* "My husband's death was like losing a major part of my life." *Nurse:* "I had a similar feeling when my husband died."
Suggestion	Posing alternatives for client consideration	*Client:* "I won't see a shrink!" *Nurse:* "Have you ever thought about…?" *Client:* "I don't like that, either." *Nurse:* "What would happen if you…?"
Confrontation	Acknowledging discrepancies in the client's verbal and nonverbal behaviors; calling attention to evasions, distortions, smoke screens, and game playing	*Client:* "I don't have a problem with alcohol." *Nurse:* "You say that alcohol hasn't created any problems for you, yet you have had two DUIs and your wife nags you about your drinking."
Concreteness	Clarifying the meaning of the client's communication; being clear, direct, and to the point	*Client:* "They said…" *Nurse:* "Who said that?"
Genuineness	Giving honest feedback when the client is ready; acting in a congruent manner with the client	*Client:* "You look bored." *Nurse:* "I'm not bored, but I do feel very tired." *Client:* "Do you think I'm weird?" *Nurse:* "Sometimes."
Immediacy	Acknowledging what's occurring between the nurse and the client as it happens	*Client:* "I think I have the right to know as much about you as you know about me." *Nurse:* "It sounds like you may not be too sure that I'll be able to understand what you're experiencing."
Empathy	Experiencing another's feelings temporarily	*Client:* "This whole thing is a mistake. I shouldn't even be here." *Nurse:* "It sounds like it's difficult for you to be here."
Respect	Conveying openness, a nonjudgmental attitude, and a desire to hear what the client has to say	*Client:* "What difference does it make? You just think I'm wrong, anyway." *Nurse:* "Try me. I'd like to hear about what's been happening."
Reflection	Paraphrasing what the client has said	*Client:* "The cop was out to get me. He had no reason to pull me over. It was a real set-up." *Nurse:* "You believe that it was unfair for the police to pull you over."
Broad opening	Using a general statement or question to encourage the client to set the direction for the session	The client enters the room, takes a seat, and looks expectantly at the nurse. *Nurse:* "How has it gone since we last met?" or "How are you today?"
Restating	Repeating what the client has said to indicate that the nurse is listening and interested (may encourage the client to elaborate)	*Client:* "I don't belong here." *Nurse:* "You don't belong here?" *Client:* "Of course not. I'm not like the others here. I'm educated and have a good job."
Focusing	Assisting the client to explore a specific topic	*Client:* "I don't know where to begin." *Nurse:* "What's your biggest problem now?" *Client:* "I can't decide about…" *Nurse:* "Let's talk about that. Perhaps more discussion will help you decide."

Nontherapeutic communication

Characteristics of nontherapeutic communication include:
- focusing on the caregiver
- giving advice, rather than seeking information
- changing the subject, rather than pursuing clarification, elaboration
- confronting the subject in an untimely or hostile manner
- failing to hear or acknowledge the client
- blaming the client (which suggests that the client is wrong)
- using trite expressions, cliches, ignoring the problem
- talking more than listening
- focusing on why instead of what we can do now.

Nursing actions
Nursing actions that promote therapeutic communication include:
- assessing the client's behavioral patterns
- diagnosing the client's underlying needs
- developing goals with the client (if the client's anxiety level permits)
- responding in a way that enhances the client's self-esteem and functioning
- using active listening skills, such as keeping an open body posture; appearing alert, relaxed, and attentive; and gesturing appropriately
- ensuring that communication is culturally sensitive, including awareness of the appropriateness of eye contact, posture, and personal space (see *Techniques that facilitate communication*)
- avoiding role conflicts
- evaluating the outcome.

See *Nontherapeutic communication,* for nursing actions that impede therapeutic communication.

Growth and development
A vital aspect of the nursing role is to understand the client's physical, cognitive, and psychosocial levels of growth and development. Renowned psychiatrists Erikson and Piaget developed theories that define personality and cognitive development.

Erikson's theory of personality development
Erik Erikson postulated a theory of personality development that begins with Freudian theory but emphasizes the healthy aspects of personality development rather than the pathologic ones, building from predictable, age-related stages. Erikson describes key conflicts or core problems from which, after successful completion or mastery of one problem, the individual moves on to the next problem. Each conflict has a favorable and unfavorable component. No core problem is ever solved in its entirety. With each new situation, the core problem demands another resolution. (See *Psychosocial development,* pages 26 and 27.)

Piaget's theory of cognitive development
Jean Piaget developed the best-known and most comprehensive theory regarding children's thinking, or cognition. The development of cognition represents a continuous and orderly process. Piaget postulated four major stages, each derived from and based on accomplishments of the previous stage.

The following information reviews psychosocial and cognitive development together with physical-motor and social-play development throughout the life span. Ages listed are approximate.

Sensorimotor: Birth to age 2
- This is a stage of simple learning.
- The child progresses from reflex activity to repetitive behavior and then to imitative behavior.
- The child displays a high level of curiosity.
- The child begins to develop a sense of self as different and separate from the environment.
- The child learns that objects have permanence and existence even if they aren't visible.

Examples of this development are the emerging social smile and differentiated cry of the infant, progressing to the self-exploration of the hands and then the feet. The infant imitates pattycake and then peek-a-boo, finally realizing that the hidden object is still there.

Preoperational: Age 2 to 7
- The young child can't empathize.
- The child interprets objects and events solely in relationship to himself.
- The child can't make deductions or generalizations. Learning and thinking embrace only what the child sees, hears, feels, or experiences.
- The child begins elaborate concepts and "correct" experiences with increasing language skills, imaginative play, questioning, and interacting.

Psychosocial development

This chart outlines key points for psychosocial development through the life span.

DEVELOPMENTAL STAGE	PSYCHOSOCIAL SKILLS	NURSING INTERVENTIONS
Birth to age 1 Sense of trust versus mistrust	<ul><li>Learns basic needs will be met</li><li>Develops self-trust and trust in others</li><li>Learns mistrust when care is inconsistent or basic needs are unmet</li></ul>	<ul><li>Educate the parents on infant care techniques.</li></ul>
Age 1 to 3 Sense of autonomy versus shame and doubt	<ul><li>Focuses on autonomy (independence) and body control (trust)</li><li>Gains physical and motor ability to be independent and can manipulate the environment and others</li><li>Holds on to or lets go such as with sphincter control</li><li>Demonstrates uncertainty with gaining mastery and control as displayed by rituals, negativism, and temper tantrums</li></ul>	<ul><li>Assess through family history the child's usual routine, physical security objects, and sensorimotor independence.</li><li>Facilitate maximum consistency in the above areas.</li><li>Assist caregivers in offering choices and in not chastising or shaming the child in response to negative behaviors.</li><li>Accept and explain regressive behaviors in response to illness and stress.</li></ul>
Age 3 to 6 Sense of initiative versus guilt	<ul><li>Displays vivid imagination, magical thinking, sense of right and wrong</li><li>Becomes increasingly aware of body parts</li><li>Displays anxiety that gives rise to night terrors, fears of bodily mutilation, physical aggression, and acting out behaviors</li></ul>	<ul><li>Provide a concrete explanation and demonstration of treatments and procedures.</li><li>Provide the opportunity for acting out participatory play.</li><li>Avoid threatening terminology, such as "cutting off," when referring to surgical procedures.</li><li>Encourage outward expression of fear, anxiety, anger, and pain.</li><li>Avoid labeling behavior as good or bad.</li></ul>
Age 6 to 12 Sense of industry versus inferiority	<ul><li>Becomes success-oriented worker and producer</li><li>Aspires to be the best at everything, doesn't like to fail</li><li>Gradually learns social skills of cooperation, compromise, negotiation, completion, and achievement</li><li>Learns to play and live by rules</li><li>Feels inadequate and inferior</li></ul>	<ul><li>Promote activities that the child can complete independently.</li><li>Foster the child's self-esteem by praising his achievements and appropriate behavior.</li></ul>
Age 12 to 19 Sense of identity versus role diffusion	<ul><li>Seeks to gain personal identity</li><li>May demonstrate negativism, ritualism, and emotional lability, reflecting emotional turmoil evolving from body changes and the question "Who am I?"</li><li>Allows peers to influence decision making</li><li>May experience role diffusion caused by unresolved answers to complex questions about adolescence</li></ul>	<ul><li>Involve the adolescent in decision making as much as possible.</li><li>Set goals together.</li><li>Encourage active participation in implementing the care plan.</li><li>Provide the supplies needed to enhance body image when possible.</li><li>Impose as few limits as possible.</li><li>Be aware of the impact of any threat to body image.</li><li>Use therapeutic communication skills.</li></ul>

Psychosocial development *(continued)*

DEVELOPMENTAL STAGE	PSYCHOSOCIAL SKILLS	NURSING INTERVENTIONS
Age 20 to 40 Sense of intimacy versus isolation	● Shares and forms commitments with other persons without fearing identity loss ● Focuses on individual needs, excluding all other interests, when intimacy isn't achieved	● Assess stresses and changes experienced. ● Provide teaching and resources to help the client to maintain health. ● Be aware that, with hospitalization, the client may face loss of employment benefits, disrupted lifestyle, and decreased self-esteem. ● Be nonjudgmental about the client's needs and lifestyle. Don't impose personal attitudes.
Age 40 to 65 Sense of generativity versus stagnation	● Helps the next generation become adults ● Assumes work, family, and community responsibility ● Becomes egocentric, caring only about himself if no responsibilities are developed ● May not develop further if the above occurs	● Consider the stresses and responsibilities that are affecting the client. ● Assess a client in relation to these stresses. ● Provide resources and emotional support to the client, his family and friends.
Age 65 and older Sense of integrity versus despair	● Reviews life events ● Displays satisfaction if content with his life ● Displays hopelessness and desperation if not content with his life	● Recognize the physical and social changes and limitations they may cause. ● Promote independence and use of the skills the client retains. ● Stimulate functioning senses. ● Treat a client as an adult even if the client behaves as an adolescent or a child. ● Provide emotional support when needed for life events such as the deaths of friends and family.

● Near the end of this stage, reasoning becomes intuitive and the child begins to work with problems of weight, length, size, and time.

Concrete operations: Age 7 to 11
● Increasingly logical and coherent thoughts are present.
● The child can sort, classify, order, and organize facts about the world.
● The child collects and saves everything from stamps to crickets and toads.
● Although containers may differ, the child realizes that weight, volume, and number may be the same.
● Problem solving proceeds in a concrete manner.
● The child can handle several aspects of a situation at one time.
● Abstractions remain incomprehensible.

● The child can now recognize other points of view, as evidenced by a stronger desire for companionship and teamwork.

Formal operations: Age 12 to 15
● This period is characterized by flexibility.
● The adolescent learns to deal with abstractions and abstract symbols.
● Arriving at answers, the adolescent may confuse the ideal world with the real world but can nevertheless solve problems, develop hypotheses, test them, and reach conclusions.
● The adolescent, working through moral, ethical, religious, and social issues, begins to achieve an adult identity.

SPOT CHECK

According to Piaget, at which stage would an individual:
A. learn that objects have permanence even when invisible?
B. learn to deal with abstractions?
C. interpret the world solely in relationship to himself?
D. learn to classify, sort, and organize?
Answers: A-sensorimotor; B-formal operations; C-preoperational;
D-concrete operations

Physical-motor and social-play development

Normal physical and motor development is usually categorized by age level, although each person's development is ongoing and unique and progress in one level may overlap into another. Such overlap is also true of social and play behaviors, which correspond with physical-motor developmental levels. The following section presents behaviors of special interest for those providing nursing care.

Birth to age 3 months
Physical-motor development
● At age 1 month, the infant's eyes follow bright, moving objects.
● At age 2 months, the crossed-eye reflex disappears.
● At age 3 months, a stimulus evokes a social smile response. The infant can rest on his forearms, keeps his head in midline, and discovers his hands and stares at them. The stepping reflex disappears and Landau reflex appears. Now able to lift his head and chest, the infant holds a rattle and stares at it and can follow any moving object with his eyes.

Social-play development
● The infant responds when a caregiver shakes a rattle or dangles a bright, moving object such as a mobile.
● The infant also responds favorably to the caregiver's smiles, caresses, and speech. When the infant is awake, the caregiver should rock, pat, and play with the infant and change his position regularly.
● The infant usually reacts positively to a busy box and enjoys the freedom to kick.
● The infant expresses demands by crying, enjoys sucking, and reacts affectionately to all who approach.
● By age 3 months, the infant coos, babbles, gurgles, and laughs aloud; responds to his name; shows pleasure; and makes sounds and faces in reaction to the social play of others.

Age 4 to 6 months
Physical-motor development
● The infant holds his head up for longer periods, displays improved eye coordination, and turns from his back to his side.
● At age 5 months, the infant can sit with support.
● At age 6 months, the infant can turn over completely.
● By age 6 months, birth weight doubles and the infant begins to turn his head toward familiar sounds.

Social-play development
● The 4-month-old infant recognizes his parents, demands attention by fussing, grasps objects with both hands, and shows excitement with his whole body.
● By age 5 months, the infant plays with his toes and smiles at a mirror image.
● At age 6 months, the infant holds out his arms to be picked up and shows definite likes and dislikes.

Age 6 months
Physical-motor development
● The 6-month-old infant can raise his chest and upper abdomen, keeping his weight on his hands.
● The infant can sit in a high chair with a straight back.
● The infant can turn from his back to his abdomen.
● The infant can hold a bottle or eat a cracker independently.
● The infant can grasp his feet and pull them to his mouth.
● Teething may begin.

Social-play development
● The infant may exhibit loud laughter.
● The infant demonstrates the ability to distinguish familiar and strange faces.
● The infant exhibits the desire to be picked up and held.
● The infant enjoys rattles and stuffed toys.
● The infant displays frequent mood swings.
● The infant begins imitating others (for instance, by coughing or sticking out his tongue).

Age 7 months
Physical-motor development
● The infant can sit and lean forward on his hands and can transfer objects from one hand to the other.
● The infant's upper central incisors typically erupt during this period.

Social-play development

● The infant begins to display a fear of strangers.
● The infant displays oral aggressiveness (biting), and he'll reject disliked foods by keeping his mouth closed.

Age 8 months
Physical-motor development

● The infant shows increased bowel and bladder regularity.
● The infant sits steadily.
● The infant releases objects at will.
● The infant exhibits a beginning pincer grasp.

Social-play development

● The infant shows his dislikes, such as for getting dressed or having a diaper changed.

Age 9 months
Physical-motor development

● The infant can typically pull to a standing position, and upper lateral incisors may erupt.

Social-play development

● The infant begins to exhibit a fear of being left alone.

Age 10 months
Physical-motor development

● Although crawling most of the time, the infant can step with one foot if supported by a person or an object.
● The infant has a neat pincer grasp but a crude release.
● New social-play behavior patterns emerge and others continue.

Social-play development

● Fear of strangers increases, and scolding elicits a strong reaction.
● The infant continues to imitate others (as when waving "bye-bye").
● The infant looks at and follows pictures in a book.

Age 11 months
Physical-motor development

● The child is creeping with his abdomen off the floor.
● The child can stroll while holding onto a person or an object.
● The child can put objects into a container and remove them

Social-play development

● The child begins to drop objects deliberately — either to marvel at their sound or to gain the attention of others.
● During this period, the child begins to learn self-feeding and helps with dressing. Playing games, such as peek-a-boo, and shaking the head "no" are common.

Age 12 months
Physical-motor development

● The child's weight has tripled from birth.
● The 1-year-old child can sit alone and can roll over.
● The child usually has eight teeth by the end of the 1st year.
● If not already evident, the child develops a fear of strangers and clings to the mother.
● The child understands simple commands.
● The child helps with dressing and points to indicate desired objects.

Social-play development

● The child discriminates in giving affection and shows fear, anxiety, and sympathy.
● Having learned to repeat behaviors that elicit laughter, the child continues to imitate, wave "bye-bye," and shake the head "no."

Age 10 to 14 months
Physical-motor development

● Creeping and crawling for locomotion, the child pulls up to a standing position independently and stands for extended periods with support.
● By the end of this stage, the child walks with a broad, stiff-legged gait.

Social-play development

● The child makes attempts at self-feeding with a spoon, poking and probing with the index finger, and develops a fondness for finger foods.

Age 13 to 15 months
Physical-motor development

● The child likes to empty containers, fill boxes, and intentionally drop objects.
● The child puts a spoon to his mouth and drinks from a cup.
● The child hands objects to people.
● The child demonstrates the ability to creep upstairs; however, he can't come down. Attempts to back down stairs begin at 15 to 16 months.

- The child can build two-block towers and put a round peg in a round hole.

Social-play development
- The child wants to be with adults but also enjoys playing alone, exploring kitchen cupboards, and imitating housekeeping duties.
- The child doesn't differentiate sex roles.
- The child displays a fondness for kissing pictures and mirrored reflections and asks for things by pointing and grunting.
- The child can remove his own shoes and perform self-feeding.
- The child wants and enjoys an audience and is capable of affection and sympathy, especially in the form of sympathetic crying.

 SPOT CHECK

At what age would a child begin to play with blocks?
13 to 15 months

Age 16 to 24 months
Physical-motor development
- The child explores his entire physical world and is all over the house.
- The child falls less frequently.
- The child walks backward with a broad-based gait; he walks forward and runs with a stiff, wide-based gait.
- The child stoops to pick up toys.
- The child can throw a ball and unzip zippers; loves to push, pull, tug, bang, carry, and hug toys; and can manage a spoon without rotation.
- By 15 to 18 months, the anterior fontanelle closes.

Social-play development
- The child continues to play alone.
- The child is profoundly ritualistic and exerts control with temper tantrums.
- At 18 months, sphincter control begins (the child controls adults through toileting). The child likes to clean up messes, flush the toilet, run water, and put things in their place.
- The child uses push-pull, noisy toys; points to body parts on request; shows sustained interest; and imitates others.
- The child finds security in thumbsucking or in a favorite blanket or toy and becomes easily frustrated and angry.

- Personal identity begins, with differentiation between "you" and "me."

Age 2
Physical-motor development
- The child puts on and takes off his shoes and clothes, washes and dries his hands, and begins to use scissors and string large beads.
- The 2-year-old child tries to dance; pinches, kicks, hits, and bites; goes up and down steps one at a time; and can turn pages.

Social-play development
- Still ritualistic, the child engages in solitary and some parallel play; imitates older children; uses three-word phrases; is shy with strangers (negativism peaks at $2\frac{1}{2}$ years); develops fears of bedwetting, animals, and being deserted; may become a fussy eater; and displays slower growth.

Age 3
Physical-motor development
- The child ascends steps with alternating feet, rides a tricycle, copies a circle, builds a nine- to ten-cube tower, and completely performs self-feeding.
- The child's pulse rate is about 95 beats/minute; respiratory rate, about 24 breaths/minute; and blood pressure, 100/67 ($\pm$25) mm Hg.

Social-play development
- The child has developed a vocabulary of about 900 words, displays telegraphic speech, and constantly asks questions.
- The child knows his own sex and identifies with it; he also engages in parallel and associative play.
- The child can better tolerate brief separation from his parents or his primary caregiver.

Age 4
Physical-motor development
- The child hops on one foot, skips, catches a ball, throws overhand, uses scissors, and can lace (but not tie) his shoes.

Social-play development
- Questioning reaches a peak during this time, and exaggerated stories and mild profanity are typical.
- The child can't conceive that, although an object's shape may change, its mass remains the same; he judges by one dimension (centering).

● The child has a developing sense of right and wrong; identifies strongly with the parent of the opposite sex; and still experiences many fears.

Age 5
Physical-motor development
● The eruption of the child's permanent teeth may begin. The child jumps rope and can tie shoelaces.

Social-play development
● The child identifies coins, can name at least four colors, and knows the days of the week.
● The child engages in cooperative play, attempts to resolve fears and anxieties through play, and tries to be brave.
● The child is independent in self-care activities, such as bathing and dressing.

Age 6
Physical-motor development
● With increased activity, the child's appetite increases; plain food, snacking, and eating on the run are favored.
● The child begins to dislike bathing.
● Possessing more poise and greater control of motor abilities, the child is in constant motion, practicing coordination of large and fine motor groups.

Social-play development
● Temper tantrums reappear at age 6.
● The child becomes more self-centered, boastful, and bossy.
● The child enjoys dramatic play to enact feelings and often is "fresh," rude, and ready to fight.
● The child develops fear concerning the supernatural, unusual noises, his mother's death, and any self-injury; persistent night terrors are common.

Age 7 to 9
Physical-motor development
● The child begins to lose his baby teeth at age 6 to 7, with his first molars coming in at around age 7.
● Physical-motor changes at ages 7, 8, and 9 are subtle, but the child develops better coordination of physical and motor skills and practices to achieve perfection.
● Less brisk and wiggly than at age 6, the child's movements are more fluid and graceful.

Social-play development
● During this time, the child is more likely to shout than act out.

● The child resists bathing less and shows little interest in clothes.
● The child prefers to play with same-sex companions; competes but doesn't like to lose; and withdraws from situations rather than resist.
● More contemplative than before, the child can be moved by sad stories and is becoming a real family member with chores and responsibilities.
● The gang stage begins; close relationships with peers begin to take shape.
● The child begins to collaborate and compromise; the major fear is failure.

Age 10 to 12
Physical-motor development
● Rapid changes in height, weight, body contour, and physiology typically coincide with an increased appetite and an awkwardness in motor ability.
● With rapid growth, the child begins to envision adulthood.
● Onset of secondary sex characteristics occurs in some boys.
● Girls can no longer compete with boys in physical strength.
● The child requires an adequate explanation of body changes; one who lags behind in physical development needs special understanding as he compares his body changes with those of classmates and friends.

Social-play development
● During this stage, girls usually seem wiser and more poised than boys.
● For both sexes, companionship becomes more important than play as a social behavior. Club membership and teamwork play increasingly significant roles, although the sexes tend to remain separated.
● The child likes to run errands, enjoys crafts and music, and seeks others' ideas and opinions.

Age 13 to 16
Physical-motor development
● The early teenager may be awkward and uncoordinated, with poor posture, and may tire easily because heart and lung growth doesn't keep pace with that of the rest of the body.
● Although the adolescent has a large appetite, a preference for fast foods and fad diets can lead to poor nutrition and lethargy.

● Physiologic problems that concern the teenager include acne, increased perspiration, and a propensity to blush easily.
● The teenager develops a full growth of pubic and axillary hair.

Social-play development
● The adolescent likes parties, dances, movies, daydreaming, telephone conversations, books, and hobbies.
● The peer group becomes extremely important.
● While beginning to become emancipated from the parents, the adolescent develops crushes on or attachments to neighbors or teachers.
● The adolescent typically shows increased interest in the opposite sex, and strong friendships develop with one or two friends.
● Concerns embrace morality, ethics, religion, and social customs.
● The adolescent requires help in adjusting to and accepting body changes.

Age 17 to 19
Physical-motor development
● A young man has a beginning beard, his structural growth is near completion, and his physique is that of a mature male, including genital size and pubic hair.
● A young woman may grow 2 to 4 inches taller after menarche; breasts and pubic hair have reached adult development, and she's capable of reproduction about 1 year after menses begin.
● Both the young man and the young woman have more energy as the growth spurt slows.

Social development
● The young adult is more mature and begins to enjoy an interdependent relationship with the parents while finding increasingly less satisfaction from the peer group.
● Learning to balance pleasure and responsibility, the young adult engages in romantic love affairs and may still daydream about adult life but also begins to establish career goals and plans how to achieve them.

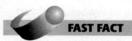 **FAST FACT**

As an adolescent passes into the 17- to 19-year-old age-group, parents may need assistance facing the loss of their dependent child.

Age 20 to 30
Physical-motor development
● Physical strength and physiologic reserve are at a maximum, and the person's health needs usually aren't significant.

Social development
● Body image and sexuality are extremely important during this time.
● Selection of a marriage partner — and perhaps the decision to have children — commonly occurs.
● Marriage and parenthood necessarily entail periods of adjustment fraught with increased stresses, such as changing one's lifestyle to accommodate children and socializing the children into the family.
● Optional lifestyles (celibacy, childless marriage, single parenthood, homosexuality, communal living) may also develop; each has inherent stresses and periods of adjustment, compromise, and change.

Age 30 to 40
Physical-motor changes
● As physical strength, physiologic reserve, and systemic functioning begin to diminish, proper nutrition becomes more important.
● The person requires fewer fats and calories in the diet and may require more vitamins and iron.
● Exercise is essential to regulate appetite, release tension, enhance rest and sleep, increase muscle tone, and improve well-being.

Social development
● Choice of vocation and career successes and failures largely determine the person's social status and roles.
● Unemployment or unsatisfying employment may lower self-esteem.
● Hectic schedules and limited income during this phase may contribute to an unhealthy diet.
● To attain career goals, the person may work or worry excessively at the expense of needed sleep and relaxation.

Age 40 to 65
Physical-motor changes
● Physical strength, physiologic reserve, and systemic functioning continue to diminish, mandating a low-calorie, high-vitamin diet with limited saturated fat.
● Exercise is still important but should be less strenuous.
● During this stage, the person may have concerns about stiff joints, wrinkles, gray hair, baldness, dentures, poor

hearing or vision, menopause, osteoporosis, nervousness, or depression.

● Angina, coronary occlusion, cancer, hypertension, peptic ulcer and, if the person smokes, respiratory disease are common.

● Stresses during this phase may lead to substance abuse or insomnia.

● Sexual problems may also develop; mutilating surgery, chronic disease, or menopause can dramatically lower the person's self-esteem, particularly if the sexual partner doesn't provide emotional support.

Social development

● Assuming more significant and varied roles at this stage than at any other stage in the life span, the adult is now responsible not only for himself, his spouse, and his children but also for his parents, coworkers, and community members.

● As children grow up and begin their own families, the adult in this stage may need to rethink his goals and consider lifestyle changes. The empty nest syndrome may occur, causing depression.

● A woman may use this period to broaden her education and enter or resume a career; a man may need to prepare for a second vocation.

Age 65 and over
Physical-motor changes

● Physical strength, physiologic reserve, and systemic functioning decline.

● Hearing and vision loss may be more pronounced, and cataracts may require surgery. Other common geriatric problems include immobility, constipation, indigestion, arteriosclerosis, stroke, peripheral vascular disease, hypertension, coronary occlusions, and cancer.

● A man may have benign prostatic hypertrophy or experience the climacteric.

● A woman may have osteoporosis, resulting in bone fractures.

● The elderly person may have multiple chronic illnesses, with accompanying exacerbations and remissions.

● Prolonged bed rest proves highly detrimental during this stage — lack of exercise can impair digestion, circulation, muscle and joint function, and mental alertness.

● Decreased sensitivity of taste buds and olfactory receptors typically causes the elderly adult to overseason foods.

● Exercise, although important, must be tailored to individual needs.

Social development

● Having worked hard to achieve career goals, the elderly adult wants to enjoy the carefree leisure of retirement.

● Pursuing hobbies, spending time with family and friends, and participating in community events can provide enjoyment and satisfaction.

● The new lifestyle usually means living on a fixed income; thus, the person with an inadequate income worries about the present and the future and may live with other persons on fixed incomes simply to make ends meet.

● Declining health and the loss of family and friends can result in grieving, loneliness, and depression during this stage; some people withdraw from society (disengagement).

● Because reconciliation is important to many elderly adults, misunderstandings may be forgotten and relationships improved.

Nutrition

Nutrition is the process by which foods are selected and ingested and their nutrients are absorbed and used by the human body. The essential nutrients are:

● carbohydrates
● fats
● protein
● vitamins
● minerals
● water.

   Water, essential to sustain life, transports nutrients throughout the body and may contribute minerals when consumed. Foods contain the nutrients and energy that the body requires for growth, activity, and health promotion and maintenance.

Food selection guidelines

Individual food preferences are influenced not only by the taste and odor of specific foods but also by the availability of foods, family economic status, cultural and religious preferences and restrictions, and the food purchaser's knowledge of nutrition. Several guidelines have been developed to help individuals plan and evaluate food intake.

Dietary reference intakes

In recent years, various agencies in the United States and Canada have been making a joint effort to develop dietary reference intakes (DRIs). These replace the periodic updates of the recommended dietary allowances (RDAs). DRIs comprise four different reference values:

Food Guide Pyramid

Each of these food groups provides some, but not all, of the nutrients you need. No one food group is more important than another for good health. Fats, oils, and sweets – the foods in the small tip of the Pyramid – should be used sparingly.

Some tips to remember when teaching clients include:

● The number of servings depends on age and degree of physical activity.

● Older children and teenagers (ages 9 to 18) and some adults over age 50 need three servings daily from the milk group. Others need two servings daily.

● During pregnancy and lactation, the recommended number of milk group servings is the same as for nonpregnant women.

● Teen boys and active men need three servings from the meat and beans group.

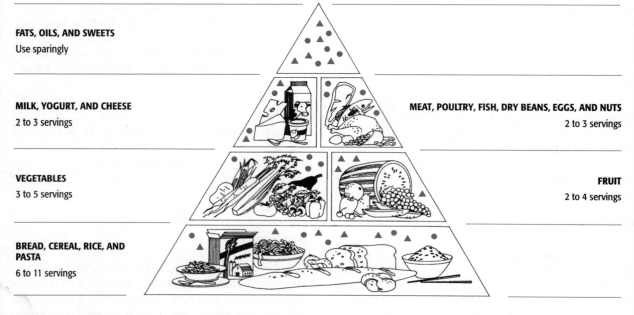

FATS, OILS, AND SWEETS
Use sparingly

MILK, YOGURT, AND CHEESE
2 to 3 servings

MEAT, POULTRY, FISH, DRY BEANS, EGGS, AND NUTS
2 to 3 servings

VEGETABLES
3 to 5 servings

FRUIT
2 to 4 servings

BREAD, CEREAL, RICE, AND PASTA
6 to 11 servings

KEY   ● Fat (naturally occurring and added)   ▲ Sugars (added)

These symbols show that fat and added sugars come mostly from fats, oils, and sweets but can be part of or added to foods from the other food groups as well.

Source: U.S. Department of Agriculture, Center for Nutrition Policy and Promotion, *Home and Garden Bulletin,* Number 252, October, 1996. Dietary Guidelines for Americans, 2000, 5E 2000. United States Department of Agriculture/United States Department of Health and Human Services, Home and Garden Bulletin #232.

● RDAs — amount of essential nutrients considered adequate for meeting the nutritional needs of 97% to 98% of the healthy population

– Daily consumption of various foods from different food groups provides the best means of meeting RDAs.

– RDAs aren't to be confused with the United States recommended daily allowances (USRDAs), separate standards used by the Food and Drug Administration for nutrition labeling purposes.

● estimated average requirement — the amount of a nutrient sufficient for 50% of individuals

● tolerable upper intake level — maximum level of daily nutrients that's unlikely to cause risks of adverse health effects in most people

● adequate intake — used for nutrient recommendations when an RDA isn't available

Food Guide Pyramid
The Food Guide Pyramid provides recommended daily servings from the basic food groups to constitute a nutritious daily food plan. (See *Food Guide Pyramid.*)

Dietary guidelines for Americans
Dietary Guidelines for Americans, most recently revised in 2000 by the U.S. Department of Agriculture and the Department of Health and Human Services, emphasize health improvement by reducing the intake of harmful foods, stressing moderation in eating habits, and encouraging physical activity. Follow these tips:
● Aim for a healthy weight.
● Be physically active each day.
● Use the Food Guide Pyramid to guide choices.
● Choose a variety of grains daily — especially whole grains.
● Choose a variety of fruits and vegetables daily.
● Keep food safe to eat.
● Choose a diet low in saturated fat and cholesterol and moderate in total fat.
● Choose beverages and foods to moderate intake of sugars.
● Choose and prepare foods with less salt.
● Drink alcohol in moderation, if at all.

Energy needs and balance
Energy is required for basal metabolism — ongoing internal processes, such as respiration, heartbeat, and glandular activity.

Basal metabolic rate
The basal metabolic rate (BMR) is influenced by sex, age, body composition, and physiologic status.

Energy value of food
The energy value of food is measured in kilocalories, commonly known as *calories.* Calories consist of carbohydrates, fats, and protein (the only nutrients that supply calories):
● Carbohydrates and protein each provide 4 calories per gram; fats provide 9 calories per gram.
● Carbohydrates and fats are the preferred energy sources, leaving protein for its important role in tissue maintenance.

● In addition to basal metabolism, calories are necessary for physical activity and for the 10% increase in BMR that occurs after eating.
When the number of calories consumed matches the number used for energy, an individual achieves energy balance. Calories in excess of energy needs are stored as fat in body adipose tissue. If insufficient calories are consumed, weight loss occurs.

Undernutrition
Resulting from a sustained deficit in nutrient intake, undernutrition depletes stored protein and compromises the immune system.

Overnutrition
Overnutrition leaves an individual vulnerable to the toxic effects of nutrient overdoses as well as to excess weight gain with associated health risks.

Energy nutrients
The essential nutrients that fuel the body are carbohydrates, protein, lipids, vitamins and minerals, and water. All of these supply the body with the necessary nutrients to sustain life.

Carbohydrates
Carbohydrates occur mainly as sugars, starches, and fiber; all carbohydrates must be modified to simple sugars before the body can absorb and use them.
The body requires at least 100 g of carbohydrates daily, the central nervous system needing a constant supply of glucose; ideally, 50% to 60% of total calories should be carbohydrates.
Although not a source of energy, fibrous plant materials provide bulk, and low fiber intake has been linked with constipation, diverticulitis, and cancer of the colon.

Sugars and starches
Sugars and starches provide the body with its primary source of energy. Glucose, also called *blood sugar,* is the form in which carbohydrates circulate in the bloodstream, providing energy to individual cells.

Lipids
Commonly known as *fats* (and chemically similar to carbohydrates), lipids provide the most concentrated source of energy to the body. Linoleic acid, the essential fatty

Reviewing selected vitamins

	MAJOR FUNCTIONS	PRIMARY SOURCES	CLINICAL DEFICIENCIES	TOXICITIES
Water-soluble vitamins				
C (ascorbic acid)	Collagen formation, wound healing, resistance to stress and infection, blood vessel elasticity	Citrus fruit, strawberries, broccoli, cabbage, green peppers	Easy bruising, bleeding gums, delayed wound healing, scurvy	GI upset, diarrhea, renal calculi
B₁ (thiamine)	Carbohydrate metabolism, nerve transmission	Pork, peanuts, whole grains	Poor appetite, leg cramps, depression	None
B₂ (riboflavin)	Carbohydrate, protein, and fat metabolism; normal appetite	Milk, meat, wheat germ	Mouth lesions, scaly skins, glossitis	None
Niacin (nicotinic acid)	Carbohydrate, protein, and fat metabolism; healthy skin	Meat, peanuts, whole grains	Pellagra, dermatitis, diarrhea, depression	Flushing, tingling, vision disturbances
B₆ (pyridoxine)	Amino acid synthesis, fatty acid metabolism	Meat, whole grains, nuts	Skin lesions, depression, seizures	None
Folic acid	Nucleic acid synthesis, amino acid breakdown, red blood cell (RBC) formation	Green, leafy vegetables; asparagus; broccoli	Slow growth, megaloblastic anemia	None
B₁₂ (cyanocoloalamin)	Formation of nucleic acids, bone marrow, and RBCs	Meat, eggs, fish	Pernicious anemia, nervousness, weakness	None
Fat-soluble vitamins				
A (retinol)	Normal vision and growth, healthy epithelium, aid to reproduction	Dark green and yellow fruits and vegetables, margarine and butter, whole milk and cheeses	Night blindness, thickened cracked skin, poor growth, reduced resistance to infection	Skin rashes, hair loss, vomiting, abnormal bone growth, increased intracranial pressure
D (cholecalciferol)	Absorption and utilization of calcium and phosphorus, bone matrix formation	Sunlight, fortified milk	Rickets (in children), osteomalacia (in adults)	Elevated serum calcium, kidney damage, growth retardation, vomiting, diarrhea
E (tocopherol)	Antioxidant (protects cell membrane)	Vegetable oils, margarine, nuts, whole grains	None	Headache, nausea, fatigue, dizziness, blurred vision
K (menadione)	Blood clotting (prothrombin formation)	Intestinal bacteria (synthesize adequate vitamin K)	Hemorrhage	Excessive breakdown of RBCs (synthetic form)

acid, must be obtained from dietary sources and is necessary for normal growth of infants. In addition to serving as an energy source, dietary fats carry fat-soluble vitamins, cushion vital body organs, insulate the body, and add a feeling of fullness and satisfaction to the completion of a meal.

Fat requirements
Ideally, fats should be limited to 30% of total calories; the requirement for linoleic acid is 3% of total calories for infants and 2% for adults. In choosing dietary fats, consider the benefits of fish (such as mackerel and tuna), which contain omega-3 fatty acids, and oils (such as peanut, canola, and olive oils), which contain monounsaturated fatty acids; both groups of fatty acids help reduce the risk of coronary heart disease.

Protein
Protein provides the foundation for all body cells. Protein is broken down by the body into its individual components, the amino acids.

Amino acids
Essential amino acids can't be made by the body and must be obtained from food. Nonessential amino acids can be synthesized within the body. The principal function of protein is to provide the amino acids needed for growth and the formation of enzymes, hormones, antibodies, muscles, hemoglobin, and other body tissues.

Protein requirements
The adult requirement for protein is 0.8 g/kg of ideal body weight. Protein is 16% nitrogen. In a healthy adult (except one who is pregnant or lactating), nitrogen intake equals nitrogen output. With disease, tissue wasting occurs, and nitrogen losses exceed nitrogen intake; this negative nitrogen balance ceases when tissue repair begins. Insufficient protein intake can compromise the immune system, impairing the body's response to stress and infection.

Vitamins and minerals
Vitamins are needed daily in small quantities to sustain growth and health; they're classified as water-soluble or fat-soluble. (See *Reviewing selected vitamins.*)

SPOT CHECK

Match the vitamin deficiency with the appropriate vitamin or nutrient.

Vitamin	Clinical deficiency
1. Vitamin A (retinol)	A. Hemorrhage
2. Vitamin B$_1$ (thiamine)	B. Scurvy
3. Vitamin B$_2$ (riboflavin)	C. None identified
4. Vitamin B$_6$ (pyridoxine)	D. Leg cramps
5. Vitamin C (absorbic acid)	E. Rickets
6. Vitamin D (cholecalciferol)	F. Mouth lesions
7. Vitamin E (tocopherol)	G. Night blindness
8. Vitamin K (menadione)	H. Pellagra
9. Niacin	I. Pernicious anemia
10. Folic acid	J. Slow growth
11. Vitamin B$_{12}$ (cyanocobalamin)	K. Skin lesions

Answers: 1-G, 2-D, 3-F, 4-K, 5-B, 6-E, 7-C, 8-A, 9-H, 10-J, 11-I

Minerals are inorganic elements that help with many vital body functions and give the body its structural strength and rigidity. (See *Reviewing selected minerals,* page 38.)

Nutrition requirements through the life cycle
Infant
The infant's nutritional needs are greater than those of any other age-group; for example:
● Protein and fluid needs are two to three times greater than those of an adult.
● Breast milk or formula alone is satisfactory for the first 5 to 6 months of life, at which time solid foods should be incorporated into the daily diet.

Childhood and adolescence
Childhood and adolescence are characterized by growth spurts that demand gradually increasing intake of all nutrients; snacking, often thought a bane, can contribute significantly to nutritional quality, particularly in adolescent years.

Adults
Nutritional needs of most adults under age 65 remain largely unchanged, with two exceptions:
● Caloric and iron requirements generally decrease.
● Pregnancy and lactation warrant special attention.
– Sound nutritional practices during pregnancy usually lead to a higher birth weight.

Reviewing selected minerals

	MAJOR FUNCTIONS	PRIMARY SOURCES	CLINICAL DEFICIENCIES
Calcium	Bone and tooth formation, blood clotting, muscle contraction, transmission of nerve impulses, normal heart rhythm	Milk, cheese, yogurt, broccoli, collards, kale, greens, canned salmon with bones	Osteoporosis, slow blood clotting, tetany, poor tooth formation
Phosphorus	Bone and tooth formation, carbohydrate and fat metabolism, pH buffer systems	Cheese, meat, milk and milk products, carbonated beverages	Osteoporosis, slow blood clotting, tetany, poor tooth formation
Magnesium	Carbohydrate, fat, and protein metabolism; adenosine triphosphate formation, nerve transmission, muscle contraction	Grains, green vegetables, milk, meat	Fluid and electrolyte imbalance, skin breakdown
Sodium	Fluid balance, nerve transmission, muscle contraction	Table salt, processed and preserved foods, milk and dairy products, protein foods	Headache, nausea, muscle spasm, mental confusion, fluid and electrolyte imbalance, cardiac disturbances, hypertension, edema
Potassium	Fluid balance, muscle activity	Widespread in all food groups, especially fruits and vegetables	Fluid and electrolyte imbalance, muscle weakness, tachycardia, cardiac arrhythmia, renal failure, severe dehydration
Trace elements			
Iron	Hemoglobin formation (as component of myoglobin)	Meats, whole grains, dried fruit, legumes	Iron deficiency anemia
Iodine	Regulation of basal metabolic rate (as component of thyroxin)	Iodized salt, saltwater fish	Goiter
Zinc	Protein synthesis, normal growth and sexual maturation, wound healing, normal senses of taste and smell, enzyme formation	Meats, legumes, nuts	Slow wound healing, altered senses of taste and smell, poor growth, delayed sexual development
Fluoride	Strengthening of tooth enamel	Fluoridated drinking water, fluoride supplementation	50% to 70% increase in tooth decay

– Daily nutritional needs include increases in calories (+300) and iron (+15 mg); protein intake increases to 60 g/day and calcium to 1,200 mg/day.

– The need for folic acid doubles during pregnancy and usually requires a vitamin supplement.
– A weight gain of 24 to 30 lb (11 to 13.5 kg) is recommended, although a gradual gain over the last two

trimesters is more important than the total amount gained.

– Lactation requires even more calories than are required during pregnancy.

– Body fat reserves accumulated during pregnancy supplement the additional 500 dietary calories needed daily for lactation.

– An additional 2 quarts (1.9 L) of fluid are needed daily to prevent dehydration and to produce an adequate milk supply.

Adults older than age 65

For those over age 65, adequate protein to maintain the immune system and muscle strength becomes increasingly important:

- Vitamin and mineral needs remain the same for an older adult.
- Energy needs may be lower because of gradual decreases in basal metabolism.
- Fluid needs are commonly overlooked because of loss of sense of thirst. It's important to prevent dehydration.

Family: The primary unit of health care

The family is the basic social unit — the primary unit of health care. Traditional definitions include:

- a group of people united by blood, marriage, or adoption who live in the same household and share a common culture
- the traditional nuclear American family consisting of husband, wife, and children.

   Example of newer concepts of family include:

- one or more people who live together, fulfilling certain roles and functions defined by the individual and the group
- those bound by blood, love, or both
- family unit without an adult.

Characteristics of families

- Loving and affectionate relationships (usually)
- Long-term associations
- Consideration of members as unique individuals

Functions of families

- Care and rearing of children
- Transmission of cultural values, traits, and rituals from one generation to another
- Socialization
- Provision of food, shelter, clothing, safety, and comfort
- Communication and decision making

Types of families

- Single adult living alone
- Beginning nuclear (husband and wife)
- Single parent
- Nuclear (husband, wife, and minor children)
- Extended (three or more generations forming a kinship network)
- Blended (husband and wife with children from previous relationships)
- Expanded (various age or kinship groups or unrelated family members)
- Communal (formed for specific ideologic or societal purposes; may comprise nuclear, extended, or expanded family units)

Developmental tasks and stages

Duvall defines families by tasks and phases.

Tasks

- Physical maintenance of the family unit
- Allocation of resources
- Division of labor
- Socialization of family members
- Reproduction or recruitment and release of family members
- Maintenance of order
- Placement of members into the larger society
- Maintenance of motivation and morale

Stages in family life cycle

There are two stages in the family life cycle — expanding families and contracting families.

Expanding families (from marriage and parenthood until children leave home)

- Childless couple establishing first home
- Expectant family or childbearing family (from first pregnancy through the first 30 months of the child's life)
- Family with preschool children
- Family with school-age children
- Family with teenagers

Contracting families
- Family with young adults
- Middle-age parent family
- Aging family

Family assessment data

In order to care for the patient, you must first assess the family using these criteria:
- family constellation (names, relationships, ages, sexes)
- education levels
- occupations
- communication patterns
- finances
- residences
- transportation needs
- family goals and functioning
- typical daily activities
- religious preferences
- avocation and recreational interests
- health resources
- strengths and coping mechanisms
- weaknesses and problems
- goals.

Rehabilitation

Rehabilitation is the restoration of a person to an optimal level of functioning in physical, mental, spiritual, and social aspects. Factors affecting rehabilitation include:
- severity or extent of injury (loss of some or all nerve pathways, muscles, bones, or circulation to a portion of the body)
- treatment and facilities (immediacy, adequacy, and continuity of medical, surgical, nutritional, and pharmacologic treatments)
- client's age, education, and psychological response to injury (all of which influence the client's ability to understand and participate in rehabilitative efforts)
- health care personnel (those skilled in various disciplines to develop and administer a rehabilitation program)
- financial resources (to pay for the facilities, treatments, and personnel services required for rehabilitation)
- legislation (to protect the rights of clients requiring rehabilitation).

Goals of rehabilitation

The short-term goals of client rehabilitation include regaining mobility, retaining remaining abilities and, when possible, preventing further incapacity or disability. The long-term goals of rehabilitation of the client include returning to a normal capacity.

Initiating therapy

Regaining and retaining the client's mobility involves initiation of various therapies, including exercise, heat or cold treatment, and the use of ambulatory and respiratory aids as well as genitourinary and speech therapy.

Additionally, the client may require occupational, physical, and nutritional therapy.

Activities of daily living
- Includes the abilities to breathe; dress, feed, bathe, move and transfer oneself; eliminate; and communicate

Exercises
- Use time and repetition to help a client regain or increase muscle tone, strength, and precision
- May involve therapists, family members, nurses, or other persons, depending on the client's needs or the expertise required
- May involve several types of exercise:
– active (performed by the client)
– active-assisted (performed by the client with therapist assistance)
– resistive-active (performed by the client with resistance provided by weights or devices)
– passive (performed without the client's active participation)
– selective or special (individualized to meet a client's needs to exercise a particular group of muscles for particular activities — for example, breathing exercises).

Heat or cold therapy
- May be moist or dry
- May involve short- or long-term application for vasoconstriction or vasodilation
- Must be intermittent to allow for tissue recovery (clients with impaired circulation have decreased tolerance for heat or cold therapy)

Ambulatory aids
- Walkers
– Lightweight, foldable, height-adjustable devices for assistance with weight bearing or mobility (the client must be cautioned about the safe degree of weight bearing and

must be taught to turn, sit, or stand to prevent falls and injury)
● Crutches
– Wood or aluminum, axillary-supported or forearm-supported, with two-, three-, or four-point gaits (the client must learn to walk, sit, rise, and go up and down stairs with one or both crutches)
● Canes
– Wood or metallic supports with one-, three-, or four-point bottoms (if using only one cane, the client holds it in the hand *opposite* the affected leg)
● Wheelchairs
– Metal or wood and metal, with detachable arm or leg rests, straps, and other supports (may be battery-operated or manually pushed; the client must learn to transfer correctly from the chair to a bed, car, and home)
● Braces
– Cloth, foam, or metallic supports for one or more joints (may be worn continuously or intermittently)
● Utensils
– Aid use by the handicapped (handles may be lengthened, enlarged, swiveled, hinged, or otherwise adapted for individual need)

Agencies for rehabilitative aid. The following agencies provide rehabilitative aid:
● Bureau of Vocational Rehabilitation for assistance in determining vocational interests, skills, and abilities and in finding aid for education and placement
● Social Security Administration for disability aid and services
● Medicare and Medicaid for primary or supplemental aid
● insurance companies for individualized coverage.

Respiratory aids
● Postural drainage to increase excretion of respiratory secretions
● Incentive spirometry to improve respiratory ventilation
● Machine-assisted breathing apparatus to increase respiratory depth and prevent atelectasis

Genitourinary rehabilitation
● Continuous bladder catheterization
● Self-catheterization and bladder training
● Bowel-training programs
● Penile prosthesis to help maintain an erection

● Sexual counseling to help the client cope with necessary adjustments

Speech rehabilitation
● Speech therapy to relearn the language or alternate speech methods
● Mechanical speech-amplifying aids

Occupational therapy
● Home management — preparation, assistance, and learning
● Craft preparation and education for muscle use
● Occupational retraining of muscles, joints, and the entire body

Physical therapy
● Specialized retraining for muscle use or muscle substitution to regain or maintain muscle strength
● Assistance in any of the previous rehabilitation techniques

Nutritional therapy
● Individualized dietary teaching for a client with a modified diet (high- or low-calorie, high-vitamin, high- or low-protein, acid ash, or low-sodium regimens or modifications, as needed)
● Modifications for home cooking and other food preparation and eating

Responses to rehabilitation
Psychological responses
Factors that influence the client's response include:
● age and personality
● severity or extent of injuries
● potential for partial or full recovery
● client's stress response pattern
● initial and continued medical, nursing, and rehabilitative care.

Common response pattern
There are five phases of the common response pattern to rehabilitation.

First phase (disbelief)
● Primary behaviors: anger, hostility, withdrawal, apathy, denial

● Other symptoms: irritability, sleeplessness, tension, numbness, fears, and vague pains (some of these behaviors may reflect the "alarm" reaction of Selye's stress response from the "onset" or "stressful event" stage of crisis intervention models)

Nursing interventions. The nurse should implement these steps:
● Allow the client to express his feelings.
● Accept dependency behaviors and provide care as needed.
● Encourage participation by the client and his family, if appropriate.
● Refer the client for vocational rehabilitation, if appropriate.

Second phase (awareness, transition, impact, and perception of the event)
● Gradual realization of the extent of injury or disability
● Possible behaviors: depression, anxiety, anger, silence, sadness, and grief (grief, sadness, and crying may or may not directly correlate with the injury or disability, but they represent the client's personal responses to developing awareness)

Nursing interventions. The nurse should implement these steps:
● Keep the lines of communication open.
● Accept the client's outward expressions of grief, sadness, anger, and guilt.
● Encourage and teach self-care as the client becomes able.
● Seek a psychiatric consultation if the client prolongs reactions.
● Refer the client for vocational rehabilitation, if appropriate.

Third phase (use of coping mechanisms – resistance, reorganization, disequilibrium, and retreat)
● Gradual realization of the disability's permanence, wavering between acceptance and rejection
● Possible behaviors: self-pity (even while actively participating in care), bargaining (for relief from pain, physical therapy, and so forth), and extreme dependence on others for detailed care

Nursing interventions. The nurse should implement these steps:

● Continue to accept the client's expressions and behaviors.
● Encourage active participation in physical therapy, occupational therapy, hydrotherapy, and so forth, as the client's condition dictates.
● Teach the client and family self-care techniques.

Fourth phase (resolution, convalescence, acknowledgment)
● Certainty of the disability's permanence, characterized by vacillation between rejection and acquiescence (client gradually leans more toward tolerance and acceptance if reactions are "normal" or "healthy")

Nursing interventions. The nurse should implement these steps:
● Accept the client's vacillations while preparing and teaching self-care.
● Allow sufficient time and opportunities for the client and family to become confident and proficient in care procedures.
● Follow up on vocational rehabilitation referrals.

Fifth phase (identity of change, restoration of equilibrium, recovery, or exhaustion; regaining as much health as possible)
● Active participation of the client in self-care and preparation for discharge
● Preparation of the family for the client's return home or transfer to a rehabilitation unit

Nursing interventions. The nurse should implement these steps:
● Ensure that the client and family can perform self-care.
● Complete continuity-of-care referrals as needed.

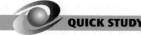 **QUICK STUDY**

How can you best remember the psychological factors that influence client responses to rehabilitation efforts?
Remember **ASPRI.**
   Age and personality
   Severity or extent of injury
   Potential for partial or full recovery
   Response to stress
   Initial and continuing care

Comparing grief and clinical depression

A client who appears to be suffering from clinical depression may actually be experiencing a phase of grieving. This chart shows the major distinctions between the two conditions.

CHARACTERISTICS OF GRIEF	CHARACTERISTICS OF CLINICAL DEPRESSION
● Healthy response	● Unhealthy response
● Self-resolution	● Self-resolution unlikely
● Little if any guilt	● Overwhelming guilt
● Self-esteem intact	● Loss of self-esteem
● Sadness	● Hopelessness, despair, and helplessness
● Ability to meet life's demands intact	● Impaired ability to meet life's demands
● No biochemical imbalance	● Possible biochemical imbalance
● Temporary loss of interest in pleasurable activities (anhedonia)	● Pervasive anhedonia

Grieving

Grieving is a normal human response to loss that may be real or perceived. Grieving may also be anticipatory such as grief when a child is terminally ill. It's a psychological process that allows one to cope with a loss and accept it as a reality and may last from 2 months to 1 year or longer.

The various phases and stages of grieving are identified by Kübler-Ross and Engel.

Phases of grief (Kübler-Ross)
- Denial and isolation
- Anger
- Bargaining
- Depression
- Acceptance

Acute stage of mourning (Engel)
- Shock and disbelief, characterized by rejection or denial
- Developing awareness, characterized by weeping and lashing out at loved ones and others
- Restitution or resolution, characterized by integration of negative and positive aspects of the lost person or object so that the individual can confront the loss comfortably

Losses that cause grief
- Client's impending death
- Loss of health, such as in cancer or another debilitating disease
- Loss of a body organ or part
- Loss or impending loss of a loved one (family member, friend, or pet)
- Major events precipitating a loss, such as job loss, divorce, loss of financial security, or one's home (see *Comparing grief and clinical depression*)

Nursing interventions
- Offer presence to the client.
- Use therapeutic communication, especially active listening.
- Encourage the client to express feelings and concerns.
- Assist the client in identifying coping mechanisms, such as significant others; and racial, cultural, religious, and spiritual support.
- Help the client to remember comfortably both negative and positive aspects of the lost person or object.

Factors that affect grieving
Some factors that may affect the grieving process include:
- developmental stage
- cultural and spiritual beliefs
- loss of a child
- gender
- cause of the loss
- unresolved issues with the deceased.

Principles of gerontologic nursing

Since the early 1970s, the number of Americans over age 65 has been increasing dramatically; the U.S. government projects that there will be 70 million Americans over age 65 by 2030. As the population ages, more demands are put on the health care delivery system by elderly clients, forcing greater focus on their special needs

The normal aging process leads to a steady deterioration in physical strength and to the development of chronic illnesses that threaten an older person's quality of life and independence. Gerontologic nursing concerns itself with the care of elderly clients and the development of processes that meet older adults' special needs.

Nursing practice focuses on helping elderly clients maintain optimum autonomy despite physiologic, pathologic, and psychosocial changes that occur during aging.

Theories of the aging process

There are many different theories regarding the aging process.

Developmental theories

● In 1963, Erikson postulated that the major developmental task of elderly clients was to choose between ego integrity and despair.
– *Ego integrity* refers to accepting one's lifestyle and the choices made during life.
– *Despair* refers to being dissatisfied with one's life and wishing for another chance to make different choices about how to live it.
● In 1972, Havighurst identified tasks that need to be completed during one's life.
– Completion leads to contentment.
– Unfulfillment leads to dejection and failure.

Social theories

● According to the ACTIVITY THEORY, satisfaction with becoming older means living a middle-age lifestyle.
● According to the CONTINUITY THEORY, adjusting successfully to the aging process requires continuing the patterns of living that have been established over one's lifetime; old habits and ethical values provide continuity as one moves from one age phase to another.

Changes associated with the aging process

With aging, the client undergoes many physiologic and psychosocial changes. You should be aware of the various changes because they affect your nursing care.

Physiologic changes

Integumentary

● Skin wrinkled, dry, thin, and pale
● Tendency toward sunburn
● Easily bruised

Cardiovascular

● Cardiac output and stroke volume decrease
● Slow pulse rate
● Increased blood pressure
● Weakened peripheral pulses, especially in the legs

Respiratory

● Increased respiratory rate
● Decreased lung expansion
● Diminished effective coughing

Musculoskeletal

● Diminished muscle mass and strength
● Trunk shortening
● Decreased joint mobility
● Bone demineralization

Neurologic

● Slowed reflexes
● Reduced ability to respond to multiple stimuli
● Reduced cerebral circulation

GI

● Dry mouth
● Swallowing difficulties
● Decreased production of digestive enzymes
● Decreased peristalsis
● Increased flatulence
● Increased constipation

Genitourinary

● Decreased kidney efficiency
● Voiding difficulties
● Urine retention
● Nocturia
● Incontinence

Reproductive

● Dyspareunia in women
● Vaginal itching and irritation
● Decreased estrogen
● Decreased size of penis and testes

- Delayed erection
- Decreased sperm count

Sensory
- Diminished hearing, taste, smell, and vision
- Reduced ability to adapt to darkness
- Increased sensitivity to glare

Psychosocial changes
- Stress about retirement and reduced income
- Development of feelings of unworthiness because of perceived loss of productivity
- Potential for social isolation
- ATTITUDINAL ISOLATION results from societal rejection because of age bias.
- PRESENTATIONAL ISOLATION results from social withdrawal because of changes in body image, mental or physical functional loss, or self-consciousness.
- BEHAVIORAL ISOLATION results from social withdrawal because of unacceptable social behavior, such as confusion, incontinence, or erratic behavior.
- Reduced memory retention
- Changes to the environment
- Moving from a house or an apartment to a retirement community
- Reorganization of one's living environment to prevent falls
- Fear of dying
- Death to an elderly person isn't always a blessing.
- Elderly people still have goals they want to achieve and aren't necessarily prepared to die until these goals are fulfilled.
- Stress from loss of a significant other

Principles of gerontologic nursing process
The nursing process includes data collection, planning and goals, interventions, and evaluation.

Data collection
- Assess the client's developmental level to identify how he feels about aging.
- Assess the client's functional level so appropriate goals and outcomes can be developed.
- Assess the client's living environment to evaluate if adjustments are needed.
- Determine if the client has health complaints that may need immediate attention to ensure optimum health.

- Note financial and support resources available to assist the client in maintaining an optimum level of independent function.
- Evaluate the client's coping skills so a realistic care plan can be developed.

Planning and goals
- Priority should be given to the client's perception of the problem's importance.
- Goals should be prioritized according to the nature of the problem.
- Goals should always be realistic and set to achieve the client's optimum level of independent function.

Interventions
- Promote socialization to help the client build secondary social relationships.
- Use therapeutic communication to build a trusting nurse-client relationship.
- Use reality orientation to maintain or restore the client's sense of awareness.
- Promote positive body image to build the client's self-confidence and to foster the willingness of others to interact with the client.
- Inform the client and family of the availability of health care services to ensure that health problems are adequately treated.
- Teach family members about respite care (short-term care given to a dependent client so that the permanent caregivers may have a break from the stress of continual-care responsibility).
- Teach the client and family how to make their home safe and comfortable; this will minimize the risk of injury from falls and maximize the client's comfort at home.
- Promote ambulation and range-of-motion exercises to maintain muscle strength, stimulate circulation, and reduce the risk of pressure ulcers.
- Promote urinary and bowel continence to foster self-esteem and minimize the risk of institutionalization.

Evaluation
- The client's response to the interventions is measured against the goals set in the care plan.
- When outcomes don't match established goals, a revised care plan is developed.
- Desired outcomes in a gerontologic nursing care plan include:

– The client maintains proper body alignment when sitting and walking.

– The client actively engages in a planned activity program with others.

– The client seeks out and maintains social contacts.

– The client maintains urinary and bowel continence.

– The client is oriented to time, place, and person.

– The client is free from bodily injury.

– The client knows how to seek health care and does so when needed.

Principles of home health care

The introduction of managed care to the U.S. health care delivery system has accelerated the need for providing more health care in the home. Reasons for this increased need include:

● Chronic health problems that used to receive periodic care in a hospital now are cared for exclusively at home.

● Early discharge of clients who have had surgery or an acute illness has raised the acuity level of clients in home care.

● Elderly clients with chronic illnesses are being treated at home with greater frequency, thereby raising the level of skills required by the caregivers.

Role of nurses

Nurses, the traditional providers of community-based care, are being called on by the federal government, through Medicare regulations, home health agencies, and insurance providers, to direct the delivery of home health care, skilled and unskilled.

Providing effective home health care requires enhanced clinical skills and an understanding of home care rules and regulations.

Home health care services

Home health care is the delivery of multidisciplinary health services to clients and their families wherever they live. The focus of home health care service is to restore the optimum level of client and family independence. There are several types of home health care services, including professional, ancillary, and equipment.

Professional home health care services

● Skilled nursing care

● Teaching health care

● Interdisciplinary collaboration among professional health care providers (ensures cooperation, continuity of care, and compliance with government eligibility requirements)

● Identification and communication of community resources (help the client and family achieve care plan outcomes)

Ancillary home health care services

● Home health aides

● Housekeepers

● Companions

Home health care equipment services

● Beds and ambulatory aids

● Portable dialysis units

● Ventilators and infusion pumps

Factors that influence effective home health care

● Thorough family education about the health problem

● Educated professionals trained in the relevant skills to deal with the health problem

● Effective social support services

● Appropriate living environment

● Reliable transportation and local emergency health facility

● Competent care managers

Home health care nursing

The clinical responsibilities of a home health nurse to the client include maintaining wound care, complying with drug therapy, maintaining nutrition, ensuring elimination needs, assisting with mobility, and controlling the spread of infection. The psychosocial responsibilities of the home health nurse include being aware of the client's psychosocial needs, understanding the legal and ethical issues, and maintaining personal safety.

Clinical responsibilities

Wound care

● Debriding and irrigating wounds

● Assessing wound healing

● Teaching wound care

Drug therapy compliance

● Teaching drug actions, adverse effects, and administration schedules

● Monitoring drug therapy effectiveness

● Monitoring client compliance

Nutrition
- Assessing the client's nutritional status
- Administering tube and parenteral feedings
- Teaching proper nutrition habits
- Monitoring diet compliance

Elimination
- Providing enterostomal care
- Teaching the client and family the use of irrigation catheters and proper skin care
- Monitoring the client for infection

Mobility
- Demonstrating the use of assistive devices
- Performing range-of-motion exercises

Infection control
- Teaching the family infection-control precautions
- Monitoring the home environment to identify areas that promote infection

Psychosocial responsibilities
- Being aware of socioeconomic factors and cultural and family dynamics in the client's home
- Recognizing that the home health nurse is a guest in the client's home
- Remaining nonjudgmental about the client's beliefs
- Accepting the client's ability to learn and willingness to follow directions

Legal and ethical responsibilities
- Complying with the laws and regulations regarding home care
- Working within an approved care plan
- Ensuring that physician collaboration on the treatment plan has been obtained
- Ensuring that the client's or family's written permission to enter the home has been obtained
- Maintaining confidentiality about the client's condition and treatment when asked by family, friends, or neighbors
- Providing documentation of care to ensure continued and optimum reimbursement for the client
- Understanding when and how to withdraw services when reimbursement authorization expires

Personal safety precautions
- Know the neighborhood and the safest route in and out.

- Carry agency, police, and emergency facility telephone numbers.
- Inform the agency of daily visit schedule, with telephone numbers of each client.
- Report in to the agency by phone after each visit.
- Don't drive an expensive automobile, wear expensive jewelry, or show a lot of money.
- Don't enter the home if anyone is intoxicated, hostile, or demonstrating obnoxious behavior.
- Never enter a home until invited, and leave if feeling unsafe.

Principles of infection control

As primary caregivers, nurses play a major role in preventing the onset and spread of infection. For an infection to occur, a series of events must be completed:
- A causative organism must be present.
- A reservoir host for the organism must exist.
- A transmission route from the reservoir host to a susceptible host must be present.
- A means of entry into the new host must exist.
- The new host must be susceptible to the organism.

  Preventing and controlling the spread of infection requires eliminating or blocking one or more of these events. (See *CDC isolation precautions*, page 48.)

  Well-established and proven interventions can prevent and control infection. Nurses need to ensure proper prevention measures, teaching methods, and the client's health and also follow an infection-control program.

Preventing transmission
- Wash hands thoroughly before and after each client contact, after handling body fluids and wastes, and after handling contaminated equipment.
- Use protective barriers:
– Use gloves when handling body substances and substances soiled with body fluids (such as open wounds, dressings, or contaminated equipment).
– Wear a mask or respirator when caring for clients with airborne infections.
– Wear a gown, goggles, and hair and shoe covers during potential exposure to sprayed body fluid.
- Use isolation techniques:
– Isolate a client suspected of or with a communicable disease or one who could endanger the immediate environment with body fluids.

CDC isolation precautions

To help hospitals maintain up-to-date isolation practices, the Centers for Disease Control and Prevention (CDC) and the Hospital Infection Control Practices Advisory Committee revised the CDC's *Guideline for Isolation Precautions in Hospitals*.

Standard precautions

The revised guidelines contain two tiers of precautions. The first—called standard precautions – are those designated for the care of all hospital clients regardless of their diagnosis or presumed infection. Standard precautions are the primary strategy for preventing nosocomial infection and take the place of universal precautions. These precautions apply to:

- blood
- all body fluids, secretions, and excretions, except sweat, regardless of whether they contain visible blood
- skin that isn't intact
- mucous membranes.

Transmission-based precautions

The second tier of precautions are known as transmission-based precautions. These precautions are instituted for clients who are known to be or suspected of being infected with a highly transmissible infection – one that needs precautions beyond those set forth in the standard precautions. There are three types of transmission-based precautions: airborne precautions, droplet precautions, and contact precautions.

Airborne precautions

Airborne precautions are designed to reduce the risk of airborne transmission of infectious agents. Microorganisms carried through the air can be dispersed widely by air currents, making them available for inhalation or deposit on a susceptible host in the same room or a longer distance away from the infected client. Airborne precautions include special air handling and ventilation procedures to prevent the spread of infection. They require the use of respiratory protection such as a mask – in addition to standard precautions – when entering an infected client's room.

Droplet precautions

Droplet precautions are designed to reduce the risk of transmitting infectious agents through large-particle (exceeding 5 micrometers) droplets. Such transmission involves the contact of infectious agents to the conjunctivae or to the nasal or oral mucous membranes of a susceptible person. Large-particle droplets don't remain in the air and generally travel short distances of 3′ (0.9 m) or less. They require the use of a mask – in addition to standard precautions – to protect the mucous membranes.

Contact precautions

Contact precautions are designed to reduce the risk of transmitting infectious agents by direct or indirect contact. Direct-contact transmission can occur through client care activities that require physical contact. Indirect-contact transmission involves a susceptible host coming in contact with a contaminated object, usually inanimate, in the client's environment. Contact precautions require the use of gloves, a mask, and a gown – in addition to standard precautions – to avoid contact with the infectious agent. Stringent hand washing is also necessary after removal of the protective items.

– Place body substances in a leakproof or puncture-proof container, and bag soiled linen.

Ensuring proper teaching on infection

- Assess the client's and family's knowledge level about infection.
- Teach control measures to use in the home to prevent transmission, such as:
– frequent hand washing
– using separate dishes and utensils
– maintaining clean environment
– keeping vaccinations current.

Maintaining the client's protective defense mechanisms

- Ensure intact, healthy skin:
– Promote regular bathing to remove organisms.
– Suggest the use of lubricants to keep skin hydrated and prevent cracking.
– Encourage the client to practice regular oral hygiene, including tartar and plaque control, to reduce oral pathogens.
- Maintain adequate nutrition and fluid intake:
– Suggest a high fluid intake to promote frequent urination, which helps flush the client's system of microorganisms.

– Encourage the client to follow a well-balanced diet, which promotes homeostasis and general resistance to infection.

Establishing an infection-control program

● An infection-control department composed of specially educated professionals administers a formal infection-control program.
● Infection-control responsibilities include:
– ensuring staff education
– establishing infection-control procedures
– conducting research on infection-control measures
– providing a liaison to community and other health agencies.

Cultural and spiritual dimensions of care

A critical part of the nursing process involves the assessment of cultural and spiritual needs, followed by appropriate planning and implementation. Too often these vital components of client care are neglected in the urgency to address critical physical needs.

Important components to address in identifying cultural and spiritual needs of clients include:
● identifying the dominant cultural and religious background of the client and family — Culture, including religion, helps to determine a person's role and status in the family and community; it influences the availability of social and material supports; how illness and health are viewed; and how individuals who are sick are expected to behave.
● performing a cultural and spiritual assessment — This may be brief or may require considerable evaluation depending on the circumstances of the patient care situation. (See *Questions for cultural and spiritual assessment.*)
● involving the client and family in planning to meet cultural and spiritual needs — Identify institutional barriers, which may need to be addressed. Identify alternate means of meeting cultural or spiritual needs when in conflict with institutional barriers. For example, when caring for a Jehovah's Witness client, be aware that blood transfusions are unacceptable, as they're considered against God's will. What alternative treatments are available and acceptable? What legal ramifications need to be considered?
● intervening as the advocate for the client and family — Ensure that cultural and religious views are taken into account as physical care is rendered. For example, when car-

---

Questions for cultural and spiritual assessment

A client's cultural and religious background can provide a powerful positive influence for healing when supported by caregivers. Taking the time to assess cultural and spiritual background can enable the practical nurse to render sensitive, effective care.
   Critical questions to ask include:
● What language is spoken by the client? Family? Is an interpreter needed?
● Is there a religious preference identified by the client? Family?
● What cultural and religious supports are available to the client and family? Have appropriate clergy been notified as requested by the client?
● How do cultural and religious views influence dietary habits? What implications does this have for treatment?
● What restrictions regarding treatment may the client and family have, based upon religious beliefs?
● What religious observances (prayers, blessings, ceremonies) might the client and family desire? Who would assist with these observances?
● What does the client do to maintain health? What religious or cultural beliefs affect health care behaviors?
● How does the client conceptualize illness? What religious or cultural beliefs may influence receptivity to medical or surgical treatment?
● What special cultural or religious medals, icons, texts, clothing, or other emblems of belief are important to the client? If not available, how can they be obtained?
● What alternate health care practices may be utilized? Are herbal or other natural remedies routinely taken? Are other nontraditional healers participating in care?

---

ing for a Latter-day Saint (Mormon) client, allowing the retention of special undergarments whenever possible will be appreciated.
● evaluating the effectiveness of the plan to include cultural and spiritual dimensions of care — Does the client feel supported and validated? Are there areas of concern or conflict? Can these be mitigated or can the difficulties be discussed sufficiently with the client and family so that they feel their concerns are understood? (See *Religious and cultural aspects of nursing care,* pages 50 and 51.)

(Text continues on page 52.)

Religious and cultural aspects of nursing care

A patient's religious beliefs can affect his attitudes toward illness and traditional medicine. By trying to accommodate the patient's religious beliefs and practices in your care plan, you can increase his willingness to learn and comply with treatment regimens. Because religious beliefs may vary within particular sects, individual practices may differ from those described here.

RELIGION	BIRTH AND DEATH RITUALS	DIETARY RESTRICTIONS	PRACTICES IN HEALTH CRISIS
Adventist	None (baptism of adults only)	Alcohol, coffee, tea, narcotics, stimulants; in many groups, meat prohibited also	Communion and baptism are performed. Some members believe in divine healing, anointing with oil, and prayer. Some regard Saturday as the Sabbath.
Baptist	● At birth, none (baptism of believers only) ● Before death, counseling by clergy member and prayer	Alcohol; in some groups, coffee and tea prohibited also	Some believe in healing by laying on of hands. Resistance to medical therapy is occasionally approved.
Christian Scientist	● At birth, none ● Before death, counseling by a Christian Science practitioner	Alcohol, coffee, and tobacco prohibited	Many members refuse all treatment, including drugs, biopsies, physical examination, and blood transfusions and permit vaccination only when required by law. Alteration of thoughts is believed to cure illness. Hypnotism and psychotherapy are prohibited. (Christian Scientist nurses and nursing homes honor these beliefs.)
Church of Christ	None (baptism at age 8 or older)	Alcohol discouraged	Communion, anointing with oil, laying on of hands, and counseling by a minister are practiced.
Eastern Orthodox	● At birth, baptism and confirmation ● Before death, last rites ● For members of the Russian Orthodox Church, arms crossed after death, fingers set in cross, and unembalmed body clothed in natural fiber	For members of the Russian Orthodox Church and usually the Greek Orthodox Church, no meat or dairy products on Wednesday, Friday, and during Lent	Anointing of the sick is practiced. For members of the Russian Orthodox Church, cross necklace is replaced immediately after surgery and shaving of a male patients is prohibited, except in preparation for surgery. For members of the Greek Orthodox Church, communion and Sacrament of Holy Unction are practiced.
Episcopalian	● At birth, baptism ● Before death, occasional last rites	For some members, abstention from meat on Friday, fasting before communion (which may be daily)	Communion, prayer, and counseling are performed by a minister.
Jehovah's Witnesses	None	Abstention from foods to which blood has been added	Typically, no blood transfusions are permitted; a court order may be required for an emergency transfusion.

Religious and cultural aspects of nursing care *(continued)*

RELIGION	BIRTH AND DEATH RITUALS	DIETARY RESTRICTIONS	PRACTICES IN HEALTH CRISIS
Judaism	● Ritual circumcision on 8th day after birth ● Burial of dead fetus ● Ritual washing of dead with burial (including organs and other body tissues) as soon as possible; no autopsy or embalming	For Orthodox and Conservative Jews, kosher dietary laws (for example, pork and shellfish prohibited); for others, usually no restrictions	Donation or transplantation of organs requires rabbinical consultation. For Orthodox and Conservative Jews, medical procedures may be prohibited on the Sabbath — from sundown Friday to sundown Saturday — and on special holidays.
Lutheran	● Baptism usually 6 to 8 weeks after birth	None	Communion, prayer, and counseling are performed by a minister.
Mormon	● At birth, none (baptism at age 8 or older) ● Before death, baptism and gospel preaching	Alcohol, tobacco, tea, and coffee prohibited; meat intake limited	Divine healing through the laying on of hands and communion on Sunday are practiced. Some members may refuse medical treatment. Many wear a special undergarment.
Moslem	● If spontaneous abortion occurs before 130 days, fetus treated as discarded tissue; after 130 days, as a human being ● Before death, confession of sins with family present ● After death, only relatives or friends permitted to touch the body	Pork prohibited; daylight fasting during 9th month of Islamic calendar	Faith healing is for the patient's morale only; conservative members reject medical therapy.
Orthodox Presbyterian	● Infant baptism ● Scripture reading and prayer before death	None	Communion, prayer, and counseling are performed by a minister.
Pentecostal Assembly of God, Foursquare Church	None (baptism only after age of accountability)	Abstention from alcohol, tobacco, meat slaughtered by strangling, any food to which blood has been added, and sometimes pork	Divine healing through prayer, anointing with oil, and laying on of hands are practiced.
Roman Catholic	● Infant baptism, including baptism of aborted fetus without sign of clinical death (tissue necrosis) ● Before death, anointing of the sick	Fasting or abstention from meat on Ash Wednesday and on Fridays during Lent; this practice usually waived for the hospitalized	Major amputated limbs (sometimes) are buried in consecrated ground. Donation or transplantation of organs is allowed if the benefit to the recipient outweigh the potential harm to the donor. Sacraments of the Sick are performed when patients are ill and just before death, sometimes shortly after admission.
United Methodist	Baptism of children and adults	None	Communion is performed before surgery or a similar crisis; donation of body parts is encouraged.

NURSING SKILLS

Various basic nursing skills are needed to provide quality care for most clients in any setting. This section covers physical assessment, blood transfusion, medication administration, cardiopulmonary resuscitation, and anticipatory guidance. These essential skills are important in the care of clients with various health needs and for promoting health and wellness for clients of all ages.

Physical assessment

Physical assessment constitutes an important part of the data collection phase of the nursing process. Physical assessment:
- must be accurate and thorough to produce appropriate nursing diagnoses
- requires effective communication techniques and interviewing skills
- should be holistic and include a comprehensive health history that explores biopsychosocial factors relevant to the client's health status
- consists of four physical examination techniques in which the nurse uses the senses to gather information about the client:
– INSPECTION uses sight and smell to collect data (for example, observing the client's gait or detecting a fruity breath odor).
– PALPATION uses touch (fingers and hands) to collect data (for example, taking a radial pulse).
– AUSCULTATION uses hearing (primarily with the aid of a stethoscope) to detect sounds produced by certain body organs (for example, taking an apical pulse).
– PERCUSSION uses the striking of one object against another to generate a vibration that produces an audible sound wave (for example, percussing the lung fields); this is the technique least likely to be used by the novice nurse.

QUICK STUDY

When trying to remember the correct order of physical assessment steps, think **IPAP.**

Inspection
Palpation
Auscultation
Percussion

Health history

The health history can provide valuable information regarding present and past health conditions as well as other factors that may affect the client's health.

General health

Identify the reason for seeking the care of the physician or nurse practitioner. During the initial examination, both the present and past health histories, including family and social histories, are assessed.

Present health history
- Allergies
- Diet
- Exercise
- Alcohol intake
- Tobacco use
- Sleep pattern
- Voiding and bowel patterns
- Medications, including prescription and nonprescription
- Appliances (for example, dentures, prostheses, glasses)

Past health history
- Childhood illnesses
- Immunizations
- Surgeries
- Injuries
- Hospitalizations
- Obstetric and menstrual history
- Adult illnesses
- Psychiatric illnesses

Family history
- Diabetes mellitus
- Heart disease
- Cancer

Social history
- Lifestyle
- Relationships with family and friends
- Occupation
- Leisure-time activities
- Residence (for example, urban or rural, one-story house or high-rise apartment, rent or own)

Perceptions of health. Finally, assess the client's perception of his own health and assess how his friends and family members perceive his health.

Physical examination

Once the health history is obtained, a general overview — including apparent state of health, signs of distress, motor activity, weight, facial expression, grooming, mood, state of awareness — should be performed. To perform the physical examination, assess the client's vital signs, body systems, and motor function.

Vital signs

● Blood pressure (assess in both arms in lying, sitting, and standing positions)
● Pulses (include carotid, abdominal aortic, femoral, tibial, and pedal and take bilaterally when possible)

Body systems

● Neurologic system (assess level of consciousness; orientation to time, place, and person; pupillary reaction to light; presence of any tics or tremors)
● Skin (inspect color, moisture, temperature, turgor, and presence of lesions, scars, ecchymosis, erythema, and moles; compare bilaterally)
● Nails (inspect capillary refill, presence of clubbing; compare bilaterally on hands and feet)
● Hair (assess amount and dry or oily texture)
● Eyes (inspect visual acuity of central and peripheral vision), noting use of glasses, contact lenses, prosthesis and the presence of eye discharge, inflammation, swelling, or redness
● Ears (assess hearing acuity, note use of hearing aid)
● Nose (palpate the nose and sinuses; note the presence of discharge)
● Mouth and pharynx (inspect the lips, the mucosa of the mouth, the gums, the teeth, the tongue, the ability to swallow and taste)
● Neck (palpate the lymph nodes [preauricular, posterior auricular, occipital, tonsillar, submaxillary, submental, superficial cervical, posterior cervical, deep cervical, and supraclavicular]; note jugular vein distention)
● Back (inspect and palpate the spine and muscles; observe for curvatures)
● Thorax and lungs (observe, percuss, and auscultate; palpate for respiratory excursion; note the presence and type of cough)
● Breasts and axillae (palpate breasts and nodes in axillae; observe for symmetry, discharge, and pain)
● Heart (auscultate; observe for palpitations, thrills, and heaves; take the heart rate at the point of maximum impulse)

● Abdomen (listen for bowel sounds; palpate for pain — note location, duration and type; note distention and symmetry)
● Genitalia (assess the penis and scrotum in men and the external genitalia and vagina in women) and groin (check for hernia)

Motor function

● Range of motion for all joints
● Coordination of movements
● Gait
● Ability to speak and write
● Sensation (assess pain and vibration in the hands, feet, arms, and legs; light touch on abdomen, arms, and legs)
● Activity level (note pain, dyspnea, fatigue, or weakness)

Blood transfusion

A blood transfusion is the I.V. infusion of blood or blood products into the bloodstream. The transfusion can be autologous (the client's blood) or homologous (donor blood).

Although a licensed PN may not be responsible for administering blood transfusions, she may be responsible for monitoring the procedure and the patient's response to it. Therefore, it's important for a PN to understand basic concepts related to blood transfusions.

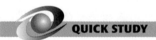

QUICK STUDY

When trying to remember the difference between autologous and homologous, just remember that:

Auto means self. Autologous blood comes from the self.
Homo means man. Homologous blood comes from any man (person).

One or more blood transfusions may be performed to replenish the client's blood volume or erythrocytes (red blood cells) or to provide platelets or other coagulation factors. The procedure carries risks that can be minimized by carefully assessing the donor's health status, following safe blood administration practices, and knowing how to recognize and manage transfusion reactions.

Donor history and screening

A donor history must be obtained, and proper screening, including blood typing and crossmatching, must be performed before a blood transfusion can take place. Donor blood is unacceptable for use if the donor's history includes:

- viral hepatitis or contact with a person who has hepatitis within the past 6 months
- blood transfusion within the past 6 months
- previous or current I.V. drug use
- exposure to the human immunodeficiency virus
- recent allergies or hives.

   Donor blood shouldn't be used if screening tests yield positive results for:

- hepatitis
- acquired immunodeficiency syndrome
- syphilis
- cytomegalovirus.

Blood typing and cross matching

ABO blood typing is a test that identifies the client's blood group (A, B, O, or AB) to check compatibility of donor and recipient blood before transfusion:

- Type A blood is that of a person whose erythrocytes contain isoagglutinin (antigen) A and antibody anti-B (about 40% of the population).
- Type B blood is that of a person whose erythrocytes contain isoagglutinin (antigen) B and antibody anti-A (about 10% of the population).
- Type O blood is that of a person whose erythrocytes contain neither isoagglutinin A nor B but do contain antibodies anti-A and anti-B (about 40% to 45% of the population, known as *universal donors*).
- Type AB blood is that of a person whose erythrocytes contain both isoagglutinins A and B but no antibodies (about 5% to 10% of the population, known as *universal recipients*).

Rh typing

Rh typing is a test that determines the presence or absence of the $Rh_o(D)$ antigen on the surface of red blood cells; an Rh-positive result indicates isoagglutinins D, C, and E in erythrocytes.

Crossmatching

Crossmatching is a test in which the donor's erythrocytes are exposed to the recipient's serum and the donor's serum is exposed to the recipient's erythrocytes; the test is performed to evaluate for agglutination.

Hazards and complications of blood transfusion

The recipient of a blood transfusion is at risk for contracting blood-borne diseases, such as serum hepatitis, syphilis, malaria, or human immunodeficiency virus.

   Transmission of incompatible or contaminated blood produces agglutination and hemolysis of the donor's erythrocytes by isoagglutination in the recipient's plasma.

   Too-rapid administration can produce circulatory overload; massive transfusions (5 L in less than 12 hours) can cause acidosis, hypothermia, citrate overload, hyperkalemia, and dilutional coagulation defects.

   Complications of blood transfusion cause about 3,000 deaths annually in the United States, primarily through serum hepatitis or hemolytic transfusion reactions. Transfusion reactions usually develop during, immediately after, or within 96 hours of the transfusion.

   Delayed complications, which may develop 10 to 120 days after the last transfusion, typically result from disease transmission or sensitization to previous transfusions.

Symptoms of transfusion reaction

Common symptoms of a transfusion reaction include:

- fever (may be as high as 103° F [39.4° C])
- chills
- itching
- flushing
- urticaria
- nausea
- vomiting
- headache
- dyspnea
- stridor
- wheezing.

   In severe cases, hemolytic reactions can develop, including:

- chest, flank, or back pain
- apprehension or feeling of impending doom
- severe hypotension
- spontaneous diffuse bleeding
- anuria.

Managing transfusion reactions

- Stop the transfusion immediately; if you have been using a Y-type set, infuse normal saline solution at a keep-vein-open rate.
- Notify the physician.
- Obtain a urine sample from the client and send it to the laboratory for analysis; continue to measure and assess urine output hourly.

● Draw a fresh sample of the client's blood and send it to the blood bank or laboratory for analysis.

● Return unused blood to the blood bank for incompatibility and contamination testing.

● Reduce the client's temperature by giving a sponge bath, administering acetaminophen, or lowering the room temperature, if necessary; measure the client's temperature every 30 minutes until it's normal.

SPOT CHECK

What should your first nursing intervention be if you suspect a transfusion reaction?

Your first priority is to stop the transfusion immediately. You should also infuse normal saline solution at a keep-vein-open rate

Medication administration

A licensed PN may be responsible for medication administration, if deemed appropriate by the state board of nursing and the requirements of the employing institution. To ensure patient safety during medication administration, many institutions require that the nurse successfully complete a medication course or pass an examination that demonstrates appropriate knowledge regarding medication policies, dosage calculations, emergency medication, and medication administration.

Nursing responsibilities

● Medication must be ordered by licensed personnel, according to the policies of the specific institution.

● The nurse is responsible for the medication administered. If the medication dosage or the administration route is inappropriate for the client, medication administration should be suspended pending further investigation of the order.

● The nurse is responsible for evaluating the client before and after administration of all medication.

● The nurse must follow proper medication administration guidelines. (See *The 5 rights of medication administration*.)

● Proper documentation of medication administration should be completed as soon as possible after administration.

● The nurse should only administer medications she has personally prepared or those that have been prepared by the pharmacist (such as I.V. piggyback antibiotics).

> ## The 5 rights of medication administration
>
> When administering a drug, remember to use the five rights of medication administration:
> 1. right client
> 2. right drug
> 3. right dose
> 4. right route
> 5. right time.

● The nurse should ensure that the client takes the medication that's administered (the nurse shouldn't leave medication at the bedside).

● The nurse should know possible drug interactions.

● Proper safety precautions should be taken before medication administration, such as checking the client's pulse and blood pressure.

● The nurse should know the reason for the medication, the average dose, and common adverse effects.

Administration guidelines

Whenever you administer medication, observe the following precautions to ensure that you're giving the right drug in the right dose to the right patient:

● **Check the order.** Check the order on the patient's medication record against the doctor's order.

● **Check the label.** Check the label on the medication three times before administering it to a patient to ensure that you're administering the prescribed medication in the prescribed dose. Check it when you take the container from the shelf or drawer, right before pouring the medication into the medication cup or drawing it into the syringe, and before returning the container to the shelf or drawer. If you're administering a unit-dose medication, check the label for the third time immediately after pouring the medication and again before discarding the wrapper. (*Remember:* Don't open a unit-dose medication until you're at the patient's bedside.)

● **Confirm the patient's identity.** Before giving the medication, confirm the patient's identity by checking his name and the identification number on his wristband. Then make sure that you have the correct medication.

● **Have a written order.** Make sure you have a written order for every medication you're supposed to administer. If you receive a verbal order, make sure the doctor signs for it within the specified time period.

● **Give labeled medication.** Don't give medication from a poorly labeled or unlabeled container. Furthermore, don't attempt to label or reinforce drug labels; this should be done only by a pharmacist.

● **Monitor medication.** Never give a medication that someone else has poured or prepared. Never let your medication cart or tray out of your sight. Never return unwrapped or prepared medications to stock containers. Instead, dispose of them, and notify the pharmacy.

● **Respond to the patient's questions.** Always explain the medication administration procedure to the patient prior to giving the medication and provide privacy. If the patient questions you about his medication or the dosage, check his medication record again. If the medication is correct, reassure him that it's correct. Be sure to tell him about any changes in his medication or dosage. Instruct him, as appropriate, about possible adverse reactions, and encourage him to report any that he experiences.

Medication administration methods
Topical

Topical drugs, such as lotions and ointments, are applied directly to the patient's skin. They're commonly used for local, rather than systemic, effects. Typically, they must be applied two or three times per day for a full therapeutic effect.

Transdermal

Given through an adhesive disk or a measured dose of ointment applied to the skin, transdermal drugs deliver constant, controlled medication directly into the bloodstream for a prolonged systemic effect.

Medications available in transdermal form include nitroglycerin, which is used to control angina; scopolamine, which is used to treat motion sickness; estradiol, which is used for postmenopausal hormone replacement; clonidine, which is used to treat hypertension; and fentanyl, which is used to control chronic pain.

Nitroglycerin ointment dilates coronary vessels for 2 to 12 hours; a nitroglycerin patch can produce the same effect for as long as 24 hours.

The scopolamine patch can relieve motion sickness for as long as 72 hours. Transdermal estradiol lasts 72 hours to 1 week; clonidine, 7 days; and fentanyl, up to 72 hours.

Ophthalmic

Ophthalmic medications — drop or ointments — serve diagnostic and therapeutic purposes. During an eye examination, eye medications can be used to anesthetize the eye, dilate the pupil, and stain the cornea to identify anomalies. Therapeutic uses include eye lubrication and treatment of such conditions as glaucoma and infections.

Otic

Otic medications may be instilled to treat infection and inflammation, to soften cerumen for later removal, to produce local anesthesia, or to facilitate removal of an insect trapped in the ear.

Nasal

Most nasal medications produce local rather than systemic effects. Nasal medications may be administered by means of drops, a spray (using an atomizer), or an aerosol (using a nebulizer). Drops can be directed at a specific area; sprays and aerosols diffuse medication throughout the nasal passages. Nasal medications include vasoconstrictors, antiseptics, anesthetics, and corticosteroids.

Oropharyngeal

Handheld oropharyngeal inhalers include the metered-dose inhaler or nebulizer, the turbo-inhaler, and the nasal inhaler. These devices deliver topical medications to the respiratory tract, producing local and systemic effects. The mucosal lining of the respiratory tract absorbs the inhalant almost immediately. Examples of inhalants include bronchodilators, which are used to improve airway patency and facilitate mucus drainage, and mucolytics, which liquefy tenacious bronchial secretions.

Vaginal

Vaginal medications include suppositories, creams, gels, and ointments. These medications can be inserted as topical treatments for infection (particularly *Trichomonas vaginalis* and candidal vaginitis) or inflammation. Suppositories melt when they come in contact with the warm vaginal mucosa, diffusing the medication topically.

Vaginal medications usually come with a disposable applicator that enables placement of medication in the anterior and posterior fornices. Vaginal administration is most effective when the patient can remain lying down afterward, aiding retention of the medication.

Oral

Most drugs are administered orally because this route is usually the safest, most convenient, and least expensive. Oral administration medications are available in many forms, including tablets, enteric-coated tablets, capsules, syrups, elixirs, oils, liquids, suspensions, powders, and granules. Some require special preparation before administration, such as mixing with juice to make them more palatable.

Oral drugs are sometimes prescribed in higher dosages than their parenteral equivalents because, after absorption through the GI system, the liver breaks them down before they reach systemic circulation.

Nasogastric tube or gastrostomy button

Besides providing an alternate means of nourishment, a nasogastric tube allows direct instillation of medication into the GI system for patients who can't ingest it orally. The gastrostomy button, inserted into an established stoma, lies flush with the skin and receives a feeding tube.

Buccal or sublingual

Certain drugs are given buccally (between the patient's check and teeth) or sublingually (under the patient's tongue) to bypass the digestive tract and facilitate their absorption into the bloodstream. When using either of these administration methods, you must observe the patient carefully to ensure that he doesn't swallow the drug or suffer mucosal irritation.

Rectal

A rectal suppository is a small, solid, medicated mass, usually cone shaped, with a cocoa butter or glycerin base. It may be inserted to stimulate peristalsis and defecation or to relieve pain, vomiting, and local irritation. An ointment is a semisolid medication used to produce local effects. It may be applied externally to the anus or internally to the rectum.

Subcutaneous injection

Subcutaneous (S.C.) injections allows slower, more sustained medication administration than intramuscular (I.M.) injections. Drugs and solutions for S.C. injections are injected through a relatively short needle, using meticulous, sterile technique.

Intradermal

Used primarily for diagnostic purposes, as in allergy or tuberculin testing, intradermal injections are administered in small amounts, usually 0.5 ml or less, into the outer layers of the skin. Because little systemic absorption takes place, this type of injection is used primarily to produce a local effect.

The ventral forearm is the most commonly used site because of its easy access and lack of hair. In extensive allergy testing, the outer aspect of the upper arms or the area of the back between the scapulae may be used.

I.M. injection

I.M. injections deposit medication deep into well-vascularized muscle for rapid systemic action and absorption of up to 5 ml.

Z-track injection

The Z-track method of I.M. injection prevents leakage, or tracking, into the S.C. tissue. Typically, it's used to administer drugs that irritate and discolor S.C. tissue — primarily iron preparations such as iron dextran. It may also be used in elderly patients who have decreased muscle mass. Lateral displacement of the skin during the injection helps to seal the drug in the muscle.

This procedure requires careful attention to technique because leakage into S.C. tissue can cause patient discomfort and may permanently stain some tissues.

Infusion through a secondary I.V. line

A secondary I.V. line is a complete I.V. set connected to the lower Y-port (secondary port) of a primary line instead of to the I.V. catheter or needle. It features an I.V. container, long tubing, and either a microdrip or macrodrip system, and it can be used for continuous or intermittent drug infusion. When used continuously, it permits drug infusion and titration while the primary line maintains a constant total infusion rate.

Medication calculation

If the available medication dosage differs from the dose of medication ordered, such as if the medication is supplied in a multidose container, it's necessary to calculate the correct amount to administer.

Basic calculations

To calculate the number of doses in a specified amount of medicine, use this equation:

$$\frac{\text{Total amount}}{\text{Size of dose}} = \text{Number of doses}$$

To calculate the size of each dose when given a specified amount of medication and the number of doses it contains, use this equation:

$$\frac{\text{Total amount}}{\text{Number of doses}} = \text{Size of dose}$$

To calculate the amount of a medicine when given the number of doses it contains and the size of each dose, use this equation:

$$\text{Total amount} = \text{Number of doses} \times \text{Size of dose}$$

You can use this short equation to determine the rate of an I.V. infusion:

$$\frac{\text{Volume of solution} \times \text{drops/ml (drip factor)}}{\text{Hours to administer} \times \text{minutes per hour (60)}} = \text{Drops/minute}$$

Dimensional analysis

Dimensional analysis (also known as *factor analysis* or *factor labeling*) is an alternative method of solving mathematical problems. It eliminates the need to memorize formulas and requires only one equation to determine an answer.

When using dimensional analysis, the problem solver arranges a series of ratios, called *factors*, in a single fractional equation. Each factor, written as a fraction, consists of two quantities and their units of measurement that are related to each other in a given problem. For example, if 1,000 ml of a drug should be administered over 8 hours, the relationship between 1,000 ml and 8 hours is expressed by the following fraction:

$$\frac{1,000 \text{ ml}}{8 \text{ hours}}$$

When a problem includes a quantity and unit of measurement that are unrelated to any other factor in the problem, they serve as the numerator of the fraction, and 1 (implied) becomes the denominator.

Some mathematical problems contain all of the information needed to identify the factors, set up the equation, and find the solution. Other problems require the use of a conversion factor. Conversion factors are equivalents (for example, 1 g = 1,000 mg) that the nurse can memorize or obtain from a conversion chart. Because the two quantities and units of measurement are equivalent, they can serve as the numerator or the denominator; thus, the conversion factor 1 g = 1,000 mg can be written in fraction form as:

$$\frac{1,000 \text{ mg}}{1 \text{ g}} \quad \text{or} \quad \frac{1 \text{ g}}{1,000 \text{ mg}}$$

The factors given in the problem plus any conversion factors necessary to solve the problem are called *knowns.* The quantity of the answer, of course, is *unknown.* When setting up an equation in dimensional analysis, work backward, beginning with the unit of measurement of the answer. After plotting all the knowns, find the solution by following this sequence:
1. Cancel similar quantities and units of measurement.
2. Multiply the numerators.
3. Multiply the denominators.
4. Divide the numerator by the denominator.

Using dimensional analysis
The doctor prescribes 0.25 g streptomycin sulfate I.M. The vial reads "2 ml = 1 g." How many milliliters should you administer?

$$\frac{0.25 \text{ g}}{1} \times \frac{2 \text{ ml}}{1 \text{ g}} = 0.5 \text{ ml}$$

Cardiopulmonary resuscitation

Cardiopulmonary resuscitation (CPR) is an emergency procedure instituted after cardiopulmonary arrest that consists of artificial respiration and external cardiac massage. CPR provides tissue oxygenation until normal cardiac function is restored. The basic principles of life support center on the ABCs of CPR: Airway, Breathing, and Circulation.

Performing CPR
Follow these steps when performing CPR:
- Determine the client's responsiveness by asking, "Are you OK?"
- If the client doesn't respond, call for help (911).
- Place the client in the supine position (flat on his back) on a hard surface, supporting the head and neck.
- Open the airway by using the head tilt–chin lift maneuver.
- Look, listen, and feel for signs of breathing.
– If the client isn't breathing, pinch the client's nose and, with your mouth, establish a tight seal over the client's mouth.
– Ventilate twice using a microshield; then pause to see whether the client's chest rises.
- If the client's breaths are blocked, reposition the head and try again. If they're still blocked, perform the Heimlich (abdominal thrust) maneuver.
- Palpate for the carotid pulse on the near side (keep the client's head tilted with your hand on the forehead).

Levels of illness prevention

LEVEL	PURPOSE	EXAMPLES OF ANTICIPATORY GUIDANCE
Primary	To prevent trauma or disease	• Child education • Infant immunization • Health screening programs • Accident prevention programs • Parent education classes
Secondary	To delay or stop the progress of an established disease or injury	• Diabetic teaching • Discharge planning • Return demonstration by the client
Tertiary	To maintain an incurably ill client at a maximal activity level	• Referral to self-help groups • Preparation of family for grieving patterns

● If the client has no pulse, begin cycles of ventilations with sternal compressions.
– Check landmarks before placing the heel of the hand on the client's sternum.
– Perform vertical compressions without bouncing.
– Try to establish a rate of 100 beats/minute by counting 4 cycles of 15 compressions to 2 ventilations.
– Make compressions and relaxations of equal duration.
– Assess each ventilation for proper chest expansion.
● Periodically assess the client for return of pulse and spontaneous breathing; don't interrupt resuscitation efforts for longer than 5 seconds.
● Continue CPR until another rescuer relieves you, the client responds, you become too exhausted to continue, or you receive instructions to terminate CPR from the appropriate authority.

Anticipatory guidance for levels of prevention

Anticipatory guidance refers to the initiation of interventions before an event occurs to prevent potential problems. Here are some facts about anticipatory guidance:
● If an event can be anticipated, guidance (teaching) increases the likelihood that the event will have a favorable outcome (for example, preparing parents for their child's impending developmental tasks or discussing the ramifications of upcoming surgery with a client).

● Anticipatory guidance is inherent in all levels of prevention related to health care. (See *Levels of illness prevention.*)
● Effective teaching strategies incorporate fundamental learning principles.

Primary client-teaching responsibilities with hospitalized clients
● Orient the client to the hospital environment.
● Explain all nursing procedures that will be performed as part of the client's care.
● Explain all diagnostic tests, treatments, and medical procedures that the client will undergo, including a discussion of what the client can expect before, during, and after the test, treatment, or procedure.
● Provide written and oral explanations and instructions.
● Determine the client's understanding and perception of health care management.
● Provide feedback as needed to clarify any concerns or correct any misconceptions the client may have.

Introduction

Homeostasis — a state of constancy or equilibrium within the body — is essential for the preservation of life. The body maintains homeostasis through a system of internal control mechanisms that regulate vital functions, including blood pressure, temperature, pH, heart rate, respiratory rate, glandular secretion, and fluid and electrolyte balance.

Contributing factors

Various factors may adversely affect homeostasis. These include:

- acute illness
- chronic illness
- trauma
- pressures of everyday life.

The degree to which these stressors alter the body's normal balance depends on the individual's adaptability and ability to cope. Typically, the body responds to stress by activating various regulatory mechanisms (primarily within the vascular system, brain, kidneys, liver, and endocrine system) that produce physiologic changes to bring the body back to normal functional levels.

Understanding physiologic responses to stress is crucial to providing appropriate nursing care. This chapter focuses on major physiologic stressors that can disrupt homeostasis as well as on the internal mechanisms by which the body responds to maintain normalcy.

INFLAMMATION

Inflammation is defined as the body's response to cellular injury. It's an immediate, defensive, and beneficial response.

Cardinal signs

- Redness (rubor) from dilation of arterioles, which increases blood flow to the injured area
- Heat (calor) from increased blood supply to and increased metabolism in the injured area
- Pain (dolor) from the release of chemicals, pH changes, and pressure on nerve endings caused by swelling and trauma
- Edema from accumulation of fluids in the interstitial tissues of the injured area
- Loss of function (functio laesa) from the accumulation of changes affecting normal functioning to the injured tissues
- Migration and extravasation of leukocytes into the injured area
- Phagocytosis (engulfing and destruction of irritants, primarily by polymorphonuclear neutrophils, monocytes, and lymphocytes)
- Walling off by leukocytes to keep the inflammation localized (by cleaning up cellular debris, leukocytes also help resolve inflammation)
- Exudate formation, produced by the accumulation of interstitial fluids (exudates dilute noxious chemicals in the inflamed area and bring antibodies to tissue defense)

 FAST FACT

Types of exudate include:
- clear (serous)
- purulent (pus-containing)
- bloody (sanguineous).

- Cellular size changes (metaplasia)
- Increased cell size or number (hypertrophy or hyperplasia)
- Decreased cell size (atrophy)
- Migration of the inflammation (metastasis) into contiguous tissues (signaled by red streaks radiating along blood vessels)

Systemic signs

- Fever (from the release of pyrogens in the body)
- Leukocytosis (increased production of white blood cells [WBCs])
- Malaise, anorexia, and disability (varies with individuals)
- Increased sedimentation rate (from changes in blood proteins and effects on red blood cells)

Factors affecting inflammation

- Blood supply (inadequate blood supply may prolong inflammation and impair healing)
- Number of leukocytes (leukocytes localize inflammation and produce phagocytosis)
- Nutritional status of the client (cellular regeneration requires adequate nutrients)
- Foreign material in the inflamed area (prevents healing and leads to infection)
- Age (children and young adults generally exhibit faster healing and recovery than older adults)
- General health status of the client (poor health would affect healing)

Complications

- Contracture (shortening or tightening of tissues, causing deformity)
- Stricture (scar tissue that encircles a tubular structure, such as the esophagus, producing a narrowing)
- Adhesion (band of granulation [or scar] tissue that binds tissues and organs, producing loss of function or other complications)
- Hernia (outward bulging of scars)
- Keloid (excessive growth of scar tissue)
- Granuloma (accumulation of scar tissue within scar tissue)

Resolution of inflammation

- Resolution (complete remission of signs and symptoms)
- Repair (replacement of lost cells with new cells)
- Scar formation (organization of connective tissue cells to form scar tissue)

Nursing interventions

- Monitor vital signs for indications of developing inflammation and report any findings to the physician, including:
- fever
- spiking temperatures
- increased pulse rate
- early signs of soreness, redness, edema, and rash
- changes in respiratory rate or breath sounds
- pain on respiration

- changes in level of consciousness (LOC), especially in the older adult (occasionally first sign noted before fever).
- Assess a wound and report any findings to the physician, including:
- color changes
- edema
- increased redness or tenderness
- increased drainage (purulent drainage signals infection).
- Assess other drainage and report any findings to the physician, including:
- yellow sputum
- cloudy urine
- diarrhea.
- Be alert for client complaints and report any findings to the physician, including:
- malaise
- fatigue
- anorexia
- increasing pain
- dysuria
- burning on urination
- frequent urination.
- Be alert for blood chemistry (signs of inflammation or infection), including:
- high WBC count
- high sedimentation rate.
- Document all data collected on the client's chart, including notification of the physician.

SHOCK

Shock is a syndrome characterized by excessive reduction of circulating blood volume, resulting in inadequate cell perfusion such as perfusion to vital organs. Cell death can occur because cells don't receive adequate nutrition and oxygen.

Shock classifications

Hypovolemic shock

- Caused by a decrease in total body fluid
- Possible factors:
- Hemorrhage
- Trauma
- Surgery
- GI ulcer
- Dehydration
- Vomiting

– Diarrhea
– Nasogastric suctioning
– Diabetes insipidus
– Hyperglycemia

Cardiogenic shock

● Caused by direct pump failure
● Possible factors:
– Myocardial infarction
– Cardiac arrest
– Ventricular arrhythmias
– Cardiomyopathies

Distributive shock

● Caused by decreased vascular volume or tone
● Possible neural-induced factors:
– Pain
– Anesthesia
– Stress
– Spinal cord injury
– Head trauma
● Possible chemical-induced factors:
– Anaphylaxis
– Sepsis
– Capillary leak
– Burns
– Extensive trauma

Obstructive shock

● Caused by indirect pump failure, including conditions that may cause an obstruction of blood flow
● Possible factors:
– Cardiac tamponade
– Pulmonary embolus
– Pulmonary hypertension
– Tension pneumothorax

Data collection findings

Some general physical changes that may be found on data collection include:
● altered LOC
● changes in skin temperature (cool, clammy or hot, flushed)
● decreased or absent bowel sounds
● decreased renal output
● elevated respiratory rate
● hypotension
● metabolic acidosis
● nausea or vomiting

> **Shared goals**
>
> The different classifications of shock share some of the same planning goals, such as:
> ● The client will have adequate cellular perfusion.
> ● The client will retain renal function.
> ● The client will suffer no complications.
> ● The client's and family's anxiety will decrease. Corresponding evaluative statements include:
> ● The client's normal blood pressure has been restored.
> ● The client's fluid and electrolyte levels fall within reference limits.
> ● The client doesn't experience complications, such as pulmonary edema or metabolic acidosis.
> ● The client's and family's anxieties have decreased satisfactorily.

● restlessness, anxiety, apprehension
● thirst. (See *Shared goals*.)

SHOCK DISORDERS

This section reviews some of the key types of shock, including anaphylaxis, cardiogenic shock, septic shock, neurogenic shock, and hypovolemic shock. Data collection, treatment, individual nursing diagnoses, and appropriate implementations of nursing interventions are provided for each example.

Anaphylaxis

ANAPHYLAXIS is a dramatic and widespread acute atopic reaction. It's a type of distributive shock that's marked by the sudden onset of rapidly progressive urticaria and respiratory distress. A severe anaphylactic reaction may cause vascular collapse, leading to systemic shock and, sometimes, death.

Possible causes

Possible causes of anaphylaxis include systemic exposure to or ingestion of sensitizing drugs or other substances, such as:
● allergen extracts
● diagnostic chemicals (such as sulfobromophthalein, sodium dehydrocholate, and radiographic contrast media)
● enzymes (such as L-asparaginase)
● food (such as legumes, nuts, berries, seafood, and egg albumin) and sulfite-containing food additives

- hormones
- insect venom (such as honeybees, wasps, hornets, yellow jackets, fire ants, mosquitoes, and certain spiders)
- local anesthetics
- penicillin and other antibiotics
- polysaccharides
- ruptured hydatid cyst (rarely)
- salicylates
- serums (usually horse serum)
- sulfonamides
- vaccines.

Data collection findings

- Cardiovascular symptoms (hypotension, shock, cardiac arrhythmias) that may precipitate circulatory collapse if untreated
- GI and genitourinary symptoms (severe stomach cramps, nausea, diarrhea, urinary urgency and incontinence)
- Persistent or delayed reaction that may occur up to 24 hours after exposure to the allergen
- Respiratory symptoms (nasal mucosal edema, profuse watery rhinorrhea, itching, nasal congestion, sudden sneezing attacks, edema of the upper respiratory tract that causes hoarseness, stridor, and dyspnea [early sign of acute respiratory failure])
- Sudden physical distress within seconds or minutes after exposure to an allergen (may include feeling of impending doom or fright, weakness, sweating, sneezing, shortness of breath, nasal pruritus, urticaria, and angioedema, followed rapidly by symptoms in one or more target organs)
- Severity of reaction inversely related to interval between exposure to an allergen and onset of symptoms — the longer the interval, the less severe the reaction

SPOT CHECK

Name two signs of physical distress a client may exhibit almost immediately after being exposed to an allergen.
The client may exhibit one or more of the following signs:

- feeling of impending doom or fright
- weakness
- sweating
- sneezing
- shortness of breath
- nasal pruritus
- urticaria
- angioedema.

Diagnostic findings

- Anaphylaxis can be diagnosed by the rapid onset of severe respiratory or cardiovascular symptoms after ingestion or injection of a drug, vaccine, diagnostic agent, food, or food additive or after an insect sting.

Nursing diagnoses

- Risk for suffocation
- Decreased cardiac output
- Anxiety

Treatment

- Cardiopulmonary resuscitation (CPR) in case of cardiac arrest
- Endotracheal tube insertion or a tracheotomy and oxygen therapy in case of laryngeal edema
- Other therapy as indicated by clinical response

Drug therapy options

- Epinephrine
- Vasopressor: norepinephrine (Levophed) and dopamine (Intropin), if hypotensive

After initial emergency

- Corticosteroid
- Antihistamine
- Epinephrine: subcutaneous; longer-acting

Nursing interventions

- In the early stages of anaphylaxis, when the client hasn't lost consciousness and is still normotensive, give epinephrine intramuscularly or subcutaneously and massage the injection site *to help the drug move into the circulation faster.*
- Maintain airway patency. Observe for early signs of laryngeal edema (stridor, hoarseness, and dyspnea), and prepare for endotracheal tube insertion or tracheotomy and oxygen therapy *to prevent cerebral anoxia.*
- In case of cardiac arrest, begin CPR, including closed-chest heart massage and assisted ventilation; initiate other therapy as indicated by the clinical response. *These measures are necessary to prevent irreversible organ damage.*
- Watch for hypotension and shock, and monitor I.V. fluids as needed *to maintain circulatory volume.* Monitor blood pressure and urine output *to monitor the client's response to treatment.*
- After the initial emergency, administer other medications (such as an antihistamine or corticosteroid) for long-term management *to prevent recurrence of symptoms.*

● When any client needs a drug with high anaphylactic potential (particularly parenteral drugs), make sure he receives each dose under close medical observation *to prevent a severe reaction.*

● Closely monitor a client undergoing diagnostic tests that use radiographic contrast dyes, such as cardiac catheterization, excretory urography, and angiography, *to detect early signs of anaphylaxis.*

● Review key teaching topics with the client *to ensure adequate knowledge about his condition and treatment,* including:

– risks of delayed symptoms and the need to report any recurrence of shortness of breath, chest tightness, sweating, angioedema, or other symptoms

– preventing anaphylaxis (avoiding exposure to known allergens, including all forms of the offending food or drug; avoiding open fields and wooded areas during the insect season in case of a reaction to an insect bite or sting; carrying an anaphylaxis kit containing epinephrine, an antihistamine, and a tourniquet)

– wearing medical identification jewelry identifying the client's allergies.

SPOT CHECK

Name three specific substances that can cause anaphylactic reactions.

Examples of substances that can cause anaphylactic reactions are:
● penicillin and other antibiotics
● salicylates
● polysaccharides
● radiographic contrast media
● seafood
● nuts.
For additional examples, see "Possible causes," on page 62.

Septic shock

SEPTIC SHOCK is usually the result of a bacterial infection. It causes inadequate blood perfusion and circulatory collapse and occurs most often among hospitalized clients, especially men over age 40 and women ages 25 to 45. It's second only to cardiogenic shock as the leading cause of shock death. About 25% of clients in whom gram-negative bacteremia develops go into shock. Unless vigorous treatment begins promptly, preferably before symptoms fully develop, septic shock rapidly progresses to death (commonly within a few hours) in up to 80% of these clients.

Possible causes
● Infection with gram-positive bacteria: *Streptococcus pneumoniae, S. pyogenes,* or *Actinomyces*
● Infection with gram-negative bacteria (in two-thirds of clients): *Escherichia coli, Klebsiella, Enterobacter, Proteus, Pseudomonas,* or *Bacteroides*

Data collection findings
Indications of septic shock vary according to the stage of the shock, the organism causing it, and the age of the client.

Early stage
● Chills
● Sudden fever (over 101° F [38.3° C])
● Oliguria
● Nausea
● Vomiting
● Diarrhea
● Prostration

Late stage
● Altered LOC
● Anuria
● Apprehension
● Hyperventilation
● Hypotension
● Hypothermia
● Irritability
● Restlessness
● Tachycardia
● Tachypnea
● Thirst from decreased cerebral tissue perfusion

FAST FACT

Infants and elderly people may have only these signs of septic shock:
● altered LOC
● hyperventilation
● hypotension.

Diagnostic findings
● Arterial blood gas (ABG) analysis indicates respiratory alkalosis (low partial pressure of carbon dioxide, low or normal bicarbonate [HCO_3^-] level, and high pH).
● Blood cultures isolate the organism.

- Blood tests show decreased platelet count and leukocytosis (15,000 to 30,000/µl), increased blood urea nitrogen (BUN) and creatinine levels, decreased creatinine clearance, and abnormal prothrombin time (PT) and partial thromboplastin time (PTT).
- Electrocardiography (ECG) findings resemble myocardial infarction (MI).

Nursing diagnoses
- Decreased cardiac output
- Deficient fluid volume
- Risk for injury

Treatment
- Removing and replacing any I.V., intra-arterial, or urinary drainage catheters that may be sources of infection
- Oxygen therapy (may require endotracheal intubation and mechanical ventilation)
- Colloid or crystalloid infusion to increase intravascular volume
- Diuretics such as furosemide (Lasix) after sufficient fluid volume has been replaced to maintain urine output above 20 ml/hour
- Blood transfusion, if anemia is present
- Surgery to drain abscesses, if present

Drug therapy options
- Antibiotic: according to sensitivity of causative organism
- Vasopressor: dopamine (Intropin) if fluid resuscitation fails to increase blood pressure

Nursing interventions
- Assist with removing I.V., intra-arterial, or urinary drainage catheters and send them to the laboratory for culture of the causative organism. New catheters will be inserted *to provide access for fluid resuscitation and to ensure accurate measurement of urine output.*
- Monitor I.V. infusion of normal saline or lactated Ringer's solution *to ensure fluid replacement.*
- Monitor the client's blood pressure and report decreases immediately *to prevent a progressive drop in blood pressure accompanied by a thready pulse, which generally signifies inadequate cardiac output from reduced vascular volume.*
- Keep accurate intake and output records. Monitor urine output (0.5 to 1 ml/kg/hour) and systolic pressure *to prevent kidney damage and fluid overload.*
- Prepare the patient for administration of I.V. antibiotics *to achieve effective blood levels quickly* and monitor drug levels *to prevent toxicity.*

- Watch closely for complications of septic shock: disseminated intravascular coagulation (abnormal bleeding), renal failure (oliguria, increased specific gravity), heart failure (dyspnea, edema, tachycardia, distended neck veins), GI ulcers (hematemesis, melena), and hepatic abnormalities (jaundice, hypoprothrombinemia, and hypoalbuminemia) *to prevent crisis.*
- Review key teaching topics with the client and family members *to ensure adequate knowledge about the condition and treatment,* including:
  – risk associated with blood transfusion
  – disease process and treatment options.

Cardiogenic shock

CARDIOGENIC SHOCK occurs when the heart fails to pump adequately, thereby reducing cardiac output and compromising tissue perfusion.

This is how cardiogenic shock progresses:
- Decreased stroke volume results in increased left ventricular volume.
- Blood pooling in the left ventricle backs up into the lungs, causing pulmonary edema.
- To compensate for a falling cardiac output, heart rate and contractility increase.
- These compensating mechanisms increase the demand for myocardial oxygen.
- An imbalance between oxygen supply and demand results, increasing myocardial ischemia and further compromising the heart's pumping action.

Possible causes
- Advanced heart block
- Cardiomyopathy
- Heart failure
- MI
- Myocarditis
- Papillary muscle rupture

Data collection findings
- Anxiety, restlessness, disorientation, and confusion
- Cold, clammy skin
- Crackles in lungs
- Hypotension (systolic pressure below 90 mm Hg), narrow pulse pressure
- Jugular venous distention
- Oliguria (urine output of less than 30 ml/hour)
- Tachycardia
- Tachypnea
- Hypoxia

● Weak, thready pulse

Diagnostic findings
● ABG levels show respiratory alkalosis initially. As shock progresses, metabolic acidosis develops.
● Blood chemistry tests show increased BUN and creatinine levels.
● ECG shows MI.

Nursing diagnoses
● Decreased cardiac output
● Ineffective tissue perfusion (cardiopulmonary, renal)

Treatment
● Intra-aortic balloon pump

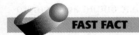
FAST FACT

An intra-aortic balloon pump helps improve coronary artery perfusion and reduce cardiac workload.

● Oxygen therapy: intubation and mechanical ventilation, if necessary
● Activity changes, including maintaining bed rest and implementing passive range-of-motion (ROM) and isometric exercises
● Continuous arteriovenous hemofiltration or continuous arteriovenous hemodialysis
● Dietary changes, including withholding food and oral fluids

Drug therapy options
● Adrenergic agent: epinephrine (Adrenalin Chloride)
● Cardiac glycoside: digoxin (Lanoxin)
● Cardiac inotrope: dopamine (Intropin), dobutamine (Dobutrex), inamrinone (Inocor), milrinone (Primacor)
● Diuretic: furosemide (Lasix), bumetanide (Bumex), metolazone (Zaroxolyn)
● Vasodilator: nitroprusside (Nitropress)
● Vasopressor: norepinephrine (Levophed)

Nursing interventions
● Assess cardiovascular status, including hemodynamic variables, vital signs, capillary refill, skin temperature, and peripheral pulses, *to monitor the effects of drug therapy and detect cardiac decompensation.*

● Assess respiratory status, including respiratory rate and breath sounds *to identify signs of pulmonary edema, such as tachypnea, crackles, and hypoxemia.*
● Monitor fluid balance, including intake and output, *to monitor kidney function and detect fluid overload leading to pulmonary edema.*
● Monitor LOC *to detect cerebral hypoxia caused by reduced cardiac output.*
● Withhold food and fluids, as directed, *to reduce the risk of aspiration due to reduced LOC.*
● Administer oxygen and medications as prescribed *to maximize cardiac, pulmonary, and renal functioning.*
● Provide suctioning *to aid in the removal of secretions and reduce the risk of aspiration.*
● Encourage the client to express his feelings, such as a fear of dying, *to reduce his anxiety.*
● Review key teaching topics with the client and family members *to ensure adequate knowledge about the condition and treatment,* including:
– recognizing early signs and symptoms of fluid overload
– maintaining activity limitations, including alternating rest periods with activity
– maintaining a low-fat, low-sodium diet.

Neurogenic shock
NEUROGENIC SHOCK is sometimes referred to as *spinal shock.* It's a form of distributive shock and causes loss of sympathetic (vasomotor) tone. Neurogenic shock may also cause:
● vasodilation
● decreased venous return
● decreased cardiac output
● decreased tissue perfusion.

Possible causes
● Nervous system damage, including damage to the medulla oblongata
● Spinal anesthesia
● Spinal cord injury
● Syncope

Data collection findings
● Bradycardia
● Warm, dry skin
● Usually normotensive (systolic blood pressure less than 90 mm Hg or 30 mm Hg less than baseline values)

Diagnostic findings
● ABG measurements may reveal a decreased pH and HCO_3^-.
● Hemodynamic monitoring may indicate a decrease in systemic vascular resistance.
● Radiographs may indicate a spinal injury.
● Computed tomography may reveal damage to the medulla.

Nursing diagnoses
● Ineffective breathing pattern
● Ineffective airway clearance
● Impaired physical mobility
● Risk for autonomic dysreflexia

Treatment
● Trauma resuscitation as indicated
● Oxygen therapy and endotracheal intubation as needed
● Maintenance of spinal immobilization

Drug therapy options
● Atropine (if bradycardia is present)
● High-dose corticosteroid: methylprednisolone (Solu-Medrol) infusion administered within 8 hours of spinal cord injury
● Vasopressor: dopamine (Intropin), phenylephrine (Neo-Synephrine), or norepinephrine (Levophed)

Nursing interventions
● Maintain a patent airway. Monitor oxygen level with pulse oximetry *to prevent hypoxemia.* If the client has experienced a trauma, maintain cervical immobilization until cleared by radiographs *to prevent injury.*
● Administer oxygen, as ordered, *to increase the amount of oxygen in the blood.* Prepare for intubation, as needed.
● Apply a cardiac monitor for continuous monitoring. *Fluid and electrolyte imbalances can cause arrhythmias.*
● Maintain the client in the supine position or, if possible, use a modified Trendelenburg's position, with the lower end of the bed elevated about 45 degrees and the client's head slightly elevated. *This promotes increased respiratory exchange and increased venous return.*
● Encourage deep breathing and coughing *to help prevent respiratory complications.*
● Apply antithrombolytic stockings. Pneumatic compression devices may also be used *to prevent deep vein thrombosis.*
● Assess the client's neurological status *to observe for autonomic hyperreflexia (autonomic dysreflexia)*, which usually begins in 3 to 6 weeks as neurogenic shock resolves.

Hypovolemic shock
HYPOVOLEMIC SHOCK is a shock state resulting from decreased intravascular volume due to fluid loss. This causes circulatory dysfunction and inadequate tissue perfusion. Without sufficient blood or fluid replacement, hypovolemic shock syndrome may lead to irreversible cerebral and renal damage, cardiac arrest and, ultimately, death.

Hypovolemic shock requires early recognition of signs and symptoms and prompt, aggressive treatment to improve the prognosis. (See *Caring for the client with shock,* page 68.)

Possible causes
● Acute blood loss (approximately one-fifth of total volume)
● Acute pancreatitis, ascites, or peritonitis
● Burns
● Diabetes insipidus
● Diarrhea or vomiting
● Severe dehydration
● Severe edema
● Surgery
● Trauma

Data collection findings
● Tachycardia
● Cold, clammy skin
● Decreased urinary output: less than 30 ml/hour
● Hypotension
● Rapid, shallow respirations
● Decreased LOC
● Thirst
● Decreased capillary refill
● Dilated, sluggish reacting pupils

Diagnostic findings
● Hemoglobin level and hematocrit decrease.
● Cardiac enzyme levels rise.
● BUN and creatinine levels increase.
● Liver enzyme and bilirubin levels increase.
● Coagulation times (PT, PPT) are prolonged.
● Urine specific gravity and urine osmolality increase.
● ABG analysis reveals metabolic acidosis.
● Gastroscopy, nasogastric (NG) tube drainage, and radiographs identify internal bleeding.

Nursing diagnoses
● Deficient fluid volume
● Decreased cardiac output

CLINICAL SITUATION

Caring for the client with shock

Evaluate the clinical situation described here. See if you're able to answer the questions as you go.

A 19-year-old male was driving home from a college fraternity party when a drunk driver struck his car. The client sustained major trauma. On assessment, the nurse finds the following injuries: laceration on the scalp, repetitive verbalization, abdominal pain with tenderness on palpation, lack of neurologic response below the nipple line, and a fractured tibia. The client could have hypovolemic shock, distributive shock, or both.

What should be included in the client data collection?
Assess, monitor, and observe the client for:
- restlessness
- anxiety
- apprehension
- altered level of consciousness
- color changes (pallor, cyanosis, flushing)
- blood pressure (systolic readings below 80 mm Hg can be caused by decreased circulating blood volume or cardiac output)
- tachycardia
- elevated respiratory rate
- urine output (output below 25 ml/hour can be caused by decreased renal perfusion)
- skin temperature (cool, cold, clammy, or flushed, hot to touch)
- bowel sounds (decreased or absent)
- nausea or vomiting
- thirst.

What would be appropriate nursing diagnoses?
- Decreased cardiac output related to left ventricular failure, volume depletion, or vasodilation
- Ineffective tissue perfusion (cardiopulmonary, cerebral, renal, GI, peripheral) related to decreased myocardial contractility, hypovolemia, or fluid shift from vascular spaces
- Deficient fluid volume related to excessive fluid loss
- Ineffective coping related to critical situation
- Compromised family coping related to critically ill family member
- Risk for injury related to sensorimotor deficits or hypotension
- Impaired gas exchange related to altered ventilation-perfusion ratio

What are appropriate goals for this client?
- The client will have adequate cellular perfusion.
- The client will retain renal function.
- The client will suffer no complications.
- The client and his family will experience less anxiety.

Questions for further thought
- What's the importance of fluid resuscitation if a client has hypovolemia?
- How can you determine if the client is getting adequate oxygenation?
- What evaluation findings would indicate that client goals are met?

- Ineffective tissue perfusion (cardiopulmonary, cerebral, or renal)

Treatment
- Blood and fluid replacement
- Control of bleeding

Drug therapy options
- Inotropic agent: dopamine (Intropin) must be used with vigorous fluid resuscitation to be effective

Nursing interventions
Management of hypovolemic shock necessitates prompt, aggressive supportive measures and careful assessment and monitoring of vital signs. Follow these priorities:

- Check for a patent airway and adequate circulation. If blood pressure and heart rate are absent, start CPR *to prevent irreversible organ damage and death.*
- Record blood pressure, pulse rate, peripheral pulses, respiratory rate, and other vital signs every 15 minutes. A systolic blood pressure lower than 80 mm Hg usually results in inadequate coronary artery blood flow, cardiac ischemia, arrhythmias, and further complications of low cardiac output. When blood pressure drops below 80 mm Hg, increase the oxygen flow rate and notify the physician immediately. A progressive drop in blood pressure accompanied by a thready pulse generally signals inadequate cardiac output from reduced intravascular volume.

- Monitor I.V. infusions of normal saline or lactated Ringer's solution *to ensure correction of the fluid volume deficit through fluid replacement.*
- An indwelling urinary catheter may be inserted *to measure hourly urine output.* Report if urine output doesn't improve.
- Administer oxygen *to ensure adequate oxygenation of tissues.*
- During therapy, assess skin color and temperature and note any changes *to identify changes in the client's condition.* Cold, clammy skin may be a sign of continuing peripheral vascular constriction, indicating progressive shock.
- Throughout these emergency measures, provide emotional support to the client and his family members *to help them cope with the overwhelming situation.*
- Review key teaching topics with the client and family members *to ensure adequate knowledge about the condition and treatment,* including causes of hypovolemia and treatment options.

PAIN

Theoretical overview

Pain is universally feared — the strongest human fear after fear of death. It serves as a bodily protective mechanism (superficial fibers are rich in pain receptors; viscera aren't). Pain is a highly complex mechanism that consists of perception and interpretation. Two theories, specificity and gate control, attempt to explain how pain is perceived and interpreted by the body.

Specificity theory

Specificity theory is the traditional theory of pain perception and interpretation. First, the onset of pain begins with a stimulus that triggers a response that's received by a receptor. A receptor, for example, responds to cold and pressure. Pain transmits to the spinothalamic tract where it travels between the spinal cord and the thalamus, where it's finally perceived. The cerebral cortex then interprets the pain. Pain pathways can be transected and pain will still occur.

Gate control theory

The gate control theory is based on the idea that only one major stimulus can be transmitted at a time. First, the onset of pain begins with a stimulus that triggers an open

and closed "gate" response within the spinal cord. Next, pain travels through the neural pathways where it's met by conflicting large fibers that close the "gate" or small fibers that open the gate. This open and close "gate" response occurs as a response to impulses from the brain stem.

Reactions to pain perception and interpretation

There are several ways that the body reacts to pain perception and interpretation.

Autonomic

- Stress response
- Increased skeletal muscle activity
- Reflexes (withdrawal from source)
- Reflex muscular rigidity over affected areas; guarding (protective reflex)
- Muscle spasms after a fracture

Voluntary

- Grimacing
- Clenching fists and teeth
- Pacing floor
- Twisting and turning
- Decreasing activity
- Altering body position

Psychological

- Anxiety, fear, and apprehension (anxiety increases the intensity of pain, which further increases anxiety)
- Anger and verbalization
- Decreased sense of control

Severe physical or psychological conditions

- Shock
- Panic
- Prolonged pain resulting from fear, depression, insomnia, anorexia, or tension

Types of pain

There are several types of pain that may be either superficial or deep.

Superficial pain characteristics

- Abrupt (sharp, prickly) or gradual (burning) onset
- Localized to one spot

Deep pain characteristics

- Dull, aching quality that persists
- Visceral — caused by spastic contraction of smooth muscle (blood vessels)
- Referred — pain of a visceral lesion gives the impression of arising in a distant area; for example, shoulder pain experienced in gallbladder disease
- Central pain — has no peripheral cause but may be caused by injury to the nerve trunk; perception of pain persists after the stimulus is gone; for example, toe pain after leg amputation (phantom limb pain)

    QUICK STUDY

When assessing pain, remember to use **PQRST.**

Provoking factors (What provokes the pain? What makes it worse? What makes it better?)

Quality of pain (How does the pain feel?)

Region or radiation (Where is the pain? Where does the pain go?)

Severity (How severe is the pain on a scale of 1 to 10?)

Time (When did the pain begin? Is the pain constant? Does it come and go?)

Pain management
Pharmacologic intervention

- Nonnarcotic analgesia (inhibits prostaglandin synthesis)
- Narcotic analgesia (acts centrally to change pain perception and interpretation)

Nonpharmacologic intervention

- Transcutaneous electrical nerve stimulation — electronic stimulation of the large fibers to close the gate to painful stimuli (based on the gate control theory)
- Acupuncture — Chinese method of inserting fine needles at certain sites on the body; how acupuncture works is uncertain
- Relaxation techniques — biofeedback, visualization, meditation, and hypnosis

ACID-BASE IMBALANCES

Key concepts
- Normal pH in the body's blood and extracellular fluids is 7.35 to 7.45.

Assessing ABG values

Arterial blood gas (ABG) analysis assesses the client's acid-base balance. See the chart here for typical adult ABG reference values based on the client's acid-base reference. Normal values may vary slightly among different institutions.

ABG REFERENCE VALUE	ADULT
pH	7.35 to 7.45
Pao_2	75 to 100 mm Hg
$Paco_2$	35 to 45 mm Hg
HCO_3^-	22 to 26 mEq/L
Sao_2	96 to 100%
Base excess	+1 to −2 mEq/L

- The concentration of carbon dioxide (CO_2) is directly related to the concentration of hydrogen (H^+) ions.
- An acid gives up H^+ in solution.
- A base binds H^+ in solution.
- Acid-base balance is regulated by chemical, respiratory, and renal mechanisms.
- Chemical buffers correct acid-base imbalances immediately.
- The lungs regulate the amount of CO_2 retained or exhaled.
- The kidneys control the amount of H^+ and HCO_3^- ions retained or excreted by the body.
- Compensation is the process by which the body uses its three regulatory mechanisms to correct changes in the pH of body fluids. (See *Assessing ABG values.*)

Key points about ABG values
- pH reflects the number of H^+ ions in the blood. The lungs and the kidneys respond to alterations in pH levels by either retaining or excreting CO_2 and HCO_3^-.
- *Pao_2* denotes the partial pressure of oxygen in arterial blood.
- *$Paco_2$* denotes the partial pressure of CO_2 in arterial blood, which is regulated by the lungs.
- HCO_3^- denotes the bicarbonate ion concentration in arterial blood, which is regulated by the kidneys.
- Oxygen saturation denotes the oxygen content of arterial blood.
- Base excess denotes the difference between the normal serum HCO_3^- level and the client's HCO_3^- level.

Respiratory acidosis

RESPIRATORY ACIDOSIS is an acid-base disturbance characterized by excess CO_2 in the blood (hypercapnia), indicated by a $Paco_2$ greater than 45 mm Hg. It results from reduced alveolar ventilation. It can be acute (from a sudden failure in ventilation) or chronic (as in long-term pulmonary disease).

Data collection findings
- Restlessness
- Dyspnea and tachypnea with papilledema and depressed reflexes
- Headaches
- Confusion
- Cardiovascular abnormalities, such as tachycardia, hypertension, irregular heart rate, and hypotension with vasodilation (in severe acidosis)
- Coma
- Fine or flapping tremor (asterixis)
- Hypoxemia

Diagnostic findings
- ABG measurements confirm respiratory acidosis. $Paco_2$ exceeds the normal level of 45 mm Hg, and pH is usually below the normal range of 7.35 to 7.45. The client's HCO_3^- level is normal in the acute stage and elevated in the chronic stage.

Nursing diagnoses
- Impaired gas exchange
- Ineffective breathing pattern
- Fear

Treatment
Treatment of respiratory acidosis is designed to correct the underlying source of alveolar hypoventilation. It may include:
- endotracheal intubation and mechanical ventilation
- dialysis to remove toxic drugs
- removal of foreign body, if appropriate.

Drug therapy options
- Antibiotic (if pneumonia is present)
- Bronchodilator
- Sodium bicarbonate (in severe cases)

Nursing interventions
- Be alert for critical changes in the client's respiratory, central nervous system (CNS), and cardiovascular functions. Maintain adequate hydration. *These measures help detect life-threatening complications.*
- Maintain a patent airway and provide adequate humidification *to ensure adequate oxygenation.* Perform tracheal suctioning regularly and vigorous chest physiotherapy if needed. Continuously monitor respiratory status.
- Closely monitor the client with chronic obstructive pulmonary disease and chronic CO_2 retention *to detect signs of acidosis.* Also, administer oxygen at low flow rates and closely monitor all clients who receive narcotics and sedatives *to prevent respiratory acidosis.*
- Instruct the client who has received a general anesthetic to turn, cough, and perform deep-breathing exercises frequently *to prevent the onset of respiratory acidosis.* Encourage the use of incentive spirometry.
- Review key teaching topics with the client and family *to ensure adequate knowledge about the condition and treatment,* including:
  – home oxygen use
  – coughing and deep-breathing exercises
  – the medication regimen and possible adverse reactions.

Evaluation
- The client doesn't have atelectasis or other respiratory complications.
- The client maintains adequate oxygenation.

Respiratory alkalosis

RESPIRATORY ALKALOSIS is characterized by a deficiency of CO_2 in the blood (hypocapnia), as indicated by a decrease in $Paco_2$. $Paco_2$ is below 35 mm Hg (normal level is 45 mm Hg). This condition is caused by alveolar hyperventilation. Elimination of CO_2 by the lungs exceeds the production of CO_2 at the cellular level, leading to CO_2 deficiency in the blood. Uncomplicated respiratory alkalosis leads to a decrease in H^+ concentration, which causes elevated blood pH.

Possible causes
Respiratory alkalosis can result from pulmonary or nonpulmonary causes.

Pulmonary causes
- Acute asthma
- Interstitial lung disease
- Pneumonia
- Pulmonary vascular disease

Nonpulmonary causes
- Anxiety
- Aspirin toxicity
- CNS disease (inflammation or tumor)
- Fever
- Hepatic failure
- Metabolic acidosis
- Pregnancy
- Sepsis

Data collection findings
- Deep, rapid breathing, possibly exceeding 40 breaths/minute (cardinal sign)
- Light-headedness or dizziness (from decreased cerebral blood flow)
- Agitation
- Circumoral or peripheral paresthesia (a prickling sensation around the mouth or extremities)
- Muscle weakness
- Carpopedal spasms (spasms affecting the wrist and foot)
- Twitching (possibly progressing to tetany)
- Seizures (severe respiratory alkalosis)
- Cardiac arrhythmias that fail to respond to conventional treatment (severe respiratory alkalosis)

Diagnostic findings
- ABG analysis confirms respiratory alkalosis and rules out respiratory compensation for metabolic acidosis. In the acute stage, $PaCO_2$ is below 35 mm Hg and pH is elevated in proportion to the fall in $PaCO_2$. pH drops toward normal in the chronic stage. HCO_3^- level is normal in the acute stage but below normal in the chronic stage.

Nursing diagnoses
- Impaired gas exchange
- Ineffective breathing pattern
- Anxiety

Treatment
Treatment seeks to eradicate the underlying condition. It may include:
- removal of ingested toxins
- treatment of CNS disease
- treatment of fever or sepsis.

In cases of severe respiratory alkalosis, the client should breathe into a paper bag, which helps relieve acute anxiety and increases CO_2 levels.

Patient care goals
- The client's respiratory status will stabilize.
- The client won't have preventable complications.
- The client and family will have decreased anxiety.
- The client's blood pH has returned to normal.

Nursing interventions
- Watch for and report changes in neurologic, neuromuscular, or cardiovascular functions *to ensure prompt recognition and treatment.*
- Remember that twitching and cardiac arrhythmias may be associated with alkalemia and electrolyte imbalances. Monitor ABG and serum electrolyte levels closely, watching for any variations *to detect early changes and prevent complications.*
- Review key teaching topics with the client and family members *to ensure adequate knowledge about the condition and treatment,* including:
– relaxation techniques
– breathing into a paper bag during an acute anxiety attack.

Evaluation
- The client maintains adequate oxygenation.
- The client has normal breath sounds.
- The client and family have decreased anxiety.

Metabolic acidosis
METABOLIC ACIDOSIS refers to a state of excess acid accumulation and deficient base HCO_3^-. It's produced by an underlying pathologic disorder. Symptoms result from the body's attempts to correct the acidotic condition through compensatory mechanisms in the lungs, kidneys, and cells.

Metabolic acidosis is more prevalent among children, who are vulnerable to acid-base imbalance because their metabolic rates are faster and their ratios of water to total body weight are lower. Severe or untreated metabolic acidosis can be fatal.

Possible causes
- Anaerobic carbohydrate metabolism
- Chronic alcoholism
- Diabetic ketoacidosis
- Diarrhea or intestinal malabsorption
- Low-carbohydrate, high-fat diet
- Malnutrition
- Renal insufficiency and failure

Data collection findings
- Headache
- Lethargy
- Drowsiness
- Kussmaul's respirations
- CNS depression
- Stupor

 FAST FACT

Kussmaul's respirations are respirations that are fast and deep without pauses. They characteristically sound labored, with deep breaths that sound like sighs. This breathing pattern develops when the respiratory centers in the medulla detect decreased blood pH, thereby triggering compensatory fast and deep breathing to remove excess CO_2 and restore pH balance.

Diagnostic findings
- ABG analysis reveals a pH below 7.35 and a HCO_3^- level less than 24 mEq/L.

Nursing diagnoses
- Ineffective breathing pattern
- Disturbed thought processes
- Decreased cardiac output

Treatment
- Correction of the underlying cause is the goal of treatment.
- Endotracheal intubation and mechanical ventilation to ensure adequate respiratory compensation (in severe cases)

Drug therapy options
- Insulin: administration and I.V. fluid administration if diabetic ketoacidosis is the cause
- Sodium bicarbonate: I.V. or orally for chronic metabolic acidosis

Patient care goals
- The client's blood pH will return to normal limits.
- The client won't have preventable complications.

Nursing interventions
- Frequently monitor vital signs and LOC *to identify changes, which can occur rapidly.*
- In diabetic acidosis, watch for secondary changes due to hypovolemia, such as decreasing blood pressure, *to prevent complications of hypoperfusion.*

- Record intake and output accurately *to monitor renal function.*
- Watch for signs of excessive serum potassium — weakness, flaccid paralysis, and irregular heart rhythm — *to detect a life-threatening situation possibly leading to cardiac arrest.* After treatment, check for overcorrection to hypokalemia *to prevent complications of potassium imbalance.*
- Prepare for possible seizures with seizure precautions *to prevent injury.*
- Provide good oral hygiene. Use sodium bicarbonate washes *to neutralize mouth acids,* and lubricate the client's lips *to prevent skin breakdown.*
- Carefully observe a client who is receiving I.V. therapy, has intestinal tubes in place, or is suffering from shock, hyperthyroidism, hepatic disease, circulatory failure, or dehydration *to prevent metabolic acidosis.*
- Review key teaching topics with the client and family members *to ensure adequate knowledge about the condition and treatment,* including:
  – testing urine for sugar and acetone
  – encouraging strict adherence to insulin or oral antidiabetic therapy

Evaluation
- The client's fluid and electrolyte levels return to normal limits.

Metabolic alkalosis

METABOLIC ALKALOSIS is a clinical state marked by decreased amounts of acid or increased amounts of base HCO_3^-. It causes metabolic, respiratory, and renal responses, producing characteristic symptoms — most notably hypoventilation. This condition always occurs secondary to an underlying cause. With early diagnosis and prompt treatment, the prognosis is good; however, untreated metabolic alkalosis may lead to coma and death.

Possible causes
- Loss of acid from vomiting, NG tube drainage, or lavage without adequate electrolyte replacement; fistulas; the use of steroids and certain diuretics (furosemide, thiazides, and ethacrynic acid); or hyperadrenocorticism
- Retention of base from excessive intake of bicarbonate of soda or other antacids (usually for treatment of gastritis or peptic ulcer), excessive intake of absorbable alkali (as in milk-alkali syndrome), administration of excessive amounts of I.V. fluids with high concentrations of bicarbonate or lactate, or respiratory insufficiency

Data collection findings

- Hypoventilation
- Irritability
- Picking at bedclothes (carphology)
- Nausea
- Vomiting
- Diarrhea
- Cyanosis
- Confusion
- Tachycardia
- Twitching
- Apnea

Diagnostic findings

- ABG analysis reveals a pH greater than 7.45 and a HCO_3^- level above 29 mEq/L.

Nursing diagnoses

- Decreased cardiac output
- Disturbed thought processes
- Risk for injury

Treatment

- Correction of the underlying cause is the goal of treatment.

Drug therapy options

- Acidifying agent: ammonium chloride I.V.
- Potassium supplement: Potassium chloride I.V.

Patient care goals

- The client's blood pH will return to normal limits.
- The client will learn how to prevent alkalosis.
- The client and family will have decreased anxiety.

Nursing interventions

- Monitor vital signs frequently, and record intake and output *to evaluate respiratory, fluid, and electrolyte status.* Respiratory rate usually decreases in an effort to compensate for alkalosis. Hypotension and tachycardia may indicate electrolyte imbalance, especially hypokalemia.
- Irrigate NG tubes with isotonic saline solution instead of plain water *to prevent loss of gastric electrolytes.*
- Review key teaching topics with the client and family members *to ensure adequate knowledge about the condition and treatment,* including:
- recognizing signs of milk-alkali syndrome (for clients with ulcers), including a distaste for milk, anorexia, weakness, and lethargy
- avoiding overuse of alkaline agents.

Evaluation

- The client's blood pH has returned to normal.
- The client knows how to prevent alkalosis.
- The client and family will have decreased anxiety.

ELECTROLYTE IMBALANCES

Electrolyte balance is the body's maintenance of normal electrolyte levels. The three electrolytes that have the most frequent imbalances are:

- sodium (135 to 145 mEq/L)
- potassium (3.5 to 5.0 mEq/L)
- calcium (8.9 to 10.1 mg/dl).

The primary extracellular electrolyte, sodium, is responsible for intracellular and extracellular movement of water, and a close relationship exists between water balance and sodium concentration. The kidneys regulate the amount of sodium excreted.

Potassium, the primary intracellular electrolyte, affects neuromuscular functioning and must be ingested daily. Serum pH directly affects the body's serum potassium concentration.

The most plentiful of the electrolytes, calcium plays a major role in bone and tooth formation, affects blood coagulation, and influences cell membrane permeability (specifically cardiac and neuromuscular functioning).

An electrolyte imbalance — an abnormally high or low level of sodium, potassium, or calcium — can result in fluid volume deficit, altered nutrition, and other complications for the client.

Sodium imbalance

Sodium is the major cation (positively charged ion) in extracellular fluid. Its functions include maintaining tonicity and concentration of extracellular fluid, acid-base balance (reabsorption of sodium ions and excretion of hydrogen ions), nerve conduction and neuromuscular function, glandular secretion, and water balance.

A sodium-potassium pump is constantly at work in every body cell. Potassium is the major cation in intracellular fluid. According to the laws of diffusion, a substance moves from an area of high concentration to an area of lower concentration. Sodium ions, normally most abundant outside the cells, want to diffuse inward. Potassium ions, normally inside the cells, want to diffuse outward. The sodium-potassium pump works to combat this ionic diffusion and maintain normal sodium-potassium balance.

During repolarization, the sodium-potassium pump continually shifts sodium into the cells and potassium out of the cells; during depolarization, it does the reverse.

The body requires only 2 to 4 g of sodium daily. However, most Americans consume 6 to 10 g daily (mostly sodium chloride, as table salt), excreting excess sodium through the kidneys and skin.

A low-sodium diet or excessive use of diuretics may induce hyponatremia (decreased serum sodium concentration); dehydration may induce hypernatremia (increased serum sodium concentration).

 SPOT CHECK

True or false? Sodium chloride is the major cation in intracellular fluid.

Answer: False. Sodium chloride is the major cation in *extra*cellular fluid. Potassium chloride is the major cation in *intra*cellular fluid.

Possible causes
Hyponatremia
- Diarrhea
- Excessive perspiration or fever
- Excessive water intake
- Low-sodium diet
- Malnutrition
- Potent diuretics
- Starvation
- Suctioning
- Trauma, wound drainage, or burns
- Vomiting

Hypernatremia
- Decreased water intake
- Diabetes insipidus
- Excess adrenocortical hormones, as in Cushing's syndrome
- Severe vomiting and diarrhea with water loss that exceeds sodium loss

Data collection findings
Hyponatremia
- Abdominal cramps
- Anxiety
- Cold, clammy skin
- Cyanosis
- Headaches
- Hypotension
- Muscle twitching and weakness

- Nausea and vomiting
- Oliguria or anuria
- Renal dysfunction
- Seizures
- Tachycardia

Hypernatremia
- Agitation and restlessness
- Circulatory disorders
- Decreased LOC
- Dry, sticky mucous membranes
- Dyspnea
- Excessive weight gain
- Fever
- Flushed skin
- Hypertension
- Intense thirst
- Oliguria
- Pitting edema
- Pulmonary edema
- Rough, dry tongue
- Seizures
- Tachycardia

Diagnostic findings
- Serum sodium level less than 135 mEq/L indicates hyponatremia.
- Serum sodium level greater than 145 mEq/L indicates hypernatremia.

Nursing diagnoses
Hyponatremia
- Deficient fluid volume
- Risk for injury

Hypernatremia
- Excessive fluid volume
- Disturbed thought processes

Treatment
Hyponatremia
- Antibiotic: demeclocycline (Declomycin)
- Saline solution: I.V. infusion
- Potassium supplement: potassium chloride (K-Lor)

Hypernatremia
- Diet: sodium restrictions
- Salt-free solution (such as dextrose in water), followed by infusion of half normal saline solution to prevent hyponatremia

---

Salty foods

Instruct the client to avoid these high-sodium foods:
- baking soda and baking powder
- bottled soft drinks, especially those with sodium or sodium saccharin
- canned soups, broth, or vegetables
- condiments, such as salted butter and margarine, ketchup, mustard, and salad dressing
- fast foods
- foods that contain monosodium glutamate
- instant foods such as cereal
- lunch meats and cheeses
- over-the-counter medications such as antacids
- pickles and pickled foods
- potato chips, pretzels, and other snack foods
- prepared foods such as TV dinners.

Patient care goals
- The client's serum sodium level will return to normal limits. (See *Salty foods.*)

Nursing interventions
For hyponatremia
- Record fluid intake and output accurately, and weigh the client daily *to guide the treatment plan.*
- Monitor administration of iso-osmolar or hyperosmolar saline solution, watch closely for signs of hypervolemia (dyspnea, crackles, engorged neck or hand veins) *to prevent respiratory distress.*
- Note conditions that may cause excessive sodium loss — diaphoresis, prolonged diarrhea or vomiting, or severe burns — *to prevent hyponatremia.*
- Refer the client receiving a maintenance dosage of diuretics to a dietitian for instruction about dietary sodium intake *to increase sodium intake and decrease the risk for hyponatremia.*
- Review key teaching topics with the client and family members with hyponatremia *to ensure adequate knowledge about the condition and treatment,* including:
  – the rationale for fluid restriction, if necessary
  – increasing dietary intake of sodium.

For hypernatremia
- Monitor vital signs for changes, especially for rising pulse rate. Watch for signs of hypervolemia, especially in the client receiving I.V. fluids, *to guide the treatment regimen.*
- Record fluid intake and output accurately, checking for body fluid loss *to prevent dehydration and accompanying hypernatremia.* Weigh the client daily *to monitor fluid volume status.*
- Review key teaching topics with the client with hypernatremia and his family *to ensure adequate knowledge about the condition and treatment,* including the importance of sodium restriction and how to plan a low-sodium diet.

Evaluation
- The client's serum sodium level rises above 138 mEq/L for hyponatremia and falls below 143 mEq/L for hypernatremia.

Potassium imbalance

Potassium is the major cation of the intracellular fluid. Because of the high concentration of potassium inside the cells, potassium exerts some control over the intracellular osmolarity and volume. Maintaining the difference in the potassium concentration between the intracellular fluid and the extracellular fluid is critical for enabling excitable tissues to generate action potentials and to transmit impulses. Because extracellular fluid potassium levels are extremely low, any alteration in the concentration is poorly tolerated by the body and profoundly affects physiologic activities.

Potassium intake averages about 2 to 20 g/day for most people. Almost all foods contain some amount of potassium. Some foods are higher in potassium than others. The healthy body keeps plasma potassium levels within the narrow range of normal values required by physiologic function.

The sodium-potassium pump within every body cell membrane is the primary controller of extracellular potassium concentration. Some potassium regulation also takes place through renal function. The kidney excretes 80% of potassium from the body. There's no identified hormone that directly controls renal reabsorption of potassium, so the kidney doesn't conserve potassium directly.

Possible causes
Hypokalemia
- Alkalosis
- Corticosteroids
- Diarrhea
- Digoxin

- Diuretics
- Inappropriate or excessive use of drugs
- No oral intake for an extended period
- Prolonged NG suctioning
- Total parenteral nutrition
- Vomiting

Hyperkalemia
- Acidosis
- Dehydration
- Overeating of potassium-containing foods
- Potassium-sparing diuretics
- Rapid infusion of potassium-containing I.V. solutions
- Renal failure

Data collection findings
Hypokalemia
- Irregular heat beat
- Nausea and vomiting
- Leg cramps
- General skeletal muscle weakness
- Orthostatic hypotension
- Constipation
- Abdominal distension
- Anxiety, lethargy, confusion, coma
- Hypoactive or absent bowel sounds
- Decreased breath sounds
- Polyuria
- Low specific gravity

Hyperkalemia
- Irregular, slow heart beat
- Muscle twitches, cramps, paresthesia (early hyperkalemia)
- Low blood pressure
- Hyperactive bowel sounds
- Diarrhea
- Ascending flaccid paralysis that progresses distal to proximal with extremities
- Profound weakness (late hyperkalemia)

Diagnostic findings
Hypokalemia
- Serum potassium level is less than 3.5 mEq/L.
- ECG reveals changes.

Hyperkalemia
- Serum potassium level is greater than 5.5 mEq/L.
- ECG reveals changes.

Nursing diagnoses
Hypokalemia
- Imbalanced nutrition: Less than body requirements
- Risk for deficient fluid volume
- Impaired physical mobility

Hyperkalemia
- Imbalanced nutrition: More than body requirements
- Diarrhea
- Activity intolerance

Treatment
Hypokalemia
- Potassium supplements (oral or I.V.)
- Potassium-sparing diuretics
- Increased potassium in diet

Hyperkalemia
- Potassium-excreting diuretics (furosemide)
- Sodium polystyrene sulfonate (Kayexalate)
- Insulin
- Dialysis, if needed

Patient care goals
- The client's serum potassium level will return to normal.
- The client will be aware of appropriate foods to include in his daily diet.
- The client won't have cardiac complications such as ventricular tachycardia.
- The client will have normal muscle function when potassium levels return to normal.

Nursing interventions
Hypokalemia
- Monitor heart beat rhythm *to assess for cardiac involvement.*
- Administer potassium supplements as needed. Oral supplements must be diluted in at least 4 oz of fluid *to prevent stomach irritations.* I.V. supplements shouldn't be infused faster than 20 mEq/hour *because this can cause life-threatening arrhythmias.*
- Review key teaching topics with the client and family *to ensure adequate knowledge about the condition and treatment,* including:
  – the importance of having potassium levels drawn at regular intervals when the client is taking diuretics
  – diet and foods high in potassium
  – awareness of problems with weakness and leg cramps
  – importance of follow-up care.

High-potassium foods

Instruct the client to avoid these high-potassium foods:
- apricots
- bananas
- dark, green leafy vegetables
- dried fruits
- oranges
- peanuts
- strawberries
- tomatoes.

Hyperkalemia

- Monitor potassium levels frequently *to guide the treatment plan.*
- Monitor for regular heat rhythm *to assess for cardiac involvement.*
- Monitor diet to ensure that client is decreasing his intake of foods high in potassium *to prevent worsening hyperkalemia.* (See *High-potassium foods.*)
- Review key teaching topics with the client and family members *to ensure adequate knowledge about the condition and treatment,* including:
  – the need to avoid salt substitutes, which usually contain potassium
  – diet and foods to avoid that contain high levels of potassium
  – the importance of follow-up evaluation.

Evaluation

- The client's potassium level is within normal limits (between 3.5 and 5 mEq/L).
- The client knows what foods are high in potassium and what diet should be followed.
- The client has no cardiovascular complications.
- The client demonstrates normal neuromuscular function.

Calcium imbalance

Calcium plays an indispensable role in cell permeability, formation of bones and teeth, blood coagulation, transmission of nerve impulses, and normal muscle contraction. Nearly all (99%) of the body's calcium is found in the bones. The remaining 1% exists in an ionized form in serum; maintaining ionized calcium in the serum is critical to healthy neurologic function.

The parathyroid glands regulate ionized calcium and determine its resorption into bone, absorption from the GI mucosa, and excretion in urine and stool. Severe calcium imbalance requires emergency treatment because a deficiency (hypocalcemia) can lead to tetany and seizures; an excess (hypercalcemia), to cardiac arrhythmias and coma.

FAST FACT

When calcium levels are too high, the thyroid releases calcitonin. High levels of calcitonin inhibit bone resorption, which causes a decrease in the amount of calcium available from bone, thereby decreasing serum calcium levels. Calcitonin may also be administered as a drug to treat hypercalcemia.

Possible causes
Hypocalcemia
- Hypomagnesemia
- Hypoparathyroidism
- Inadequate intake of calcium and vitamin D
- Malabsorption or loss of calcium from the GI tract
- Overcorrection of acidosis
- Pancreatic insufficiency
- Renal failure
- Severe infections or burns

Hypercalcemia
- Hyperparathyroidism
- Hypervitaminosis D
- Multiple fractures and prolonged immobilization
- Multiple myeloma
- Other causes (milk-alkali syndrome, sarcoidosis, hyperthyroidism, adrenal insufficiency, and thiazide diuretics)
- Tumors

Data collection findings
Hypocalcemia
- Perioral paresthesia
- Twitching
- Carpopedal spasm
- Tetany
- Seizures
- Irregular heart beat

Hypercalcemia
- Muscle weakness
- Decreased muscle tone
- Anorexia
- Constipation
- Nausea
- Vomiting

- Polydipsia
- Dehydration
- Polyuria
- Irregular or life threatening heart rhythm and eventual coma with severe hypercalcemia (serum calcium levels that exceed 5.7 mEq/L).

Diagnostic findings
- A serum total calcium level less than 4.5 mEq/L confirms hypocalcemia; a level greater than 5.5 mEq/L, hypercalcemia. (Because approximately one-half of serum calcium is bound to albumin, changes in serum protein must be considered when interpreting serum calcium levels.)
- Sulkowitch urine test shows increased urine calcium precipitation in hypercalcemia.
- ECG reveals a lengthened QT interval, a prolonged ST segment, and arrhythmias in hypocalcemia; in hypercalcemia, a shortened QT interval and heart block.

Nursing diagnoses
Hypocalcemia
- Imbalanced nutrition: Less than body requirements
- Acute pain

Hypercalcemia
- Impaired physical mobility
- Impaired urinary elimination

Treatment
Hypocalcemia
- Diet: adequate intake of calcium, vitamin D, and protein

Drug therapy options
- Ergocalciferol (vitamin D_2), cholecalciferol (vitamin D_3), calcitriol, dihydrotachysterol (synthetic form of vitamin D_2) for severe deficiency
- Immediate correction with I.V. calcium gluconate or calcium chloride for acute hypocalcemia (an emergency)
- Vitamin D in multivitamin preparation for mild hypocalcemia
- Vitamin D supplements to facilitate GI absorption of calcium to treat chronic hypocalcemia

Hypercalcemia
- Hydration with normal saline solution to eliminate excess serum calcium through urine excretion
- Diet: Low calcium with increased oral fluid intake

Drug therapy options
- Calcitonin (Calcimar) (for hypocalcemia)
- Corticosteroid: prednisone (Deltasone) and hydrocortisone (Solu-Cortef), for treating sarcoidosis, hypervitaminosis D, and certain tumors
- Loop diuretic: ethacrynic acid (Edecrin) and furosemide (Lasix) to promote calcium excretion (thiazide diuretics are contraindicated in hypercalcemia because they inhibit calcium excretion)
- Plicamycin (Mithracin) to lower serum calcium level (especially against hypercalcemia secondary to certain tumors)
- Sodium phosphate solution administered by mouth or by retention enema (promotes calcium deposits in bone and inhibits absorption from the GI tract)

Patient care goals
For hypocalcemia
- The client will identify food sources rich in calcium and vitamin D.
- The client will consume a diet high in calcium and vitamin D.
- The client will attain a total serum calcium level within the reference range.
- The client will state and carry out appropriate interventions for pain relief.
- The client will experience relief from muscle cramps.

For hypercalcemia
- The client will have a total serum calcium level within the reference range.
- The client will maintain a normal balance between intake and output.
- The client will show no evidence of complications related to impaired physical mobility, such as contractures, venous stasis, thrombus formation, or skin breakdown.
- The client will adhere to his treatment regimen, which will prevent or minimize further elevations in serum calcium level.

Nursing interventions
For the client with hypocalcemia
- Watch for hypocalcemia in clients receiving massive transfusions of citrated blood and in those with chronic diarrhea, severe infections, and insufficient dietary intake of calcium and protein (especially elderly clients). *Identifying clients at risk can ensure early treatment intervention.*

Calcium sources

Instruct the client to eat these calcium-rich foods:
- broccoli
- turnip greens
- spinach
- dairy products such as low-fat yogurt
- tofu
- dried beans and apricots
- salmon
- sardines.

- When monitoring calcium solutions, watch for anorexia, nausea, and vomiting, *which are possible signs of overcorrection to hypercalcemia.*
- Monitor the client closely for a possible drug interaction if he's receiving cardiac glycosides with large doses of oral calcium supplements. *Administration of digoxin concomitantly with calcium supplements may cause synergistic effects of digoxin that precipitate arrhythmias.* Watch for signs of digoxin toxicity (anorexia, nausea, vomiting, yellow vision, and cardiac arrhythmias). Administer oral calcium supplements 1 to $1\frac{1}{4}$ hours after meals or with milk *to promote absorption.*
- Provide a quiet, stress-free environment for the client with tetany *to prevent seizure activity.* Observe seizure precautions for clients with severe hypocalcemia (may lead to seizures) *to prevent client injury.*
- Review key teaching topics with the client and family *to ensure adequate knowledge about the condition and treatment,* including:
– the importance of calcium for normal bone formation and blood coagulation
– eating foods rich in calcium, vitamin D, and protein, such as fortified milk and cheese (see *Calcium sources*)
– avoiding chronic laxative use and overuse of antacids.

For the client with hypercalcemia

- Watch for signs of heart failure in clients receiving normal saline solution diuresis therapy. *Infusion of large volumes of normal saline solution may cause fluid volume excess, leading to heart failure.*
- Administer loop diuretics (not thiazide diuretics) *to promote diuresis and rid the body of excess calcium.* Monitor intake and output, and check the urine for renal calculi and acidity. Provide acid-ash drinks, such as cranberry or prune juice, because calcium salts are more soluble in acid than in alkali.

- Check the client's vital signs frequently to assess for changes in the client's condition. In the client receiving cardiac glycosides, watch for signs of toxicity, such as anorexia, nausea, vomiting, and bradycardia (commonly with arrhythmia). Fatal arrhythmias may result when digoxin is administered in hypercalcemia.
- Help the client walk as soon as possible *to promote mobility.* Handle the client with chronic hypercalcemia gently *to prevent pathologic fractures.*
- If the client is bedridden, reposition him frequently *to monitor for changes in the client's condition* and encourage range-of-motion exercises *to promote circulation and prevent urinary stasis and calcium loss from bone.*
- Review key teaching topics with the client and family members *to ensure adequate knowledge about the condition and treatment,* including:
– the importance of calcium for normal bone formation and blood coagulation
– eating a low-calcium diet and increasing fluid intake to prevent recurrence of hypercalcemia.

Evaluation

- The client's calcium level is within reference limits (4.5 to 5.5 mEq/L).
- The client can identify foods rich in calcium and vitamin D and verbalizes the appropriate foods to include in his daily diet.
- The client demonstrates an absence of muscle discomfort with the return of calcium to a normal level.
- The client demonstrates no complications as a result of impaired physical mobility.

FLUID IMBALANCES

Sodium balance vitally affects fluid balance. Equivalent amounts of sodium and water that are lost or gained won't change serum osmolarity (tonicity), but the client may show signs of fluid volume deficit or overload.

Fluid volume deficit

Fluid volume deficit (dehydration) results from excessive loss of water and electrolytes from extracellular fluid.

Possible causes

- Excessive fluid loss through secretions or excretions
- Insufficient intake of water and electrolytes

Both of these causes can occur simultaneously. A third possible cause is third-space shifting.

Data collection findings
- Collapsed neck and hand veins
- Dizziness, syncope, and weakness
- Dry skin
- Decreased skin turgor
- Dry mucous membranes

FAST FACT

To assess skin turgor in an adult, pick up a small fold of skin over the sternum or the arm. (In an infant, roll a fold of loosely adherent skin on the abdomen between your thumb and forefinger.) Then release it. Normal skin will immediately return to its previous contour. In decreased skin turgor, the fold of skin will "hold" for up to 30 seconds.

- Hypotension
- Increased thirst
- Nausea and vomiting
- Oliguria
- Orthostatic blood pressure differences
- Tachycardia

Diagnostic findings
- BUN reveals creatinine greater than 10:1.
- Complete blood count reveals increased hematocrit levels.
- Serum sodium is increased (hypertonic), decreased (hypotonic), or normal (isotonic).
- Serum and urine osmolality are increased (hypertonic), decreased (hypotonic), or normal (isotonic).
- Urine specific gravity is elevated (may not occur for several hours).

Nursing diagnoses
- Deficient fluid volume

Treatment
- Depends on the cause; may vary from the treatment used for shock (see "Shock," page 61) to replacment of fluids by oral supplementation and I.V. therapy (see "Acid-base imbalances," page 70, and "Electrolyte imbalances," page 74.)

Drug therapy options
- Albumin
- Blood transfusion
- Dextrose 5% in normal saline solution
- Vasopressors

Patient care goals
- The client will achieve and maintain adequate hydration.

Nursing interventions
- Monitor intake and output *to assess fluid balance.* Normally, the body maintains a balance of about 2,300 ml of intake as fluids and food and 2,300 ml of output as sensible or insensible fluid loss.
- Weigh the client daily at the same time and on the same scale with the same amount of linens or clothes *to ensure accurate measurements.* Each 2 lb (0.9 kg) weight loss reflects a 1-L fluid loss.
- Measure urine specific gravity as needed *to evaluate the client's fluid status and response to therapy.*

SPOT CHECK

If a client is being treated for deficient fluid volume and the nurse notes that his urine specific gravity has decreased, is this client responding to treatment?
Answer: Yes. Deficient fluid volume causes the urine specific gravity to increase. A decrease indicates a positive response to treatment.

- Assess hemodynamic parameters, such as central venous pressure, pulmonary artery pressure, and cardiac output, *to monitor the client's fluid status and response to therapy.*
- Review key teaching topics with the client and family *to ensure adequate knowledge about the condition and treatment,* including:
  – diet instruction regarding sodium-containing foods
  – signs of fluid volume deficit.

Evaluation
- The client voids at least 30 ml/hour.

Fluid volume overload

Fluid volume overload (excess) reflects an increased accumulation of water and electrolytes in the extracellular fluid; it usually results from an increase in total sodium concentration, causing more water to be drawn into the extracellular fluid to reestablish the proper sodium-water ratio.

Possible causes
- Diminished homeostatic mechanisms, such as those occurring in heart failure, cirrhosis, or excessive corticosteroid therapy
- Fluid overload
- Sodium overload

Data collection findings
- Bounding pulses
- Crackles on auscultation
- Dependent edema (such as pedal, sacral, or scrotal edema)
- Dyspnea
- Hypertension
- Neck vein distension

Diagnostic findings
- BUN level is decreased.
- Hematocrit level is decreased.
- Serum sodium level is normal or decreased.
- Serum and urine osmolality are decreased in clients with normal renal function.

Nursing diagnoses
- Excess fluid volume

Treatment
Drug therapy options
- Diuretics act to increase the excretion of water and sodium and other electrolytes through the kidneys, such as:
– loop diuretic: bumetanide (Bumex), furosemide (Lasix)
– osmotic: mannitol (Osmitrol)
– potassium-sparing: spironolactone (Aldactone)
– thiazide: chlorothiazide (Diuril), hydrochlorothiazide (HydroDIURIL).

Patient care goals
- The client's circulating blood volume will be within reference limits.

Nursing interventions
- Administer diuretics, as ordered, *to decrease fluid volume.*
- Maintain fluid restrictions *to promote fluid balance.*

- Monitor intake and output hourly *to assess for changes in fluid status.*
- Measure urine specific gravity as needed *to evaluate the client's fluid status and response to therapy.*
- Weigh the client daily at the same time and on the same scale with the client wearing the same amount of clothing *to evaluate fluid balance.* Significant weight gain reflects fluid volume overload.
- Assess the client for engorged neck and hand veins, *which indicate fluid volume overload.*
- Monitor the client for signs of heart failure or pulmonary edema *to identify changes in physical condition.*
- Review key teaching topics with the client and family members *to ensure adequate knowledge about the condition and treatment,* including:
– diet instruction regarding sodium-containing foods
– signs of fluid volume excess, including weight gain, shortness of breath, and swelling of the feet or ankles.

Evaluation
- The client maintains a stable body weight.
- The client displays no overt signs of edema or dehydration.

IMMOBILITY

IMMOBILITY is a temporary or permanent decrease in the client's ability to move all or part of the body easily or comfortably. Types of immobility include:
- loss of motor function
- loss of sensory function
- combined loss of motor and sensory function.
    The client can also lose proprioception (awareness of one's position, weight, posture, or equilibrium).

Loss of motor function
Loss of motor function can produce weakness or paralysis of the muscles, as in quadriplegia (paralysis of all extremities), paraplegia (paralysis of the legs), and hemiplegia (paralysis of one side of the body).

Loss of sensory function
Loss of sensory function can result in blindness, hemianopsia (blindness in half of the field of vision in one or both eyes), agnosia (inability to comprehend or recognize

an object), deafness, anesthesia (inability to feel pain or touch), and aphasia (inability to speak intended words or to understand words).

Possible causes

● Anoxia (loss of oxygen to cells, resulting in cell death; may accompany hemorrhage or blood loss, excessive swelling, or acid-base imbalances)
● Certain medications (such as anesthetics) and poisons
● Degenerative conditions (such as myasthenia gravis and amyotrophic lateral sclerosis) that gradually cause tissues to lose function
● Infectious agents (microorganisms exerting toxic effects on cells, either from the organisms themselves or from the toxins they produce)
● Severe anxiety
● Trauma (cutting or transection of nerve pathways or muscle fibers to or from affected tissues)
● Treatment for a medical condition (such as surgery or cast application)

Data collection findings

● Possible involvement of all major body systems
● Respiratory and cardiovascular changes that affect the rate, depth, and strength of respiratory effort, predisposing the client to anoxia, atelectasis, and pneumonia
● Integumentary effects resulting from pressure and stasis: atrophy, tissue breakdown, and pressure ulcers
● Decreased energy expenditure, predisposing the client to anorexia, altered intake, and altered nutrient use and metabolism, which result in diarrhea, hemorrhoids, and malnutrition
● Decreased fluid intake and urinary stasis, predisposing the client to urinary tract infections and formation of renal calculi
● Loss of innervation and sensation, predisposing the client to muscle spasticity or flaccidity, with neurologic consequences, such as altered pain perception, autonomic dysreflexia, confusion, and disorientation
● Endocrine metabolic effects of immobility: predisposition to weight loss; acid-base, fluid, and electrolyte imbalances; stress ulcers; anemia; osteoporosis; pathologic fractures; prolonged healing; amenorrhea; impotence; and loss of libido
● Psychological effects: anxiety, fear, depression, death (may result from inability to obtain employment or develop and maintain social relationships [especially in chronic immobility])

SPOT CHECK

Name three adverse effects of immobility.
Answer: A few examples of adverse effects of immobility include atelectasis, pneumonia, muscle atrophy, tissue breakdown, pressure ulcers, urinary tract infections, and muscle spasticity. For a more complete list, see "Data collection findings".

Diagnostic findings

● The suspected source of the sensory loss guides the evaluation. If a neurological cause is suspected, electromyography shows nerve disease.

Nursing diagnoses

● Impaired physical mobility

Treatment

● Treatment focuses on preventive measures and the treatment of specific complications that arise.

Patient care goals

● The client will maintain function in unaffected tissues.
● The client will regain maximal function in affected tissues.
● The client will fulfill usual or new roles within the family and society.

Nursing interventions

● Instruct the client to perform regular deep-breathing and coughing exercises and use incentive spirometry *to prevent pulmonary complications.*
● Initiate ROM exercises to affected areas *to help maintain muscle tone.*
● Frequently change the client's position and position the client *to maintain joint and body functions.* Turn the client from side to side by logrolling if the spinal cord has been damaged. Perform proper hygiene, including baths and use of lotions, and use padding, mattresses, protective barriers, and rails *to prevent skin breakdown or tissue trauma.*
● Provide appropriate nutritional and fluid intake *to ensure adequate nutrition.*
● Encourage increased intake of fluids (unless contraindicated), especially fruit juices, and of foods that increase dietary bulk (unless contraindicated) *to prevent constipation.*
● Administer a fecal softener or laxative, if ordered, *to maintain adequate elimination.* If ordered, administer an

enema if the client doesn't have a bowel movement within 3 days.

● Monitor the client's weight *to ensure adequate nutrition.*

● If appropriate, reduce diet calcium levels, as ordered, *to prevent renal calculi.*

● Regularly observe the client for adverse effects of immobility *so the need for prompt early interventions is identified.*

● Provide emotional support to the client and family members *to decrease anxiety.* The client needs emotional support and reassurance from both the family and health professionals. Psychiatric consultation may help during prolonged anxiety and depression.

● Include family members in the client's care, as feasible, and teach them client care before discharge *to facilitate home support of the client.*

Evaluation

● The client demonstrates no adverse effects from immobility.

● Interventions have been taken to treat any adverse effects.

● The client verbalizes ways to avoid effects of immobility after discharge.

5 Perioperative nursing

Introduction

Perioperative nursing — nursing care provided for a surgical client — encompasses three phases:
- preoperative period (before surgery)
- intraoperative period (during surgery)
- postoperative period (after surgery).

Because clients experience varying degrees of anxiety and deficient knowledge related to surgery, careful planning by the nurse can help ensure a positive outcome.

Standards of perioperative nursing practice based on the nursing process have been developed to provide guidance to those who work in this important nursing specialty. This section, therefore, uses the nursing process to review the three phases of perioperative nursing.

PREOPERATIVE PERIOD

The preoperative period begins when the client decides to have surgery and ends when the client is transferred to the operating room. This period is used to physically and psychologically prepare the client for surgery. The nurse plays a major role in client teaching and in relieving the client's and the family's anxieties.

Data collection findings
- Assess the client for signs of anxiety, including:
– anger
– elevated pulse and respiratory rates
– increased verbalization
– quiet or withdrawn behavior
– restlessness
– sleeplessness
– sweating.

All of these are signs of increased anxiety. Virtually every client about to undergo surgery experiences anxiety in some form, from mild to severe.
- Assess the client's knowledge about the upcoming surgery and solicit questions about the procedure. Questions are normal: knowledge will help speed the client's recovery. Depending on the surgical procedure, the client may experience various stages of loss, including depression and anger.

Diagnostic findings
- A complete blood cell count is obtained to check for anemia, polycythemia, or infection.
- A urinalysis is obtained to ensure that the client doesn't have a urinary tract infection, renal disorder, or diabetes mellitus.
- Blood chemistry is examined to ensure that the client doesn't have liver disease, diabetes mellitus, or renal problems.
- Chest radiography may be performed to evaluate for pulmonary disease.
- Electrocardiography may be performed especially if the client has a history of heart disease or hypertension.

Nursing diagnoses
- Anxiety
- Deficient knowledge (client)

Patient care goals
- The client will express concerns freely.
- The client will be calm and relaxed.
- The client will verbalize an understanding of the perioperative routine.
- The client will demonstrate activities and exercises to promote postoperative recovery.

NURSING PROCEDURE

Using an incentive spirometer

Purpose
The purpose of incentive spirometry is for the patient to achieve maximum ventilation. Maximum ventilation is necessary to help prevent and reverse alveolar collapse, which can cause atelectasis and pneumonitis.

Implementation
- Assess the client's condition.
- Explain the procedure and the importance of regularly performing incentive spirometry to maintain alveolar inflation.
- Position the client in a comfortable sitting or semi-Fowler position to promote optimal lung expansion
- Instruct the client to insert the sterile mouthpiece and to close his lips tightly around it to create a seal.
- Tell the client to exhale normally and then inhale as slowly and deeply as possible; instruct him to retain the entire volume of air inhaled for 3 seconds or, if he's using a device with a light indicator, until the light turns off.
- Tell the client to remove the mouthpiece and exhale normally. Repeat this sequence 5 to 10 times during every waking hour.
- Document the client's response and tidal volumes.

Nursing interventions
- Increase the time spent privately with the client, and encourage the client to express feelings openly. *A nurse's presence indicates a concern for the client's well-being, which reduces the client's anxiety.*
- Encourage the client to participate in decision making *to increase the his sense of control and help maintain his self-esteem.*
- Touch the client, if appropriate, while communicating *to express caring and to have a calming effect.*
- Provide the client with necessary information about surgery *to promote trust and also to ensure that the client's rights are being upheld.*
- Provide teaching, as indicated, related to postoperative exercises, such as breathing and leg exercises, use of incentive spirometry, and splinting of the anticipated surgical area *to decrease the client's anxiety, which helps create well-being and comfort.* Usually, a client who knows what to expect and how to comply has fewer complications. (See *Using an incentive spirometer.*)

- Teach the client about preoperative hygiene, such as a shower or bath and skin preparation.
- Inform the client about special preparations for the procedure, such as an enema, suppository, or other bowel preparation, if necessary.
- Administer sedatives or antianxiety agents as ordered the night before surgery *to decrease anxiety and allow the client to sleep restfully.* Observe the client for adverse reactions.
- Administer preoperative medications, such as narcotics (morphine, meperidine) and anticholinergics (atropine, glycopyrrolate), as ordered. *Narcotics sometimes are given to decrease anxiety and tension and to aid anesthetic induction. Anticholinergic agents decrease secretions, vomiting, laryngospasm, and bronchospasm.*

QUICK STUDY

The word **TEACH** is a good way to remember information to include in preoperative teaching.

    Turn, cough, and deep-breathe
    Exercises to perform after surgery
    Administration of medication for pain and nausea
    Concerns of the client should be addressed
    Healing of the wound

Evaluation
- The client approaches surgery with only mild anxiety and freely expresses concerns.

INTRAOPERATIVE PERIOD

The intraoperative period begins when the client enters the surgical suite and ends with the completion of the surgical procedure.

In the operating room, the client usually is sedated and under the care of anesthesia personnel. Depending on the surgical procedure, regional or general anesthetic is administered. Expect to assist anesthesia personnel or to monitor the client when conscious sedation, local, and certain regional anesthesia techniques are used. (See *Types of anesthesia.*)

Types of anesthesia

Regional anesthesia

Effects on the client
- Loss of motor and sensory perception to a particular area of the body
- Intact consciousness

Common types
- *Spinal*—injection of a local anesthetic into the subarachnoid space between the second and third or the third and fourth lumbar vertebrae.
- *Epidural*—injection of a local anesthetic into the epidural space

Uses
- Surgical procedures involving the legs, lower abdomen, or perineum

Potential complications
- Sympathetic preganglionic block of fibers in the anterior root of the spinal cord, causing vasodilation and reduced venous blood return to the heart
- Spinal headache
- Respiratory depression (if thoracic, intercostal, or accessory muscles are inadvertently anesthetized)
- Overanesthetization of the spinal cord (resulting in the client's inability to breathe; oxygen and ventilatory support are required)
- Other complications: low blood pressure, depressed myocardium, anaphylactic reaction, seizures, ringing in the ears, facial numbness or twitching, nausea and vomiting

Nursing implementations
- Assess the client for hypotension; have a vasopressor, such as ephedrine sulfate (Pretz-D) or phenylephrine (Neo-Synephrine), available.
- Record the client's respiratory rate and depth.
- Protect anesthetized area until full sensation has returned.
- Assess for return of sensation and motor function below the level of anesthesia; ask the client to move the anesthetized part and to report any perception of touch.

- Keep the client flat in bed for about 8 hours after regional anesthesia to prevent spinal fluid leakage into the epidural space, which is thought to cause spinal headache.
- Tell the client not to strain when moving in bed or having a bowel movement; straining increases intracranial pressure, which can exacerbate loss of cerebrospinal fluid.
- If spinal headache occurs, administer an analgesic, keep the client flat, and report the headache to the physician.
- Provide adequate hydration to help replace spinal fluid and prevent venous stasis. Note that oral intake is often avoided during the early postoperative period.
- Have resuscitation equipment available at all times.
- Know the toxic dose of each local anesthetic used during a procedure.

General anesthesia

Effects on the client
- Produces unconsciousness
- Blocks motor and sensory pathways to major nerve and muscle groups

Administration methods
- Inhalation gas
- I.V. injection

Nursing implementations
- Close operating room doors. Check for proper positioning of the safety belt. Have suction equipment available and working. Minimize room noise.
- Stay with the client.
- Avoid stimulating the client. Be available to provide protection or restraint.
- Be available to assist anesthesia personnel with intubation. Confirm with them the appropriate times for positioning and scrubbing the client. To prevent impaired circulation, make sure that the client's feet aren't crossed.
- Be ready to assist in treating cardiac or respiratory arrest. Have emergency drugs and defibrillation equipment available. Document the drug administration.

Nursing responsibilities
- Positioning the patient to avoid injury
- Monitoring physiologic responses to surgery
- Keeping the client comfortable
- Meeting the client's physical needs
- Meeting the client's needs for safety and dignity

POSTOPERATIVE PERIOD

The postoperative period begins with the completion of the surgical procedure and continues after discharge from the hospital or ambulatory surgical facility. Usually clients are transferred from the surgical suite to the postanesthesia care unit (PACU) until their condition stabilizes and consciousness returns. Clients in the PACU require intensive care, and nursing actions must maintain basic priorities that are applicable to all clients.

FAST FACT

Potential complications for postoperative clients include:
- altered respiratory function
- decreased mental status
- altered mental status
- discomfort and pain
- altered GI function
- decreased urine output
- impaired skin integrity
- impaired peripheral circulation.

This section covers routine postoperative nursing care for all surgical clients. It includes potential postoperative problems and complications, with appropriate nursing diagnoses and interventions listed for each potential problem.

Routine postoperative care
Nursing interventions
- Check the client's airway regularly, and position the client *to prevent aspiration*. The side-lying position (unless contraindicated) best prevents aspiration.

- Check the client's circulation; measure vital signs every 15 minutes until the client is stable *to identify labile vital signs after surgery.*
- Check the client's neurologic status *to identify return of neurologic function*. Note orientation to person, place, and time; check reflexes, sensations, and motor functions. *The client can't be discharged from the PACU until neurologic functions have returned to normal.*
- Check the client's dressing and bedclothes, including underneath the client, *for evidence of hemorrhage.* Gravity may carry drainage under the client. *Careful inspection of dressings and bedclothes can detect hemorrhage and ensure prompt treatment.*
- Connect all tubes and catheters *to ensure drainage and proper tube functioning.*
- Promote client comfort and relieve pain as needed *to decrease pain and discomfort.* Don't overlook pain unrelated to the surgical procedure. In addition to surgery, the client's discomfort may be caused by body position, a full bladder, flatus, hypoxemia, and tight dressings, casts, or bandages.
- Ensure the client's safety by keeping the side rails up at all times until the client is fully recovered from anesthesia *to prevent the risk of falling out of bed.*

POTENTIAL PROBLEMS FOR POSTOPERATIVE CLIENTS

During the postoperative period, the client must be monitored carefully for complications, some of which can be life-threatening. The following entries focus on nursing care of a postoperative client following major surgery. Nursing activities are separated to differentiate the various complications that may occur.

Altered respiratory function
Ensuring an open airway and efficient respiratory function are imperative. An endotracheal tube or an oral airway may be in place until consciousness returns.

Causes
- Airway obstruction
- Anesthesia
- Atelectasis
- Chronic obstructive pulmonary disease
- Pain

Data collection findings

- Dyspnea, which indicates impaired ventilation
- Tachycardia, which may indicate hypoxia
- Decreased breath sounds, which may indicate atelectasis because of alveolar collapse.
- Crackles, rhonchi, and stertorous respirations, which indicate airway secretions and possibly an airway obstruction
- Pallor, which indicates poor oxygenation and a reduced hemoglobin level
- Anxiety and restlessness, which are early signs of hypoxia caused by cerebral irritability
- Temperature greater than 100.4° F (38° C), which can may indicate atelectasis

 FAST FACT

Atelectasis is the most common cause of increased body temperature during the first 24 hours after surgery.

Diagnostic findings

- Arterial blood gas (ABG) analysis checks for hypoxemia, hypercapnia, and metabolic or respiratory acidosis or alkalosis.
- A pulse oximetry sensor placed on a finger, toe, or earlobe determines hemoglobin saturation.

Nursing diagnoses

- Impaired gas exchange
- Ineffective airway clearance

Patient care goals

- The client will be free from postoperative respiratory complications.

Nursing interventions

- Review preoperative teaching of deep-breathing exercises, incentive spirometry, and how and when to change positions *to promote the client's participation in recovery to avoid postoperative complications.*
- Tell the client to turn and perform deep-breathing exercises and to use the incentive spirometer every 1 to 2 hours. Be sure to splint the incision during these exercises by holding a pillow over the dressing and applying slight pressure to the incision site. *Turning, using the incentive spirometer, and breathing deeply prevent atelectasis and ventilate the distal alveoli. External splinting decreases pain and allows for increased chest expansion.*
- Ensure that the client gets out of bed and ambulates, as tolerated, *to facilitate full chest expansion.*

- Administer analgesics as ordered, splint the incision site, and reposition the client *to relieve the client's pain.* The client will be unable to perform deep-breathing exercises, cough, or ambulate if the pain is too severe.

Evaluation

- The client is free from pulmonary complications.
- The client's pulse oximetry readings, ABG levels, and pulmonary function remain within reference limits.

Decreased cardiac output

Maintaining adequate cardiac output is essential to prevent shock. Shock may be classified as cardiogenic, distributive, or hypovolemic. (For more information, see the discussion on shock in chapter 4, Maintaining homeostasis.)

Causes

- Fluid volume deficit
- Hemorrhage
- Vasodilation

Data collection findings

- Monitor the client for decreased blood pressure — less than 80 mm Hg indicates shock and inadequate tissue perfusion.
- Monitor the client's urine output and note any decrease, which indicates hypovolemia or poor renal perfusion.
- Observe the client for a weak, thready, rapid pulse. As stroke volume decreases, heart rate increases to maintain the same cardiac output.
- Monitor the client for decreased heart sounds, which indicate hypovolemia.
- Observe the client's skin for pallor, which indicates decreased peripheral circulation.
- Observe the client for restlessness, which is an early sign of hypoxia from cerebral irritability.
- Monitor the client for profuse perspiration and increased drainage from dressings, which may indicate fluid loss.
- Monitor for signs of hemorrhage, such as:
- bleeding
- decreased blood pressure
- increased pulse rate
- pallor. The greatest risk of hemorrhage is during the first 48 hours after surgery.

Nursing diagnoses

- Decreased cardiac output
- Deficient fluid volume

● Ineffective tissue perfusion (cardiopulmonary, cerebral, renal, GI, peripheral)

Patient care goals
● The client's blood pressure will stabilize 1 to 2 hours after surgery.
● The client's pulse rate will remain at 60 to 100 beats/minute.
● The client's urine output will be 30 to 50 ml/hour.

Nursing interventions
● Check vital signs every 15 minutes until the client is stable, then every half hour for 2 hours, and then every 4 hours for 24 hours to identify changes in the client's condition. *Shock may occur as a result of anesthesia, blood loss, or medication. As vital signs become more stable, changes occur less frequently.*

QUICK STUDY

When caring for a postoperative client, remember your **ABC**s:
    Airway
    Breathing
    Circulation

● Encourage the client to ambulate as soon as prescribed *to stimulate cardiovascular function.*
● Check the client's dressing and bedclothes, including underneath the client, for evidence of hemorrhage. *Hemorrhage or fluid loss may lead to shock. Gravity may carry drainage under the client.*

Evaluation
● Vital signs are stable and urine output is adequate.

Altered mental status
Regardless of the type of surgical procedure, the client's mental status will be affected. Protecting the client from injury is important while the mental status is altered.

Causes
● Anesthesia
● Hypoxia
● Sedatives

Data collection findings
● Level of consciousness — a client who can't be aroused hasn't fully recovered from the anesthesia or may have nervous system damage

● Decreased reflexes (gag, cough, swallow, and deep tendon) — can indicate the client's state of alertness
● Decreased pupillary response — normally, pupils are the same size and constrict equally to light
● Neuromuscular irritability — after surgery and anesthesia, the client will have an increased response to stimuli
● Decreased neuromuscular response to stimuli — indicates that the client may not have recovered fully from anesthesia and requires safety precautions to be taken

Nursing diagnoses
● Ineffective tissue perfusion (cerebral)
● Disturbed sensory perception (kinesthetic)

Patient care goals
● The client will be mentally alert and oriented after surgery.
● The client will regain all reflex activity.

Nursing interventions
● Assess the client's orientation and neuromuscular reflex response *to help determine whether the client has fully recovered from anesthesia.*
● Withhold narcotics or administer them in small doses, as ordered, *to prevent further depression of the central nervous system (CNS). Until fully recovered from anesthesia, the client doesn't usually require a full narcotic dose. Narcotics can depress respirations, decrease blood pressure, and alter mentation.*

Evaluation
● The client is oriented to time, place, and person.
● The client's reflexes return.

Discomfort and pain
The postoperative client almost always reports some discomfort or pain. Surgical pain usually peaks on the 2nd postoperative day when the client has fully recovered from anesthesia.

Causes
● Client position
● Distended bladder
● Edema
● Flatus
● Surgical incision
● Tissue trauma

Data collection findings

● Discomfort and its source, such as a catheter, dressing, or cast (postoperative discomfort may have many causes that the nurse should rule out before assuming that the incision is the primary source of pain)
● Pain rating on a scale of 1 to 10, which allows comparison of the client's level of pain from one time to another

Nursing diagnoses

● Acute pain

Patient care goals

● The client's postoperative pain will be minimal.

Nursing interventions

● Reposition the client as necessary, at least every 2 hours, *to help relieve pain. The client's position may be a source of discomfort. Repositioning the client and explaining its purpose usually helps.*
● If appropriate, relieve tension on the urinary catheter, loosen bedclothes, and reposition the nasogastric (NG) tube. *Relieving these sources of discomfort helps achieve the nurse's primary goal: to minimize the client's postoperative pain.*
● Provide comfort measures and other nonpharmacologic interventions, such as gentle back massage, encouraging participation in diversional activities, teaching relaxation techniques, and reducing external stimuli, *to reduce anxiety and to allow the client to relax and rest.*
● Administer narcotics or other analgesics, as appropriate. Make sure the client understands how to use patient-controlled analgesia (PCA), if ordered. *Narcotics act on the CNS to reduce pain perception.* Many clients who use PCA fear giving themselves too much medication and need reinforcement about the correct use of PCA.

Evaluation

● The client's pain is relieved.

Altered GI function

The usual intake of food and fluids is disrupted for almost all surgical procedures. For some clients, maintaining fluid and electrolyte balance can be a challenge.

Causes

● Anesthesia
● Bacterial overgrowth
● Bowel manipulation
● Infection
● Obstruction

● Paralytic ileus
● Surgery
● Total cessation of bowel function

Data collection findings

● Anorexia — decreased peristalsis from stress increases the potential for poor nutrition
● Nausea and vomiting caused by decreased peristalsis and oral fluids given too soon after surgery
● Abdominal distention and gas pain (common postoperative problems as peristalsis returns)
● Absence of bowel sounds, which indicates a lack of peristalsis and may signal paralytic ileus
● Diarrhea and incontinence, which result from increased peristalsis or bacterial overgrowth
● Dehydration, which is indicated by dry mucous membranes and "tenting" of skin

Diagnostic findings

● Blood is drawn to check potassium, sodium, chloride, and magnesium electrolyte levels.

Nursing diagnoses

● Diarrhea
● Bowel incontinence
● Deficient fluid volume
● Imbalanced nutrition: Less than body requirements

Patient care goals

● The client's GI function will resume a normal pattern.
● The client's fluid and electrolyte balance will be restored.

Nursing interventions

● Withhold food and fluids until bowel sounds return (possibly 2 to 3 days after abdominal surgery) *to prevent complications of decreased peristalsis caused by anesthesia, narcotics, and the stress response, particularly after abdominal surgery.*
● Monitor I.V. access and fluids as ordered *to allow for fluids and electrolytes to be administered until the client's oral intake is adequate.*
● Gradually change the client's diet from clear to regular *to provide nutrition consistent with the return of normal bowel functions.*
● Ensure that the client drinks 2 to 3 L of fluid daily *to provide adequate hydration for bowel movement.*
● Ensure that the client ambulates as tolerated *to help prevent constipation and other problems caused by immobility.*

● Note signs and symptoms of paralytic ileus: absence of bowel sounds, abdominal distention and discomfort, and nausea and vomiting. *Clients with altered GI function are at risk for paralytic ileus.* Measures designed to provide rest for the GI tract include food and fluid restrictions, NG tube drainage, and I.V. therapy.

Evaluation
● The client's bowel sounds return.
● The client passes stool.
● The client's electrolyte levels are within reference limits.

Decreased urine output
The nothing-by-mouth status required for surgery as well as fluid loss due to surgery can impact urinary output. Accurately recording all intake and output while the client is at risk for fluid imbalances is critical.

Causes
● Anesthesia
● Hypovolemia
● Increased antidiuretic hormone (ADH) levels
● Poor position for voiding
● Urine retention
● Stress

Data collection findings
● Urine output, which should resume within 6 to 10 hours after surgery or after an indwelling urinary catheter is discontinued, and greater than or equal to 30 ml/hour with voiding (if the client is well hydrated, allow voluntary control of urine output)
● Distention found on palpation of the bladder above the symphysis pubis (a bladder that isn't palpable isn't distended)

Nursing diagnoses
● Impaired urinary elimination

Patient care goals
● The client's voluntary control of urine output will resume within 6 to 10 hours after surgery.

Nursing interventions
● Provide eight to twelve 8-oz glasses (2,000 to 3,000 ml) of fluid daily *to provide adequate hydration, which prevents urinary stasis.* Initially, urine output may be less than 1,500 ml because of body fluid losses and increased ADH levels; however, it should stabilize within 48 hours.

● Institute measures to induce voiding if urine retention occurs. Running water stimulates voiding, as does pouring warm water over the perineum, which relaxes the sphincter.
● Insert an indwelling urinary or straight catheter, as ordered, *to perform catheterization if urine retention occurs.*

Evaluation
● The client's urine output is greater than 30 ml/hour.
● The client voids without difficulty.

Impaired skin integrity
The preoperative health status for the client will impact the healing of the surgical incision. Clients who smoke, are over age 65, are obese, or have impaired immune systems may have more problems with impaired skin integrity.

Causes
● Surgical incision

Data collection findings
● Wound healing — the clean surgical wound heals by primary intention and may take more than 1 year
● Infection, which is indicated by fever and incisional redness and swelling after the third postoperative day
● Signs of insufficient wound healing, including dehiscence (separation of surgical wound layers, producing pink serous drainage; the client feels a pull at the wound site) and evisceration (such as outright protruding of abdominal contents) — a client with poor nutrition, cancer, or wound infection is prone to ineffective wound healing; dehiscence and evisceration indicate a complete separation of the wound edges, a medical emergency

Nursing diagnoses
● Impaired skin integrity
● Risk for infection

Patient care goals
● The client's incision will heal without complications.

Nursing interventions
● Keep the incision clean and dry *to help prevent bacterial infection. Bacteria thrive in a moist environment.*
● Encourage ambulation. *Movement stimulates vascular perfusion, which promotes wound healing.*
● Instruct the client to splint the incision when coughing or moving to avoid putting stress on the incision, *which could impair healing or cause wound dehiscence or evisceration.*

● If dehiscence or evisceration occurs, notify the physician immediately and cover the wound with sterile normal saline solution. Stay with the client and tell him not to move or cough. Administer antibiotics if ordered. Evisceration is a medical emergency. *Covering the evisceration prevents drying and necrosis of abdominal contents. Antibiotics prevent infection.*

SPOT CHECK

Which statement by a client indicates that additional discharge teaching is needed after surgery?
A. "I'm really looking forward to going outside for short walks."
B. "I can hardly wait to get home and pick up my 18-month-old baby."
C. "I'll call my physician if I have a fever or notice drainage from my incision."
D. "I'll clean my incision every morning in the shower and pat it dry with a clean towel."
Answer: B. Lifting an 18-month-old child would place stress on the incision and should be avoided.

Evaluation
● The client's wound heals without infection.

Impaired peripheral circulation

Immobility during and after surgery is a predisposing factor to impaired peripheral circulation. A potentially dangerous situation can occur if a clot forms, dislodges, and travels to the lungs.

Causes
● Phlebitis
● Thrombosis

Data collection findings
● Homans' sign, which indicates phlebothrombosis (clotting without inflammation)
● Pain, warmth, and tenderness in the calf muscles, which indicates thrombophlebitis

FAST FACT

The steps for testing for Homans' sign are:
● support the client's thigh with one hand and his foot with the other
● bend the leg slightly at the knee
● firmly and abruptly dorsiflex the ankle.

Nursing diagnoses
● Ineffective tissue perfusion (peripheral)
● Risk for injury

Patient care goals
● The client will have adequate peripheral circulation.

Nursing interventions
● Take the following preventive antithrombus measures *to promote peripheral circulation:*
– Provide elastic stockings and an antiembolitic compression hose *to compress the superficial veins, increase blood flow through the deep veins, and prevent venous pooling.*
– Don't put pressure on the popliteal space, *which causes blood stasis.*
– Don't massage the client's legs, *which may dislodge a clot.*
– Ensure that the client exercises and ambulates soon after surgery, *which can prevent venous stasis.*
● Treat thrombophlebitis with bed rest, heat, elastic bandages or hose, and anticoagulant drugs. *Bed rest promotes healing and prevents clot dislodgment. Heat and elastic bandages increase circulation to the area. Anticoagulant drugs prevent blood clotting.*

Evaluation
● The client shows no signs of circulatory stasis.

DISCHARGE INSTRUCTIONS

Early discharge, which has become common, typically increases client teaching needs. Be sure to provide information about wound care, activity restrictions, dietary management, medication administration, symptoms to report, and follow-up care.

A client recovering from same-day surgery in an outpatient surgical unit must be in stable condition before discharge. This client must not drive home; make sure a responsible adult takes the client home.

7 Maternal-neonatal nursing 147

8 Pediatric nursing   199

9 Adult nursing   269

6   Mental health nursing

Introduction

When experiencing the stressors of life, a person tends to respond in a characteristic manner. The person's overall flexibility or rigidity in using this characteristic behavior determines whether the behavior is healthful, unhealthful, or somewhere in between.

A healthy person uses many diverse behaviors to manage daily stressors; a person with compromised mental health doesn't. Instead, the unhealthy person responds to stress by exhibiting a narrow range of behaviors in a manner symptomatic of psychopathology. Using the principles of the nursing process and therapeutic communication as outlined in chapter 3, Nursing concepts and skills, this chapter focuses on clients who demonstrate various types of psychopathology or behavioral problems. After reviewing this chapter, you'll be better prepared to apply mental health concepts and principles in any clinical setting.

Therapeutic communication

The nurse who provides care for a client with a mental illness uses therapeutic communication to convey acceptance, preserve the client's self-esteem, and gain a greater understanding of how the client perceives the situation. Therapeutic responses encourage the client to continue talking. Examples include:
- "Tell me about…"
- "What happened after…"
- "I'm not sure what you're saying."
- "And then…?"

In contrast, evaluative statements ("You must have felt sad" or "I'll bet you miss your children") close off communication and convey lack of understanding. (For a more detailed review of therapeutic communication, see chapter 3.)

Research and technology

As health care professionals strive to understand what causes mental illness, research and technology continue to play significant roles. Despite advances, a simple explanation for mental illness hasn't been revealed; causation appears to be multidimensional, with psychological, biological, social, and cultural factors affecting human behavior.

The nurse-client relationship

Any therapeutic relationship, including the nurse-client relationship, passes through three phases:
- beginning (orientation) phase — During the orientation phase, the nurse establishes certain parameters for the relationship, such as the time and duration of nurse-client visits, the responsibilities that each must bear, and the types of issues that they'll address.
- middle (working) phase — During the working phase, the client actively works on issues germane to managing daily affairs. Although this phase may be emotionally painful, the client must be willing to examine issues with the nurse.
- ending (termination) phase — During the termination phase, the client and the nurse summarize their work and the client plans for the future. If the client and the nurse have become emotionally attached, the termination phase may be painful for both of them. Ideally, termination begins during the first meeting with the nurse, when the parameters of the relationship are negotiated.

Working with groups

Nurses are expected to have group skills so that they can work therapeutically with clients in a group setting. Nurses can facilitate educational groups, skills in living groups, parenting groups, support groups, and socialization groups.

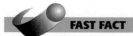

Working with clients in small groups has many benefits for both the nurse and client. Because the nurse works with several clients simultaneously, the technique is cost effective. Also, it allows the nurse to observe interaction patterns and permits situation repetition. Being in a group allows clients to:
- receive feedback from peers
- learn information about themselves
- practice new interactional and coping skills
- express their feelings
- see that others have had similar experiences.

It also helps them meet unfulfilled needs for belonging and acceptance and gives them a chance to network.

To work with groups, the nurse must understand group dynamics and therapeutic communication. The nurse also must establish group standards or rules — for example, who has access to what group members say (confidentiality), who's responsible for determining content and keeping the group focused (leadership and responsibility), and will smoking, eating, drinking, interrupting, or swearing be permitted (norms). What's said in a group is referred to as *group content.* The meeting of individual needs while meeting group goals is called *group process.*

Standard group protocol
When setting up a group, consider the following:
- designated group leaders
- purpose and goals of the group
- framework to guide the group
- content for discussion
- methods for keeping the group working
- determining appropriate participants
- measuring outcomes by specific evaluation methods
- documenting group work and participant progress.

Roles of group members
Group members may take on the following roles:
- opinion giver or seeker
- information giver or seeker
- initiator
- elaborator
- coordinator
- evaluator
- summarizer.

Goals of group therapy
According to some practitioners, the goals of group therapy are achieved in four phases:
1. Boundaries and dependence on the group leader are established.
2. Conflict emerges.
3. The group becomes cohesive and new behaviors begin.
4. Support for group members becomes evident as roles change, effective work is done, and goals are accomplished.

Some goals of group therapy include:
- reducing or modifying symptoms
- mitigating disturbed behavior patterns
- promoting positive behaviors.

Leading a group
The group leader, or facilitator, has multiple functions:
- to keep the group focused
- to monitor established group rules or norms
- to facilitate the group process (how members respond to each other and the topic being discussed), when appropriate
- to address problems that occur in the group
- to screen group members, when appropriate
- to evaluate outcomes.

Group facilitation
To facilitate a therapeutically oriented group, the nurse can use various strategies. For example, to start a new session, briefly review the last session, and then ask how things have gone since then. When appropriate, respond to themes. For instance, say, "At least three people have talked about staying balanced. Perhaps it would be useful to examine what staying balanced means to each of us."

Dealing with problems within a group
When a group is cohesive, members have the potential to experience maximal growth because they're committed to themselves as well as to fellow participants. This commitment allows members to risk dealing with sensitive issues within the group. Threats to group cohesion include:
- transient group members
- poorly selected group members
- cliques
- competition
- transference and countertransference
- unacknowledged conflict

Problem behaviors in a group

Common problems encountered within groups are listed here along with possible causes. It's important for the nurse to remember that these behaviors are intended to protect the person who's engaging in them.

PROBLEM BEHAVIOR	POSSIBLE CAUSE
Conflict	<ul><li>Attempt to focus attention elsewhere</li><li>Lack of knowledge as to how to resolve issues in a healthy manner</li><li>Highly charged issue</li><li>Transferences and countertransferences</li></ul>
Group gets sidetracked	<ul><li>Unclear focus</li><li>Group members with limited intellectual capacity or inability to consider a wide range of ideas</li><li>Lack of group structure</li><li>Avoidance of painful issues</li><li>Leader doesn't effectively assist group members in analyzing what's happening within the group</li></ul>
Member approaches group leader outside group to discuss group business	<ul><li>Inability to confront issues directly</li><li>Attempt to manipulate leader to gain power</li><li>Lack of understanding about how groups work</li><li>Lack of clarity about group rules</li><li>Testing behavior</li><li>Fear of reprisal within group</li><li>Attempt to seek attention to fill inner void</li></ul>
Member uses strong or offensive language	<ul><li>Attempt to control others</li><li>Testing behavior</li><li>Self-protection</li><li>Poor communication skills</li></ul>
Member exhibits minimal or no active participation	<ul><li>Anxiety</li><li>Past experience (previously squelched)</li><li>Uncertainty regarding group rules</li><li>Fear that expressed ideas may lead to more work</li></ul>
Dominating member	<ul><li>Anxiety with silence</li><li>Feeling of being overly responsible for outcome</li><li>Attempt to feel important</li><li>Avoidance of painful issues</li><li>Attempt to control outcome through bulldozing</li><li>Frequent compulsive speaking as attempt to decrease anxiety</li></ul>

- lack of privacy
- irregular meetings.

Many individuals find that participating in therapeutic groups designed to examine their own behavior threatening. To protect themselves, these individuals may respond by exhibiting signs of resistance or problem behaviors. (See *Problem behaviors in a group.*)

Common signs of resistance include:
- missing sessions
- rescuing others

CLINICAL SITUATION

Caring for the client who has been raped

Evaluate the clinical situation described here. See if you're able to answer the questions as you go.

A deeply religious 24-year-old woman is brought in to the emergency department by the police. During triage, she sits stiffly, clutching her coat tightly around her and keeping her head down. "I'm so ashamed," she says in a barely audible voice. "It's all my fault." She doesn't raise her head to answer questions. She repeatedly says, "I don't know what to do." The nurse finds out that the client lives alone, that her parents live in a nearby city, and that she has a married sister who lives within 5 miles of the hospital. She has few friends.

During the medical examination (performed using the hospital's rape protocol), the client tries to maintain her composure, but she can't help crying at times. The examination reveals small lacerations of the external genitalia and vagina as well as scratches on her face, throat, breasts, arms, and legs.

Following completion of the rape protocol examination, the client tells the nurse she's afraid to leave the hospital and return to her apartment because the rapist has her purse, which contains her identification and house keys. After much persuasion on the nurse's part, the client agrees to contact her sister.

While waiting for her sister to arrive, the client sits in her cubicle crying softly. She says that she can't understand how God could let this happen to her, that she was a virgin, and now she's "nothing more than a dirty rag that no one would ever want."

"I guess it doesn't make any difference what happens now," she says. "No one will ever want me."

What key elements should be established during assessment?

● The client's physical condition

When a client presents with a physical condition and a psychological one, the physical condition (lower-level need) must be assessed before psychological intervention can take place.

● The client's level of anxiety

This will help establish which nursing interventions are required. Nursing interventions will change as the client's anxiety level fluctuates.

● The presence of balancing factors:
– realistic perception of the event
– adequate social supports
– adequate coping skills

Absence of any of the balancing factors will prolong the crisis.
● The availability of a rape counselor and survivor group referrals for continued support while back in the community

Nurses in the emergency department don't provide support after the client leaves the hospital. Follow-up counseling will help the client put the rape into perspective and move on with her life.

What are appropriate interventions for the initial treatment of this client?

● Don't leave the client alone. *A calming presence can prevent the client from becoming more overwhelmed by the rape experience.*
● Ask the client where she's experiencing pain *to help the client focus on something specific and to communicate your caring and concern.*
● Assist the client with completing the hospital's rape protocol *to allow her to concentrate on the tasks at hand.* Because of her traumatic experience, the client's anxiety level will fluctuate. The client will need assistance with completing the hospital's rape protocol, which includes documenting her condition and obtaining laboratory specimens and potential legal evidence.
● Offer the client a cleansing shower, mouthwash, and other supplies after all evidence has been gathered; help her clean up if she can't care for herself *to help decrease her level of anxiety.* The client may feel the need to wash away the traumatic experience. Symbolically, this cleaning can help the client decrease her high level of anxiety. The nurse's assistance conveys caring and concern.
● When her anxiety level is at or below the moderate level, ask the client to tell you about the rape, allowing her to set the pace. Phrase your questions and comments with care and sensitivity. *This approach promotes the client's eventual cognitive mastery over the rape experience, decreasing her tendency to withdraw and to feel guilt and shame.* Thoughtlessly worded comments and questions ("Were you really raped?") convey doubt and project blame. In contrast, a carefully worded statement ("I'd like to hear about what happened") conveys the nurse's desire to understand the client's experience.
● Help the client to identify her most immediate concern, *which provides a concrete focus to her thoughts.* This allows the client to begin regaining control of her life.
● Ask the client to name someone who can stay with her for the next 24 to 48 hours, which may ease her anxiety, help her feel safe, and help her cope with periodic waves of anxiety and fear.

(continued)

Caring for the client who has been raped *(continued)*

● Provide the names and telephone numbers of appropriate community resources. If possible, introduce the client to a rape counselor *before* she leaves the emergency department. Explaining about community resources lets the client know that she won't be abandoned. Giving her the information in writing increases the probability that she'll contact someone for rape counseling. Establishing contact with the rape counselor before leaving the emergency department will decrease the client's sense of aloneness and better assure that she'll seek follow-up rape counseling. In the weeks after the rape, the counselor explores the event with her and works with her to strengthen her coping skills.

What interventions would be appropriate during the counseling sessions?
● Encourage the client to recall how she has dealt with past traumatic events, *which help demonstrate to the client that she'll be able to cope with this unwanted experience just as she has coped with others.*
● Help the client talk about the rape and vent her feelings, *which can decrease her sense of helplessness, powerlessness, and self-doubt.* Talking about the rape helps the client put the traumatic experience into perspective, permitting self-growth and healing. Unexpressed feelings may lead to depression and other symptoms in the future.
● Help the client examine any differences in her lifestyle that have resulted from the rape to help the client determine whether she's

giving this experience more power in her life than she would like, which helps her gain a realistic perception of the rape.
● Allow the client to express negative thoughts and feelings. Encouraging the person to sort out thoughts and feelings enables her to determine the reality of the situation.
● Talk with the client about her spiritual beliefs. If appropriate, consider seeking pastoral assistance for her as the client's spiritual condition shouldn't be ignored. For the deeply religious client, restoration of her faith in God may enhance healing.
● Discuss the client's thoughts and feelings about prosecuting her attacker. This discussion conveys that the client has the option to take direct action against her attacker. Under no circumstances, however, should the nurse coerce the client into filing charges.
● Encourage the client to participate in group therapy, individual therapy, or a support group. Group or individual therapy can assist the client to develop coping skills and promote optimal level of functioning. Support can enable the person to decrease anxiety and increase feelings of well-being.
● Encourage the client to engage in problem solving. Using problem-solving skills decreases anxiety levels and promotes the person's sense of control.

Questions for further thought
● What would be appropriate nursing diagnoses for this client?
● What evaluation findings would indicate that the client is able to function with minimal posttraumatic stress symptoms?

● projecting blame
● showing up late
● engaging in small talk
● changing the subject
● forming cliques
● verbally attacking other members or the leader
● becoming overinvolved or focused on social behaviors.

Crisis intervention
An event that disrupts a person's usual manner of coping with stress can precipitate a crisis. Such an event may be situational (such as divorce), maturational (occurring when a person enters a new developmental phase of his life or career), or adventitious (caused by uncontrolled events, such as flood, war, or assault). An event that triggers a crisis in one person may not in another.

According to some practitioners, three balancing factors offset a crisis:
● realistic perception of the event
● adequate emotional support
● adequate coping mechanisms.

Absence of any of these factors predisposes a person to crisis. This section reviews the key phases of a crisis and then provides an in-depth look at an adventitious crisis, namely rape-trauma syndrome.

 FAST FACT

The types of crises are:
● adventitious crisis
● maturational crisis
● situational crisis.

Phases of a crisis

A crisis develops in four phases:

● Phase 1 — The person responds with increased anxiety and tries to problem solve to decrease anxiety.

● Phase 2 — Problem solving is unsuccessful and anxiety increases; the person becomes very distressed and may use a trial-and-error approach to handle the situation.

● Phase 3 — The person's attempts to cope fail; the person must find behaviors that bring relief and may flee from the situation or refine the event to make it understandable to prevent maladaptive responses such as violence to self or to others.

● Phase 4 — The crisis resolves; work begins to return to one of three levels of functioning (precrisis level, higher level, or lower level). The person can learn adaptive coping and sets goals to recover from the event.

Crisis intervention aims to restore at least a precrisis level of functioning and to prevent untoward emotional sequelae. (See *Caring for the client who has been raped,* pages 105 and 106.)

ANXIETY AND MOOD DISORDERS

ANXIETY is unexplained discomfort, apprehension, or uneasiness. The energy generated by anxiety can be used constructively or destructively.

Anxiety can be precipitated in several ways:

● unmet expectations that are important to one's self-worth

● an actual or perceived threat to one's values, status, prestige, biological integrity, or body image

● psychological or physiologic stress

● an adverse reaction to chemical substances (for example, a bad trip after taking D-lysergic acid diethylamide).

Anxiety has emotional, cognitive, and physical manifestations, which the nurse must consider when planning care. (See *Responses to anxiety.*) Defense mechanisms are used to cope with anxiety. They operate on an unconscious level (except for suppression) and allow the client to deny or distort reality.

Regardless of the underlying psychopathology, the nurse must assess the client's anxiety level because this guides the choice of nursing interventions. For example, a client with a moderate anxiety level is able to solve problems with assistance and commonly benefits from relaxation techniques. In contrast, a client with severe or panic-level anxiety can't problem-solve and needs more guidance, support, and structure from the nurse. (See *Anxiety levels and nursing implications,* page 108.)

Here are client behavior characteristics at different anxiety levels:

● A client with mild anxiety can function well and needs no assistance from the nurse.

● A client with moderate anxiety will require some assistance because of selective inattention and an inability to provide the self-structure needed to remain focused.

Responses to anxiety

A client may have emotional, cognitive, and physical responses to anxiety. This chart lists examples of each type.

EMOTIONAL RESPONSES	COGNITIVE RESPONSES	PHYSICAL RESPONSES
● Worry	● Rumination	● Restlessness
● Irritability, hypersensitivity	● Forgetfulness	● Tremulousness
● Apprehension	● Poor concentration	● Increased pulse and respiratory rates
● Vague discomfort	● Blocking of thoughts	● Elevated blood pressure
● Expectation of danger	● Inattentiveness	● Muscle tightness
● Tendency to cry easily	● Distractibility	● Nausea
● Lack of self-confidence	● Preoccupations	● Dizziness
● Strong startle response		● Fatigue
		● Urinary urgency or frequency or both
		● Constipation or diarrhea

Anxiety levels and nursing implications

This chart presents manifestations of and nursing implications for the four primary levels of anxiety.

ANXIETY LEVEL	MANIFESTATIONS	NURSING IMPLICATIONS
Mild	<ul><li>Alertness</li><li>Maximal ability to solve problems</li><li>Enhanced learning</li></ul>	<ul><li>Client can be fully responsible for himself.</li></ul>
Moderate	<ul><li>Selective inattention</li><li>Impaired ability to solve problems</li><li>Complaints of feeling uptight, on edge, or nervous</li></ul>	<ul><li>Help the client talk through the situation and label his feelings.</li><li>Use relaxation techniques.</li></ul>
Severe	<ul><li>Narrowed attention span</li><li>Inability to grasp meanings</li><li>Inability to solve problems</li><li>Distorted view</li><li>Self-absorption</li><li>Inability to connect events or details</li><li>Clingy or demanding behavior</li><li>Physiologic signs, including increased blood pressure, dry mouth, restlessness, and muscular tightness</li></ul>	<ul><li>The client needs structure and direction.</li><li>Don't force the client to make decisions.</li><li>Provide one-on-one supervision.</li><li>Give as-needed medication for escalating anxiety, as ordered.</li><li>Provide a nonstimulating environment.</li><li>Use touch carefully. Don't physically touch the client without first obtaining permission or explaining what you're doing; a severely anxious client may misinterpret touch as an attack.</li><li>Maintain a calm, soothing tone of voice.</li><li>Act as a focal point, taking over the interaction and actively directing the client's attention to you. This usually has a calming effect on the client.</li><li>Dress conservatively to maintain a soothing environment; bright coloring can overstimulate severely anxious and manic clients.</li></ul>
Panic	<ul><li>Inability to solve problems</li><li>Client feeling detached from his body or feeling "unreal"</li><li>Physiologic signs, such as those previously mentioned in severe anxiety and breathing problems</li><li>Loss of contact with reality or withdrawal</li><li>Inability to communicate</li><li>Insomnia</li><li>Inability to recognize familiar objects, persons, or environment</li><li>Erratic behavior</li><li>Sense of terror</li></ul>	<ul><li>See the nursing implications for severe anxiety.</li></ul>

● A client with severe anxiety will require much assistance from the nurse because of an inability to solve problems and a preoccupation with internal experience.
● A client at the panic level of anxiety is at risk for harming himself or others because of distortions of reality.

The client with an anxiety disorder experiences overwhelming anxiety, which interferes with his quality of life. To relieve the anxiety, the client develops a variety of symptoms, which may or may not control the anxiety. Defenses used in anxiety disorders include:

Comparing anxiety disorders

The different types of anxiety disorders are described briefly in the chart here. A combination of drug therapy and behavioral or cognitive approaches is used to treat these disorders.

DISORDER	DESCRIPTION	TREATMENT
Generalized anxiety disorder	Excessive worry about many life circumstances; anxiety that persists during most waking hours	• Relaxation exercises • Cognitive reframing • Benzodiazepines
Obsessive-compulsive disorder	Overwhelming need to carry out a stereotypical act to relieve anxiety precipitated by an obsessive thought	• Behavioral techniques, such as response prevention and thought stopping • Antidepressant drugs
Panic disorder	Unpredictable attacks of intense anxiety lasting a few minutes to several hours	• Benzodiazepines • Antidepressant drugs • Relaxation exercises
Posttraumatic stress disorder	Re-experiencing the original traumatic event; may be acute, delayed, or chronic	• Benzodiazepines • Antidepressant drugs • Cognitive therapy • Group therapy • Hypnosis
Simple phobia	Avoidance of something that in reality is harmless	• Benzodiazepines • Desensitization • Distraction
Social phobia	Avoidance of social situations that in reality aren't life-threatening	• Social skills training • Benzodiazepines

---

• displacement
• reaction formation
• intellectualization
• undoing
• repression.
   Types of anxiety and mood disorders include:
• bipolar disorder
• generalized anxiety disorder
• major depression
• obsessive-compulsive disorder
• panic disorder
• phobias
• posttraumatic stress disorder. (See *Comparing anxiety disorders.*)

Bipolar disorder

BIPOLAR DISORDER, also known as manic depression, is a severe disturbance in affect, manifested by episodes of extreme sadness alternating with episodes of euphoria. Severity and duration of episodes vary. The exact biological basis of bipolar disorder remains unknown.

   Two common patterns of bipolar disorder include:
• bipolar I, in which depressive episodes alternate with full manic episodes (hyperactive behavior, delusional thinking, grandiosity and, commonly, hostility)
• bipolar II, characterized by recurrent depressive episodes and occasional manic episodes.

   During the manic phase, the client commonly exhibits excessive motor activity and may become highly irritable if caregivers place limits on his behavior. The client also demonstrates disturbed thought processes that lead to socially inappropriate behavior. Because the client lacks self-pacing and problem-solving abilities, care and treatment focus on slowing the client's movements and activities. Otherwise, a manic client can die of self-induced exhaustion or injury. The potential for suicide increases when the client's mood is changing from mania to depression or from depression to mania; suicide precautions may be needed.

SPOT CHECK

Which bipolar pattern is characterized by depressive episodes alternating with full manic episodes?
Answer: Bipolar I is characterized by alternating depressive and full manic episodes.

Contributing factors
- Concurrent major illness
- Environment
- Heredity
- History of psychiatric illnesses
- Seasons and circadian rhythms that affect mood
- Sleep deprivation
- Stressful events (may produce limbic system dysfunction)

Data collection findings
During periods of mania
- Bizarre and eccentric appearance
- Cognitive manifestations, such as difficulty concentrating, flight of ideas, delusions of grandeur, and impaired judgment
- Motor agitation
- Decreased sleep
- Deteriorated physical appearance
- Dry mouth
- Euphoria or hostility
- Feelings of grandiosity
- Increased libido
- Increased social contacts
- Inflated sense of self-worth
- Lack of inhibition
- Recklessness
- Rapid, jumbled speech
- Tremors
- Tachycardia
- Labored respirations

During periods of depression
- Altered sleep patterns
- Amenorrhea
- Anorexia and weight loss
- Confusion and indecisiveness
- Constipation
- Decreased alertness
- Delusions and hallucinations
- Difficulty thinking logically
- Guilt, helplessness, sadness, and crying
- Impotence and lack of interest in sex
- Inability to experience pleasure
- Irritability
- Pessimism
- Lack of motivation
- Low self-esteem
- Poor hygiene and posture

Diagnostic findings
- Abnormal dexamethasone suppression test results indicate bipolar I disorder.
- Cortisol secretion increases during manic episodes of bipolar I disorder.
- The electroencephalogram is abnormal during the depressive episodes of bipolar I disorder and major depression.

Nursing diagnoses
- Disturbed thought processes
- Risk for injury
- Disturbed sleep pattern
- Impaired social interaction

Treatment
- Electroconvulsive therapy, if drug therapy fails
- Individual therapy
- Family therapy

Drug therapy options
- Anticonvulsant agent: carbamazepine (Tegretol), divalproex sodium (Depakote)
- Antimanic agent: lithium carbonate (Eskalith), lithium citrate (Cibalith-S)
- Selective serotonin reuptake inhibitor: paroxetine (Paxil)

Patient care goals
- The client won't harm himself.
- The client will control his thought processes.

● The client will demonstrate a stable mood and a normal sleep pattern and will practice self-care activities such as eating.

● The client will interact adequately with others.

Nursing interventions
During the client's manic phase

● Decrease environmental stimuli by behaving consistently and supplying external controls *to promote relaxation and enable sleep.*

● Ensure a safe environment *to protect the client from himself.*

● Channel the client's energy in one direction and pace activities, *which may decrease his energy expenditure, prevent overstimulation and, sometimes, have a soothing effect.*

● Define and explain acceptable behaviors and then set limits *to begin a process in which the client will eventually define and set his own limits.*

● Monitor drug levels, especially lithium, *to keep the dosage within the therapeutic range.*

● If a mood swing to depression seems imminent, implement suicide precautions for the client. *The client is at increased risk for suicide during mood swings.*

During the client's depressive phase

● Assess the level and intensity of the client's depression *to obtain baseline information essential for effective nursing care.*

● Ensure a safe environment for the client *to protect him from self-inflicted harm.*

● Assess the risk for suicide and formulate a safety contract with the client, as appropriate, *to ensure his well-being and to open lines of communication.*

● Observe the client for medication compliance and adverse effects; *without compliance, there's little hope for progress.*

● Encourage the client to identify current problems and stressors *so that he can begin therapeutic treatment.*

● Promote opportunities for increased involvement in activities through a structured, daily program *to help the client feel comfortable with himself and others.*

● Select activities that ensure success and accomplishment *to increase self-esteem.*

● Help the client to modify negative expectations and think more positively *because positive thinking will help him begin a healing process.*

● Spend time with the client, even if he's too depressed to talk, *to enhance the therapeutic relationship.*

Evaluation

● The client engages in goal-directed activity and no longer exhibits disturbed thinking.

● The client sleeps through the night.

● The client doesn't harm himself or others.

● The client is adequately maintained on medication, expresses a desire to follow the medication regimen, understands why he must take the drug, knows its adverse effects and how to manage them, and has a plan for getting serum drug levels analyzed once a month.

● The client maintains adequate nutrition.

● The client expresses understanding of the illness and states how to obtain assistance or support from others.

Generalized anxiety disorder

A client with GENERALIZED ANXIETY DISORDER worries excessively and experiences tremendous anxiety almost daily. He experiences moderate to severe levels of anxiety during most waking hours. He can't feel calm or relaxed in situations that most persons don't perceive as particularly stressful. The worry lasts for longer than 6 months and is usually disproportionate to the situation. Adults and children can be diagnosed with generalized anxiety disorder, although the content of the worry may differ. Because the client's anxiety is so pervasive, it affects most areas of his life.

Contributing factors

● Family history of anxiety

● Preexisting psychiatric problems, such as social phobia, panic disorder, and major depression

Data collection findings

● Excessive worry and anxiety

● Excessive attention to surroundings

● Distractibility

● Fatigue

● Sleep disorder

● Motor and muscle tension

● Pounding heart

● Repetitive thoughts

● Strained expression

● Tingling of the hands or feet

● Easy startle reflex

● Fears of grave misfortune or death

● Autonomic hyperactivity

Diagnostic findings
● Laboratory tests exclude physiologic causes.

Nursing diagnoses
● Anxiety
● Ineffective coping
● Deficient knowledge (disease process and treatment)

Treatment
● Individual therapy focusing on coping skills

Drug therapy options
● Antihypertensive agent: clonidine (Catapres)
● Anxiolytic agent: alprazolam (Xanax), lorazepam (Ativan), clonazepam (Klonopin), buspirone (BuSpar)
● Beta-adrenergic blocker: propranolol (Inderal)
● Monoamine oxidase inhibitor: phenelzine (Nardil), tranylcypromine (Parnate)
● Selective serotonin reuptake inhibitor: fluoxetine (Prozac), paroxetine (Paxil), sertraline (Zoloft)
● Tricyclic antidepressant: desipramine (Norpramin), imipramine (Tofranil)

Patient care goals
● The client will verbalize signs and symptoms of increasing anxiety.
● The client will identify coping mechanisms to manage the physical, emotional, and behavioral signs and symptoms of anxiety.

Nursing interventions
● Help the client identify and explore coping mechanisms used in the past — *establishing a baseline for the level of current functioning will enable the nurse to build on the client's knowledge.*
● Observe for signs of mounting anxiety *to direct measures to moderate it.*
● Negotiate a contract to work on goals *to give the client control of his situation.*
● Alter the environment *to reduce the client's anxiety or to meet his needs.*
● Monitor diet and nutrition; reduce caffeine intake *to reduce anxiety.*
● Review key teaching topics with the client and family members *to ensure adequate knowledge about the condition and treatment,* including:
– recognizing signs of anxiety
– altering diet when receiving monoamine oxidase inhibitors (caffeine can cause arrhythmias; foods containing tyramine, such as fava beans, yeast-containing and fer-

mented foods, and avocados, can cause a hypertensive crisis)
– reviewing coping behaviors.

Evaluation
● The client exhibits decreased signs and symptoms of anxiety.
● The client verbalizes coping strategies to use to manage increased anxiety levels.

Major depression
Major depression is a syndrome of persistent sad, dysphoric mood accompanied by disturbances in sleep and appetite from lethargy and an inability to experience pleasure. This disorder can profoundly alter social functioning, but the most severe complication of major depression is the potential for suicide. (See *Forms of depression and nursing implications.*)

Effective emergency intervention should be based on an assessment of the client's lethality. For this, the nurse uses a lethality scale, which considers such factors as the client's age, employment status, availability of support systems, and intended manner of committing suicide. Adolescents and young adults (ages 15 to 24) and elderly white males over age 80 are the two groups at highest risk for suicide. (For indicators of suicidal behavior, see *Identifying a suicidal client,* page 114, and *Classifying suicidal behavior,* page 115.)

Contributing factors
● Current substance abuse
● Deficiencies in the receptor sites for some neurotransmitters: norepinephrine, serotonin, dopamine, acetylcholine
● Family history of depressive disorders
● Hormonal imbalances
● Lack of social support
● Nutritional deficiencies
● Previous episode of depression
● Significant medical problems
● Stressful life events

Data collection findings
● Sadness and crying
● Lack of motivation
● Low self-esteem
● Inability to experience pleasure
● Feelings of guilt, helplessness, and pessimism
● Confusion and indecisiveness

Forms of depression and nursing implications

Use this chart to review commonly observed forms of depression and related nursing implications.

FORM	CHARACTERISTICS	NURSING IMPLICATIONS
Seasonal affective disorder	• Onset between mid-October and mid-November • Remission between mid-February and mid-April • Signs and symptoms of dysthymia	• Advise the client to use bright lights and to go outdoors as much as possible. • If possible, advise the client to purchase full-spectrum lights designed specifically to treat this disorder. • Suggest that the client vacation in the winter, rather than the summer, in a place with longer daylight hours.
Dysthymia	• Depressed mood • Poor appetite • Low energy level or fatigue • Feelings of hopelessness • Poor concentration • Sleep pattern disturbances • Low self-esteem • Difficulty making decisions	• Help the client identify activities that promote well-being. • Help the client establish a healthy daily routine. • Assist the client in setting realistic goals.
Severe depression	• Severe manifestations of dysthymia, plus limited ability to respond to stimuli • Severe psychomotor retardation or agitation • Limited ability to perform life-sustaining activities • Severe anhedonia • Feelings of worthlessness • Excessive guilt • Morbid thoughts and preoccupation with death	• Provide a structured daily routine. • Don't give the client choices. • Make the client engage in activities. • Use compliments sparingly. Ill-timed compliments indicate insensitivity to the client's inner pain and may precipitate regression or a suicide attempt. • Assist the client with self-care activities until his energy returns. • Make decisions for the client until his energy returns.
Psychotic depression	• Characteristics of severe depression as well as hallucinations, delusions, or both	• Intervene as for a severely depressed client. • Orient a hallucinatory or delusional client to reality, as needed. • Provide a consistent environment.

- Altered sleep patterns
- Anorexia and weight loss
- Decreased alertness
- Difficulty thinking logically
- Amenorrhea
- Irritability
- Poor hygiene
- Poor posture
- Impotence or lack of interest in sex
- Constipation
- Delusions and hallucinations

Diagnostic findings
- Thyroid test results are abnormal in major depression.
- Beck depression inventory indicates depression.

Nursing diagnoses
- Hopelessness
- Impaired social interaction
- Chronic low self-esteem

Identifying a suicidal client

In hospitalized clients, the nurse should stay alert for these signs, which suggest suicidal tendencies:
- unexpected calmness
- insistence on obtaining or using grounds privileges
- change in behavior patterns
- verbal threats.

    If the client has any of these signs, be prepared to intervene as follows:
- If the client's behavior has changed, ask him what these changes mean.
- Place the client on suicide precautions.
- Ask the client, "Are you suicidal?"
- Consult with nurse-colleagues, other health care team members, and the client's physician.
- Document your observations and actions.
- Don't promise to keep secrets. Sometimes, a client will ask a nurse to keep something confidential in advance; if the information needs to be shared, the promise can cause problems.

Treatment
- Electroconvulsive therapy
- Individual therapy
- Family therapy
- Phototherapy

Drug therapy options
- Monoamine oxidase inhibitor: phenelzine (Nardil)
- Selective serotonin reuptake inhibitor: paroxetine (Paxil), fluoxetine (Prozac), sertraline (Zoloft)
- Tricyclic antidepressant: amitriptyline (Elavil), desipramine (Norpramin), imipramine (Tofranil)

Patient care goals
- The client will remain safe from suicidal impulses.
- The client will develop a positive attitude about himself, other people, and the future by the time of discharge.
- The client will initiate interactions with peers, staff, and family members by the time of discharge.
- The client will learn to cope with problems, stressors, and losses.

Nursing interventions
- Assess the level and intensity of the client's depression *because baseline information is essential for effective nursing care.*

- Ensure a safe environment for the client *to protect him from self-inflicted harm.*
- Assess the risk for suicide and formulate a safety (no-suicide) contract with the client, as appropriate, *to ensure his well-being and open lines of communication.* This is an agreement that the client will seek out someone to talk out suicidal feelings with rather than act on them.

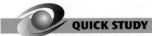
QUICK STUDY

When assessing different aspects of a suicide plan, remember **SLAP**:

> **S**pecific details of a plan
> **L**ethality of method
> **A**vailability of method
> **P**roximity of help

- Reorient the client undergoing electroconvulsive therapy as needed; *clients commonly have temporary memory loss.*
- Observe the client for medication compliance and adverse effects; *without compliance, there's little hope of progress.*
- Encourage the client to identify current problems and stressors *so that therapeutic treatment can begin.*
- Promote opportunities for increased involvement in activities through a structured, daily program *to help the client feel comfortable with himself and others.*
- Select activities that ensure success and accomplishment *to increase self-esteem.*
- Help the client to modify negative expectations and to think more positively; *positive thinking will help the client begin a healing process.*
- Spend time with the client, even if he's too depressed to talk *to enhance the therapeutic relationship.*
- Review key teaching topics with the client and family members *to ensure adequate knowledge about the condition and treatment,* including:
– learning relaxation and sleep methods
– complying with therapy
– if taking monoamine oxidase inhibitors, avoiding tyramine-containing foods, such as wine, beer, cheese, preserved fruits, meats, and vegetables.

Evaluation
- The client doesn't attempt suicide while receiving treatment.
- The client interacts spontaneously with staff, peers, and visitors.

Classifying suicidal behavior

A brief method of classifying the suicide risk for a given client is shown here. No matter how low the risk assessed, all threats of suicide must be taken seriously.

LOW RISK	MODERATE RISK	HIGH RISK
● Verbal threat	● Verbal threat	● Verbal threat
● No specific plan	● Specific plan	● Specific plan
● Relationship problems	● Relationship conflicts	● Cut off from others or in abusive relationships
● Minimal support	● Inconsistent support	● Social isolation with lack of support
● Gesture with no threat to life	● Lethal plan	● Lethal plan
	● Attempt made where rescue is possible	● Attempt made where rescue is highly unlikely

● The client develops specific and realistic expectations for himself and for significant others.
● The client practices positive coping skills, which help to decrease the chance of engaging in self-destructive behaviors.

Obsessive-compulsive disorder

OBSESSIVE-COMPULSIVE DISORDER is characterized by recurrent obsessions (intrusive thoughts, images, and impulses) and compulsions (repetitive behaviors in response to an obsession). The obsessions and compulsions cause intense stress and impair the client's functioning. The client spends a great deal of emotional energy containing his underlying anxiety and maintaining control of himself and life situations. He frequently uses the defense mechanisms of denial, isolation, reaction formation, and undoing. Some clients have simultaneous symptoms of depression.

Fear of losing control and the esteem of others are central issues for persons with obsessive-compulsive disorder. Perfectionistic, overly conscientious, and filled with self-doubt, they typically have trouble being spontaneously emotional because of their intense underlying need to stay "in control" and not make waves. They have intense needs for love, affection, and belonging.

Common obsessions
● Germs
● Illness
● Self doubts

Common compulsions
● Checking
● Counting
● Washing
● Avoiding

Contributing factors
● Brain lesions
● Childhood trauma
● Lack of role models to teach coping skills
● Multiple stressors

Data collection findings
● Obsessive thoughts (which may include thoughts of contamination, repetitive worries about impending tragedy, and repeating and counting images or words)
● Compulsive behavior (which may include repetitive touching, counting, doing and undoing, or other repetitive activity)
● Social impairment

Diagnostic findings
● Positron emission tomography shows increased activity in the frontal lobe of the cerebral cortex.

Nursing diagnoses
● Anxiety
● Ineffective coping
● Chronic low self-esteem

Treatment
● Behavioral therapy
● Individual therapy

Drug therapy options
● Benzodiazepine: alprazolam (Xanax), clonazepam (Klonopin), lorazepam (Ativan)

CLINICAL SITUATION

Caring for the client with obsessive-compulsive disorder

Evaluate the clinical situation described here. See if you're able to answer the questions as you go.

A 40-year-old female client is seeing a nurse on an outpatient basis at a community mental health center. Although her colleagues consider her a top-notch travel agent, she seldom feels she has done her job well enough.

For the past 6 weeks, the resulting anxiety has greatly interfered with her ability to eat and sleep. She sleeps only 3 hours at a time and can't eat more than a few bites of food at each meal. She also spends a great deal of time thinking and talking about what she should have done or should be doing. An exceptionally neat person, she spends about 1½ hours each morning dressing and applying makeup. She calls her husband at work throughout the day to make sure he's all right, and she calls the children when they get home from school to check on them. She says she becomes tense when things don't go well or when she has to make spur-of-the-moment changes.

The client tells the nurse she's a super-organized person who easily becomes upset if the house is messy or if her three high-school–age children fail to follow the daily schedule she establishes for them. She came to the mental health clinic because she felt exhausted and believed her life was getting out of control.

What key points should be established during data collection?

● The client's anxiety level and underlying needs, *which allows the nurse to assist in planning appropriate care*
● Identifying obsessive-compulsive behaviors and the types of events in the client's environment that precipitate her obsessive-compulsive behavior, *which will enable the nurse to engage in anticipatory planning with the client to manage her anxiety*
● The client's eating and sleeping patterns, *which indicates the amount of anxiety she's experiencing*

● The client's expectations of her meetings with you and what goals should be set, *which enables the nurse and the client to monitor the client's progress and provides clues about the appropriateness of the client's expectations of herself and others*
● The client's expectations of her family: Does she see family members as autonomous individuals? How does she feel when family members don't behave as she expects? *This helps to evaluate whether there are inappropriate expectations of others. This can reflect an individual's problems with autonomy and feelings of self-worth.* The obsessive-compulsive client typically feels a great need to control everyone around her and derives her sense of worth from being perfect. For example, she may not be satisfied with the way others do their jobs.

The following nursing diagnoses have been established:
● Anxiety related to fear of losing control of the environment
● Disturbed sleep pattern related to the client's underlying anxiety.

What are appropriate goals to include when planning this client's care?

● The client will verbalize her feelings of anxiety and distress and how these feelings influence her ability to function.
● The client will discuss the unhealthy consequences of her thoughts and actions.
● The client will discuss self-esteem issues or feelings she has about herself.
● The client will develop new coping skills.
● The client will identify factors that precipitate her obsessive-compulsive behavior and plan accordingly.
● The client will relinquish her need to control others.
● The client will sleep for at least 6 hours at a time and feel rested on arising.

● Monoamine oxidase inhibitor: phenelzine (Nardil), tranylcypromine (Parnate)
● Selective serotonin reuptake inhibitor: paroxetine (Paxil)
● Tricyclic antidepressant: desipramine (Norpramin), imipramine (Tofranil)

Patient care goals
● The client will verbalize signs and symptoms of increasing anxiety.
● The client will learn coping strategies to decrease obsessive thinking and compulsive behavior.
● The client will develop and maintain an enhanced self-esteem and increased sense of competency.

Nursing interventions

● Encourage the client to express his feelings *to decrease his level of stress.*
● Help the client assess how his compulsive behaviors affect his functioning. *The client needs to realistically evaluate the consequences of his behavior.*
● Instruct the client to keep a daily journal of thoughts, feelings, and actions to identify those that immediately precede the onset of his obsessive-compulsive behavior. *A journal helps the client identify anxiety-precipitating factors and can provide a sense of being in control.*

FAST FACT

When caring for a client diagnosed with obsessive-compulsive disorder, remember that compulsions shouldn't be forbidden or interrupted because doing so escalates the client's anxiety.

● Help the obsessive-compulsive client engage in anticipatory planning, *which helps him feel in control of potentially anxiety-producing situations.*
● Help the client identify expectations of self and others *to avoid unrealistic expectations.* Obsessive-compulsive people typically set themselves up for failure because their unrealistically high expectations mean they can't accept anything less than perfection in themselves or others.
● Encourage the client to identify situations that produce anxiety and precipitate obsessive-compulsive behavior *to help him evaluate and cope with his own condition.*
● Work with the client to develop appropriate coping skills, such as response prevention and thought stopping, *to reduce anxiety and interrupt automatic obsessive-compulsive behavior.*
● Review key teaching topics with the client and family members *to ensure adequate knowledge about the condition and treatment,* including understanding anxiety and obsessive-compulsive disorder.

Evaluation

● The client identifies situations and activities that may precipitate obsessive-compulsive behavior.
● The client demonstrates a decreased reliance on negative coping mechanisms, such as rituals, and demonstrates new coping strategies.
● The client verbalizes thoughts openly and has realistic expectations of himself and others. (See *Caring for the client with obsessive-compulsive disorder.*)

Panic disorder

While everyone experiences some level of anxiety, clients with PANIC DISORDER experience a nonspecific feeling of terror and dread, accompanied by symptoms of physiologic stress. Attacks can be unpredictable and paralyzing. Many can't identify trigger events and live in constant fear of having an attack. To avoid public embarrassment, they may refuse to leave home and may then concurrently develop agoraphobia (fear of public and open places). This level of anxiety makes it difficult, if not impossible, for the client to carry out the normal functions of everyday life.

Contributing factors

● Agoraphobia (fear of being alone or in public places)
● Asthma
● Cardiovascular disease
● Familial pattern
● GI disorders
● History of anxiety disorders
● History of depression
● Neurologic abnormalities: abnormal activity on the medial portion of the temporal lobe in the parahippocampal area and significant asymmetric atrophy of the temporal lobe
● Neurotransmitter involvement
● Stressful lifestyle

Data collection findings

● Physical tension and uneasiness
● Chest pressure, lump in throat, or choking sensation
● Decreased ability to relate to others
● Diminished ability to focus, even with direction from others
● Edginess and impatience
● Fidgeting or pacing
● Eyelid twitching
● Flushing or pallor
● Generalized weakness
● Tremors
● Increased or decreased blood pressure
● Insomnia
● Loss of appetite or revulsion toward food
● Loss of objectivity
● Palpitations and tachycardia
● Avoidance (client refusal to encounter situations that may cause anxiety)
● Confusion
● Abdominal discomfort or pain, nausea, heartburn, or diarrhea

- Potential for dangerous, impulsive actions
- Rapid, shallow breathing or shortness of breath
- Severely impaired rational thought
- Rapid speech
- Startle reaction
- Sudden urge and frequent urination
- Sweating
- Itching

Diagnostic findings
- Medical tests eliminate physiologic cause.
- Urine and blood tests check for presence of psychoactive agents.

Nursing diagnoses
- Anxiety
- Ineffective coping
- Powerlessness

Treatment
- Individual therapy
- Group therapy

Drug therapy options
- Tricyclic antidepressant: desipramine (Norpramin), imipramine (Tofranil)
- Selective serotonin reuptake inhibitor: paroxetine (Paxil)
- Monoamine oxidase inhibitor: phenelzine (Nardil); in clients with severe panic disorder, tranylcypromine (Parnate)
- Benzodiazepine: alprazolam (Xanax), lorazepam (Ativan), clonazepam (Klonopin)

Patient care goals
- The client will identify life stressors — specific situations, events, or activities that initiate a panic attack — and will be able to identify signs and symptoms of a panic attack.
- The client will recognize which situations can and can't be changed and will demonstrate coping skills that can decrease anxiety.

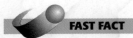 **FAST FACT**

According to research, there's a correlation between lactic acid buildup and panic attacks; aerobic exercise can precipitate panic attacks in some people.

Nursing interventions
- During panic attacks, distract the client from the attack *to alleviate the effects of panic.*
- Discuss other methods of coping with stress *to make the client aware of alternatives.*
- Approach the client calmly and unemotionally *to reduce the risk of further stressing the client.*
- Use short, simple sentences *because the client's ability to focus and to relate to others is diminished.*
- Administer medications as needed *to ensure a therapeutic response.*
- Review key teaching topics with the client and family members *to ensure adequate knowledge about the condition and treatment,* including:
  – learning decision-making and problem-solving skills
  – learning relaxation techniques.

Evaluation
- The client can identify situations or activities that initiate a sense of panic.
- The client verbalizes steps to take to manage a panic attack.
- The client has less anxiety and verbalizes a feeling of increased control.

Phobias

A phobia is an irrational fear of something that in reality can cause little if any harm. It's a fear that persists, even though the client recognizes its irrationality. Phobias may be social, such as performance-related phobias, or simple, such as a fear of dogs, water, or blood.

Phobias serve the purpose of externalizing anxiety. When the anxiety has been projected onto the unconsciously chosen object, anxious feelings can be displaced onto the object, which can then (ideally) be avoided. Forced contact with the phobic object or situation may precipitate panic. Persons experiencing phobias have underlying needs for love, affection, and belonging.

Phobias become problems if they expand or if the object can't be successfully avoided. When this happens, the person's ability to meet daily commitments is impaired. Phobias are resistant to insight-oriented therapies. Behavioral techniques, such as desensitization and distraction, have provided relief for clients with phobias.

SPOT CHECK

Name two types of behavioral therapy that are effective in the treatment of clients with phobias.

Two types of behavioral therapy that are effective in the treatment of clients with phobias are:

- desensitization
- distraction.

Contributing factors

- Biochemical, involving neurotransmitters
- Familial patterns
- Traumatic events

Data collection findings

- Panic when confronted with the feared object
- Persistent fear of specific things, places, or situations
- Displacement (shifting of emotions from their original object) and symbolization
- Disruption in social life or work life

Diagnostic findings

- No specific test is used to diagnose phobias.

Nursing diagnoses

- Anxiety
- Fear
- Powerlessness

Treatment

- Individual therapy
- Systematic desensitization

Drug therapy options

- Benzodiazepine: alprazolam (Xanax), clonazepam (Klonopin), lorazepam (Ativan)
- Beta-adrenergic blocker: propranolol (Inderal) for phobia related to public speaking
- Monoamine oxidase inhibitor: phenelzine (Nardil), tranylcypromine (Parnate)
- Selective serotonin reuptake inhibitor: paroxetine (Paxil)
- Tricyclic antidepressant: desipramine (Norpramin), imipramine (Tofranil)

Patient care goals

- The client will become desensitized to the phobic object or situation.
- The client will discuss fears and anxiety related to the phobic object or situation.

Nursing interventions

- Collaborate with the client to identify the feared object or situation *to develop an effective treatment plan.*
- Assist in desensitizing the client *to diminish his fear.*
- Remind the client about resources and personal strengths *to build his self-esteem.*
- Review key teaching topics with the client and family members *to ensure adequate knowledge about the condition and treatment,* including:
– learning assertiveness techniques
– learning relaxation techniques
– participating in the desensitizing process.

Evaluation

- The client identifies situations, activities, or objects that increase anxiety.
- The client verbalizes signs and symptoms of increasing anxiety.
- The client engages in desensitization activities and exhibits decreased symptoms of anxiety.

Posttraumatic stress disorder

POSTTRAUMATIC STRESS DISORDER (PTSD) is a group of symptoms that develop after a traumatic event. This traumatic event may involve death, injury, witnessing an event that results in serious injury or death of another person, or a threat to physical integrity. In PTSD, ordinary coping behaviors fail to relieve the anxiety. The client may experience reactions that are acute, chronic, or delayed.

Acute PTSD resolves spontaneously; chronic or delayed PTSD requires intervention. The nurse plays an essential role in assessing the client with PTSD and in making appropriate referrals. Regardless of the cause, a crucial component of intervention is encouraging the client to express and share emotions associated with the trauma.

Contributing factors

- High anxiety
- Low self-esteem
- Personal experience of threatened injury or death
- Preexisting psychopathology
- Witnessing trauma to a close friend or family member

Data collection findings

Physical symptoms

- Diaphoresis
- Dyspnea
- GI upset
- Hypertension
- Tachycardia
- Muscle tension

Psychological symptoms

- Anger and self-hatred
- Anxiety
- Depression
- Avoidance of people involved in the trauma
- Avoidance of places where the trauma occurred
- Chronic tension
- Intrusive thoughts
- Detachment and emotional numbness
- Difficulty concentrating and hyperalertness
- Difficulty falling or staying asleep
- Flashbacks of the traumatic experience
- Inability to recall details of the traumatic event
- Nightmares about the traumatic experience
- Poor impulse control
- Social isolation
- Survivor guilt

Diagnostic findings

- No specific tests identify or confirm PTSD.

Nursing diagnoses

- Posttrauma syndrome
- Powerlessness
- Chronic low self-esteem

Treatment

- Alcohol and drug rehabilitation, when indicated
- Individual therapy
- Group therapy
- Progressive relaxation
- Systematic desensitization

Drug treatment options

- Benzodiazepine: alprazolam (Xanax), clonazepam (Klonopin), lorazepam (Ativan)
- Beta-adrenergic blocker: propranolol (Inderal)
- Monoamine oxidase inhibitor: phenelzine (Nardil), tranylcypromine (Parnate)
- Tricyclic antidepressant: amitriptyline (Elavil), imipramine (Tofranil)

Patient care goals

- The client will discuss the traumatic event and feelings related to it.
- The client will experience less anxiety with intrusive thoughts and memories.
- The client will regain control over his feelings, behaviors, and symptoms related to PTSD.
- The client will have enhanced self-esteem and an increased ability to handle frustrations and problems.

Nursing interventions

- Work with the client to identify stressors *to initiate effective coping.*
- Provide for client safety *because the client's ineffective coping, coupled with the intensity of the reaction and poor impulse control, increases his risk for injury.*
- Encourage the client to explore the traumatic event and the meaning of the event *to promote effective coping.*

FAST FACT

The client with PTSD must acknowledge the experience and his feelings or he won't be able to gain cognitive mastery over them. Through active listening, the nurse can help the client gain objectivity.

- Assist the client with problem solving and resolving guilt *to help him understand that circumstances beyond his control probably played a larger part in the trauma than did his personal actions, decisions, or inactions.*
- Review key teaching topics with the client and family members *to ensure adequate knowledge about the condition and treatment,* including:
  – information about PTSD
  – joining support groups
  – learning relaxation techniques
  – promoting social interaction.

Evaluation

- The client acknowledges his experience and feelings and verbalizes less anxiety regarding intrusive thoughts and memories.
- The client reports a sense of control over his feelings and behaviors and exhibits the ability to manage emotional reactions.

- The client verbalizes positive statements regarding himself.

COGNITIVE DISORDERS

COGNITIVE DISORDERS result from any condition that alters or destroys brain tissue and, in turn, impairs cerebral functioning. Symptoms include cognitive impairment, behavioral dysfunction, and personality changes.

Cognitive mental disorders are characterized by the disruption of cognitive functioning. Clinically, they're manifested as mental deficits in clients who had not previously exhibited such deficits.

Cognitive disorders are difficult to identify and treat. The key to diagnosis lies in the discovery of an organic problem with the brain's tissue. They may result from:
- a primary brain disease
- the brain's response to a systemic disturbance such as a medical condition
- the brain tissue's reaction to a toxic substance (as in substance abuse).

Delirium

Delirium is commonly caused by the disruption of brain homeostasis. When the source of the disturbance is eliminated, cognitive deficits generally resolve.

Common causes of delirium include postoperative conditions, metabolic disorders, withdrawal from alcohol and drugs, and toxic substances. Toxic substances are especially difficult to deal with, as they can have residual effects. Drugs present another problem — a medication may be innocuous by itself but deadly when taken with another medication or food. Elderly clients are especially susceptible to the toxic effects of medication.

Dementia

Unlike delirium, dementia is caused by primary brain pathology. Consequently, reversal of cognitive defects is less likely. Dementia can easily be mistaken for delirium, so the cause needs to be thoroughly investigated.

Alzheimer's type dementia

A client with Alzheimer's type dementia suffers a global impairment of cognitive functioning, memory, and personality. The dementia occurs gradually but with continuous decline. Damage from Alzheimer's type dementia is irreversible. Because of the difficulty of obtaining direct pathological evidence of Alzheimer's disease, the diagnosis can be made only when other etiologies for the dementia have been eliminated.

Contributing factors

- Alterations in acetylcholine (a neurotransmitter)
- Altered immune function, with autoantibody production in the brain
- Familial history such as a first-degree relative with Alzheimer's disease or Down syndrome
- Increased brain atrophy, with wider sulci and cerebral ventricles than that seen in normal aging
- Neurofibrillary tangles and beta-amyloid neuritic plaques, mainly in the frontal and temporal lobes

Data collection findings
Stage I
- Decline in recent memory and an inability to retain new memories
- Decreased concentration
- Disorientation regarding time
- Decline in personal appearance
- Agitated or apathetic mood
- Depression
- Attempts to cover up symptoms
- Disturbed sleep
- Susceptibility to falls
- Wandering
- Transitory delusions of persecution

Stage II
- Inability to retain new information
- Diminishing ability to understand or use language
- Disorientation to person, place, and time
- Confabulation (unconscious filling of gaps in memory with fabricated facts and experiences)
- Inability to recognize family members
- Continuous, repetitive behaviors
- Socially unacceptable behavior
- Tantrums
- Increased appetite with no weight gain
- Need for assistance with activities of daily living
- Hoarding
- Bowel and bladder incontinence

Stage III
- Severe decline in cognitive functioning
- Compulsive touching and examination of objects

Key nursing considerations in Alzheimer's disease

Alzheimer's disease has an insidious onset. At first, changes are barely perceptible, but they gradually lead to serious problems. This table provides some key interventions the nurse can perform to assist the client and caregiver as the symptoms of this disease progress.

SIGNS AND SYMPTOMS	NURSING CONSIDERATIONS
• Forgetfulness	• Provide support for the client's concerns regarding forgetfulness. • Encourage the client to discuss his feelings with family members.
• Noticeable changes in mental status and personal appearance • Attempts to hide symptoms • Decreased recall of current events • Difficulty performing job • History of wandering, getting lost	• Encourage the client to verbalize his feelings about his deteriorating status. • Discuss ways to help the client function at work and at home, such as writing notes to himself. • As condition progresses, encourage the client's caregiver to allow the client to perform simple household tasks as tolerated as his condition declines.
• Decreasing ability to understand or use language • Inability to complete activities of daily living • Difficulty recognizing family members, gaps in memory • Socially unacceptable behavior	• Instruct the caregiver to keep the demands on the client to a minimum to decrease stress. • Encourage the caregiver to set up a daily routine that meets the caregiver's and the client's needs. • Discuss the need to provide observation with the caregiver to promote client safety and decrease wandering episodes. • Discuss the availability of local support groups with the client's caregiver and ways for the caregiver to get some relief (such as consulting a home health care agency and family members). • Support the caregiver's decisions regarding the care and placement of the client.
• Decreased response to stimuli • Deterioration in motor ability • Nonresponsiveness	• Perform skin care and range-of-motion exercises if the client is bedridden. • Assist with other aspects of the client's care (such as elimination), as the client's condition warrants. • Allow the caregiver the opportunity to verbalize feelings and to grieve for the client.

• Deterioration in motor ability
• Emaciation
• Decreased response to stimuli
• Nonresponsiveness
(See *Key nursing considerations in Alzheimer's disease.*)

Diagnostic findings
• Cognitive assessment scale demonstrates cognitive impairment.
• Functional dementia scale shows degree of dementia.
• Magnetic resonance imaging (MRI) shows apparent structural and neurologic changes.
• Mini–Mental Status Examination reveals disorientation and cognitive impairment.
• Spinal fluid contains increased beta amyloid.

 SPOT CHECK

During what stage of Alzheimer's type dementia does confabulation occur?
Answer: Confabulation occurs during stage 2.
During what stage does a decrease in recent memory occur?
Answer: Decrease in recent memory occurs during stage 1.

Nursing diagnoses
• Impaired memory
• Bathing or hygiene self-care deficit
• Caregiver role strain

Treatment
• Group therapy
• Hyperbaric oxygen treatment

- Palliative medical treatment
- Tissue transplantation (currently being studied)

Drug therapy options
- Anticholinesterase agent: donepezil (Aricept), tacrine (Cognex)
- Antipsychotic agent: haloperidol (Haldol), risperidone (Risperdal) in low doses
- Benzodiazepine: alprazolam (Xanax)

Patient care goals
- The client will maintain the ability to engage in familiar activities and to meet personal safety needs and hygiene and grooming needs as long as possible.
- The caregiver will take steps to help preserve the client's memory as long as possible.
- The caregiver will seek out information about Alzheimer's type dementia and will engage in healthy grieving about the significant other's illness.

Nursing interventions
- Remove hazardous items and potential obstacles from the client's environment *to maintain a safe environment.*
- Monitor food and fluid intake *to ensure that the client is meeting his nutritional needs.*
- Provide verbal and nonverbal communication that's consistent and structured *to prevent added confusion.*
- State expectations simply and completely *to orient the client.*
- Increase social interaction *to provide stimuli for the client.*
- Encourage the use of community resources; make appropriate referrals as necessary *to find outside support for the caregiver.*
- Promote physical activity and sensory stimulation *to alleviate symptoms of the disorder.*
- Review key teaching topics with the client and family members *to ensure adequate knowledge about the condition and treatment,* including:
  – finding support and education (for caregivers)
  – learning stress-relief techniques (for caregivers).

Evaluation
- The client demonstrates the ability to meet physical, safety, and hygiene needs with minimal assistance.
- The caregiver relates steps taken to help promote the client's memory.
- The caregiver joins an Alzheimer's disease support group.

- The caregiver maintains his social network and uses family and community resources for help when needed. (See *Caring for the client with Alzheimer's disease,* page 124.)
- The caregiver copes with the client's ongoing deterioration of health and loss of self-care ability.

Delirium
Delirium is a disturbance of consciousness accompanied by a change in cognition that can't be attributed to preexisting dementia. It's characterized by an acute onset and may last from hours to a number of days. It's potentially reversible but can be life-threatening if not treated.

Contributing factors
- Cerebral hypoxia
- Effects of medication
- Fever
- Fluid and electrolyte imbalances
- Infection (especially of the urinary tract and upper respiratory system)
- Metabolic disorders
- Multiple drug use, especially anticholinergics
- Neurotransmitter imbalance
- Pain
- Sensory overload or deprivation
- Sleep deprivation
- Stress
- Substance intoxication

Data collection findings
- Distractibility
- Impaired decision making
- Disorganized thinking
- Disorientation (especially to time and place)
- Visual and auditory illusions
- Inability to complete tasks
- Insomnia or daytime sleepiness
- Altered psychomotor activity, such as apathy, withdrawal, and agitation
- Altered respiratory depth or rhythm
- Picking at bed linens and clothes
- Poor impulse control
- Rambling, bizarre, or incoherent speech
- Bizarre, destructive behavior that worsens at night
- Tremors and generalized seizures

CLINICAL SITUATION

Caring for the client with Alzheimer's disease

Evaluate the clinical situation described here. See if you're able to answer the questions as you go.

A 65-year-old female lives at home with her husband; their four children are grown. The client is a florist with her own business. During the past year, her husband relates, she has become forgetful and absent-minded and has had occasional outbursts of anger, which are atypical for her.

One month ago, the client started withdrawing from social activities and began refusing to go to the florist shop. She said she was tired and didn't need to waste her time in meaningless activities. Her husband has noticed that she frequently misidentifies people, doesn't remember simple things unless prompted, makes up stories about events, and rarely uses people's names. Sometimes at night the client becomes agitated and wanders around the house. If the client's husband asks what she's doing, the client tells him it's none of his business. The client has been diagnosed with Alzheimer's type dementia.

The client's husband has decided that his wife will remain at home until he can no longer care for her, but he confided to the office nurse that he feels inadequate to care for his wife because he knows so little about her illness. A referral to a visiting nurse association has been made.

After data collection, the following nursing diagnoses were established:

- Risk for injury related to impaired cognition
- Anticipatory grieving related to loss of ability to function
- Interrupted family processes related to role changes necessitated by the client's condition.

What are appropriate interventions the nurse can implement for this client and caregiver?

- Have the client's husband establish a daily routine for the client, *which can help preserve her memory function so she stays reality-oriented and functional.*

- Label and color-code any objects that the client has difficulty identifying, *which can help her use it appropriately and avoid confusion.*
- Ensure that someone is available to help the client with grocery lists, cleaning, and other home tasks *to promote healthy functioning and to enhance the client's self-esteem.*
- Write down the client's routines and procedures, put a large clock in a prominent spot, and hang signs showing the day and date *to help the client stay reality-oriented and functional.*
- Teach the client's husband the predictable progression of Alzheimer's disease *to allow him to make sound decisions about disease management.*
- Help the client's husband identify areas in which he needs assistance managing his wife at home, such as respite care, meal preparation, and toileting, *to reduce the husband's anxiety and enhance his ability to remain in control of the situation.*
- Give the social worker's or case manager's contact information to the client's husband so that he may find out about Alzheimer's disease support groups and community resources available to help him, such as weekend respite care, day care for persons with Alzheimer's disease, and home health aide services. *Support groups and community resources can help the client's spouse manage care so that the client need not enter an extended-care facility until the late stage of her illness.*

Questions for further thought

- What type of communication skills would be helpful when the nurse makes her home visits?
- How can the nurse evaluate whether the client's husband is engaging in anticipatory problem-solving to meet the client's needs?

Diagnostic findings
- Laboratory results indicate that the delirium is a result of a physiologic condition, intoxication, substance withdrawal, toxic exposure, prescribed medicines, or a combination of these factors.

Nursing diagnoses
- Risk for injury
- Impaired verbal communication
- Disturbed sensory perception

Treatment
- Correction of underlying physiologic problem
- Individual therapy

Drug therapy options
- Tranquilizer: droperidol (Inapsine)
- Benzodiazepine: low-dose lorazepam (Ativan)
- Cholinesterase inhibitor: physostigmine (Antilirium)
- Antipsychotic agent: risperidone (Risperdal)

Patient care goals
- The client will remain free from injury and have a safe environment.
- The client will have minimal anxiety over misperceptions regarding his care and environment.

Nursing interventions
- Determine the degree of cognitive impairment *to understand and treat the client.*
- Create a structured and safe environment *to prevent self-harm.*
- Institute comfort measures *to help the client relax and fall asleep.*
- Keep room lit *to allay the client's fears and prevent visual hallucinations.*
- Monitor the effects of medications *to prevent exacerbating symptoms.*

Evaluation
- The client remains free from injury.
- The client demonstrates calm behavior regardless of cognitive impairment.

ATTENTION DEFICIT AND DISRUPTIVE BEHAVIOR DISORDERS

Attention deficit and disruptive behavior disorders can manifest in various settings, such as in the home, school, work, and social settings. One of the major neurologic disorders in pediatric clients is ATTENTION DEFICIT HYPERACTIVITY DISORDER.

Attention deficit hyperactivity disorder

The child with attention deficit hyperactivity disorder (ADHD), previously called attention deficit disorder, displays long-term behaviors, such as hyperactivity, impulsiveness, and inattention. These behaviors occur in all facets of the child's life and frequently worsen when sustained attention is required. When a child is involved in an activity for a long time or one in which sustained attention is required, the symptoms are exacerbated. Males are affected by this disorder more frequently than females.

FAST FACT

The symptoms of ADHD are commonly determined when the child has difficulty adjusting to elementary school. This is when symptoms are likely to manifest.

To qualify as having ADHD, behaviors must be present in two or more settings, be present before age 7, and result in a significant impairment in social or academic functioning.

Chaotic family life and parents who struggle with their parenting skills are factors that accentuate the difficulties of a child with ADHD.

Possible causes
- The cause of ADHD is believed to be a deficit in neurotransmitters, specifically dopamine and norepinephrine, and serotonin.

Data collection findings
- Climbs, runs, or talks excessively
- Decreased attention span
- Difficulty organizing tasks and activities
- Difficulty waiting for his turn
- Easily distracted
- Failure to give close attention to school work or activity
- Failure to listen when spoken to directly
- Fidgets or squirms in seat
- Frequent forgetfulness; frequently loses things needed for tasks
- Impulsive behavior
- Inability to follow directions

Diagnostic findings
- Complete psychological, medical, and neurologic evaluations rule out other problems, such as epilepsy, lead poisoning, and preexisting conditions such as child abuse.
- To diagnose ADHD, the findings are combined with data from several sources, including parents, teachers, and the child.

Nursing diagnoses
- Impaired social interaction
- Compromised family coping
- Risk for injury
- Risk for impaired parenting

Treatment
- Behavioral modifications
- Individual therapy
- Family therapy
- Interdisciplinary interventions: pathologic assessment and diagnosis of specific learning needs

Drug therapy options
- Amphetamine: dextroamphetamine (Dexedrine), methylphenidate (Ritalin) to help the child concentrate
- Antidepressant: imipramine (Tofranil)
- Antihypertensive: clonidine (Catapres)

Patient care goals
- The client will learn new coping skills, acknowledge strengths, and demonstrate beginning social skills.
- The client and family members will learn strategies to assist the child in coping with the condition.

Nursing interventions
- Monitor growth. *If the child is receiving methylphenidate, growth may be slowed.*
- Give one simple instruction at a time so the child can successfully complete the task; *this promotes self-esteem.*
- Give medications in the morning and at lunch *to avoid interfering with sleep.*
- Ensure adequate nutrition; *medications and hyperactivity may cause increased nutrient needs.*
- Reduce environmental stimuli *to decrease distraction.*
- Formulate a schedule for the child *to provide consistency and routine.*
- Develop situations and assist the child with performing the steps necessary to complete a task without getting distracted *to allow the child to feel good and to set the stage for continued successful behaviors.*
- Teach the child strategies to get along with other children without taking on the role of class clown. *By knowing the correct ways of behaving and interacting with peers, the client doesn't have to resort to attention-seeking behaviors.*
- Encourage the child to identify strengths *to enhance self-esteem.*

- Give positive reinforcement for the child's attempts to change negative behaviors, *which contributes to his desire and motivation to change disruptive behaviors.*
- Teach family members how to avoid overstimulation of the child to handle disruptive behaviors, *which permits the family to cope and to handle problematic situations in an effective manner.*
- Discuss the family's method of disciplining the child *to establish a framework for reinforcing positive strategies already being used and to teach additional disciplinary techniques.*
- Review key teaching topics with the client and family members *to ensure adequate knowledge about the condition and treatment,* including:
- allowing the child to expend energy after being in restrictive environments such as school
- monitoring for adverse reactions to medications
- structuring learning to minimize distractions
- taking breaks from caregiving to avoid strain
- teaching important material in the morning (when medication levels peak).

Evaluation
- The client participates in healthy interactions with peers.
- The client practices effective coping skills.
- The client's family members verbalize understanding of the child's diagnosis and the child's strengths and learn how to effectively handle their child.

PERSONALITY DISORDERS

Clients with personality disorders control anxiety by adopting behavior patterns that interfere with their ability to adapt to daily stressors and establish healthy relationships. Personality disorders fall into three major groups:
- cluster A — odd or eccentric behavior
- cluster B — dramatic or emotional behavior
- cluster C — anxious or fearful behavior. (See *Characterizing personality disorders.*)

Borderline personality disorder
BORDERLINE PERSONALITY DISORDER results in a pattern of instability in a person's mood, interpersonal relationships, self-esteem, self-identity, behavior, and cognition. Impulsiveness is its most prominent characteristic, and it appears to originate in early childhood.

Characterizing personality disorders

Personality disorders fall into three groups, or clusters, as shown in this chart. Clients with cluster A personality disorders are characteristically aloof and restrained in relationships; others may describe them as odd or strange. Clients with cluster B disorders typically are dramatic, unrestrained, and unpredictable. Those with cluster C disorders are overly apprehensive about the present and future and worry about failing.

PERSONALITY DISORDER	CLIENT DESCRIPTION
Cluster A	
Schizotypal personality disorder	<ul><li>Has some cognitive and perceptual distortion</li><li>May be viewed as odd or eccentric in speech and behavior</li><li>Has poorly developed social skills</li><li>Has strained and uncomfortable relationships</li><li>Is easily overwhelmed by too much social or interpersonal stimuli</li></ul>
Paranoid personality disorder	<ul><li>Uses projection</li><li>Is extremely suspicious of others' motives</li><li>Is very guarded in relationships and finds hidden meanings</li><li>Is very private</li><li>Expects to be exploited or harmed by others</li><li>Questions others' loyalty</li><li>Reads hidden meaning into harmless remarks or events</li><li>Doesn't forgive slights, insults, or injuries</li></ul>
Schizoid personality disorder	<ul><li>Is emotionally cold and detached</li><li>Is withdrawn and controlled</li><li>Can't form warm, spontaneous relationships</li><li>Usually lives alone or in parents' home</li><li>Has little need for friendship or intimacy</li><li>Has a solitary lifestyle</li><li>Seems indifferent to praise or criticism</li></ul>
Cluster B	
Narcissistic personality disorder	<ul><li>Can't empathize with others because of intense need for love and admiration</li><li>Demands much time and attention from others</li><li>Feels entitled or special</li><li>Is arrogant, haughty, and envious</li><li>Expects to be recognized as superior without commensurate achievements</li></ul>
Histrionic personality disorder	<ul><li>Controls anxiety through dramatic presentation of self</li><li>Uses attention-seeking behaviors and flattery to get others to meet needs</li><li>Is overly concerned with physical attractiveness</li><li>Can't tolerate delayed gratification</li><li>Has a seductive appearance or behavior</li><li>Becomes anxious when limits are placed on attention-seeking behaviors</li></ul>
Borderline personality disorder	<ul><li>Has a poorly developed sense of self and is easily influenced by others</li><li>Struggles with overwhelming feelings of anger and anxiety</li><li>Views situations in extremes (all good or all bad)</li><li>Has intense fear of abandonment</li><li>Feels empty and devoid of substance</li><li>Needs others around to maintain a sense of self (you + me = self)</li></ul>

(continued)

Characterizing personality disorders (continued)

PERSONALITY DISORDER	CLIENT DESCRIPTION
Antisocial personality disorder	• Is aggressive and impulsive • Acts out conflicts within social contexts • Has no regard for rules and norms • Lacks remorse • Takes no responsibility for outcomes of own behavior • Blames others when things go wrong • Believes others are unreliable • Must have immediate gratification • Disregards the truth • Has a poor work history • Can't sustain a monogamous relationship

Cluster C

PERSONALITY DISORDER	CLIENT DESCRIPTION
Dependent personality disorder	• Is unable to be assertive • Remains in abusive situations • Falls apart if significant other leaves or dies • Doesn't trust own judgment • Feels incapable of managing on own • Needs excessive reassurance and advice • Lacks self-confidence • Will go to extremes to get nurturing from others
Obsessive-compulsive personality disorder	• Controls anxiety through extreme orderliness, cleanliness, and punctuality • Needs to be in control • Is excessively devoted to work and productivity • Is overly conscientious • Is unable to discard worn or useless objects • Is reluctant to delegate tasks to others • Hoards supplies for future catastrophes
Avoidant personality disorder	• Remains aloof in relationships • Wants friendships but can form them only if assured of not getting hurt or shamed • Doesn't like surprises • Is preoccupied with fear of being criticized or rejected in social situations • Feels inferior to others

Most clients with personality disorders are treated as outpatients. However, a client with borderline personality disorder may be hospitalized after a self-destructive act such as a suicide attempt. Typically, clients with borderline personality disorder attempt suicide when feeling abandoned; their goal is to get others to take care of them.

Contributing factors
• Brain dysfunction in the limbic system or frontal lobe
• Decreased serotonin activity
• Early parental loss or separation
• Increased activity in alpha-2 noradrenergic receptors
• Major losses early in life
• Physical abuse
• Sexual abuse
• Substance abuse

Data collection findings
• Inability to maintain relationships
• Inability to develop a healthy sense of self
• Compulsive behavior
• Destructive behavior

- Emotional reactions, with few coping skills
- Dissociation (separating objects from their emotional significance)
- Dysfunctional lifestyle
- High self-expectations
- Impulsive behavior
- Extreme fear of abandonment
- Moodiness
- Self-directed anger
- Paranoid ideation
- Self-mutilation
- Shame
- Suicidal behavior
- View of others as either extremely good or bad

Diagnostic findings
- Standard psychological tests reveal a high degree of dissociation.

Nursing diagnoses
- Impaired social interaction
- Risk for self-directed violence
- Chronic low self-esteem

Treatment
- Alcohol and drug rehabilitation, as indicated
- Milieu therapy
- Group therapy
- Family therapy
- Individual therapy

Drug therapy options
- Antimanic agent: carbamazepine (Tegretol), lithium carbonate (Eskalith)
- Anxiolytic agent: buspirone (BuSpar)
- Monoamine oxidase inhibitor: phenelzine (Nardil)
- Narcotic detoxification adjunct agent: naltrexone (ReVia)
- Selective serotonin reuptake inhibitor: fluoxetine (Prozac), paroxetine (Paxil)

Patient care goals
- The client will learn how to process experiences before and after taking action.
- The client will refrain from self-destructive behaviors or destructive behavior toward others.
- The client will learn new coping skills.

Nursing interventions
- Recognize behaviors that the client uses to manipulate others *to avoid unconsciously reinforcing these behaviors.*
- Set appropriate expectations for social interaction and praise the client when these expectations are met *to create a healthy therapeutic environment.*
- Teach the client how to engage in anticipatory planning *to aid the development of new coping skills.*
- Respect the client's sense of personal space *to increase trust.*
- Review key teaching topics with the client and family members *to ensure adequate knowledge about the condition and treatment,* including:
  – developing problem-solving skills
  – developing therapeutic communication skills
  – implementing relaxation techniques.

Evaluation
- The client exhibits the ability to see how his behavior affects others.
- The client develops new coping skills, which can provide a sense of empowerment and improve self-esteem.
- The client exhibits the ability to identify and plan for situations that precipitate acting out.
- The client doesn't exhibit behavior that's harmful to himself or others.

Paranoid personality disorder
PARANOID PERSONALITY DISORDER is characterized by extreme distrust of others. Paranoid people avoid relationships in which they aren't in control or have the potential of losing control.

Contributing factors
- Genetic predisposition
- Neurochemical alteration
- Parental antagonism

Data collection findings
- Feelings of being deceived
- Suspiciousness and mistrust of friends and relatives
- Refusal to confide in others
- Hostility
- Emotional reactions, including nervousness, jealousy, anger, or envy
- Self-righteousness
- Social isolation
- Sullen attitude
- Lack of social support systems

- Hyperactivity, especially in children
- Irritability, especially in children
- Bad temper, especially in children
- Delusional thinking
- Hypervigilance
- Lack of humor
- Major distortions of reality
- Need to be in control

Diagnostic evaluation
- There are no specific tests for paranoid personality disorder.

Nursing diagnoses
- Anxiety
- Ineffective coping
- Chronic low self-esteem
- Social isolation

Treatment
- Possible drug-free treatment to reduce the chance of causing increased paranoia
- Individual therapy

Drug therapy options
- Antipsychotic agent: chlorpromazine (Thorazine), fluphenazine (Prolixin), haloperidol (Haldol), olanzapine (Zyprexa), risperidone (Risperdal), thioridazine (Mellaril)

Patient care goals
- The client will identify feelings that impede social interaction.
- The client will learn new coping skills to decrease anxiety in social interactions.
- The client will feel safe about changing behaviors when coping with situations.

Nursing interventions
- Establish a therapeutic relationship by listening and responding to the client *to initiate therapeutic communication.*
- Encourage the client to take part in social interactions *to introduce other people's perceptions and realities to the client.*
- Help the client to identify negative behaviors that interfere with relationships *so he can see how his behavior impacts others.*
- Instruct and help the client practice strategies that facilitate the development of social skills *so he can gain confidence and practice interacting with others.*

- Review key teaching topics with the client and family members *to ensure adequate knowledge about the condition and treatment,* including:
  - learning coping strategies
  - understanding the disorder (for family members and client).

Evaluation
- The client verbalizes what factors cause impaired social interactions.
- The client identifies strategies for improving behaviors during social interactions.
- The client verbalizes decreased anxiety when socializing with others and participates in group or social interactions.

EATING DISORDERS

Anorexia nervosa and bulimia nervosa, two major forms of eating disorders, result in death for 5% to 15% of the people they affect. The incidence of eating disorders is particularly high among adolescent girls from highly competitive, upwardly mobile families.

Persons with these eating disorders share many characteristics, including:
- excessive concern about food and weight control
- use of extreme measures to control weight (starvation, purging)
- perfectionistic self-expectations
- concern about how one is viewed by others
- eagerness to please and make a good impression
- underdeveloped sense of personal identity
- discomfort in social situations
- unresolved issues of autonomy
- underlying needs for love, affection, and belonging.

The anorexic client and the bulimic client also display distinct behavioral differences. For example, when the client is finally hospitalized for treatment of anorexia nervosa, malnutrition is apparent. (See *Anorexia nervosa and bulimia nervosa: Client behaviors.*) It isn't unusual for a client with anorexia nervosa to weigh as little as 70 to 80 lb (32 to 36 kg). In most cases, the client must weigh at least 90 lb (41 kg) before psychotherapy can be initiated successfully.

Anorexia nervosa and bulimia nervosa: Client behaviors

ANOREXIA NERVOSA	BULIMIA NERVOSA
● Denies that the eating pattern is abnormal	● Recognizes that the eating pattern is abnormal
● Loses significant amounts of body weight	● Keeps weight within a normal range; preoccupied with weight gain
● Is introverted and perfectionistic	● Appears extroverted with poor impulse control
● Copes with stress by starving self	● Copes with stress by bingeing
● Denies feeling fatigued	● Admits feeling fatigued
● Exercises compulsively	● May exercise strenuously
● Tightly controls food intake	● Is unable to control food intake
● Is unlikely to abuse alcohol	● May abuse alcohol
● Feels powerful after abstaining from food	● May be suicidal after bingeing
● Secretive and self-absorbed	● Secretive with food
● Overwhelmed by fear of losing control	● Overwhelmed and feels out of control
● High achiever	● Low self-esteem can prevent achievement

Anorexia nervosa

In anorexia nervosa, the client deliberately starves herself or engages in binge eating and purging. A client with anorexia nervosa wants to become as thin as possible and refuses to maintain an appropriate weight. There are two categories of anorexia nervosa — the restricting type (where the amount of food intake is restricted) and the binge-eating–purging type.

A key clinical finding is a refusal to sustain weight at or above the minimum requirements for the client's age and height. If left untreated, anorexia nervosa can cause the client's death.

Contributing factors
- Age (most prominent in adolescents)
- Distorted body image
- Gender (primarily affects females)
- Genetic predisposition
- Low self-esteem
- Neurochemical changes
- Poor family relations
- Preoccupation with weight and dieting
- Sexual abuse

Data collection findings
- A decrease in a person's body weight to less than 85% of the weight considered normal for the person's age and height
- Amenorrhea, fatigue, loss of libido, infertility
- Body image disturbance
- Cognitive distortions, such as overgeneralization, dichotomous thinking, or ideas of reference
- Compulsive behavior
- Decreased blood volume, evidenced by lowered blood pressure and postural hypertension
- Dependency on others for self-worth
- Electrolyte imbalance, evidenced by muscle weakness, seizures, or arrhythmias
- Emaciated appearance
- Denial of hunger and guilt associated with eating
- Exercising to excess despite fatigue
- GI complications, such as constipation or laxative dependence
- Impaired decision making
- Need to achieve and please others
- Obsessive rituals concerning food
- Overly compliant attitude
- Perfectionist attitude
- Refusal to eat and severe curtailment of intake
- Fear of gaining weight

Diagnostic findings
- Eating Attitude test suggests an eating disorder.
- Electrocardiogram reveals nonspecific ST interval, prolonged PR interval, and T-wave changes.
- Laboratory test results show elevated blood urea nitrogen and electrolyte imbalances.
- Female clients exhibit low estrogen levels.
- Leukopenia and mild anemia are apparent.
- Male clients exhibit low serum testosterone levels.

CLINICAL SITUATION

Caring for the client with anorexia nervosa

Evaluate the clinical situation described here. See if you're able to answer the questions as you go.

A 17-year-old female client has been admitted to your unit in the hospital for treatment of severe weight loss. The client is 5'6" (168 cm) tall and weighs 85 lb (38.6 kg). She has been in counseling at a community mental health center for the past 2 months but was hospitalized when her weight dropped below 90 lb (40.8 kg).

The client, who lives with her parents and three younger siblings, is an honor student and president of the student council. She works hard to please her teachers and her parents.

According to her history, 6 months ago the client decided to lose 25 lb (11.3 kg) so others would find her more attractive and she would look slimmer in her graduation pictures. When she attained her goal of 110 lb (50 kg), she decided to continue dieting in the firm belief that her ability to lose weight and remain thin would demonstrate her self-discipline and ability to succeed.

On your unit, the client becomes extremely upset when anyone tries to get her to eat, saying that the sight of food nauseates her. When she does eat, she complains of feeling bloated and needs to go to the bathroom immediately. The client says she doesn't understand why everyone is so concerned about her weight. She just feels fat and doesn't want to be any heavier. The client rarely socializes with the other teenagers on the unit, preferring to spend time in solitary activity. When she does socialize, she appears uncomfortable and sometimes makes tactless remarks.

What are appropriate nursing diagnoses for this situation?
● Ineffective denial related to uncertainty about the future
● Imbalanced nutrition: Less than body requirements related to fear of becoming fat
● Disturbed body image related to distorted perception of body size

What interventions are appropriate to promote intake of nutritious foods?
● Offer highly nutritious foods every 3 hours in small amounts *because the client isn't able to ingest large quantities of food at one time.*
● Observe the client for at least 90 minutes after she eats a meal or snack *to prevent unobserved actions, such as vomiting, to keep her weight down.*

Questions for further thought
● How would a therapy group consisting of clients with similar problems help the client?
● How would assertiveness skills assist the client?

Nursing diagnoses
● Imbalanced nutrition: Less than body requirements
● Disturbed body image
● Chronic low self-esteem

Treatment
● Behavioral modification
● Group therapy
● Individual therapy
● Nutritional therapy

Drug therapy options
● Antianxiety agent: alprazolam (Xanax), lorazepam (Ativan)
● Antidepressant: amitriptyline (Elavil), imipramine (Tofranil)
● Selective serotonin reuptake inhibitor: fluoxetine (Prozac), paroxetine (Paxil)

Patient care goals
● The client will increase weight according to established goals.
● The client will formulate a healthy self-concept and engage in independent behaviors.
● The client's physiologic processes will be within normal limits.
● The client will learn coping techniques to deal with anxiety.

Nursing interventions
● Obtain a complete physical assessment *to identify complications of anorexia nervosa.*
● Contract for amount to be eaten *to avoid arguments and conflict between the staff and client.*
● Provide one-on-one support before, during, and after meals *to foster a strong nurse-client relationship and to ensure that the client is eating.*

● Prevent the client from using the bathroom for 90 minutes after eating *to break the purging cycle.*

● Encourage verbal expression of feelings *to foster open communication about body image.*

● Help the client identify coping mechanisms for dealing with anxiety *to promote healthy coping techniques.*

● Help the client learn ways to satisfy personal, unmet needs *to facilitate developing a healthy lifestyle. The client needs to learn the coping skills and strategies to meet physiologic and emotional needs.*

● Weigh the client once or twice a week at the same time of day using the same scale *to accurately monitor weight gain.*

● Help understand the anorectic cycle *to prevent future anorectic behavior.*

● Discuss the client's perception of her appearance. Help her understand how arbitrary social standards for beauty have affected her self-perception. Point out that she doesn't have to accept society's equation of thinness and beauty. Explain that she has a right to think of herself as beautiful regardless of how she compares with others *to build self-esteem.*

● Discuss the client's progress with her *to increase awareness of achievements and promote continued effort.*

● Review key teaching topics with the client and family *to ensure adequate knowledge about the condition and treatment,* including:

– need for gradual weight gain

– nutritional support measures

– treatment options

– support services and community resources.

Evaluation

● The client's vital signs, electrolyte levels, and fluid intake and output are within reference limits.

● The client verbalizes that she's pleased with her appearance and expresses self-confidence.

● The client is able to maintain a healthy food intake and her weight has reached the established goal.

● The client relates the coping strategies that can be used when anxiety level is increased. (See *Caring for the client with anorexia nervosa.*)

Bulimia nervosa

Bulimia nervosa is characterized by episodic bingeing on food, followed by purging in the form of vomiting. The client's weight may remain normal or close to normal. The severity of the disorder depends on the frequency of the binge and purge cycle as well as physical complica-

tions. The client commonly views food as a source of comfort.

Contributing factors

● History of sexual abuse

● Low self-esteem

● Neurochemical changes

● Few family relations

Data collection findings

● Alternating periods of binge eating and purging

● Anxiety

● Avoidance of conflict

● Cognitive distortions such as those with anorexia nervosa

● Constant preoccupation with food

● Disruptions in interpersonal relationships

● Dissatisfaction with body image

● Extreme need for acceptance and approval

● Feelings of helplessness

● Focus on changing a specific body part

● Frequent lies and excuses to explain behavior

● Guilt and self-disgust

● Irregular menses

● Perfectionist attitude

● Parotid and salivary gland swelling

● Pharyngitis

● Physiologic problems as in anorexia nervosa (amenorrhea, fatigue, loss of libido, infertility, electrolyte imbalance, GI complications)

● Possible use of amphetamines or other drugs to control hunger

● Problems caused by frequent vomiting

● Repression of anger and frustration

● Russell sign (bruised knuckles or abrasions on the back of the hand due to induced vomiting)

● Sporadic, excessive exercise

Diagnostic findings

● Beck Depression Inventory may reveal depression.

● Eating Attitudes test suggests eating disorder.

● Metabolic acidosis may occur from diarrhea caused by enemas and excessive laxative use.

● Metabolic alkalosis (the most common metabolic complication) may occur from frequent vomiting.

Nursing diagnoses

● Imbalanced nutrition: Less than body requirements

● Anxiety

● Powerlessness

Treatment
● Cognitive therapy (to identify triggers for bingeing and purging)
● Family therapy

Drug therapy options
● Selective serotonin reuptake inhibitor: fluoxetine (Prozac), paroxetine (Paxil)
Note: Drug therapy is most effective when combined with cognitive therapy.

Patient care goals
● The client will learn coping techniques to deal with increased anxiety.
● The client will increase her weight according to the established goals and will maintain normal eating habits.
● The client will formulate a healthy self-concept.
● The client's physiologic processes will be within normal limits.

Nursing interventions
● Perform a complete physical assessment *to identify complications associated with bulimia nervosa.*
● Explain the purpose of a nutritional contract *to encourage a dietary change without initiating argument or struggle.*
● Avoid power struggles around food *to keep the focus on establishing and maintaining positive self-image and self-esteem.*
● Prevent the client from using the bathroom for 2 hours after eating *to help avert the purging behavior.*
● Provide one-on-one support before, during, and after meals *to monitor and assist the client with eating.*
● Encourage the client to express her feelings *to facilitate conversation and promote understanding.*
● Weigh the client once or twice a week at the same time of day using the same scale *to accurately monitor weight.*
● Help the client identify the cause of the disorder *to help her gain understanding and work toward wellness.*
● Point out cognitive distortions *to help identify sources of the problem.*
● Discuss the client's perception of her appearance. Help her understand how arbitrary social standards for beauty have affected her self-perception. Point out that she doesn't have to accept society's equation of thinness with beauty. Explain that she has a right to think of herself as beautiful regardless of how she compares herself with others *to build self-esteem.*

● Discuss the client's progress with her *to increase her awareness of her achievements and to promote continued effort.*
● Review key teaching topics with the client and family *to ensure adequate knowledge about the condition and treatment,* including:
– need to gain weight gradually
– treatment options
– support services and community resources.

Evaluation
● The client's vital signs, electrolyte levels, and fluid intake and output are within reference limits.
● The client can maintain a healthy food intake, and weight has reached the established goal.
● The client relates the coping strategies that can be used when anxiety level is increased.

SCHIZOPHRENIC AND DELUSIONAL DISORDERS

People with major distortions in ego functioning experience serious disturbances in all areas of their lives, having impaired reality testing and a compromised ability to relate with others. Common signs of impairment in reality testing include bizarre behaviors, inability to assume responsibility for oneself, and misinterpretation of environmental stimuli.

Major disturbances in ego functioning can result from functional causes, such as acute psychosis, or from underlying organic causes related to drug ingestion, high fever, an accumulation of toxins in the body, or dementia.

SCHIZOPHRENIA is a brain disease characterized by neurotransmitter imbalances and structural changes within the brain. Distorted thought processes make living with this disease a challenge. Symptoms from schizophrenia may be characterized as positive or negative. Positive symptoms focus on a distortion of normal functions; negative symptoms focus on a loss of normal functions. (See *Symptom classification of schizophrenia.*)

Catatonic schizophrenia
Clients with CATATONIC SCHIZOPHRENIA show little reaction to their environments. Catatonic behavior involves remaining completely motionless or continuously repeating one motion. This behavior can last for hours. Catatonic schizophrenia is the least common type of schizophrenia.

Symptom classification of schizophrenia

Here are examples of positive and negative symptoms of schizophrenia.

POSITIVE SYMPTOMS	NEGATIVE SYMPTOMS
● Bizarre, disorganized, or catatonic behavior ● Delusions ● Disorganized speech ● Hallucinations ● Loose associations ● Paranoia	● Disorganized thinking process ● Flat affect ● Inability to have pleasure (anhedonia) ● Lack of motivation ● Lack of self-initiated behaviors (avolition) ● Poverty of speech (alogia) ● Social withdrawal

Contributing factors
● A fragile ego, which can't withstand the demands of reality
● Brain abnormalities
● Developmental abnormalities
● Genetic factors
● Hyperactivity of the neurotransmitter dopamine
● An infectious agent or autoimmune response (unproven cause)
● Social or environmental stress, interacting with the person's inherited biological makeup

Data collection findings
● Agitation at times, which may be unexpected and dangerous
● Bizarre postures, waxy flexibility (posture held in odd or unusual fixed positions for extended periods), resistance to being moved
● Childlike, regressed behavior
● Clang association
● Displacement (switching emotions from their original object to a more acceptable substitute)
● Dissociation (separation of things from their emotional significance)
● Echolalia (repetition of another's words)
● Echopraxia (involuntary imitation of another person's movements and gestures)
● Episodes of impulsiveness
● Fantasy
● Inability to trust
● Little reaction to environment
● Mutism
● Neologism
● Projection
● Purposeless overactivity or underactivity
● Ritualistic mannerisms
● Social isolation
● Speech resembling a word salad (string of words that aren't connected in any way)

Diagnostic findings
● MRI shows possible enlargement of lateral ventricles, enlarged third ventricle, and enlarged sulci.
● The client shows impaired performance on neuropsychological and cognitive tests.

Nursing diagnoses
● Disturbed thought processes
● Ineffective coping
● Bathing or hygiene self-care deficit

Treatment
● Electroconvulsive therapy
● Family therapy
● Milieu therapy
● Outpatient group therapy
● Psychoeducational programs
● Social skills training
● Stress management
● Supportive psychotherapy

Drug therapy options
● Antiparkinsonian agent: benztropine (Cogentin) for adverse effects of antipsychotic agents
● Antipsychotic agent: fluphenazine (Prolixin), haloperidol (Haldol), olanzapine (Zyprexa), risperidone (Risperdal), thioridazine (Mellaril)

Patient care goals
- The client will regain control of thought processes.
- The client will perform self-care without assistance.
- The client won't experience physical harm.
- The client will establish a relationship with the primary nurse, refer to other clients by name, and make eye contact when talking with others.
- The client will develop healthy ways to handle anxiety, fears, and other threats to self.

Nursing interventions
- Provide skin care *to prevent skin breakdown.*
- Monitor intake and output. *Body weight may decrease as a result of inadequate intake.*
- Monitor the client for adverse effects of antipsychotic drugs, such as dystonic reactions and tardive dyskinesia. *Early identification of extrapyramidal effects can help diminish or eliminate the client's anxiety about these symptoms.*
- Be aware of the client's personal space; use gestures and touch judiciously. *Invading the client's personal space can increase his anxiety.*
- When discussing care, give short, simple explanations at the client's level of understanding *to increase cooperation.*
- Provide appropriate measures *to ensure the client's safety and explain why you're doing so. Implementing and explaining safety measures can promote trust and decrease anxiety while increasing the client's sense of security.*
- Promote a trusting relationship *to create a safe environment in which the client can practice social interaction skills and prepare for social interaction.*
- Briefly explain procedures, routines, and tests *to allay the client's anxiety.*
- Collaborate with the client to identify anxious behavior as well as probable causes. *Involving the client in examination of behavior can increase his sense of control.*
- Provide opportunities for the client to learn adaptive social skills in a nonthreatening environment. *Learning new social skills can enhance the client's adjustment after discharge.*
- Review key teaching topics with the client and family members *to ensure adequate knowledge about the condition and treatment,* including:
  – accepting that feelings are valid
  – recognizing extrapyramidal effects of antipsychotic medications
  – preventing photosensitivity reactions to drugs by avoiding exposure to sunlight.

Evaluation
- The client experiences less confusion in thinking or thought processes.
- The client talks about situations and issues that reinforce reality.
- The client independently manages daily care.
- The client doesn't place himself at risk for harm.
- The client interacts appropriately with staff, selected peers, and visitors.

Delusional disorder
A delusion is a false belief to which a person adheres despite contradictory evidence. Clients with DELUSIONAL DISORDER hold firmly to false beliefs despite contradictory information. The client with delusional disorder tends to be intelligent and can have a high level of competence but has impaired social and personal relationships. One indication of delusional disorder is an absence of hallucinations.

 FAST FACT

The most common types of delusions include:
- *delusions of grandeur* – belief that one is highly important, famous, or powerful
- *delusions of persecution* – belief that one is being persecuted or harmed by others
- *delusions of reference* – belief that one is connected to events unrelated to oneself

Contributing factors
- Brain abnormalities
- Developmental involvement
- Family history of schizophrenic, avoidant, and paranoid personality disorders
- Lower socioeconomic status
- Neurotransmitter abnormalities
- Social or environmental stress, interacting with the person's inherited biological makeup

Data collection findings
- Antagonism
- Brushes with the law
- Delusions that are visual, auditory, or tactile
- Denial
- Ideas of reference (everything in the environment takes on a personal significance)

- Inability to trust
- Irritable or depressed mood
- Marked anger and violence
- Projection
- Stalking behavior or erotomania (the belief one is loved by a prominent person)

Diagnostic findings

- Blood and urine testing eliminates an organic or chemical cause.
- Endocrine function tests rule out hyperadrenalism, pernicious anemia, and thyroid disorders.
- Neurologic evaluations rule out an organic cause.

Nursing diagnoses

- Impaired social interaction
- Ineffective coping
- Risk for self-directed violence
- Risk for other-directed violence

Treatment

- Family therapy
- Group therapy
- Milieu therapy
- Psychoeducational programs
- Stress management
- Supportive psychotherapy

Drug therapy options

- Antiparkinsonian agent: benztropine (Cogentin) for adverse effects of antipsychotic medications
- Antipsychotic agent: chlorpromazine (Thorazine), fluphenazine (Prolixin), haloperidol (Haldol), olanzapine (Zyprexa), risperidone (Risperdal), thioridazine (Mellaril)

Patient care goals

- The client won't harm himself or others.
- The client will learn alternative coping strategies.
- The client will regain a normal level of functioning.

Nursing interventions

- Assist in formulating realistic, modest goals with the client *to help diminish suspicion while increasing his self-esteem and sense of control.*
- Establish a therapeutic relationship *to foster trust.*
- Work as a team with other staff members to allow one nurse to communicate with the client and to supervise other staff members with regard to the client's care *to build trust and to minimize opportunities for the client to exhibit hostility.*

- Explore events that trigger delusions *to help you understand the dynamics of the client's delusional system.* Discuss anxiety associated with triggering events.
- Don't directly attack the delusion *to avoid increasing the client's anxiety.* Instead, be patient in formulating a trusting relationship.
- Once the dynamics of the delusions are understood, discourage repetitious talk about delusions and refocus the conversation on the client's underlying feelings. *As the client identifies and explores feelings, he'll decrease his reliance on delusional thought.*
- Recognize the delusions as the client's perception of the environment. Avoid getting into arguments with the client regarding the content of delusions *to foster trust.*
- Teach the client alternative coping mechanisms *to handle periods of increased anxiety and enhance his self-esteem and self-control.*
- Review key teaching topics with the client and family members *to ensure adequate knowledge about the condition and treatment,* including:
– learning decision-making, problem-solving, and negotiating skills
– understanding potential adverse effects of medication.

Evaluation

- The client doesn't harm himself or others.
- The client demonstrates less suspicious behavior.
- The client can identify signs and symptoms of anxiety.
- The client identifies factors that precipitate delusions and alternative coping mechanisms to handle anxiety.

Paranoid schizophrenia

Clients with PARANOID SCHIZOPHRENIA have delusions unrelated to reality. Clients commonly display bizarre behavior, are easily angered, and are at high risk for violence. The prognosis for independent functioning is better in most cases than for other types of schizophrenia.

Contributing factors

- A fragile ego, which can't withstand the demands of external reality
- Brain abnormalities
- Developmental involvement
- Genetic factors
- Neurotransmitter abnormalities
- Social or environmental stress, interacting with the person's inherited biological makeup

Data collection findings

- Anxiety
- Argumentativeness
- Delusions and auditory hallucinations
- Displacement
- Dissociation
- Easily angered
- Inability to trust
- Potential for violence
- Projection
- Withdrawal or aloofness

Diagnostic findings

- MRI shows possible enlargement of ventricles and enlarged sulci. The presence of the enlarged sulci suggests cortical loss, particularly in the frontal lobe.
- Neuropsychological and cognitive tests indicate impaired performance.

Nursing diagnoses

- Disturbed thought processes
- Social isolation
- Disturbed sensory perception (auditory)

Treatment

- Family therapy
- Group therapy
- Milieu therapy
- Psychoeducational programs
- Social skills training
- Stress management
- Supportive psychotherapy

Drug therapy options

- Antiparkinsonian agent: benztropine (Cogentin) for adverse effects of antipsychotic drugs
- Antipsychotic agent: chlorpromazine (Thorazine), clozapine (Clozaril), fluphenazine (Prolixin), haloperidol (Haldol), olanzapine (Zyprexa), risperidone (Risperdal), thioridazine (Mellaril)

Patient care goals

- The client will regain control of thought processes.
- The client will establish a relationship with the primary nurse, refer to other clients by name, and make eye contact when talking with others.
- The client will no longer experience delusions.

Nursing interventions

- Inform the client that you'll help him control his behavior *to promote feelings of safety.*
- Set limits on aggressive behavior and communicate your expectations to the client *to prevent injury to the client and others.*
- Work as a team with other staff members to allow one nurse to communicate with the client and to direct other staff members who care for the client *to foster trust and a stable environment and to minimize opportunities for the client to exhibit hostility.*
- Maintain a low level of stimuli *to minimize the client's anxiety, agitation, and suspiciousness.*
- Be flexible — allow the client some control. Approach him in a calm and unhurried manner. Let the client talk about anything he wishes, but keep the conversation light and social *to avoid entering into power struggles.*
- Don't let the client put you on the defensive, and don't take his remarks personally. If he tells you to leave him alone, leave but return soon. *Brief contacts with the client may be most useful at first.*
- Don't make attempts to combat the client's delusions with logic. Instead, respond to feelings, themes, or underlying needs — for example, "It seems you feel you've been treated unfairly." *Combating delusions may increase feelings of persecution or hostility.*
- If the client is taking clozapine, stress the importance of returning weekly to the facility or an outpatient setting to have his blood checked *to monitor for adverse effects and to prevent toxicity.*
- Teach the client the importance of complying with the medication regimen. Tell him to report adverse reactions instead of discontinuing the drug *to maintain therapeutic drug levels.*
- If he takes a slow-release formula, make sure that he understands when to return for his next dose *to promote compliance.*
- Review key teaching topics with the client and family *to ensure adequate knowledge about the condition and treatment,* including:
– avoiding exposure to sunlight (to prevent photosensitive reactions to antipsychotic drugs)
– reporting adverse affects of antipsychotic medication
– visiting the hospital weekly to have blood chemistry monitored.

Evaluation

- The client regains control of thought processes.

- The client establishes a relationship with the primary nurse, refers to other clients by name, and makes eye contact when talking with others.
- The client no longer has delusions or can take action to control delusions.

SOMATOFORM DISORDERS

A SOMATOFORM DISORDER is the literal transference of inner conflict onto a body part, commonly resulting in crippling. Individuals with somatoform disorders channel anxiety through a body system. Channeling anxiety in this manner usually succeeds because the person is unaware of uncomfortable amounts of anxiety.

Symptoms of a somatoform disorder aren't under voluntary control and suggest a physical disorder with a psychogenic origin. Physical symptoms aren't consistent with the presence or degree of underlying pathophysiology. At an affective level, persons with somatoform disorders don't experience emotional distress over life events but are keenly aware of uncomfortable somatic sensations, for which they seek treatment.

Two examples of somatoform disorders, hypochondriasis and conversion reaction, are presented in this section. Most people who experience conversion reactions accept their condition with a complacency known as *la belle indifference.*

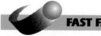

FAST FACT

Forcing a client with a somatoform disorder to renounce his symptoms heightens his anxiety and prolongs the condition.

Conversion disorder

The client with CONVERSION DISORDER exhibits symptoms that suggest a physical disorder, but evaluation and observation can't determine a physiologic cause. The onset of symptoms is preceded by psychological trauma or conflict, and the physical symptoms are a manifestation of the conflict.

Contributing factors
- Psychological conflict
- Overwhelming stress

Data collection findings
- Aphonia (inability to produce sound)
- Blindness
- Deafness
- Dysphagia
- Impaired balance and impaired coordination
- La belle indifference (a lack of concern about the symptoms or limitation on functioning)
- Loss of touch sensation
- Lump in the throat
- Paralysis
- Seizures
- Urinary retention

Diagnostic findings
- Test results are inconsistent with physical findings.
- The absence of expected diagnostic findings can confirm the disorder.

Nursing diagnoses
- Ineffective coping
- Anxiety

Treatment
- Individual therapy

Drug therapy options
- Benzodiazepine: alprazolam (Xanax), lorazepam (Ativan)

Patient care goals
- The client will demonstrate new coping skills.
- The client will identify signs and symptoms of anxiety.

SPOT CHECK

What precedes the onset of symptoms in a conversion disorder?
Answer: Psychological trauma or conflict precedes the onset of symptoms in a conversion disorder.

Nursing interventions
- Ensure and maintain a safe environment *to protect the client.*
- Establish a supportive relationship that communicates acceptance of the client but keeps the focus away from symptoms *to help him learn to recognize and express anxiety.*
- Review all laboratory and diagnostic study results *to ascertain whether any physical problems are present.*

● Encourage the client to identify emotional conflicts that may have occurred before the onset of physical symptoms *to make the relationship between the conflict and the symptoms more clear.*
● Promote social interaction *to decrease the client's level of self-involvement.*
● Identify constructive coping mechanisms *to encourage the client to use practical coping skills and relinquish the role of being sick.*
● Review key teaching topics with the client and family members *to ensure adequate knowledge about the condition and treatment,* including:
– setting limits on the client's sick role behavior while continuing to provide support
– instituting stress-reduction methods
– recognizing the importance of REM and NREM sleep; some individuals may have increased amounts of slow-wave sleep.

Evaluation
● The client identifies signs and symptoms of increased anxiety.
● The client demonstrates acquired coping strategies when dealing with increased anxiety.
● The client focuses less attention on sick role and physical symptoms.

Hypochondriasis

In HYPOCHONDRIASIS, the client is preoccupied by fear of a serious illness, despite medical assurance of good health. The client with hypochondriasis interprets all physical sensations as indications of illness, impairing his ability to function normally.

Contributing factors
● Death of someone close to the individual
● Family member with a serious illness
● Previous serious illness

Data collection findings
● Abnormal focus on bodily functions and sensations
● Anger, frustration, and depression
● Frequent visits to doctors and specialists despite assurance from health care providers that the client is healthy
● Intensified physical symptoms around sympathetic people
● Rejection of the idea that symptoms are stress-related
● Use of symptoms to avoid difficult situations
● Vague physical symptoms

Diagnostic findings
● Test results are inconsistent with client's complaint and physical findings.

Nursing diagnoses
● Ineffective coping
● Ineffective health maintenance

Treatment
● Individual therapy

Drug therapy options
● Benzodiazepine: alprazolam (Xanax), lorazepam (Ativan)
● Tricyclic antidepressant: amitriptyline (Elavil), doxepin (Sinequan), imipramine (Tofranil), phenelzine (Nardil)

Patient care goals
● The client will become aware of how emotional issues affect physiologic functioning.
● The client will learn coping strategies for emotional issues.
● The client will demonstrate a decreased focus on symptoms.

Nursing interventions
● Assess the client's level of knowledge about how emotional issues can impact physiologic functioning *to promote understanding of the condition.*
● Encourage emotional expression *to discourage emotional repression, which can have physical consequences.*
● Respond to the client's symptoms in a matter-of-fact way *to reduce the secondary gain he achieves from talking about his symptoms.*
● Review key teaching topics with the client and family *to ensure adequate knowledge about the condition and treatment,* including:
– practicing relaxation and assertiveness techniques
– initiating conversations that focus on something other than physical maladies.

Evaluation
● The client identifies coping strategies to use when dealing with emotional issues.
● The client initiates conversations unrelated to physical complaints.

SUBSTANCE ABUSE DISORDERS

Some people discover that certain chemical substances appear to relieve their anxiety, boredom, depression, or feelings of inadequacy. Over time, continual intake of a chosen substance becomes abusive, tolerance develops, and the person must ingest increasingly larger quantities to obtain the desired effects.

Continued substance abuse leads to physiologic and psychological changes. Some family members, friends, and coworkers may notice these changes and protect the abuser, either by excusing misbehavior at home or by taking on extra work to make up for the abuser's decreased productivity on the job. Others may be slow to recognize that substance abuse is adversely affecting the abuser as well as his family members, friends, and associates.

Health professionals typically see a substance abuser for the first time when the client seeks treatment for a related health problem, such as gastric ulcers, malnutrition, or hepatitis. The abuser may be admitted to a general hospital directly or through the emergency department — for example, following an accident or overdose.

Lack of cause-and-effect insight makes treating such a client a challenge for nurses. Because most substance abusers don't view themselves as having a problem, they don't initiate treatment for their abusive behavior. Furthermore, they overuse the defense mechanisms denial, rationalization, and projection, and they make considerable use of negative manipulation. (See *Selected substances of abuse*, pages 142 and 143.)

Alcohol abuse disorder

Although alcohol abuse is considered a substance abuse disorder, assessment findings and treatment differ somewhat from that for other substances. Alcohol is a sedative but creates a feeling of euphoria. Sedation increases with the amount ingested.

Possible causes
- Familial tendency
- Gender (males have increased likelihood of addiction)
- History of abuse, depression, or anxiety
- Influence of nationality and ethnicity
- Personality disorders
- Religious or family taboos regarding alcohol consumption

Data collection findings
- Adrenocortical insufficiency
- Alcoholic cardiomyopathy
- Alcoholic cirrhosis
- Alcoholic hepatitis
- Alcoholic paranoia
- Blackouts
- Erection problems
- Esophageal varices
- Gastritis or gastric ulcers
- Hallucinations
- Korsakoff's psychosis
- Liver damage
- Muscular myopathy
- Pancreatitis
- Pathologic intoxication
- Peripheral neuropathy
- Wernicke's encephalopathy

Diagnostic findings
- Positive blood and urine drug screenings confirm the diagnosis.
- Standard alcoholism screening tools, such as the CAGE questionnaire and the Michigan Alcoholism Screening test, indicate alcoholism.

Nursing diagnoses
- Ineffective denial
- Ineffective coping
- Risk for injury

Treatment
- Alcoholics Anonymous
- Individual therapy
- Rehabilitation

Drug therapy options
- Antidepressant agent: bupropion (Wellbutrin)
- Benzodiazepine: chlordiazepoxide (Librium), diazepam (Valium), or lorazepam (Ativan)
- Disulfiram (Antabuse) to prevent relapse into alcohol abuse (client must be alcohol-free for 12 hours before administering this drug)
- Naltrexone (Trexan) to prevent relapse into alcohol abuse
- Selective serotonin reuptake inhibitor: fluoxetine (Prozac), paroxetine (Paxil) (see *Treating alcohol abuse*, page 144)

(Text continues on page 144.)

Selected substances of abuse

This chart lists various substances of abuse, signs of withdrawal, and corresponding nursing interventions. During the acute withdrawal stage (detoxification), the nurse may administer medications intended to prevent or minimize the severe consequences of withdrawal, such as seizures or delirium.

SUBSTANCE	WITHDRAWAL SIGNS	NURSING INTERVENTIONS
Alcohol (beer, wine, liquor)		
	• Mild tremors • Diaphoresis • Nervousness • Increased blood pressure • Increased heart rate	• Monitor the client's vital signs. • Obtain order for benzodiazepines to relieve withdrawal signs. • Remain with the client and monitor his behavior. • Promote sleep and rest.
	• Moderate to severe tremors • Appetite loss • Disorientation • Hallucinations • Delusions	• Monitor the client's vital signs. • Administer benzodiazepines, as ordered. • Maintain a quiet environment. • Remain with the client.
	• Persistent hallucinations • Grand mal seizures	• Monitor the client's vital signs. • Remain with the client. • Administer anticonvulsants, as ordered. • Take seizure precautions. • Minimize environmental stimulation. • Offer foods and fluid when the client is lucid.
	• Withdrawal delirium • Sleeplessness • Tachycardia • Hallucinations	• Monitor the client's vital signs. • Remain with the client. • Minimize environmental stimulation. • Offer foods and fluids, as tolerated.
Opiates (such as morphine and heroin)		
	• Lacrimation • Runny nose • Yawning • Diaphoresis • Tachycardia • Fever • Insomnia • Muscle aches • Drug craving • Nausea or vomiting • Dilated pupils • Chills	• Monitor the client's vital signs. • Remain with the client. • Offer foods and fluids, as tolerated. • Provide a soothing environment. • If ordered, wean the client by offering small doses of opiate. • If ordered, administer methadone.
Inhalants		
	• Anxiety • Central nervous system damage • Renal failure or other problems • Respiratory damage • Sleep problems	• Monitor the client's vital signs. • Evaluate and monitor physiological condition. • Promote rest.

Selected substances of abuse *(continued)*

SUBSTANCE	WITHDRAWAL SIGNS	NURSING INTERVENTIONS
Sedatives		
	• Anxiety • Diaphoresis • Hallucinations • Seizures • Tachycardia	• Monitor the client's vital signs. • Attend to physiologic and safety needs, especially if seizures occur. • Promote rest and calm environment.
Central nervous system stimulants		
Amphetamines	• Depression • Fatigue • Agitation • Suicidal thoughts • Paranoia • Disorientation • Insomnia or hypersomnia	• Monitor the client's vital signs. • Monitor the client for suicidal ideation. • Promote sleep and rest. • Administer antidepressants, if ordered. • Remain with the disoriented or frightened client; orient him to reality.
Cocaine, crack cocaine	• Depression • Fatigue • Agitation • Suicidal thoughts • Paranoia • Insomnia or hypersomnia • Craving for drug • Increased appetite	• Monitor the client's vital signs. • Monitor the client for suicidal ideation. • Promote sleep and rest. • Administer antidepressants, if ordered. • Remain with the disoriented or frightened client; orient him to reality.
Hallucinogens		
Lysergic acid diethylamide (LSD)	• Flashbacks at a later time • Apprehension • Panic	• Administer diazepam if the client has severe anxiety during flashbacks, as ordered.
Phencyclidine (PCP)	• Depression • Lethargy • Craving • Hypertension • Seizures • Bizarre behavior	• Monitor the client's vital signs and safety. • Monitor the client for suicidal ideation. • Promote sleep and rest. • Administer antidepressants, if ordered. • Remain with the disoriented or frightened client; orient him to reality.
Marijuana (cannabis)	• Insomnia • Irritability • Anorexia • Agitation • Restlessness • Tremors • Depression • Chronic respiratory problems	• If the client is depressed, attend to physiologic and safety needs. • Know that physicians rarely order medication to ease withdrawal. • Monitor respiratory problems.

Treating alcohol abuse

TREATMENT RECOMMENDATIONS	ASSESSMENT FACTORS	RATIONALES
Monitor alcohol intake	● Consumes fewer than 6 drinks/week ● Blood alcohol content (BAC) levels over the legal limit ● Benign scores on CAGE or other screening tests ● Benign family history	● Increased awareness of intake may prevent future problems.
Limit alcohol intake	● BAC over the legal limit ● Benign CAGE scores ● History of exceeding the legal blood alcohol limit more than four times/year ● History of consuming more than 10 drinks/week	● The client is at risk for developing alcohol dependency; limiting intake now helps to prevent increased future intake.
Abstain from alcohol; use support and counseling services (Alcoholics Anonymous, inpatient treatment, family counseling)	● BAC significantly over the legal limit ● Significant alcohol abuse screening test scores ● History of daily alcohol consumption ● History of consuming more than 15 drinks/week ● Family history of alcohol abuse ● Extreme defensiveness about alcohol use ● Multiple drug use ● Presence of blackouts, personality changes, other problems related to alcohol use ● Inability to control alcohol intake ● Previous conviction for driving while intoxicated or previous treatment for alcohol abuse ● Presence of family problems related to the client's alcohol abuse	● Data indicative of addiction, which is best controlled by abstinence. ● Abstinence is best maintained with the help of a support group. ● Inpatient treatment may be indicated for the client assessed as at high risk for dying or for doing harm to self or others. ● Alcohol abuse potentiates problems within the family (alcoholism is a family disease).

Patient care goals
● The client will recognize that alcohol is creating problems in his life.
● The client will develop specific plans for abstinence from alcohol and for managing stress.
● The client will experience an uncomplicated recovery from alcohol withdrawal.

Nursing interventions
● Monitor the client for signs of alcohol withdrawal. *During withdrawal, protective nursing measures, such as one-on-one care, should be implemented if the client's symptoms progress beyond mild tremors, diaphoresis, nausea, nervousness, tachycardia, and increased blood pressure.* (See *Recognizing alcohol withdrawal syndrome.*)

● Assess the client's use of denial as a coping mechanism *to begin a therapeutic relationship.*
● Encourage the verbalization of anger, fear, inadequacy, grief, and guilt *to promote healthy coping behaviors.*
● Set limits on denial and rationalization *to help the client gain control and perspective.*
● Have the client formulate goals for maintaining a drug-free lifestyle *to help avoid relapses.*
● Review key teaching topics with the client and family members *to ensure adequate knowledge about the condition and treatment,* including:
– understanding substance abuse and relapse prevention
– maintaining good nutrition.

Recognizing alcohol withdrawal syndrome

Use this chart to review alcohol withdrawal syndrome, keeping in mind that the client should have one-on-one care as symptoms worsen. **For** nursing management, use restraints only as a last resort; restraining the client will heighten anxiety and increase agitation.

SIGNS AND SYMPTOMS	ONSET AND DURATION	NURSING MANAGEMENT
Mild tremors, diaphoresis, nausea, nervousness, tachycardia, increased blood pressure	Signs and symptoms may occur within 4 to 6 hours after the last drink.	• Carefully monitor the client's behavior. • Seek the physician's order for medication to relieve withdrawal symptoms. • Talk to the client about symptoms, and remain with him when withdrawal begins. • Monitor the client's vital signs.
Increased tremors, hyperactivity, insomnia, anorexia, disorientation, delusions, transient visual hallucinations, tachycardia	Signs and symptoms commonly occur 8 to 10 hours after the last drink.	• Administer medications, as ordered, to relieve withdrawal symptoms. • Remain with the client and orient him to reality. • Keep the room free from distractions and unnecessary noise. • Monitor the client's vital signs as able.
Same as those listed above plus persistent hallucinations, nausea, and vomiting; withdrawal seizures may also occur 7 to 48 hours after last drink	Signs and symptoms occur 12 to 48 hours after the last drink.	• Remain with the client. • Monitor the client's vital signs as able. • Institute seizure precautions. • Administer anticonvulsant medications as ordered. • Offer fluids and light foods, as tolerated, during periods of lucidity. • Maintain a peaceful environment.
Withdrawal delirium (lasts 2 to 3 days), disorientation, fluctuating consciousness, hallucinations, agitation, and low-grade fever	Signs and symptoms most commonly occur 48 to 72 hours after the last drink, but may not arise until 7 days after.	• Remain with the client. • Monitor the client's vital signs as able. • Maintain a peaceful environment. • Offer fluids and light foods, as tolerated, during periods of lucidity. • Administer medications, as ordered.

Evaluation
• The client freely acknowledges the problems created by alcohol ingestion and makes plans for restitution.
• The client participates in stress-management group sessions and identifies specific strategies for managing stress.
• The client exhibits no signs of adverse effects from alcohol withdrawal.
• The client identifies and takes care of physical health problems.

Substance abuse disorder
SUBSTANCE ABUSE DISORDER includes all patterns of abuse excluding alcohol and cocaine. Abuse disorders have a great deal in common, although symptoms vary depending on the abused substance.

Contributing factors
• Familial tendency
• Gender (females have increased likelihood of abusing prescription drugs; males have increased likelihood of addiction)

- History of abuse, depression, or anxiety
- Influence of nationality and ethnicity
- Personality disorders

Data collection findings

- Attempts to avoid anxiety and other emotions
- Attempts to avoid conscious feelings of guilt and anger
- Attempts to meet needs by influencing others
- Blaming others for problems
- Development of biological or psychological need for a substance
- Dysfunctional anger
- Feelings of grandiosity
- Impulsiveness
- Manipulation and deceit
- Need for immediate gratification
- Pattern of negative interactions
- Possible malnutrition
- Symptoms of withdrawal
- Use of denial and rationalization to explain consequences of behavior

Diagnostic findings

- Positive blood and urine drug screening results confirm the diagnosis.
- Standard alcoholism screening tools, such as the CAGE questionnaire and the Michigan Alcoholism Screening test, indicate alcoholism.

Nursing diagnoses

- Ineffective health maintenance
- Imbalanced nutrition: Less than body requirements
- Risk for self-directed violence
- Risk for other-directed violence

Treatment

- Behavior modification
- Employee assistance programs
- Family counseling
- Group therapy
- Halfway houses
- Individual therapy
- Informal social support
- Self-help groups

Drug therapy options

- Clonidine (Catapres) for opiate withdrawal symptoms
- Methadone maintenance for opiate addiction detoxification

Patient care goals

- The client will learn the adverse effects of substance abuse on the body.
- The client will have adequate nutritional intake
- The client won't harm himself or others.
- The client will commit to a recovery program and get assistance to maintain abstinence and coping skills.

Nursing interventions

- Ensure a safe, quiet environment free from stimuli *to provide a therapeutic setting and to alleviate withdrawal symptoms.*
- Monitor for withdrawal symptoms, such as delirium, tremors, seizures, or anxiety, *to provide the most comfortable environment possible.*
- Assess the client for polysubstance abuse *to plan appropriate interventions.*
- Help the client understand the ultimate consequences of substance abuse *to assist recovery.*
- Provide measures to induce sleep *to help the client manage the discomfort of withdrawal.*
- Encourage the client to vent fear and anger *to facilitate the healing process.*
- Review key teaching topics with the client and family members *to ensure adequate knowledge about the condition and treatment,* including:
– contacting addiction support agencies
– learning healthy coping mechanisms.

Evaluation

- The client relates the adverse effects of substance abuse and verbalizes plans for lifestyle changes and getting follow-up support.
- The client has sufficient nutritional intake.
- The client doesn't harm himself or others during hospitalization.

7

Maternal-neonatal nursing

Introduction

Maternal and neonatal nursing care involves application of the nursing process during family planning as well as during the antepartum, intrapartum, postpartum, and neonatal periods.

FAMILY PLANNING

Family planning involves exercising choices to prevent or achieve pregnancy and to control the timing and number of pregnancies, lifestyle, and partner support. Effectiveness, cost, contraindications, and adverse reactions for all contraceptives should be presented to the client.

Information from the client's menstrual and obstetric history is used for determining the safety of using oral contraceptives and which contraceptive method is best for the client. (See *Comparing contraceptives,* pages 148 and 149.)

The nurse uses information obtained during the interview to plan appropriate teaching. The effectiveness and safety of oral contraceptives depend greatly on the client's knowledge of and compliance with the chosen method. Inability to understand the proper use of the contraceptive device or unwillingness to use it correctly or consistently may result in pregnancy.

Family planning data collection

Data collection for family planning involves collecting a reproductive history, including:
- interval between periods (See *Menstrual cycle,* page 150.)
- duration and amount of flow
- problems occurring during menstruation
- number of pregnancies
- number of births (date of each)
- duration of each pregnancy

- type of each delivery
- gender and weight of children when delivered
- problems occurring during pregnancy
- problems occurring after delivery.

Complications

Information obtained from the client's history may identify that the client is at risk for complications:
- Contraindications for oral contraceptives include malignancy of the reproductive system, hypertension, pregnancy, and liver dysfunction. A client older than age 35 is at increased risk for a fatal heart attack if she smokes more than 15 cigarettes per day and takes oral contraceptives.
- Oral contraceptive use affects the reproductive system. Use of oral contraceptives is contraindicated in the presence of malignant cell growth. A Papanicolaou (Pap) test may be performed to detect cellular abnormalities.
- If the client's sexual partner is infected with human immunodeficiency virus, acquired immunodeficiency syndrome, or hepatitis B, she must use the condom method of contraception to prevent transmission of the infection.
- For a breast-feeding client, the physician may prescribe progesterone alone or a low-dose combination of oral contraceptives. This may cause the client's milk supply to decrease.
- Low-dose oral contraceptives may be prescribed for a client who has diabetes with no vascular complications.
- The Food and Drug Administration recently revised its position on oral contraceptives, stating that for healthy, nonsmoking women older than age 40, the benefits (such as decreased menstrual cramps and increased cycle regularity) may outweigh the risks.

Nursing diagnoses

Information obtained during data collection is also used to develop nursing diagnoses for family planning. Nursing diagnoses may include:
- Imbalanced nutrition: Less than body requirements

(Text continues on page 150.)

Comparing contraceptives

When discussing contraception with clients, emphasize the importance of history, physical examination, diagnostic tests, and follow-up examinations. Use the following chart to review the methods and proper use of contraception, their effectiveness against sexually transmitted diseases, and the possible adverse reactions that can occur.

METHOD AND ACTIONS	CONTRAINDICATIONS	POTENTIAL PROBLEMS	CLIENT TEACHING
Intrauterine device (IUD) Not fully understood: may cause an inflammatory process that interferes with implantation; 95% effective	Pelvic infections, uterine abnormalities, cancer of the reproductive organs	May cause increased menstrual flow, abdominal cramps, expulsion, infection, ectopic pregnancy, uterine perforation (many have been withdrawn from the market)	● Teach the client to check string placement after each menstrual period and before coitus. ● Advise her to follow the manufacturer's timetable for replacement.
Diaphragm Mechanical barrier; 81% effective within 4 hours of placement	Cervicitis	May be allergenic	● Teach the client to keep the diaphragm clean and dry and to check it for holes. ● Tell her to leave it in place for at least 6 hours after coitus. ● Advise her to use a spermicidal agent along with the diaphragm. ● Caution her that she must have the diaphragm refitted after significant weight gain or loss and after childbirth.
Spermicidal agent (jelly, cream, foam, suppository) Chemical barrier; 82% effective	Cervicitis	May be allergenic	● Instruct the client to insert the agent high into the vagina not more than 1 hour before coitus and to remain supine after insertion. ● Advise her to use the agent with a condom. ● Tell her to avoid douching.
Male condom Mechanical barrier; 90% effective	None	May be allergenic; may tear	● Advise the client to make sure her partner leaves a small space in the tip of the condom when applying. ● Instruct her on proper condom use to avoid tears. ● Emphasize that the condom must be held in place during withdrawal to prevent spillage.
Female condom Mechanical barrier; 95% effective	None	May break or become dislodged	● Teach insertion procedure (inner ring covers the cervix, second ring remains outside the vagina). ● Tell her the condom may be inserted 8 hours before intercourse. ● Advise her that a female condom shouldn't be used with a male condom.

Comparing contraceptives *(continued)*

METHOD AND ACTIONS	CONTRAINDICATIONS	POTENTIAL PROBLEMS	CLIENT TEACHING
Fertility awareness methods Abstinence during the fertile period, determined by one or more methods (calendar method, basal body temperature graph, and cervical mucus test); 75% effective	None	Has low reliability because of difficulty in determining the fertile period; may reduce spontaneity	● Calendar (rhythm) method: Tell the client to document the duration of her periods and to presume that ovulation occurs 14 days before menses. ● Basal body temperature graph: Tell the client to document her body temperature over time and to presume that a drop in temperature followed by a sustained increase indicates ovulation. ● Cervical mucus test: Teach the client that the spinnbarkeit is high at ovulation. The client must be self-disciplined, keep accurate records, and be prepared to cope with unexpected pregnancy.
Oral contraceptives (such as estrogen and progestin combination) Prevents ovulation; 98% effective	Reproductive system cancers, hypertension, pregnancy, liver dysfunction	May cause spotting, nausea, vomiting, breast tenderness, hyperglycemia, thrombophlebitis	● Inform the client of health benefits, such as decreased menstrual cramps and increased cycle regularity.
Medroxyprogesterone acetate (Depo-Provera; 150 mg administered I.M. every 3 months) Suppresses release of gonadotropic hormones and prevents ovulation; 99% effective	Pregnancy, liver disease, undiagnosed vaginal bleeding, breast cancer, blood clotting disorders, cardiovascular disease	May cause changes in menstrual cycle, weight gain, headache, nervousness, fatigue	● Teach the client that this drug prevents pregnancy for 3 months. ● Inform her that most women can conceive within 12 months after last dose.
Levonorgestrel (Norplant System; subdermal implant consisting of six Silastic capsules) Prevents ovulation and stimulates production of thick cervical mucus, which inhibits sperm penetration; 99% effective	Pregnancy, liver disease, undiagnosed vaginal bleeding, breast cancer, blood clotting disorders, cardiovascular disease	May cause irregular menstruation, spotting, amenorrhea, weight gain, headache	● Inform the client that capsules must be replaced every 5 years. ● Counsel the client about potential adverse effects such as menstrual irregularities.
Tubal ligation Interruption of fallopian tube passageways; 99.6% effective (40% to 75% reversible)	Client-specific surgical risks	May cause menstrual disorders; discomfort from carbon dioxide during laparoscopy; problems of laparotomy, such as infection, hemorrhage, and anesthesia complications	● Advise the client to approach the procedure as irreversible. ● Demonstrate aseptic incision care. ● Inform her that the procedure can be reversed in 40% to 75% of clients.
Vasectomy Interruption of vas deferens passageways; 99.6% effective (29% to 85% reversible)	Client-specific surgical risks	May cause autoimmune response; surgical complications	● Advise the client to approach the procedure as irreversible (although reversal may be possible). ● Suggest an alternative contraceptive method until a sperm count confirms the procedure's effectiveness. ● Teach incision care.

Menstrual cycle

The menstrual cycle (female reproductive cycle) typically lasts 28 days. Throughout the cycle, hormones influence the release of a mature ovum from a graafian follicle in the ovary. Hormones also stimulate changes in the endometrial layer of the uterus, preparing it for ovum implantation.

Hormones involved in this cycle are estrogen, progesterone, follicle-stimulating hormone (FSH), and luteinizing hormone (LH). The diagram below illustrates how hormones relate to various phases of the menstrual cycle.

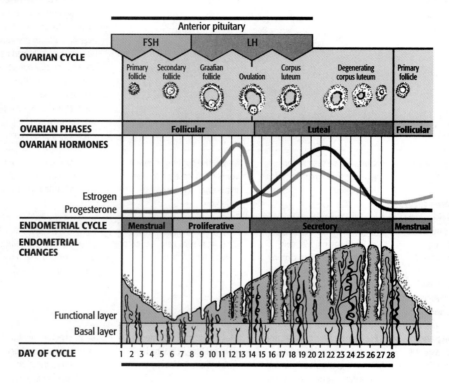

- Noncompliance with family planning
- Deficient knowledge related to family planning
- Risk for injury

Patient care goals

Significant aspects of the client's health history are identified during data collection and used to develop planning and goals, such as:
- All questions will be answered in a manner understood by the client and the procedure for the chosen contraceptive method will be described accurately by the client.
- Possible adverse reactions to contraceptive use will be identified.
- Follow-up appointments will be kept.
- The client will express satisfaction and success with the chosen contraceptive method.

Nursing interventions

- Nursing interventions in family planning consist mainly of client teaching. The implementation and rationales for such teaching include:
– Teach the proper use of the selected contraceptive method *to obtain desired effects of contraception and to minimize adverse effects.*
– Inform the client about possible adverse reactions to contraceptives, especially oral contraceptives (fluid retention, weight gain, breast tenderness, headache, breakthrough bleeding, chloasma, acne, yeast infection, nausea, and fatigue), and direct the client to report adverse reactions to the physician. *It may be necessary to change the type of contraceptive or the dosage of an oral contraceptive to relieve adverse reactions.*

– Instruct the client on the dietary needs of a woman taking an oral contraceptive. Tell her to increase her intake of foods high in vitamin B_6 (wheat, corn, liver, meat) and folic acid (liver; green, leafy vegetables). About 20% to 30% of oral contraceptive users have dietary deficiencies of vitamin B_6 (pyridoxine) and folic acid. Moreover, health care professionals increasingly speculate that oral contraceptive users should increase their intake of vitamins A, B_2, B_{12}, and C and niacin.
– Encourage compliance with follow-up appointments, and explain their importance. *During follow-up visits, evaluation of contraceptive use and adverse reactions can occur as well as repeating a Pap test and addressing the client's questions.*

Evaluation

● The client cooperates in providing health history information.
● The client describes the use of the selected contraceptive correctly.
● The client describes adverse reactions to the selected contraceptive and states her responsibility to report any that occur.
● The client makes an appointment for her next visit (if indicated).
● The client states that the current method of birth control is acceptable.

ANTEPARTUM PERIOD

The antepartum period extends from conception to the onset of labor. During this time, care of both the mother (client) and fetus focuses on health maintenance and the prevention of complications. Nursing care during the normal antepartum period includes taking a thorough maternal history, performing a complete physical examination, and educating the client about antepartum health.

Gametogenesis and conception

Gametogenesis is the production of specialized sex cells called *gametes:*
● The male gamete (spermatozoon) is produced in the seminiferous tubules of the testes during spermatogenesis.
● The female gamete (ovum) is produced in the graafian follicle of the ovary during oogenesis.
● As gametes mature, the number of chromosomes they contain is halved (through meiosis) from 46 to 23.

Conception, or fertilization, occurs with the fusion of a spermatozoon and an ovum (oocyte) in the ampulla of the fallopian tube.
● The fertilized egg is called a *zygote.*
● The diploid number of chromosomes (a pair of each chromosome; 44 autosomes and 2 sex chromosomes) is restored when the zygote is formed.
● A male zygote is formed if a spermatozoon carrying a Y chromosome fertilizes the ovum.
● A female zygote is formed if a spermatozoon carrying an X chromosome fertilizes the ovum.

Implantation and fetal development

Implantation occurs when the cellular wall of the blastocyst (trophoblast) implants itself in the endometrium of the anterior or posterior fundal region about 7 to 9 days after fertilization.
● Primary villi appear within weeks after implantation.
● After implantation, the endometrium is called the *decidua.*

Fetal structures

Structures unique to the fetus include fetal membranes, the umbilical cord, the placenta, and amniotic fluid. During placentation, chorionic villi invade the decidua and become the fetal portion of the future placenta. By the 4th week of gestation, a normal fetus begins to show noticeable signs of growth.

Fetal membranes

Two fetal membranes are unique to the fetus:
● The chorion is the fetal membrane closest to the uterine wall; it gives rise to the placenta.
● The amnion is the thin, tough, inner fetal membrane that lines the amniotic sac.

Three different embryonic germ layers generate fetal tissues:
● The ectoderm generates the epidermis, nervous system, pituitary gland, salivary glands, optic lens, lining of the lower portion of the anal canal, hair, and tooth enamel.
● The endoderm generates the epithelial lining of the larynx, trachea, bladder, urethra, prostate gland, auditory canal, liver, pancreas, and alimentary canal.
● The mesoderm generates the connective and sclerous tissues; the blood and vascular system; the musculature; teeth (except enamel); mesothelial lining of the pericardial, pleural, and peritoneal cavities; and kidneys and ureters.

Umbilical cord

The umbilical cord serves as the lifeline from the embryo to the placenta. At term, it measures 20″ to 22″ (51 to 56 cm) in length and about ¾″ (2 cm) in diameter. The umbilical cord contains two arteries, one vein, and Wharton's jelly (which prevents kinking of the cord in utero). Blood flows through the cord at about 400 ml/minute.

Fetal circulation

Fetal circulation structures include the:
- umbilical vein, which carries oxygenated blood to the fetus from the placenta
- umbilical arteries, which carry deoxygenated blood from the fetus to the placenta
- foramen ovale, which serves as the septal opening between the atria of the fetal heart
- ductus arteriosus, which connects the pulmonary artery to the aorta, allowing blood to shunt around the fetal lungs
- ductus venosus, which carries oxygenated blood from the umbilical vein to the inferior vena cava, bypassing the liver.

Placenta

The placenta weighs about 1 to 1.3 lb (455 to 590 g), measures 6″ to 10″ (15 to 25 cm) in diameter and, at term, is 1″ to 1¼″ (2.5 to 3 cm) thick. It contains 15 to 20 subdivisions called *cotyledons*. Rough in texture, the placenta appears red on the maternal surface and shiny and gray on the fetal surface. The placenta:
- functions as a transport mechanism between the mother and the fetus
- has a life span and function that depend on oxygen consumption and maternal circulation (circulation to the fetus and placenta improves when the mother lies on her left side)
- receives maternal oxygen by way of diffusion
- produces hormones, including human chorionic gonadotropin (HCG), human placental lactogen, gonadotropin-releasing hormone, thyrotropin-releasing factor, corticotropin, estrogen, and progesterone
- supplies the fetus with carbohydrates, water, fat, protein, minerals, and inorganic salts
- carries end products of fetal metabolism to the maternal circulation for excretion
- transfers passive immunity by way of maternal antibodies.

Amniotic fluid

The amniotic fluid prevents heat loss, preserves constant fetal body temperature, cushions the fetus, and facilitates fetal growth and development. Amniotic fluid is replaced every 3 hours.

At term, the uterus contains 800 to 1,200 ml of amniotic fluid, which is clear and yellowish and has a specific gravity of 1.007 to 1.025 and a pH of 7.0 to 7.25. Maternal serum provides amniotic fluid in early gestation, with increasing amounts derived from fetal urine late in gestation. Amniotic fluid contains:
- albumin
- bilirubin
- creatinine
- enzymes
- fat
- lanugo
- lecithin
- leukocytes
- sphingomyelin
- urea.

Antepartum data collection

The client's general health history and family health history may identify abnormal conditions that place the client at high risk for pregnancy-related complications. The client's menstrual history may be used to identify potential problems and to determine the client's expected date of delivery. (See *Estimating delivery dates and gestational age.*)

The client's obstetric history may reveal potential problems. Useful information from previous pregnancies includes *gravida* (the number of pregnancies, including the current one; also the term used for a pregnant woman) and *para* (the number of past pregnancies of at least 20 weeks' gestation; also the term used for a woman who has given birth to a viable fetus or infant). For each pregnancy, identify the type of delivery, the length of gestation, the length of labor, the size of the newborn, and information about problems that occurred. Many hospitals use the GTPAL system to document previous pregnancies:
- G stands for the number of pregnancies.
- T stands for the number of term infants born.
- P stands for the number of preterm infants born.
- A stands for the number of pregnancies ending in spontaneous or elective abortion.
- L stands for the number of living children. Multiple gestation doesn't change G (gravida) or P (para).

Family data collection

Health status and risk behaviors of the client's family members may reveal potential transmission of disease to the pregnant client and her fetus. Genetically transmitted diseases should be identified and considered in the care plan for the pregnant client.

Psychosocial assessment of the client and her partner discloses the couple's needs. The client's learning needs disclose deficient knowledge of changes that will occur in the upcoming months. Evaluation of the client's support systems discloses emotional support available to the client. Assessment of the client's economic status may reveal potential problems in meeting basic needs for a healthy pregnancy and delivery. Assessment of the family's ethnic and cultural values, beliefs, and practices reveal variations in family members' understanding of adaptations to pregnancy.

Cardiovascular changes

Cardiovascular system changes that occur due to pregnancy include:
- cardiac hypertrophy from increased blood volume and cardiac output
- displacement of the heart upward and to the left from pressure on the diaphragm
- progressive increase in blood volume, peaking in the third trimester at 30% to 50% more than prepregnancy levels
- resting pulse rate fluctuations, with increases ranging from 0 to 15 beats per minute at term
- pulmonic systolic and apical systolic murmurs resulting from decreased blood viscosity and increased blood flow
- increased femoral venous pressure caused by impaired circulation in the lower extremities (from pressure of the enlarged uterus on the pelvic veins and inferior vena cava)
- decreased cerebrospinal fluid space from enlargement of the vessels surrounding the spinal cord's dura mater
- increased fibrinogen levels (up to 50% at term) from hormonal influences
- increased levels of blood coagulation factors VII, IX, and X, leading to a hypercoagulable state
- increase of approximately 33% in total red blood cell (RBC) volume, despite hemodilution and decreasing erythrocyte count
- decrease in hematocrit (HCT) of about 7%
- increase in total hemoglobin (Hb) level of 12% to 15%, which is less than the overall plasma volume increase, thus reducing Hb concentration and leading to physiologic anemia of pregnancy

---

Estimating delivery dates and gestational age

- Nägele's rule is used to determine the estimated date of delivery by subtracting 3 months from the first day of the last menstrual period and adding 7 days; for example, October 5 – 3 months = July 5 + 7 days = July 12.
- Quickening is described as light fluttering and usually is felt between 16 and 22 weeks' gestation.
- Fetal heart sounds can be detected at 12 weeks' gestation with a Doppler ultrasound and can be auscultated with a fetoscope at 16 to 20 weeks' gestation.
- Fetal crown-to-rump measurements, determined by ultrasonography, can be used to assess the fetus's age until the head can be defined.
- Biparietal diameter is the widest transverse diameter of the fetal head. Measurements can be made by about 12 to 13 weeks' gestation.
- McDonald's rule uses fundal height to determine the duration of pregnancy in either lunar months or weeks. To use this rule, place a tape measure at the symphysis pubis and measure up and over the fundus. Fundal height in centimeters $\times$ $^2/_7$ = duration of pregnancy in lunar months; fundal height in centimeters $\times$ $^8/_7$ = duration of pregnancy in weeks.

- leukocyte production equal to or slightly greater than blood volume increase (average leukocyte count is 10,000 to 11,000/µl; this peaks at 25,000/µl during labor, possibly through an estrogen-related mechanism).

GI changes

GI system changes that occur due to pregnancy include:
- gum swelling from increased estrogen levels (gums may be spongy and hyperemic)
- lateral and posterior displacement of the intestines
- superior and lateral displacement of the stomach
- delayed intestinal motility and gastric and gallbladder emptying time from smooth-muscle relaxation caused by high placental progesterone levels
- nausea and vomiting, which usually subside after the first trimester
- hemorrhoids late in pregnancy from venous pressure
- constipation from increased progesterone levels, resulting in increased water absorption from the colon
- displacement of the appendix from McBurney's point (making diagnosis of appendicitis difficult).

Hormonal changes

Endocrine system (hormonal) changes that occur due to pregnancy include:

- increased basal metabolic rate (up 25% at term) caused by demands of the fetus and uterus and by increased oxygen consumption
- increased iodine metabolism from slight hyperplasia of the thyroid caused by increased estrogen levels
- slight hyperparathyroidism from increased requirement for calcium and vitamin D
- elevated plasma parathyroid hormone levels, peaking between 15 and 35 weeks' gestation
- slightly enlarged pituitary gland
- increased production of prolactin by the pituitary gland late in pregnancy
- increased estrogen levels and hypertrophy of the adrenal cortex
- increased cortisol levels to regulate protein and carbohydrate metabolism
- possibly decreased maternal blood glucose levels
- decreased insulin production early in pregnancy
- increased production of estrogen, progesterone, and human chorionic somatomammotropin by the placenta and increased levels of maternal cortisol, which reduce the mother's ability to use insulin, thus ensuring an adequate glucose supply for the fetus and placenta.

Respiratory changes

Respiratory system changes that occur due to pregnancy include:

- increased vascularization of the respiratory tract caused by increased estrogen levels
- shortening of the lungs caused by the enlarged uterus
- upward displacement of the diaphragm by the uterus
- increased tidal volume, causing slight hyperventilation
- increased chest circumference (by about 2³⁄₈″ [6 cm])
- altered breathing, with abdominal breathing replacing thoracic breathing as pregnancy progresses
- slight increase (2 breaths per minute) in respiratory rate
- lowered threshold for carbon dioxide due to increased levels of progesterone.

Metabolic changes

Metabolic system changes that occur due to pregnancy include:

- increased water retention caused by higher levels of steroidal sex hormones, decreased serum protein levels, and increased intracapillary pressure and permeability
- increased levels of serum lipids, lipoproteins, and cholesterol

- increased iron requirements caused by fetal demands
- increased carbohydrate needs
- increased protein retention from hyperplasia and hypertrophy of maternal tissues
- weight gain of 25 to 30 lb (11.5 to 13.5 kg).

FAST FACT

Maternal weight gain is commonly estimated at 3, 12, and 12 lb (1.4, 5.4, and 5.4 kg) for the first, second, and third trimesters, respectively.

Skin changes

Integumentary system changes that occur due to pregnancy include:

- hyperactive sweat and sebaceous glands
- changing pigmentation from the increase of melanocyte-stimulating hormone caused by increased estrogen and progesterone levels (darkened line from symphysis pubis to umbilicus known as linea nigra)
- darkening of the nipples, areola, cervix, vagina, and vulva
- pigmentary changes, known as facial chloasma, on the nose, cheeks, and forehead.

Genitourinary changes

Genitourinary system changes that occur due to pregnancy include:

- dilated ureters and renal pelvis caused by progesterone and pressure from the enlarged uterus
- increased glomerular filtration rate (GFR) and renal plasma flow (RPF) early in pregnancy; elevated GFR until delivery, but a near-normal RPF level by term
- increased clearance of urea and creatinine due to increased renal function
- decreased blood urea and nonprotein nitrogen values due to increased renal function
- glucosuria due to increased glomerular filtration without an increase in tubular reabsorptive capacity
- decreased bladder tone
- increased sodium retention due to hormonal influences
- increases in dimensions of the uterus from approximately 2¹⁄₂″ to 12¹⁄₂″ (6.5 to 32 cm) in length; 1¹⁄₂″ to 9¹⁄₂″ (4 to 24 cm) in width; 8⁵⁄₈″ to 10″ (22 to 25 cm) in depth; 2 to 42 oz (57 to 1,191 g) in weight; and ¹⁄₈ to 170 oz (3.5 to 5,028 ml) in volume (see *Typical uterine changes during pregnancy*)
- hypertrophied uterine muscle cells (5 to 10 times normal size)

Typical uterine changes during pregnancy

Beginning at the 20th week, fundal height equals gestational age, plus or minus 2 cm.

UTERUS	NONPREGNANT	PREGNANT (AT TERM)
Length	6.5 cm	32 cm
Width	4 cm	24 cm
Depth	2.5 cm	22 cm
Weight	50 g	1,000 g

FUNDAL HEIGHT RELATED TO GESTATIONAL WEEKS

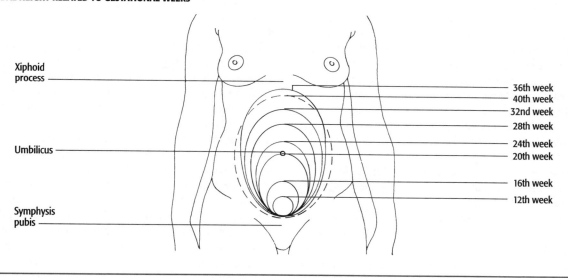

Signs and symptoms of pregnancy

- increased vascularity, edema, hypertrophy, and hyperplasia of the cervical glands
- increased vaginal secretions with a pH of 3.5 to 6
- discontinued ovulation and maturation of new follicles
- thickening of vaginal mucosa, loosening of vaginal connective tissue, and hypertrophy of small muscle cells.

Signs and symptoms of pregnancy

Presumptive (early) signs and symptoms of pregnancy may include:
- AMENORRHEA or slight, painless spotting of unknown cause in early gestation
- breast enlargement and tenderness
- fatigue
- increased skin pigmentation
- nausea and vomiting

- quickening (the first recognizable movement of the fetus)
- thinning and softening of fingernails
- urinary frequency and urgency.

Signs and symptoms of a probable pregnancy include:
- ballottement (passive fetal movement in response to tapping of the lower portion of the uterus or cervix)
- Braxton Hicks contractions (painless uterine contractions that occur throughout pregnancy)
- Chadwick's sign (change in color of the vaginal walls from normal light pink to deep violet)
- Goodell's sign (softening of the cervix)
- Hegar's sign (softening of the lower uterine segment) that may be present at 6 to 8 weeks' gestation
- positive pregnancy test results
- uterine enlargement.

Signs and symptoms of a definite pregnancy include:
● detection of fetal heartbeat (by 17 to 20 weeks' gestation)
● detection of fetal movements (after 16 weeks' gestation)
● ultrasonography findings (as early as 6 weeks' gestation).

Diagnostic findings

● Blood type, Rh, and abnormal antibodies identify whether the fetus is at risk for erythroblastosis fetalis or hyperbilirubinemia.
● Immunologic tests, such as rubella antibodies, detect the presence of rubella; rapid plasma reagin detects untreated syphilis; and hepatitis B surface antigen detects hepatitis B.
● Urine tests measure HCG to confirm pregnancy.
● Hematologic studies involve the use of blood samples to analyze and measure RBCs, white blood cells (WBCs), erythrocyte sedimentation rate (ESR), prothrombin time (PT), partial thromboplastin time (PTT), platelets, Hb level, and HCT. (See *Maternal and neonatal laboratory values.*)
● Genital cultures, such as a gonorrhea smear and chlamydia test, are used to detect sexually transmitted diseases (STDs).
● Triple screen between 15 and 20 weeks' gestation is used to identify a fetus at increased risk for Down syndrome and neural tube defect.
● High maternal serum alpha-fetoprotein levels may suggest fetal neural tube defects, such as spina bifida and anencephaly.
● Amniocentesis is usually performed after the 14th week of gestation, when amniotic fluid is sufficient and the uterus has moved into the abdominal cavity. This procedure involves transabdominal insertion of a spinal needle into the uterus to aspirate amniotic fluid. This procedure is used to:
– determine gestational age and fetal lung maturity by analyzing the lecithin-sphingomyelin ratio, two key components of surfactant
– measure creatinine levels
– diagnose genetic disorders, such as chromosomal aberrations, sex-linked disorders, inborn errors of metabolism, and neural tube defect
– diagnose and evaluate isoimmune disease, including Rh sensitization and ABO blood type incompatibility.
● Chorionic villi sampling can be performed as early as 8 weeks' gestation. It involves removal and analysis of a small tissue specimen from the fetal portion of the placenta. This test helps determine the genetic makeup of the fetus, providing earlier diagnosis and allowing earlier and safer abortion if the fetus carries the risk of spontaneous abortion, infection, hematoma, fetal limb defects, and intrauterine death.
● Ultrasonography, a noninvasive and painless procedure, uses ultrasonic waves reflected by tissues of different densities to visualize deep structures of the body. Reflected signals are then amplified and processed to produce a visual display, providing immediate results without harm to the fetus or mother. Ultrasound can be used to detect:
– fetal death
– malformation
– malpresentation
– placental abnormalities
– multiple gestation
– hydramnios or oligohydramnios.
● The nonstress test (NST) is used to detect fetal heart accelerations in response to fetal movement. This noninvasive test provides simple, inexpensive, immediate results without contraindications or complications. It may be indicated for a client at risk for uteroplacental insufficiency or for altered fetal movements. The NST can be performed between 32 and 34 weeks' gestation. A nonreactive test result indicates the possibility of fetal hypoxia, fetal sleep cycle, or the effects of drugs. The results may be inconclusive if the client is extremely obese.
● The oxytocin challenge test (OCT) is used to evaluate fetal ability to withstand an oxytocin-induced contraction. This test, given after a nonreactive NST result, requires I.V. administration of oxytocin in increasing doses every 15 to 20 minutes until three high-quality uterine contractions are obtained within 10 minutes. The OCT is performed on a client at risk for uteroplacental insufficiency or fetal compromise from diabetes, heart disease, hypertension, or renal disease or on a client with a history of stillbirth. The OCT isn't indicated for those with previous classic cesarean section or third-trimester bleeding or for those at high risk for preterm labor.
● The nipple stimulation stress test induces contractions by activating sensory receptors in the areola, triggering the release of oxytocin by the posterior pituitary gland. The receptors are activated by rolling the nipple manually or by applying a warm washcloth. This test has the same reactive pattern as the reactive NST result.
● The vibroacoustic stimulation test uses vibration and sound to induce fetal reactivity during an NST. Vibration is produced by an artificial larynx or a fetal acoustic stimulator (over the fetus's head for 1 to 5 seconds). This test is noninvasive, quick, and convenient.

Maternal and neonatal laboratory values

TEST	NONPREGNANT WOMEN	PREGNANT WOMEN	POSTPARTUM WOMEN	TERM NEONATES
Hemoglobin (Hb)	12 to 16 g/dl	11 to 15 g/dl	11 to 15 g/dl	15 to 20 g/dl
Hematocrit	37% to 48%	36% to 46% (32% to 35% indicates physiologic anemia)	32% to 46%	43% to 61%
Red blood cells	4 to 5 million/µl	5 to 6.25 million/µl	5 to 6.25 million/µl	5 to 6 million/µl
White blood cells	5,000 to 10,000/µl	5,000 to 12,000/µl	5,000 to 16,000/µl (possibly up to 25,000/µl)	10,000 to 30,000/µl
Platelets	150,000 to 400,000/mm³	150,000 to 400,000/mm³	150,000 to 400,000/mm³	100,000 to 280,000/mm³
Serum glucose	65 to 105 mg/dl	Below 120 mg/dl	Below 120 mg/dl	First 24 hours: 40 to 100 mg/dl
Glucola screen	Below 140 to 150 mg/dl	Below 140 to 150 mg/dl	(Not performed)	(Not performed)
3-hour glucose tolerance test (3GTT)	1-hour: below 190 mg/dl 2-hour: below 165 mg/dl 3-hour: below 145 mg/dl	1-hour: below 190 mg/dl 2-hour: below 165 mg/dl 3-hour: below 145 mg/dl	(Not performed)	(Not performed)
Hb A₁C	6% to 8%	6% to 8%	(Not performed)	(Not performed)
Serum bilirubin (total)	(Not performed)	(Not performed)	(Not performed)	Cord blood: Below 2.8 mg/dl At 24 hours: 2 to 6 mg/dl At 3 to 5 days: 4 to 6 mg/dl
Urine protein	Negative	Negative or trace	Negative to +1 False positive may occur due to lochia	Negative
Urine glucose	Negative	Negative or 1+	Negative to +1 False positive may occur due to lochia	Negative

● The biophysical profile assesses four to six parameters — fetal breathing movements, body movements, muscle tone, amniotic fluid volume, heart rate reactivity, and placental grade — using real-time ultrasound. This test is noninvasive and quick and can detect central nervous system depression.

● Fetal blood flow studies use umbilical or uterine Doppler velocimetry to evaluate vascular resistance, especially in clients with hypertension, diabetes, isoimmunization, and lupus. These studies are useful when congenital anomalies or cardiac arrhythmias are suspected.

● Percutaneous umbilical blood sampling (PUBS) is an invasive procedure that involves inserting a spinal needle into the umbilical cord to obtain fetal blood samples or to transfuse the fetus in utero. Usually performed during the second or third trimester, PUBS is indicated when the fetus is at risk for congenital and chromosomal abnormalities, congenital infection, or anemia. It carries a 1% to 2% risk of fetal loss.

Nursing diagnoses
● Ineffective health maintenance
● Risk for deficient fluid volume

Patient care goals
● The results of the client's health history and physical and diagnostic examinations will be within normal limits.
● The client will be able to describe the warning signs of pregnancy complications.
● The client will discuss concerns about her pregnancy related to personal and family psychosocial needs.
● The client will return for routine follow-up visits.

Nursing interventions
● Teach the warning signs of pregnancy-related complications: vaginal bleeding, gush of fluid from the vagina, persistent vomiting, chills and fever, abdominal pain, visual disturbances, severe headache, and swelling of the face and hands. *These warning signs indicate complications, such as spontaneous abortion, fluid and electrolyte imbalance, pregnancy-induced hypertension (PIH), and infection.*
● Explain that only prescribed medication should be taken. *Many medications are teratogenic, especially in the first trimester, when the fetal organs are developing.*
● Explain the suggested treatment for nausea and vomiting (morning sickness). *Nausea and vomiting can be managed by eating dry crackers before rising; eating small, frequent, high-protein meals; and avoiding spicy and fried foods.*
● Stress the importance of regular health supervision during pregnancy. *The quality of prenatal care has a great impact on the well-being of the mother and fetus. In addition to enabling the physician to detect and treat problems promptly, prenatal visits provide an opportunity for teaching the client about pregnancy, labor and delivery, and postpartum and neonatal care.*

● Provide the opportunity for the client to ask questions and talk about expectations. *Listening to the client helps to establish an open, positive, caring nurse-client relationship. It also provides an opportunity to evaluate individual needs and provide appropriate care.*

Evaluation
● The results of the client's health history and physical and diagnostic examinations are within normal limits.
● The client describes the warning signs of pregnancy complications and the importance of reporting them.
● The client verbalizes gradual acceptance of body changes of early pregnancy.
● The client identifies sources of emotional and material support adequate to meet personal and family needs during the pregnancy.
● The client has made an appointment for her next visit.

ANTEPARTUM COMPLICATIONS

During the antepartum period, the client must be monitored carefully for complications, some of which can be life threatening for the mother and fetus. The following entries focus on nursing care of the antepartum client with complications.

Abortion, spontaneous

SPONTANEOUS ABORTION, or simply abortion, is the term used to describe termination of a pregnancy when gestation is less than 20 weeks. (See *Care during threatened or inevitable abortion; Complications of early pregnancy,* page 160; and *Preterm labor,* page 161.)

Possible causes
● Hormonal imbalances
● Infection
● Reproductive tract abnormalities
● Use of abnormal conception products

Data collection findings
● Bleeding, abdominal cramps or pain, cervical dilation, and rupture of membranes, which may indicate inevitable abortion
● Alteration in vital signs, which may indicate shock or infection
● Change in emotional status that may reflect fear, guilt, and anxiety

Care during threatened or inevitable abortion

TYPE	SYMPTOMS	NURSING CONSIDERATIONS
Threatened abortion	Vaginal bleeding, cramping, cervix remains closed	• Maintain the client on bed rest with a light diet. • Instruct the client to avoid any kind of straining. • Administer a mild sedative as ordered. • Keep a perineal pad count to determine blood loss. • Tell the client to restrict sexual intercourse.
Inevitable abortion	Vaginal bleeding, cramping, cervical dilation	*Complete abortion* • Keep a complete perineal pad count and save all tissue samples. • Monitor blood or fluid replacement as necessary. *Incomplete abortion* • Use the same considerations as for complete abortion. • Prepare for dilatation and curettage.

Diagnostic findings
• The amount of bleeding can be assessed through a pad count.
• Examination of any tissue expelled vaginally may reveal products of conception and can be used to determine if the abortion was complete or incomplete.

Nursing diagnoses
• Risk for injury
• Dysfunctional grieving

Treatment
• Bed rest until bleeding is controlled
• Dilatation and curettage (D&C) if incomplete abortion occurs

Patient care goals
• The client won't develop complications, such as infection and shock.
• The client will express knowledge of her condition and of the procedures being performed.
• The client won't exhibit signs of extreme anxiety and fear.
• The client will have an opportunity to begin grieving.
• The client will identify her support system and available resources.

Nursing interventions
• Explain all procedures *to promote the client's trust and to help reduce anxiety.*

• Estimate blood loss, recording the number of perineal pads used, the degree of pad saturation, and a description of pad contents *to estimate the client's blood loss and risk for hemorrhagic shock.*
• Evaluate pad contents *to determine whether an abortion has occurred and whether all the products of conception were expelled (complete abortion) or only a portion (incomplete abortion).*
• Obtain a type and crossmatch blood specimen *in preparation for replacement of blood or blood products, if necessary.*
• Monitor vital signs frequently *to detect complications, such as infection and hemorrhage.*
• If the abortion is incomplete, prepare the client for D&C *to remove the risk of hemorrhage and infection.*
• Allow verbalization *to assist with acceptance of the loss of pregnancy.*

Evaluation
• The client doesn't develop complications.
• The client verbalizes understanding of what happened with her pregnancy.
• The client begins to use positive coping strategies to deal with her anxiety and begins to express her feelings about the loss of her pregnancy.

Abruptio placentae
ABRUPTIO PLACENTAE is premature separation of the placenta from the uterine wall after 20 to 24 weeks' gestation. It may occur as late as the first or second stage of

Complications of early pregnancy

CONDITION	DEFINITION	SIGNS AND SYMPTOMS	TREATMENT	NURSING CONSIDERATIONS
Ectopic pregnancy	Pregnancy outside the uterine cavity (the fallopian tube is the most common site)	• Signs and symptoms of pregnancy • Rupture at 6 to 12 weeks (usually) • Possible vaginal bleeding • Severe pain in lower abdomen • Vaginal tenderness • Shock	• Salpingectomy • Salpingostomy and tubal repair	• Assess the client for bleeding and pain. • Prepare the client for abdominal surgery. • Provide emotional support to the client.
Hydatidiform mole	Abnormal pregnancy that results in a grapelike cluster of vesicles	• Incidence in two age groups: under 20 and over 40 • Rapid uterine growth • Nausea and vomiting • Elevated levels of chorionic gonadotropin • Uterine bleeding in first and second trimesters • Symptoms of preeclampsia	• Hysterotomy • Hysterectomy • Dilatation and curettage	• Prepare the client for the procedures. • Allow the client to verbalize her feelings. • Stress the importance of follow-up care (a high incidence of choriocarcinoma is associated with hydatidiform mole). • Plan birth control for at least 1 year.
Hyperemesis gravidarum	Persistent vomiting during pregnancy, thought to be caused by high chorionic gonadotropin levels or psychological problem	• Nausea and vomiting • Weight loss • Fatigue • Signs of dehydration • Signs of starvation	• Antiemetics • I.V. fluids (vitamins and electrolytes) • Quiet environment • Sedation • Counseling	• Provide treatment as ordered. • Allow the client to verbalize her feelings.
Incompetent cervix	Failure of the cervix to remain closed, resulting in abortion at 18 to 20 weeks' gestation	• Signs and symptoms of inevitable abortion	• Cerclage of the cervix (using Shirodkar operation or McDonald maneuver) for future pregnancies	• Assist with the procedure. • Provide emotional support to the client. • Maintain bed rest for 24 hours after cerclage.

labor. Placental separation is measured by degree (from grades 0 to 3) to determine the fetal and maternal outcome. (See *Grading abruptio placentae,* page 162.)

Perinatal mortality depends on the degree of placental separation and the fetal level of maturity. Most serious complications stem from hypoxia, prematurity, and anemia. The maternal mortality rate is about 6% and depends on the severity of the bleeding, the presence of coagulation defects, hypofibrinogenemia, and the time lapse between placental separation and delivery.

Possible causes
• Abdominal trauma
• Cocaine use

Preterm labor

Preterm labor begins between 20 and 37 weeks' gestation. This quick-reference overview of preterm labor outlines its incidence and etiology, symptoms, risk factors, treatments, and associated nursing care.

Incidence and etiology
- From 8% to 19% of all births
- From 75% to 80% of all neonatal mortality and morbidity
- Pathophysiology related to increased estrogen, fetal stress, increased stretch of uterine muscle, increased prostaglandins, increased maternal oxygen

Symptoms
- Palpable uterine contractions, more than 4 per hour, greater than 30 seconds in duration
- Effaced and dilated cervix
- Increased vaginal drainage

Risk factors
- Medical and pregnancy history factors (such as previous preterm delivery, diethylstilbestrol exposure, cervical shortening)
- Current pregnancy problems (such as multiple gestation, pregnancy-induced hypertension, infection, premature rupture of membranes)
- Socioeconomic factors (such as age extremes, insufficient prenatal care, education)
- Lifestyle habits (such as poor nutrition or substance abuse)

Treatment
- Tocolytics (magnesium sulfate, ritodrine, terbutaline)
- Glucocorticoids (betamethasone)
- Medical therapy (cervical cerclage, bed rest)

Nursing care
- Discuss risks related to preterm delivery with the client and her support system.
- Teach self-care measures:
  – Increase fluid intake to 2 to 3 qt (2 to 3 L)/day.
  – Empty bladder every 2 hours while awake.
  – Follow activity restrictions (bed rest, lay on left side).
  – Avoid nipple stimulation.
  – Use home monitoring techniques.

- Decreased blood flow to the placenta
- Hydramnios
- Multifetal pregnancy
- Other risk factors (low serum folic acid levels, vascular or renal disease, PIH)

Data collection findings
- Acute abdominal pain, which may indicate placental abruption
- Hemorrhage, either concealed or apparent, with dark red vaginal bleeding, which indicates intrauterine bleeding
- Rigid abdomen, which indicates high uterine tonicity resulting from hemorrhage
- Altered vital signs, which may indicate shock
- Frequent, low-amplitude contractions (noted with external fetal monitor), which may occur as the uterus attempts to contract or constrict blood vessels and control bleeding
- Uteroplacental insufficiency as evidenced by fetal distress

Diagnostic findings
- Ultrasonography locates the placenta and a clot or hematoma may be apparent.
- Hematology may show disseminated intravascular coagulation (DIC) as indicated by increased PTT and PT, elevated level of fibrinogen degradation products, decreased fibrinogen level, or decreased platelet count.

Nursing diagnoses
- Ineffective tissue perfusion (cardiopulmonary)
- Risk for deficient fluid volume
- Acute pain
- Anxiety

Treatment
- Transfusion of packed RBCs, platelets, and fresh frozen plasma, if necessary
- Cesarean delivery

Patient care goals
- The client will remain hemodynamically stable.
- The fetus will maintain an adequate heart rate and perfusion until delivery.

Grading abruptio placentae

Separation of the placenta from the uterine wall is classified as minimal, moderate, or extreme. Hemorrhaging may or may not be apparent, even with complete separation.

GRADE	CRITERIA
0	Maternal and fetal signs don't indicate difficulty. Premature separation isn't apparent until the placenta is examined after delivery.
1	Minimal separation causes vaginal bleeding and alterations in maternal vital signs, but hemorrhagic shock and fetal distress don't appear.
2	Moderate separation produces signs of fetal distress. The uterus is tense and painful when palpated.
3	Extreme separation occurs, possibly causing maternal shock and fetal death in the absence of immediate intervention.

- The client won't exhibit signs of extreme anxiety and fear.
- The client will indicate a decrease in pain.

Nursing interventions

- Monitor maternal vital signs, fetal heart rate (FHR), uterine contractions, and vaginal bleeding *to assess maternal and fetal well-being.*
- Monitor fluid and electrolyte balance *to assess kidney function.*
- Avoid pelvic or vaginal examinations and enemas *to prevent further placental disruption.*
- Maintain an I.V. line for administration of fresh whole blood, packed RBCs, platelets, or plasma *to replace blood volume.*
- Provide oxygen by mask *to minimize fetal hypoxia.*
- Obtain maternal laboratory values *to assess for DIC.*
- Position the client in a left lateral recumbent position *to help relieve pressure on the vena cava from an enlarged uterus, which could further compromise fetal circulation, and to promote comfort.*
- Provide emotional support *to allay the client's anxiety.*

Evaluation

- The client has stable vital signs.
- The fetus maintains a strong heartbeat until delivery and is adequately perfused.
- The client remains calm.
- The client is more comfortable.

Adolescent pregnancy

A teenage mother is at risk for such complications as PIH, cephalopelvic disproportion, anemia, and nutritional deficiencies. Teenagers also have a high incidence of STDs, posing a concern for the mother and neonate.

Infants born to teenage mothers are at risk for such complications as prematurity and low birth weight.

Possible causes

Contributing factors for adolescent pregnancy include:
- desire to gain love, adulthood, and independence through pregnancy
- fear of reporting sexual activity to parents
- high level of adolescent sexual activity
- lack of appropriate role models
- limited access to contraceptives
- low level of education correlated with incorrect use of contraceptives
- lack of knowledge about ability to become pregnant
- sporadic use of contraception.

Data collection findings

- Amenorrhea
- Denial of pregnancy, which may delay the client from seeking medical attention early in pregnancy

Diagnostic findings

- Pregnancy test is positive.
- Ultrasound confirms presence of fetus.

Nursing diagnoses
- Deficient knowledge (client) about pregnancy and related responsibilities
- Imbalanced nutrition: Less than body requirements
- Interrupted family processes

Treatment
- Diet with calorie intake sufficient to support the growing adolescent and her developing fetus

Drug therapy options
- Antibiotic for STDs (if necessary)

Patient care goals
- The client will increase her knowledge concerning pregnancy and related responsibilities concerning the fetus.
- The client will follow a nutritious diet.
- The client will receive support from family members.

Nursing interventions
- Monitor the client's weight gain *to assess for nutritional deficiencies.*
- Monitor urine protein *to detect possible PIH* and glucose levels *to detect possible gestational diabetes.*
- Obtain fundal height *to detect how the pregnancy is progressing.*
- Monitor fetal heart sounds *to monitor fetal well-being.*
- Assess the client's knowledge of her pregnancy *to determine the need for further teaching.*
- Assess the client's family and available support *to determine the need for referrals.*
- Provide nutritional support and encouragement *to promote the well-being of the mother and fetus.*
- Stress the importance of attending scheduled prenatal appointments *to promote the well-being of the mother and fetus.*
- Advise the client of her options, including terminating the pregnancy, continuing the pregnancy and giving up the infant for adoption, and continuing the pregnancy and keeping the infant *to promote informed decision making.*
- Allow the client to express her feelings about her pregnancy and herself *to promote mental and emotional well-being.*

Evaluation
- The client participates in prenatal care.
- The client follows a nutritious diet and has appropriate weight gain.
- The client receives support during pregnancy.

Ectopic pregnancy

ECTOPIC PREGNANCY is implantation of the fertilized ovum outside the uterine cavity. Most commonly, ectopic pregnancy occurs in a fallopian tube; other sites include the cervix, ovary, and abdominal cavity. It's the second most frequent cause of vaginal bleeding early in pregnancy.

Possible causes
- Hormonal factors
- Malformed fallopian tubes
- Ovulation induction drugs
- Progestin-only oral contraceptives
- Tubal atony
- Tubal damage from pelvic inflammatory disease
- Tubal damage from previous pelvic or tubal surgery
- Tubal spasms
- Use of intrauterine devices

Data collection findings
- Irregular vaginal bleeding and dull abdominal pain on the affected side early in pregnancy
- Rupture of tubes, causing sudden and severe abdominal pain, syncope, and referred shoulder pain as the abdomen fills with blood
- Unstable blood pressure and rapid, thready pulse, possibly indicating shock secondary to hemorrhage

 FAST FACT

Signs of possible early ectopic pregnancy are irregular vaginal bleeding and dull abdominal pain. Signs of possible ruptured ectopic pregnancy are severe abdominal pain, orthostatic hypotension, tachycardia, and dizziness.

Diagnostic findings
- HCG titers are abnormally low.
- Ultrasound is positive for ruptured tube and collective pelvic fluid.
- Vaginal examination reveals a palpable tender mass in Douglas's cul-de-sac.

Nursing diagnoses
- Deficient fluid volume
- Risk for infection
- Acute pain

Treatment
- Laparotomy to ligate the bleeding vessels and remove or repair damaged fallopian tube

● Transfusion therapy, including packed RBCs (if bleeding is uncontrolled)

Drug therapy options
● Methotrexate (Folex) followed by leucovorin (Wellcovorin) to stop the trophoblastic cells from growing (therapy continues until negative HCG levels are achieved), if the fallopian tube hasn't ruptured

Patient care goals
● The client will remain hemodynamically stable.
● The client will have the ectopic pregnancy resolved safely.
● The client will verbalize understanding of the possible cause and required treatment of the ectopic pregnancy.
● The client will verbalize feelings over the termination of the pregnancy.

Nursing interventions
● Monitor vital signs and intake and output *to assess for intense blood loss and shock.*
● Monitor for severe abdominal pain, orthostatic hypotension, tachycardia, and dizziness, *which may indicate rupturing ectopic pregnancy.*
● Monitor WBC count and ESR *for signs of infection.*
● Administer I.V. fluid replacement *to accommodate for blood loss.*
● Maintain a patent I.V. line for administration of blood products *to replace volume loss.*
● Administer $Rh_o D$ immune globulin *to combat isoimmunization in the client who's Rh-negative.*
● Provide routine postoperative care if surgical intervention is necessary.
● Provide emotional support for parents grieving over the loss of the pregnancy.

Evaluation
● The client maintains stable vital signs.
● The ectopic pregnancy is resolved without injury to the client.
● The client verbalizes understanding of the ectopic pregnancy.
● The client demonstrates appropriate coping mechanisms in dealing with the loss of the pregnancy.

Gestational diabetes mellitus

In GESTATIONAL DIABETES MELLITUS, the client's pancreas, stressed by the normal adaptations to pregnancy, can't meet the increased demands for insulin. A client may have preexisting diabetes or may develop gestational diabetes while she's pregnant. Gestational diabetes is associated with an increased risk of congenital anomalies, hydramnios, macrosomia, PIH, spontaneous abortion, and fetal death. Additionally, the infant of a client with diabetes is at risk for developing sacral agenesis, a congenital anomaly characterized by incomplete formation of the vertebral column. The client with gestational diabetes has an increased risk of developing diabetes mellitus.

Possible causes
● Stress of pregnancy

Risk factors
● Chronic hypertension
● Family history of diabetes
● Gestational diabetes in previous pregnancies
● Maternal age older than 25

Data collection findings
● Glycosuria
● Ketonuria
● Polyuria
● Possible monilial infection (vaginal yeast infection)

Diagnostic findings
● One-hour glucose tolerance test reveals a glucose level greater than 140 mg/dl.
● Three-hour glucose tolerance test reveals a fasting serum glucose level of 105 mg/dl or greater.
● Three-hour glucose tolerance test reveals a 1-hour serum glucose level of 190 mg/dl or greater.
● Three-hour glucose tolerance test reveals a 2-hour serum glucose level of 165 mg/dl or greater.
● Three-hour glucose tolerance test reveals a 3-hour serum glucose level of 145 mg/dl or greater.

Nursing diagnoses
● Imbalanced nutrition: More than body requirements
● Risk for deficient fluid volume
● Ineffective coping

Treatment
● 1,800- to 2,200-calorie diet, divided into three meals and three snacks that should also be low in fat and cholesterol and high in fiber
● Oral antidiabetic agents contraindicated because of adverse effects on the fetus

Drug therapy options
● Insulin

Patient care goals
● The client will describe the responsibility related to insulin administration and blood glucose regulation.
● The client will understand the recommended diet and the importance of following it.
● The client will demonstrate coping mechanisms to deal with the complications of gestational diabetes mellitus.
● The client will verbalize understanding of the potential effects diabetes mellitus may have on her fetus.

Nursing interventions
● Teach the client to use the glucose monitoring system and administer insulin correctly *to adequately control her blood sugar level.*
● Encourage adherence to dietary regulations *to maintain euglycemia.*
● Encourage the client to exercise moderately *to reduce blood glucose levels and decrease the need for insulin.*
● Prepare the client for antepartum fetal surveillance testing, including OCT, nipple stimulation stress testing, amniotic fluid index, biophysical profile, and NST *to assess fetal well-being.*
● Encourage the client to verbalize her feelings *to allay her fears.*
● Provide emotional support *to reduce anxiety.*

Evaluation
● The client appropriately performs serum glucose monitoring and insulin regulation and administration.
● The client follows the recommended diet appropriately.
● The client demonstrates coping mechanisms that address the occurrence of diabetes mellitus.
● The client asks appropriate questions about the diagnostic assessments of the fetus's well-being.

Hydatidiform mole

HYDATIDIFORM MOLE (also known as gestational trophoblastic disease or molar pregnancy) is a developmental anomaly of the placenta that converts the chorionic villi into a mass of clear vesicles (hydatid vesicles). There are two types:
● complete mole, in which there's neither an embryo nor an amniotic sac
● partial mole, in which there's an embryo (usually with multiple abnormalities) and an amniotic sac.

Possible causes
● Poor maternal nutrition
● Defective ovum

Data collection findings
● Intermittent or continuous bright red or brownish vaginal bleeding by 12 weeks' gestation
● Passage of clear fluid-filled vesicles and vaginal bleeding
● Disproportionate enlargement of the uterus
● Absence of fetal heart tones
● Excessive nausea and vomiting
● Symptoms of pregnancy-induced hypertension before 20 weeks' gestation

Diagnostic findings
● HCG levels are extremely high for early pregnancy.
● Ultrasonography fails to reveal a fetal skeleton.

Nursing diagnoses
● Risk for deficient fluid volume
● Anticipatory grieving
● Deficient knowledge (client and partner)

Treatment
● Therapeutic abortion (suction and curettage) if a spontaneous abortion doesn't occur
● Pelvic examinations and chest X-rays at regular intervals
● Weekly monitoring of HCG levels until they remain normal for 3 consecutive weeks
● Periodic follow-up for 1 to 2 years because of the increased risk of neoplasm

Drug therapy options
● Methotrexate (Folex) prophylactically (the drug of choice for choriocarcinoma)

Patient care goals
● The client will remain stable and the molar pregnancy will be resolved safely.
● The client will verbalize feelings over the loss of the pregnancy.
● The client will express knowledge about the cause and treatment of molar pregnancy.

Nursing interventions
● Monitor and record vital signs and intake and output *to assess for changes that may indicate complications.*
● Provide emotional support for the grieving couple *to assist in coping with pregnancy loss.*

● Monitor vaginal bleeding *to assess for hemorrhage.*
● Send the contents of the uterine evacuation to the laboratory for analysis *to assess for the presence of hydatid vesicles.*
● Advise the client to avoid pregnancy until HCG levels are normal (may take up to 2 years*) to avoid future complications.*

Evaluation

● The client's condition is stable and the pregnancy is resolved safely.
● The client demonstrates appropriate coping mechanisms in dealing with pregnancy loss.
● The client verbalizes understanding of the cause of and treatment for hydatidiform mole.

Hyperemesis gravidarum

HYPEREMESIS GRAVIDARUM is persistent, uncontrolled vomiting that begins in the 1st weeks of pregnancy and may continue throughout pregnancy. Unlike "morning sickness," hyperemesis can have serious complications, including severe weight loss, dehydration, and electrolyte imbalance. (See *Comparing morning sickness and hyperemesis gravidarum.*)

Possible causes
● Gonadotropin production
● Psychological factors
● Trophoblastic activity

Data collection findings
● Continuous, severe nausea and vomiting
● Jaundice
● Dehydration
● Electrolyte imbalance

● Dry skin and mucous membranes
● Nonelastic skin turgor
● Oliguria
● Metabolic acidosis

Diagnostic findings
● Arterial blood gas analysis reveals alkalosis.
● Hb level and HCT are elevated.
● Serum potassium level reveals hypokalemia.
● Urine ketone levels are elevated.
● Urine specific gravity is increased.

Nursing diagnoses
● Imbalanced nutrition: Less than body requirements
● Deficient fluid volume
● Risk for injury to mother and fetus
● Anxiety

Treatment
● Removal of potential vomiting triggers
● Total parenteral nutrition (TPN)
● Restoration of fluid and electrolyte balance through diet strategies or supplements

Drug therapy options
● Antiemetics for vomiting

Patient care goals
● The client will maintain proper hydration and nutrition.
● The client will have decreased episodes of vomiting.
● The client will verbalize feelings regarding potential fetal injury.

Nursing interventions
● Monitor vital signs and fluid intake and output *to assess for fluid volume deficit.*

Comparing morning sickness and hyperemesis gravidarum

MORNING SICKNESS	HYPEREMESIS GRAVIDARUM
● Onset occurs in first trimester and resolves in second trimester.	● Onset occurs in first trimester and continues throughout pregnancy.
● Weight is maintained or increased.	● Weight loss occurs.
● Serum electrolytes remain normal.	● Serum electrolytes are abnormal.
● Ketosis doesn't develop.	● Ketosis occurs.
● Skin turgor remains hydrated.	● Skin turgor is dehydrated.
● Serum thyroid levels remain normal.	● Serum thyroid levels are abnormal.
● Skin color remains normal.	● Jaundice may occur.

- Obtain blood samples and urine specimens for laboratory tests *to evaluate nutritional and hydration status.*
- Provide small, frequent meals *to maintain adequate nutrition.*
- Encourage liquids between meals instead of with meals *to maintain adequate hydration.*
- Recommend the client maintain an upright position for 1 to 2 hours after eating *to decrease gastric reflux.*
- Maintain I.V. fluid replacement and TPN *to reduce fluid deficit and pH imbalance.*
- Provide emotional support *to help the client cope with her condition.*

Evaluation
- The client increases her weight during pregnancy.
- The client remains adequately hydrated.
- The client and fetus maintain stable conditions throughout the pregnancy.
- The client demonstrates coping mechanisms regarding continual illness.

Placenta previa

In PLACENTA PREVIA, the placenta is implanted in the lower uterine segment (low implantation). The placenta can occlude the cervix partially or totally.

Risk factors
- Maternal age older than 35
- Multiple pregnancies
- Placental villi torn from the uterine wall as the lower uterine segment contracts and dilates in the third trimester
- Uterine fibroid tumors
- Uterine scars from surgery
- Uterine sinuses exposed at the placental site and bleeding

Data collection findings
- Painless, bright red vaginal bleeding, especially during the third trimester (possibly increasing with each successive incident)

Diagnostic findings
- Early ultrasound evaluation reveals the placenta implanted in the lower uterine segment.

Nursing diagnoses
- Risk for injury to mother and fetus
- Risk for deficient fluid volume
- Anxiety

Treatment
- Surgical intervention (by cesarean delivery), depending on the placental placement and maternal and fetal stability (treatment of choice)
- If gestational age is less than 34 weeks, hospitalization of the client and restriction to bed rest to avoid preterm labor
- Administration of supplemental iron if anemia is present
- Restriction of maternal activities (for example, avoiding lifting heavy objects, long-distance travel, and sexual intercourse)
- Transfusion of packed RBCs if Hb level and HCT are low

Drug therapy options
- betamethasone to increase fetal lung maturity if preterm labor can't be halted

Patient care goals
- The client and fetus will remain hemodynamically stable.
- The client will verbalize anxiety related to potential pregnancy loss.

Nursing interventions
- Monitor maternal vital signs, including uterine activity, *to assess for maternal well-being.*
- Monitor for vaginal bleeding *to estimate blood loss.*
- Monitor fetal heart rate, using electronic fetal monitoring, *to assess for complications.*
- Don't perform rectal or vaginal examinations unless equipment is available for vaginal and cesarean delivery *to avoid stimulating uterine activity.*
- Obtain blood samples for HCT, Hb level, PT, PTT, fibrinogen level, platelet count, and typing and crossmatching *to assess for complications.*
- Provide routine postoperative care, if cesarean delivery is performed, *to ensure the client's well-being.*
- Monitor for postpartum hemorrhage *because a client with placenta previa is more prone to hemorrhage.*
- Provide emotional support *to reduce anxiety.*
- Provide I.V. fluids as ordered *to reduce fluid loss.*

Evaluation
- The client and fetus maintain stable vital signs; the fetus is delivered safely.
- The client demonstrates appropriate coping mechanisms in dealing with anxiety over fetal injury.

Pregnancy-induced hypertension

PIH is characterized by hypertension, proteinuria, and edema. The client is at risk for cerebral hemorrhage, circulatory collapse, heart failure, hepatic rupture, and renal failure. If delivery occurs before term, fetal prognosis is poor because of hypoxia, acidosis, and immaturity. (See *Caring for the pregnant client with a cardiovascular disorder,* for related information.)

Uncontrolled PIH may progress to seizures (ECLAMPSIA). The maternal mortality from eclampsia is 10% to 15%, usually resulting from intracranial hemorrhage and heart failure.

Risk factors

- Adolescent mother
- Antiphospholipid antibodies
- Diabetes mellitus
- Familial tendency
- Hydatidiform mole
- Hydramnios
- Hydrops fetalis
- Hypertension
- Malnutrition
- Maternal age older than 35
- Multifetal pregnancy
- Obesity
- Renal disease

Data collection findings

PIH usually appears between 20 and 24 weeks' gestation and disappears within 42 days after delivery. It's classified as gestational hypertension, mild eclampsia, severe preeclampsia, or eclampsia, depending on the degree of hypertension and other symptoms. (See *Caring for the client with preeclampsia,* page 170.)

Gestational hypertension

- Blood pressure of 140/90 mm Hg or a systolic pressure elevated 30 mm Hg above the prepregnancy level
- No proteinuria

Mild eclampsia

- Blood pressure of 140/90 mm Hg, systolic pressure elevated more than 30 mm Hg above prepregnancy level, or diastolic pressure elevated 15 mm Hg above prepregnancy level
- Proteinuria of 1 + to 2 +
- Weight gain of more than 2 lb (0.9 kg) per week in the second trimester and 1 lb (0.5 kg) per week in the third trimester

- Mild edema in the upper extremities or face

Severe preeclampsia

- Blood pressure of 160/110 mm Hg (noted on two readings taken 6 hours apart while on bed rest)
- Proteinuria of 3 + to 4 +
- Oliguria (500 ml or less in 24 hours)
- Pulmonary edema with shortness of breath
- Peripheral edema or severe facial edema
- Frontal headaches
- Blurred vision
- Hyperreflexia
- Nausea and vomiting
- Irritability
- Cerebral disturbances
- Epigastric pain
- Presence of HELLP syndrome (hemolysis, elevated liver enzymes, and low platelet count)

Eclampsia

- Blood pressure higher than 160/100 mm Hg
- Tonic-clonic seizures

Diagnostic findings

- Blood chemistry reveals increased blood urea nitrogen, creatinine, and uric acid levels and elevated liver function studies.
- Hematology reveals thrombocytopenia (HELLP syndrome).

Nursing diagnoses

- Excess fluid volume
- Risk for injury
- Activity intolerance
- Ineffective coping

Treatment

- Bed rest in a lateral position
- Delivery (in mild preeclampsia, after the fetus is mature and safe induction is possible; in severe preeclampsia, regardless of gestational age)
- High-protein diet with restriction of excessively salty foods
- Restriction of I.V. fluid administration during labor

Drug therapy options

- Antihypertensive (in severe preeclampsia): betamethasone (Celestone) to accelerate fetal lung maturation, diazoxide (Hyperstat), hydralazine (Apresoline)

Caring for the pregnant client with a cardiovascular disorder

CONDITION	IMPLICATIONS
Vena cava syndrome (supine hypotensive syndrome)	Vena cava syndrome occurs when something interferes with blood flow to the right atrium. This may occur if the near-term or full-term pregnant woman lies on her back, with the weight of the uterus compressing the inferior vena cava. The symptoms are dizziness, tingling of the extremities, circumoral pallor, and faintness. The client should lie on her side to relieve pressure on the inferior vena cava and restore circulation.
Chronic hypertension	Although a client with chronic hypertension develops the condition before pregnancy, her blood pressure will rise with each pregnancy and won't return to the prepregnancy level. Because it interferes with oxygen supply, chronic hypertension poses a danger to the mother and fetus.
Anemia ● First trimester: Hemoglobin (Hb) level below 12 g/dl Hematocrit (HCT) below 37% ● Second and third trimesters: Hb below 11 g/dl HCT below 35%	Maternal problems associated with anemia include abortion, infection, preeclampsia, premature labor, and heart failure. Fetal problems associated with anemia include growth retardation, morbidity, and mortality. Treatment includes an iron-rich diet, vitamin C, and folic acid. Additionally, the physician may prescribe an iron supplement (for example, ferrous sulfate). If so, teach the client to take the supplement between meals with a source of vitamin C and to include roughage and fluids in her diet because iron may cause constipation. Also caution the client that iron will make her stools black.
Heart disease	The normal physiologic changes of pregnancy are stressful to the client with heart disease. Periods of increased risk include: ● around 28 weeks' gestation, when the blood volume increase peaks, resulting in additional stress on the heart ● during the second trimester, when an elevated basal metabolic rate increases maternal-fetal oxygen requirements ● during labor and delivery, at which time epidural or caudal anesthesia is recommended (forceps may be used to prevent pushing) ● during the 1st postpartum week as body fluid levels return to normal. Care focuses on adequate rest, prevention of infection, diet management, and controlled, cautious weight loss.

● Magnesium sulfate to reduce the amount of acetylcholine produced by motor nerves, thereby preventing seizures

Patient care goals
● The client will describe the warning signs that indicate the need for immediate medical attention.
● The client will describe the required alterations to her diet and activity.
● The client will exhibit decreased severity of signs and symptoms of preeclampsia.
● The client will verbalize concerns and fears over her blood pressure problems.

Nursing interventions
All clients
● Assess the client for edema and proteinuria, *which may indicate impending eclampsia.*
● Monitor daily weight *to identify sodium and water retention.*
● Maintain a high-protein diet with moderate sodium restriction *as a measure against PIH.*
● Maintain seizure precautions *to ensure the client's safety.*
● Encourage bed rest in a left lateral recumbent position *to improve uterine and renal profusion.*
● Monitor FHR continuously during labor *to assess fetal well-being.*

CLINICAL SITUATION

Caring for the client with preeclampsia

A 38-year-old primigravida is in her 8th month of pregnancy. During a routine checkup today, the nurse notes a weight gain of 8 lb (3.6 kg) since the client's last visit. The client remarks that she has had to remove her rings because her fingers are swollen. Her blood pressure is 144/92 mm Hg.

What should be included in the data collection?

● Evaluation of blood pressure: elevated blood pressure (140/90 mm Hg), systolic measurement 30 mm Hg above normal, or diastolic measurement 15 mm Hg above normal; blood pressure of 160/110 mm Hg indicates a more severe problem
● Testing for protein in urine: protein is a sign of preeclampsia
● Weight measurement: weight gain greater than 1 lb (0.5 kg) per week may indicate fluid weight gain
● Review of client's diet: excessive sodium intake can cause fluid weight gain
● Evaluation of serum electrolytes: to assess nutritional and hydration status as well as renal function
● Monitoring of fetal heart tones: to determine fetal well-being

What initial interventions are appropriate to prevent preeclampsia from progressing?

● Recommend bed rest in the left side-lying position to promote better circulation.
● Provide a quiet environment to enhance relaxation.
● Provide a high protein and moderate salt diet to replace protein loss and control fluid retention.
● Measure weight daily to evaluate fluid retention.
● Report signs and symptoms of possible progression to severe preeclampsia: generalized edema, decreased urine output, headache, visual disturbances, nausea, vomiting, epigastric pain, and hyperreflexia.
● Schedule follow-up visits as recommended, usually twice weekly.

Questions for further thought

● What evaluation findings would indicate that this client is compliant with recommended interventions?
● What support measures would assist this client in maintaining maternal and fetal safety?

Severe preeclampsia

● Monitor maternal blood pressure every 4 hours, or more frequently if unstable, *to assess for abnormalities.*
● Monitor FHR *to assess for decreased variability after magnesium sulfate administration.*
● Monitor serum magnesium levels *to assess for toxicity.*
● If necessary, prepare the client for amniocentesis *to assess fetal maturity.*
● Administer I.V. fluids, as prescribed (restricted to 60 to 150 ml/hour in the client in labor with preeclampsia) *to replace fluids.*
● Obtain blood samples for complete blood count, platelet count, and liver function studies and to determine serum levels of blood urea nitrogen, creatinine, and fibrin degradation products *to assess for DIC.*
● Be prepared to obtain a blood sample for typing and crossmatching *because the client is at risk for developing placenta previa.*
● Obtain urine specimens to determine urine protein levels and specific gravity, and perform 24-hour urine collection for protein and creatinine, as ordered, *to evaluate renal function.*
● Maintain a patent I.V. line for administration of I.V. magnesium sulfate *to evaluate for toxicity evidenced by deep tendon reflexes.*
● Be prepared to obtain blood samples to monitor serum blood levels while the client is receiving I.V. magnesium sulfate *to assess for magnesium sulfate toxicity.*
● Monitor urine output *to assess for complications.*
● Maintain a patent I.V. line *to prepare for calcium gluconate administration (antidote to magnesium sulfate) in case of magnesium sulfate toxicity (elevated serum levels, decreased deep tendon reflexes, muscle flaccidity, central nervous system depression, and decreased respiratory rate and renal function).*
● Promote relaxation *to reduce fatigue.*
● Encourage the client to verbalize her feelings *to allay anxiety.*

Evaluation

● The client appropriately identifies situations requiring immediate medical attention.
● The client effectively manages her diet as recommended.
● The client maintains a stable blood pressure, edema decreases, and renal function is stable.
● The client demonstrates effective coping mechanisms in dealing with PIH.

INTRAPARTUM PERIOD

The intrapartum period includes labor and delivery. During the intrapartum period, monitor the stages of labor as well as fetal posture and positioning.

Intrapartum data collection

Nursing care in the intrapartum period depends on which signs and symptoms are present at the onset of labor and the client's physiologic and psychosocial responses to labor. Care may involve basic obstetric procedures and methods of monitoring the client and fetus. To intervene effectively during the birthing process (considered a normal process), the nurse must understand not only the physiology of labor and delivery but also the impact of sociocultural and personal factors on the client's childbearing experience.

Fetal posture and positioning

The posture and positioning of the fetus may be monitored during labor and delivery.

Fetal habitus

The term *fetal habitus*, or *fetal attitude*, is used to describe the relationship of fetal parts. The relationship usually is one of flexion; that is, legs flexed against the trunk, arms flexed across the chest, and so on. Any extended part presents a potential problem for labor and delivery.

The fetal head is the most significant body part because it's the least malleable. (See *Fetal head diameters.*) Suture lines allow for molding of the fetal head during labor and delivery. They meet to form the anterior and posterior fontanels; the location of the fontanels is helpful in assessing fetal position. Suture lines also allow for rapid growth during the infant's 1st year.

Fetal lie

Fetal lie is the relationship of the long axis (spine) of the fetus to the long axis of the mother — that is, whether the fetus is lying in a horizontal (transverse) or vertical (longitudinal) position. Approximately 99% of fetuses assume a longitudinal lie (long axis parallel to the long axis of the mother).

Fetal presentation and presenting part

Fetal presentation refers to the part of the fetus closest to the internal os of the mother's cervix, or the portion of the fetus that enters the pelvic passageway first. Various fetal

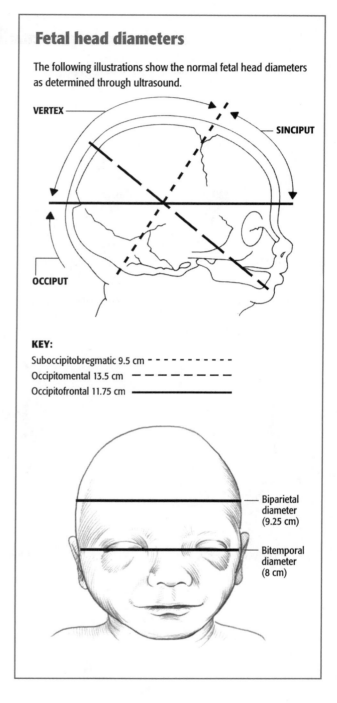

Fetal head diameters

The following illustrations show the normal fetal head diameters as determined through ultrasound.

VERTEX

SINCIPUT

OCCIPUT

KEY:
Suboccipitobregmatic 9.5 cm – – – – – – – – – –
Occipitomental 13.5 cm — — — — — — —
Occipitofrontal 11.75 cm ——————

Biparietal diameter (9.25 cm)

Bitemporal diameter (8 cm)

presentations are possible (see *Fetal positions and variations in presentation,* page 172):
● In a cephalic presentation, any part of the head can present, including the occiput or vertex, brow, or face.
● In a transverse presentation, the back or shoulders present, and vaginal delivery isn't possible.

Fetal positions and variations in presentation

These illustrations depict the four fetal positions and the variations in presentation as the fetus enters the pelvic passageway.

Fetal positions

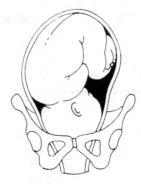

RIGHT OCCIPITAL ANTERIOR

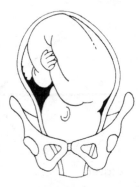

LEFT OCCIPITAL INTERIOR

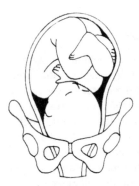

RIGHT OCCIPITAL POSTERIOR

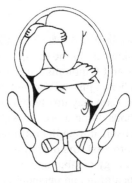

LEFT OCCIPITAL POSTERIOR

Variations in presentation

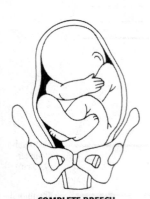

COMPLETE BREECH

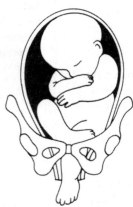

FOOTING BREECH

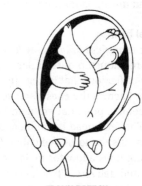

FRANK BREECH

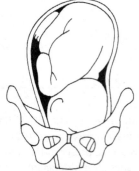

FACE OR BROW

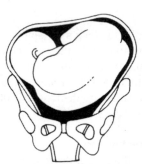

SHOULDER OR TRANSVERSE

- In a breech presentation, the buttocks (frank breech), one or both feet (footling breech), or both the buttocks and feet (complete breech) are the presenting parts.

Fetal position

Fetal position describes the relationship of the presenting part of the fetus to the four quadrants of the mother's pelvis (front, back, and sides).

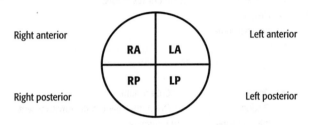

Right anterior   Left anterior

RA   LA

RP   LP

Right posterior   Left posterior

The examiner can determine fetal position through vaginal examination, location of fetal heart tones, Leopold's maneuvers, and ultrasonography or X-ray. During a vaginal examination, the examiner first determines the presenting part (location of the suture lines and fontanels) and then determines whether the presenting part is directed toward the right or left side of the mother and toward the symphysis pubis (anterior) or the sacral area (posterior). For example, in the left occipital anterior (LOA) position, the presenting part is the occiput, and it's directed toward the left side of the pelvis and toward the symphysis pubis. (The middle initial represents the presenting part.) Occipital anterior is the preferred delivery position because the fetal head can extend under the arch of the symphysis pubis; LOA is the ideal position because, with the fetus lying on the mother's left side, oxygen supply to the client and the fetus is maximized. With occipital posterior, the occiput attempts to extend into the sacral area.

Fetal station

FETAL STATION, also called *degree of engagement,* is the location of the presenting part in relation to the mother's ischial spines. Fetal station can be determined by vaginal examination.

Labor and delivery

Preliminary signs that indicate the onset of labor include:
- lightening, or fetal descent into the pelvis, which usually occurs 2 to 3 weeks before term in a primiparous client and later or during labor in a multiparous client

- Braxton Hicks contractions, which can occur irregularly and intermittently throughout pregnancy and may become uncomfortable and produce false labor
- cervical changes, including softening, effacement, and slight dilation several days before the initiation of labor
- bloody show as the mucus plug is expelled from the cervix
- membrane rupture, occurring before the onset of labor in about 12% of clients and within 24 hours for about 80% of clients
- sudden burst of energy before the onset of labor, commonly demonstrated by house cleaning activities and called the *nesting instinct.*

Passage, passenger, and power

Three important components of labor are the passage, passenger, and power. These components must work together for labor to progress normally.

Passage

Passage refers to the maternal pelvis and soft tissues, the passageway through which the fetus exits the body. This area is affected by the shape of the inlet, structure of the pelvis, and pelvic diameters.

Passenger

Passenger refers to the fetus and its ability to move through the passage. This ability is affected by such fetal features as:
- size of the fetal skull
- lie
- presentation
- position.

The fetal head can flex or extend 45 degrees and rotate 180 degrees, allowing its smallest diameters to move down the birth canal and pass through the maternal pelvis. Pressure exerted by the maternal pelvis and birth canal during labor and delivery causes the sutures of the skull to allow the cranial bones to shift, resulting in molding of the fetal head.

Power

Power refers to uterine contractions, which cause complete cervical effacement and dilation.

Other factors

Other factors that affect labor are:
- accomplishment of the tasks of pregnancy
- coping mechanisms

Stages of labor

STAGE	CONTRACTION CHARACTERISTICS	MATERNAL PHYSICAL CHANGES	FETAL POSITION CHANGES	NURSING CARE
First: Dilation				
Starts with first true labor contraction and ends with complete cervical effacement and dilation	See contraction characteristics for individual stage 1 phases below.	● Percent of effacement (0% to 100%) ● Dilation (1 to 10 cm)	● Engagement ● Descent ● Flexion ● Internal rotation	See nursing care for individual first stage phases below.
Phases *Early* (latent, inactive): Cervix dilates 1 to 4 cm; longest, least uncomfortable phase	● Every 5 to 20 minutes for 15 to 40 seconds ● Mild to moderate, increasing in frequency, duration, and intensity		● Descent ● Flexion ● Internal rotation	● Collect data. ● Orient the client to the environment and equipment. ● Establish a nurse-client relationship. ● Welcome the support person. ● Provide comfort measures. ● Encourage ambulation. ● Measure vital signs and fetal heart rate per protocol. ● Teach or review breathing methods.
Active: Cervix dilates 4 to 8 cm	● Every 2 to 4 minutes for 60 seconds ● Moderate to strong ● Most effacement and dilation in shortest period			● Reinforce breathing techniques. ● Keep the client informed of her progress. ● Change the client's position frequently. ● Encourage the client to void every 2 hours. ● Provide ice chips and lip moisturizer.
Transitional: Cervix dilates 8 to 10 cm; shortest, most uncomfortable phase	● Every 2 minutes for up to 60 seconds ● Increase in strength and duration; may decrease in frequency			● Provide positive reinforcement to support person. ● Encourage the client to rest between contractions. ● Keep an emesis basin nearby.
Second: Expulsion				
Starts with complete cervical effacement and dilation and ends with delivery	● Strong ● Upper part of uterus is active; lower part is passive	● Perineal bulging ● Crowning of fetal head ● Delivery of fetus	● Extension ● External rotation ● Expulsion	● Assist the client to push. ● Praise the client, and keep her informed of her progress. ● Maintain the client's privacy.

Stages of labor *(continued)*

STAGE	CONTRACTION CHARACTERISTICS	MATERNAL PHYSICAL CHANGES	FETAL POSITION CHANGES	NURSING CARE
Third: Placental stage				
Starts with delivery of baby and ends with delivery of placenta and membranes	• Strong • Every 3 minutes	• Placental separation 5 minutes after delivery • Gush of blood • Descent of umbilical cord • Uterus rises in the abdomen and becomes globular • Placental expulsion		• Measure the client's blood pressure. • Monitor blood loss. • Praise the client, and provide information about her status and the infant's status. • Administer oxytocin, as ordered.
Fourth: 1st hour postdelivery				
	Not applicable	• Uterus contracted and usually midway between umbilicus and symphysis pubis • Lochia present		• Monitor the client's vital signs, lochia, and fundus every 15 minutes. • Provide comfort measures, including warm blankets and perineal ice. • Introduce the neonate to the family, and encourage attachment behaviors.

• mother's ability to bear down (voluntary use of abdominal muscles to push during the second stage of labor)
• past experiences
• placental positioning
• preparation for childbirth
• psychological readiness
• support systems.

Stages of labor

The labor process is divided into four stages, ranging from the onset of true labor, through delivery of the fetus and placenta, to the 1st hour after delivery. (See *Stages of labor.*) Nursing care may be specific to the stage of labor that the client is experiencing. (See *Nursing care during labor and delivery,* page 176.)

First stage

The first stage is measured from the onset of true labor to complete dilation of the cervix. This period lasts from 6 to 18 hours in a primiparous client and from 2 to 10 hours in a multiparous client. There are three phases of stage one:

• During the latent phase, the cervix is dilated 0 to 3 cm, contractions are irregular, and the client may experience anticipation, excitement, or apprehension.
• During the active phase, the cervix is dilated 4 to 7 cm. Contractions are about 5 to 8 minutes apart and last 45 to 60 seconds with moderate to strong intensity. During this phase, the client becomes serious and concerned about the progress of labor; she may ask for pain medication or use breathing techniques. If the membranes haven't ruptured spontaneously, amniotomy may be performed.
• During the transitional phase, the cervix is dilated 8 to 10 cm. Contractions are about 1 to 2 minutes apart and last 60 to 90 seconds with strong intensity. During this phase, the client may lose control, thrash in bed, groan, or cry out.

Second stage

The second stage of labor extends from complete dilation to delivery. This stage lasts an average of 40 minutes (20 contractions) for the primiparous client and 20 minutes (10 contractions) for the multiparous client. It may last longer if the client has had epidural anesthesia.

Nursing care during labor and delivery

Nursing actions include interventions that correspond to all stages of labor as well as those that apply only to certain stages.

Care during all stages of labor
● Monitor and record vital signs, I.V. fluid intake, and urine output.
● Provide emotional support to the client and her coach.
● Assess the need for pain medication, and evaluate the effectiveness of pain-relief measures.
● Maintain aseptic technique and standard precautions.
● Maintain the client's comfort by offering mouth care, ice chips, and a change of bed linen.
● Explain the purpose of all nursing actions and medical equipment.

Care during first, second, and third stages
● Assist with breathing techniques.
● Encourage rest between contractions.

Care during the fourth stage
● Assess lochia and the location and consistency of the fundus.
● Encourage bonding.
● Initiate breast-feeding.

The client may become exhausted and dehydrated as she moves from coping with contractions to actively pushing. During this stage, the fetus is moved along the birth canal by the mechanisms of labor listed below:
● The fetus's head is considered to be engaged when the biparietal diameter passes the pelvic inlet.
● The movement of the presenting part through the pelvis is called descent.
● During flexion, the head flexes so that the chin moves closer to the chest.
● Internal rotation is the rotation of the head to pass through the ischial spines.
● Extension is when the head extends as it passes under the symphysis pubis.
● External rotation involves the external rotation of the head as the shoulders rotate to the anteroposterior position in the pelvis.

Third stage
The third stage of labor extends from delivery of the neonate to expulsion of the placenta and lasts from 5 to 30 minutes. During this period, the client typically focuses on the neonate's condition. The client may experience discomfort from uterine contractions before expelling the placenta.

Fourth stage
The fourth stage of labor is the 1st hour after delivery, when the primary activity is the promotion of maternal-neonatal bonding.

 SPOT CHECK

A client is admitted to the hospital with contractions that are about 1 to 2 minutes apart and last for 60 seconds. Vaginal examination reveals that her cervix is dilated 8 cm. The client is in what stage of labor?
A. Latent phase
B. Active phase
C. Third phase
D. Transitional phase
Answer: D. The client is in the transitional phase of labor, which is characterized by cervical dilation of 8 to 10 cm and contractions that are about 1 to 2 minutes apart and last for 60 to 90 seconds with strong intensity.

Measuring contractions
Phases of uterine contractions include increment (buildup and longest phase), acme (peak of the contraction), and decrement (letting-down phase). Contractions are measured by duration, frequency, and intensity. Here's how to measure each:
● Duration is measured from the beginning of the increment to the end of the decrement and averages 30 seconds early in labor and 60 seconds later in labor.
● Frequency is measured from the beginning of one contraction to the beginning of the next and averages 5 to 30 minutes apart early in labor and 2 to 3 minutes apart later in labor.
● Intensity is assessed during the acme phase and can be measured with an intrauterine catheter or by palpation (normal resting pressure when using an intrauterine catheter is 5 to 15 mm Hg; pressure increases to 30 to 50 mm Hg during the acme).

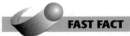

Key terms related to contractions include increment, acme, decrement, duration, frequency, and intensity.

Labor also prompts a series of responses throughout the mother's body, including changes in the cardiovascular, respiratory, and GI systems. (See *Maternal responses to labor.*)

Pain relief during labor and delivery

Pain relief is an important element of client care during labor and delivery. Pain relief during labor includes nonpharmacologic methods, analgesics, and general and regional anesthetics.

Nonpharmacologic pain relief

● Effleurage, a light abdominal stroking with the fingertips in a circular motion, is effective for mild to moderate discomfort.
● Distraction can divert attention from mild discomfort early in labor.
● Three patterns of controlled chest breathing, called Lamaze breathing, are used primarily during the active and transitional phases of labor.
● The stimulation of key trigger points with needles (acupuncture) or finger pressure (acupressure) can reduce pain and enhance energy flow.

Analgesic

● An opioid, such as meperidine (Demerol), can be used to relieve pain. If medication is given within 2 hours of delivery, it can cause neonatal respiratory depression, hypotonia, and lethargy.

Anesthetic

● General anesthetics can be administered I.V. or through inhalation, resulting in unconsciousness. General anesthetics should be used only if regional anesthetics are contraindicated or in a rapidly developing emergency.
    I.V. anesthetics, which are usually reserved for clients with massive blood loss, include:
● thiopental (Pentothal)
● ketamine (Ketalar).
    Inhalation anesthetics include:
– nitrous oxide
– isoflurane (Forane)
– halothane (Fluothane).

Maternal responses to labor

During labor, the mother undergoes various physiologic changes. Monitor changes in fluid and electrolyte balance as well as the cardiovascular, respiratory, hematopoietic, GI, and renal systems to avoid serious complications.

Cardiovascular system
● Increased intrathoracic pressure during pushing in the second stage
● Increased peripheral resistance during contractions, which elevates blood pressure and decreases pulse rate
● Increased cardiac output

Fluid and electrolyte balance
● Increased water loss from diaphoresis and hyperventilation
● Increased evaporative water volume from increased respiratory rate

Respiratory system
● Increased oxygen consumption
● Increased respiratory rate

Hematopoietic system
● Increased plasma fibrinogen level and leukocyte count
● Decreased blood coagulation time and blood glucose levels

GI system
● Decreased gastric motility and absorption
● Prolonged gastric emptying time

Renal system
● Forward and upward displacement of the bladder base at engagement
● Possibly proteinuria from muscle breakdown
● Possibly impaired blood and lymph drainage from the bladder base, resulting from edema caused by the presenting fetal part
● Decreased bladder sensation if epidural anesthetic has been administered

---

● Lumbar epidural anesthesia requires an injection of medication into the epidural space in the lumbar region, leaving the client awake and cooperative. An epidural provides analgesia for the first and second stages of labor and anesthesia for delivery without adverse fetal effects. Hypotension is uncommon, but its incidence increases if the

client doesn't receive a proper fluid load before the procedure. Epidural anesthesia may decrease the woman's urge to push.
- Spinal anesthesia involves an injection of medication into the cerebrospinal fluid in the spinal canal. Because of its rapid onset, spinal anesthesia is useful for urgent cesarean deliveries.
- Local infiltration involves an injection of anesthesia into the perineal nerves. It offers no relief from discomfort during labor but relieves pain during delivery.
- A pudendal block involves blockage of the pudendal nerve. This procedure is used only for delivery.
- A paracervical block involves the blockage of nerves in the peridural space at the sacral hiatus, which provides analgesia for the first and second stages of labor and anesthesia for delivery. This procedure increases the risk of forceps delivery.

INTRAPARTUM COMPLICATIONS

During the intrapartum period, the client must be monitored carefully for complications, some of which can be life-threatening for the mother or fetus.

Dystocia
Dystocia is a difficult or abnormal labor. In many cases, surgical intervention is required to safely deliver the fetus.

Possible causes
- Contracted pelvis
- Obstructive tumors
- Malpresentation of the fetus
- Malformation of the fetus
- Hypertonic uterine patterns
- Hypotonic uterine patterns

Data collection findings
- Arrested descent
- Hypertonic contractions
- Hypotonic contractions
- Prolonged active phase
- Prolonged deceleration phase
- Protracted latent phase
- Uncoordinated contractions

Diagnostic findings
- Contraction monitoring reveals hypotonic or hypertonic contractions and progression of labor.
- Abdominal and vaginal examinations are used to determine fetal presentation.
- Ultrasonography confirms fetal presentation.

Nursing diagnoses
- Risk for injury
- Anxiety
- Deficient knowledge (client and family members)

Treatment
- Amniotomy (artificial rupture of membranes)
- Fluid hydration
- Cesarean delivery

Drug therapy options
- Analgesic (or to relax hypertonic contractions): morphine sulfate
- Labor augmentation: oxytocin (Pitocin)

Patient care goals
- The client will have decreased fear during labor because of health care and personal support.
- The mother and fetus will remain hemodynamically stable during labor and delivery.
- The mother will have increased knowledge of all circumstances of labor and delivery.

Nursing interventions
- Monitor I.V. fluids *to maintain adequate hydration of the mother and fetus.*
- Monitor fetal heart tones and vital signs *to evaluate hemodynamic status.*
- Tell the mother to remain in a side-lying position *to provide increased perfusion to the fetus.*
- Answer all questions and provide information to the mother regarding all procedures and findings *to decrease anxiety and to assist her and family members in understanding the status of labor and planned treatment.*
- Provide support to the mother and family *to decrease fear over complications.*

Evaluation
- The client experiences less fear.
- The client and fetus remain hemodynamically stable.
- The client has increased knowledge regarding her labor.

Emergency birth

Emergency delivery of the fetus may become necessary when the well-being of the mother or fetus is in jeopardy.

Possible causes

● Contributing factors vary for each emergency birth situation.

Prolapsed umbilical cord

A prolapsed umbilical cord occurs when the umbilical cord descends into the vagina before the presenting part. It may be caused by:
● fetus at high fetal station
● hydramnios (excess of amniotic fluid)
● multifetal pregnancy
● small fetus or breech presentation
● transverse lie.

Uterine rupture

A uterine rupture occurs when the uterus undergoes more strain than it can bear. It can be caused by:
● prolonged labor
● faulty presentation
● obstructed labor
● blunt abdominal trauma
● high parity with thin uterine wall
● intense uterine contractions (natural or oxytocin-induced), especially with fetopelvic disproportion
● previous uterine surgery.

Amniotic fluid embolism

In amniotic fluid embolism, amniotic fluid escapes into the maternal circulation. During labor (or during the post-partum period), solid particles, such as skin cells, enter the maternal circulation and reach the lungs as small emboli, forcing a massive pulmonary embolism. It may be caused by:
● a defect in the membranes after rupture
● partial abruptio placentae
● fetal particulate matter (skin, hair, vernix, cells, meconium) in the fluid that obstructs the maternal pulmonary vessels.

Data collection findings

Assessment findings vary for each emergency birth situation.

Prolapsed umbilical cord

● Cord palpable during vaginal examination
● Cord visible at the vaginal opening
● Variable decelerations or bradycardia noted on fetal monitor strip

Uterine rupture

● Abdominal pain and tenderness especially at the peak of a contraction or the feeling that "something ripped"
● Excessive external bleeding
● Late decelerations, reduced FHR variability, tachycardia and bradycardia, cessation of FHR
● Hypovolemic shock caused by hemorrhage
● Chest pain or pain on inspiration
● Cessation of uterine contractions
● Palpation of the fetus outside the uterus

Amniotic fluid embolism

● Chest pain
● Sudden dyspnea
● Tachypnea
● Coughing with pink, frothy sputum
● Increasing restlessness and anxiety
● Hemorrhage
● Shock disproportionate to blood loss
● Cyanosis

Diagnostic findings
Prolapsed umbilical cord

● Ultrasonography confirms that the cord is prolapsed.

Uterine rupture

● Urinalysis can detect gross hematuria.
● Ultrasonography may reveal the absence of the amniotic cavity within the uterus.

Amniotic fluid embolism

● Arterial blood gas analysis reveals hypoxemia.
● Hematology reveals thrombocytopenia, decreased fibrinogen level and platelet count, prolonged PT, and a PTT consistent with DIC.

Nursing diagnoses

● Ineffective tissue perfusion (fetal cardiopulmonary)
● Acute pain
● Risk for infection
● Ineffective coping

Treatment

● Administration of I.V. fluids.
● Administration of oxygen by nasal cannula or mask (endotracheal intubation and mechanical ventilation may be necessary in the case of amniotic fluid embolism)

Cesarean delivery

Cesarean delivery is the planned or emergency removal of the neonate from the uterus through an abdominal incision. The surgical incision may be midline and vertical (classic), allowing easy access to the fetus, and is usually the approach of choice in emergency situations. A low-segment, transverse, or Pfannenstiel's (bikini) incision is usually chosen in a planned cesarean birth.

Nursing actions

During a cesarean birth, you should:
- provide emotional support and reassurance to the patient and family, including reassurance about the well-being of the fetus
- record fetal heart rate, maternal vital signs, and intake and output
- maintain I.V. fluid replacement, as necessary
- prepare the patient for surgery, including shaving of the abdomen and perineal area as necessary
- insert an indwelling urinary catheter, as ordered
- provide preoperative teaching, as necessary
- administer preoperative sedation as ordered
- provide immediate postoperative care after surgery.

- Emergency cesarean delivery (see *Cesarean delivery*)
- Emergency hysterectomy (with uterine rupture)
- Possible transfusion of packed RBCs, fresh frozen plasma, or platelets

Patient care goals
- The fetus will maintain adequate cardiopulmonary perfusion.
- The client will remain free from infection.
- The client will verbalize understanding of the complication, its treatment, and potential outcomes.
- The client will demonstrate decreased anxiety.
- The client will experience decreased pain.

Nursing interventions
- Position the client in the knee-chest or Trendelenburg's position *to decrease pressure on the umbilical cord and promote fetal cardiopulmonary perfusion.*
- Monitor maternal vital signs, pulse oximetry, intake and output, and FHR *to assess for complications.*
- Administer maternal oxygen by cannula or mask at 8 to 10 L/minute *to maintain uteroplacental oxygenation.*
- Maintain I.V. fluid replacement *to replace volume loss.*

- Provide emotional support and reassurance to the client *to allay her fears and reduce anxiety.*
- Obtain blood samples to determine HCT, Hb level, PT, PTT, fibrinogen level, and platelet count and type and crossmatch blood *to establish baseline values.*
- Maintain a patent I.V. line for administration of blood products as necessary *to replace volume loss.*
- Prepare the client and her family for the possibility of cesarean delivery *to reduce anxiety.*

Evaluation
- The fetus is delivered safely.
- The client is free from infection.
- The client has decreased pain and anxiety.

Laceration

Laceration refers to tears in the perineum, vagina, or cervix from the stretching of tissues during delivery. A laceration is classified as first, second, third, or fourth degree:
- A first-degree laceration involves the vaginal mucosa and the skin of the perineum and fourchette.
- A second-degree laceration involves the vagina, perineal skin, fasciae, levator ani muscle, and perineal body.
- A third-degree laceration involves the entire perineum and the external anal sphincter.
- A fourth-degree laceration involves the entire perineum, rectal sphincter, and portions of the rectal mucosa.

Possible causes
- Delivery of a large fetus
- Rapid delivery
- Use of forceps or vacuum extractor during delivery

Data collection findings
- Increased vaginal bleeding after delivery of placenta
- Visualization of the tear

Diagnostic findings
- Inspection of the affected area will reveal the extent of the laceration.

Nursing diagnoses
- Risk for deficient fluid volume
- Acute pain

Treatment
- Surgical repair
- Administration of appropriate pain medication

Patient care goals
- The client will remain hemodynamically stable.
- The client will have relief from pain.

Nursing interventions
- Monitor vital signs after delivery *to evaluate signs of shock.*
- Monitor the amount of vaginal bleeding *to determine if surgical repair is warranted (if not done) or if the client needs blood replacement.*
- Administer appropriate pain medication *to make the client more comfortable.*

Evaluation
- The client remains hemodynamically stable.
- The client has an expected amount of postdelivery vaginal bleeding.
- The client verbalizes relief from pain.

Premature rupture of membranes
In premature rupture of membranes, rupture occurs 1 or more hours before the onset of labor. Chorioamnionitis may occur if the time between rupture of the membranes and onset of labor is longer than 24 hours.

Possible causes
- Infection
- Fetal distress
- Malpresentation of the fetus
- Incompetent cervix

Data collection findings
- Fetal tachycardia
- Foul-smelling amniotic fluid
- Maternal fever
- Uterine tenderness

Diagnostic findings
- Vaginal examination reveals fluid leakage from the cervical os when the client bears down.
- Amniotic fluid testing, which is obtained by vaginal examination, confirms nonintact membranes.

Nursing diagnoses
- Risk for infection
- Anxiety
- Deficient knowledge (client and family members)

Treatment
- Bed rest
- Administration of I.V. fluids
- Emergency cesarean section

Patient care goals
- The client will remain hemodynamically stable and free from infection.
- The client will demonstrate decreased anxiety.
- The client will verbalize understanding of procedures and findings related to premature rupture of membranes.

Nursing interventions
- Monitor vital signs *to evaluate signs of infection and fetal distress.*
- Obtain WBC count *to determine the presence of infection.*
- Monitor amniotic fluid for color and meconium *to detect fetal infection or distress.*
- Provide education about treatment and potential complications *to promote client understanding.*
- Provide emotional support *to decrease anxiety regarding unexpected complications.*

Evaluation
- The client and fetus remain free from infection.
- The client verbalizes understanding of the procedure and treatment.
- The client demonstrates decreased anxiety over unexpected events of pregnancy.

Preterm labor
Preterm labor, also known as premature labor, occurs before the end of the 37th week of gestation. Preterm labor can place the client and fetus at high risk.

Possible causes
- Causes of preterm labor can be maternal or fetal.

Maternal causes
- Abdominal surgery or trauma
- Cardiovascular or renal disease
- Dehydration
- Diabetes mellitus
- Incompetent cervix
- Infection
- Placental abnormalities
- PIH
- Premature rupture of membranes

Fetal causes
- Hydramnios
- Infection
- Multifetal pregnancy

Data collection findings
- Feeling of pelvic pressure or abdominal tightening
- Menstrual-like cramps
- Persistent, low, dull backache
- Vaginal spotting
- Intestinal cramping
- Increased vaginal discharge
- Uterine contractions that result in cervical dilation and effacement

Diagnostic findings
- Electronic fetal monitoring confirms uterine contractions.
- Vaginal examination confirms cervical effacement and dilation.

Nursing diagnoses
- Risk for injury
- Anxiety
- Deficient knowledge (client and family members)

Treatment
- Suppression of preterm labor (if fetal membranes are intact, there's no evidence of bleeding, the well-beings of the fetus and mother aren't in jeopardy, cervical effacement is no more than 50%, and cervical dilation is less than 4 cm)

Drug therapy options
- Betamethasone (Celestone) administered I.M. at regular intervals over 48 hours to increase fetal lung maturity in a fetus expected to be delivered preterm
- Calcium channel blocker: nifedipine (Procardia) to decrease the production of calcium, a substance associated with the initiation of labor; adverse maternal effects include dizziness, nausea, bradycardia, and flushing
- Indomethacin (Indocin) to decrease the production of prostaglandins and lipid compounds associated with the initiation of labor; adverse maternal effects include nausea, vomiting, and dyspepsia; premature closure of the fetus's ductus arteriosus can occur if indomethacin is given before 32 weeks' gestation
- Magnesium sulfate to prevent reflux of calcium into the myometrial cells, thereby maintaining a relaxed uterus

- Tocolytic agent: ritodrine (Yutopar) or terbutaline sulfate (Brethine) to inhibit uterine contractions

Patient care goals
- Preterm contractions will cease or the fetus will be delivered safely.
- The client will verbalize understanding of the treatment and potential outcomes of preterm labor.
- The client will demonstrate decreased anxiety over the unexpected complication of preterm labor.

Nursing interventions
- Monitor maternal vital signs, contractions, and FHR every 15 minutes during tocolytic therapy (otherwise, provide continuous fetal monitoring) *to assess maternal and fetal well-being.*
- Assess the mother's respiratory status *to assess for pulmonary edema, an adverse effect associated with tocolytic therapy.*
- Monitor for maternal adverse reactions to terbutaline or ritodrine *to detect possible tachycardia, diarrhea, nervousness, tremors, nausea, vomiting, headache, hyperglycemia, hypoglycemia, hypokalemia, or pulmonary edema.*
- Notify the physician if the maternal pulse rate exceeds 120 beats per minute or the FHR exceeds 180 beats per minute *to expedite medical evaluation of maternal and fetal status.*
- Provide emotional support to the mother *to ease anxiety and establish a therapeutic relationship.*
- Monitor laboratory results *to detect abnormalities and initiate early intervention.*
- Place the client in the lateral position *to increase placental perfusion.*
- Prepare the client for possible administration of propranolol (Inderal) *to counteract an adverse reaction or an overdose of terbutaline or ritodrine.*
- Monitor for magnesium sulfate toxicity, which causes central nervous system depression in the mother and fetus; make sure calcium gluconate is available *to reverse these effects.*
- Assess the neonate for possible adverse effects if indomethacin was administered before 32 weeks' gestation *to identify signs of premature closure of the ductus arteriosus.*
- Administer nifedipine and monitor the client for adverse effects, such as dizziness, nausea, bradycardia, and flushing, *which may compromise maternal and fetal well-being.*

Evaluation

- Preterm labor subsides.
- The fetus is delivered safely.
- The client verbalizes decreased anxiety.
- The client verbalizes understanding of treatments and follows all medical advice appropriately.

SPOT CHECK

A client in the 28th week of gestation comes to the emergency department because she thinks that she's in labor. To confirm a diagnosis of preterm labor, the nurse would expect physical examination to reveal:

A. irregular uterine contractions with no cervical dilation.

B. painful contractions with no cervical dilation.

C. regular uterine contractions with cervical dilation.

D. regular uterine contractions with no cervical dilation.

Answer: C. Regular uterine contractions (every 10 minutes or more) along with cervical dilation before 36 weeks' gestation or rupture of fluids indicate preterm labor. Uterine contractions without cervical change don't indicate preterm labor.

POSTPARTUM PERIOD

The postpartum period, or puerperium, begins with the fourth stage of labor and lasts approximately 6 weeks. During this period, the woman's reproductive organs return to their nonpregnant state. Knowledge of normal physiologic and psychologic changes during the postpartum period enables the nurse to recognize deviations and intervene early.

Physiologic changes after delivery

In the vascular system, blood volume decreases and HCT increases after vaginal delivery. Excessive activation of blood-clotting factors also occurs. Blood volume returns to prenatal levels within 3 weeks.

In the reproductive system, uterine involution occurs rapidly immediately after delivery. Progesterone production ceases until the client's first ovulation. Endometrial regeneration begins after 6 weeks. The cervical opening is permanently altered from a circle to a jagged slit.

GI system changes include:

- increased hunger after labor and delivery

- delayed bowel movement from decreased intestinal muscle tone and perineal discomfort
- increased thirst from fluids lost during labor and delivery.

   Genitourinary system changes include:
- increased urine output during the first 24 hours after delivery due to increased GFR and a drop in progesterone levels
- increased bladder capacity
- proteinuria caused by the catalytic process of involution (in 50% of women)
- decreased bladder-filling sensation caused by swollen and bruised tissues
- return of dilated ureters and renal pelvis to prepregnancy size after 6 weeks.

SPOT CHECK

Which of the following is a normal physiologic response in the early postpartum period?

A. Urinary urgency and dysuria

B. Rapid diuresis

C. Decrease in blood pressure

D. Increased motility of the GI system

Answer: B. In the early postpartum period, there's an increase in the GFR and a drop in progesterone levels, which result in rapid diuresis. There should be no urinary urgency, although a woman may be anxious about voiding. There's minimal change in blood pressure following childbirth and a residual decrease in GI motility.

In the endocrine system, thyroid function and the production of anterior pituitary gonadotropic hormones are increased. Simultaneously, the production of other hormones, including estrogen, aldosterone, progesterone, HCG, corticoids, and ketosteroids, decreases.

Psychological changes after pregnancy

More than 50% of women experience transient mood alterations immediately after pregnancy. This mood change is called postpartum depression, or the "baby blues," and signs and symptoms include sadness, crying, fatigue, and low self-esteem. Possible causes include hormonal changes, genetic predisposition, and adjustment to an altered role and self-concept.

Teach the client that mood swings and bouts of depression are normal postpartum responses; they typically occur during the first 3 weeks after delivery and subside within 1 to 10 days.

Maternal behavior after delivery is divided into three phases:

● taking-in phase
● taking-hold phase
● letting-go phase.

During the taking-in phase (1 to 2 days after delivery), the mother is passive and dependent, directing energy toward herself instead of toward her infant. She may relive her labor and delivery experience to integrate the process into her life and may have difficulty making decisions. During the taking-hold phase (about 2 to 7 days after delivery), the mother has more energy and begins to act independently and initiate self-care activities. Although she may express a lack of confidence in her abilities, she accepts responsibility for her neonate and becomes receptive to infant care and teaching about self-care activities.

During the letting-go phase (about 7 days after delivery), the mother begins to readjust to family members, assuming the mother role and the responsibility that comes with it. She relinquishes the infant she has imagined during her pregnancy and accepts her real infant as an entity separate from herself.

Postpartum data collection

The period immediately after labor and delivery is crucial to good postpartum nursing care. An understanding of normal and abnormal assessment findings is essential. Expected findings are listed here.

Vital signs

● The client's respiratory rate should return to normal after delivery.
● The client's temperature may be elevated to 100.4° F (38° C) from dehydration and the exertion of labor.
● Blood pressure is usually normal within 24 hours after delivery.
● Bradycardia of 50 to 70 beats per minute is common during the first 6 to 10 days after delivery because of reductions in cardiac strain, stroke volume, and the vascular bed.

Nursing interventions

● Monitor vital signs every 15 minutes for the first 1 to 2 hours, then every 4 hours for the first 24 hours, and then during every shift.

Fundus

Check the tone and location of the fundus (the uppermost portion of the uterus) every 15 minutes for the first 1 to 2 hours after delivery and then during every shift. The involuting uterus should be at the midline. The fundus is usually:

● midway between the umbilicus and symphysis 1 to 2 hours after delivery
● 1 cm above or at the level of the umbilicus 12 hours after delivery
● 3 cm below the umbilicus by the 3rd day after delivery
● firm to the touch.

The fundus will continue to descend about 1 cm per day until it isn't palpable above the symphysis (about 9 days after delivery). The uterus shrinks to its prepregnancy size 5 to 6 weeks after delivery.

A firm uterus helps control postpartum hemorrhage by clamping down on uterine blood vessels. The physician may prescribe oxytocin (Pitocin), ergonovine maleate (Ergotrate), or methylergonovine (Methergine) to maintain uterine firmness. (See *Fundal assessment and massage.*)

Nursing interventions

● Massage a boggy (soft) fundus gently; if the fundus doesn't respond, use a firmer touch.
● Be aware that the uterus may relax if it's overstimulated by massage or medications.
● Suspect a distended bladder if the uterus isn't firm at the midline. A distended bladder can impede the downward descent of the uterus by pushing it upward and, possibly, to the side.
● Assess maternal-infant bonding by observing how the mother responds to her neonate.
● Assess for excessive vaginal bleeding.

Lochia

Lochia is discharge from the sloughing of the uterine decidua. There are different types of lochia:

● Lochia rubra is the vaginal discharge that occurs for the first 2 to 3 days after delivery; it has a fleshy odor and is bloody with small clots.
● Lochia serosa refers to the vaginal discharge that occurs during days 3 through 9; it's pinkish or brown with a serosanguineous consistency and fleshy odor.
● Lochia alba is a yellow to white discharge that usually begins about 10 days after delivery; it may last from 2 to 6 weeks.

Some lochia characteristics may indicate the need for further intervention, for example:

● Foul-smelling lochia may indicate an infection.

NURSING PROCEDURE

Fundal assessment and massage

Purpose

Fundal assessment is done to evaluate the evolutional progress of the uterus after birth. It identifies uterine size, firmness, and descent. Fundal massage helps to maintain or stimulate uterine contractions, which are essential in preventing postpartum hemorrhage.

Implementation

- Explain fundal assessment and massage to the client and answer any questions. Provide privacy.
- Perform massage and assessment every 15 minutes for the 1st hour after delivery, every 30 minutes for the next 2 hours, every hour for the next 4 hours, and then every 4 hours for the 1st postpartum day.
- Place the client in the supine position or with her head slightly elevated.
- Expose the abdomen and perineum.
- Gently compress the uterus between your hands to evaluate firmness and position in relation to the umbilicus (in fingerbreadths or centimeters).
- If the fundus seems soft and boggy, massage it gently in a circular motion until it's firm.
- Observe lochia flow during massage.
- Document the client's position, firmness of the fundus, and the response to massage (if performed).

- Continuous seepage of bright red blood may indicate a cervical or vaginal laceration.
- Lochia that saturates a sanitary pad within 45 minutes usually indicates an abnormally heavy flow.
- Lochia may diminish after a cesarean delivery.
- Numerous large clots should be evaluated further; they may interfere with involution.
- Lochia may be scant but should never be absent; absence may indicate postpartum infection.

Nursing interventions

- Assess the lochia during every shift and note its color, amount, odor, and consistency.

Breasts

Assess the size and shape of the client's breasts every shift, noting reddened areas, tenderness, and engorge-

ment. Check the nipples for cracking, fissures, and soreness.

Nursing interventions

- Tell the client that she can relieve discomfort from engorged breasts by wearing a support bra, applying ice packs, and taking prescribed medications.
- If the client is breast-feeding, advise her that she can relieve breast engorgement by eating frequent meals, applying warm compresses, and expressing milk manually.

Elimination

Assess the client's elimination patterns. The client should void within the first 6 to 8 hours after delivery. Observe for a distended bladder, which can interfere with elimination, within the first few hours after delivery.

Nursing interventions

- The client may use pain medication before urination. Pour warm water over the perineum to eliminate the fear of pain.
- The client who can't void may require catheterization.
- Encourage the client to have a bowel movement within 1 to 2 days after delivery to avoid constipation.
- The client with hemorrhoids may require ice packs or analgesic preparations.
- Encourage the client to increase her fluid and roughage intake.
- Alleviate maternal anxieties regarding pain from or damage to the site of episiotomy (surgical incision into the perineum and vagina).
- The client may require laxatives, stool softeners, suppositories, or enemas.
- A client with a fourth-degree laceration should never have a rectal temperature reading nor should she be administered an enema.

Episiotomy

The site of episiotomy should be assessed every shift to evaluate healing, noting erythema, intactness of stitches, edema, and odor or drainage. Twenty-four hours after delivery, the edges of an episiotomy are usually sealed. This assessment can be performed during perineal care. (See *Postpartum perineal care*, page 186.)

Nursing interventions

- Administer medications to relieve discomfort from the episiotomy, uterine contractions, incisional pain, or engorged breasts, as prescribed. Medications may include

NURSING PROCEDURE

Postpartum perineal care

Purpose
Vaginal birth (which stretches and sometimes tears the perineal tissues) and episiotomy (which may minimize tissue injury) usually leave the patient with perineal edema and tenderness. Postpartum perineal care aims to relieve edema and tenderness, promote healing, and prevent infection.

Implementation
- This procedure can be done by the nurse or client.
- Tell the client to lie on the bedpan or sit on the commode.
- If using a water-jet irrigation system, insert the prefilled cartridge containing antiseptic or medicated solution into the handle, and push the disposable nozzle into the handle until it audibly clicks into place. Place the nozzle parallel to the perineum and turn on the unit. Rinse the perineum for at least 2 minutes from front to back. Then turn off the unit, remove the nozzle, and discard the cartridge. Dry the nozzle, and store it appropriately for later use.
- If using a peri-bottle, fill it with cleaning solution and pour it over the perineal area.
- Apply a new perineal pad front to back to avoid infection.
- Be alert for such signs of infection as unusual swelling, pain, and foul-smelling drainage.
- Document perineum and wound appearance.

analgesics, stool softeners and laxatives, or oxytocic agents.

QUICK STUDY

To remember what to assess in the postpartum client, remember **BE BLUE:**

Bladder
Elimination
Breasts
Lochia
Uterus
Episiotomy

POSTPARTUM COMPLICATIONS

Common postpartum complications include mastitis, postpartum hemorrhage, psychological maladaptation, and puerperal infection.

Mastitis
Mastitis is an infection of the lactating breast. It most commonly occurs during the 2nd and 3rd weeks after birth but can occur at any time.

Possible causes
- *Staphylococcus aureus* (the most common causative pathogen)
- Altered immune response
- Constriction from a bra that's too tight (may interfere with complete emptying of the breast)
- Engorgement and stasis of milk (usually precede mastitis)
- Injury to nipple, which may allow a causative organism to enter through an injured area of the nipple, such as a crack or blister

Data collection findings
- Localized area of redness and inflammation
- Temperature of 101.1° F (38.4° C) or higher
- Purulent drainage
- Chills
- Fatigue
- Headache
- Aching muscles
- Malaise

Diagnostic findings
- Culture of the purulent discharge may test positive for *S. aureus* bacteria.

Nursing diagnoses
- Acute pain
- Ineffective coping
- Situational low self-esteem

Treatment
- Incision and drainage if abscess occurs
- Moist heat application
- Breast pumping to preserve breast-feeding ability

Drug therapy options
● Analgesic: acetaminophen (Tylenol), ibuprofen (Advil)
● Antibiotic: cephalexin (Keftab), cefaclor (Ceclor), clindamycin (Cleocin)

Patient care goals
● The client will positively respond to treatment, with resolution of the infection.
● The client will report relief from pain.
● The client will have her self-esteem restored.

Nursing interventions
● Monitor vital signs *to assess for complications.*
● Administer antibiotic therapy *to treat infection.*
● Apply moist heat *to increase circulation and reduce inflammation and edema.*
● Be supportive of alternate feeding for the infant and include other family members in infant care *to foster improved client self-esteem.*

Evaluation
● The client is free from infection.
● The client verbalizes relief from pain.
● The client demonstrates improved self-esteem.

Postpartum hemorrhage
Postpartum hemorrhage is maternal blood loss from the uterus greater than 500 ml within a 24-hour period. It can occur immediately after delivery (within the first 24 hours) or later (during the remaining days of the 6-week puerperium). (See *Caring for the client with postpartum hemorrhage.*)

Possible causes
● Administration of magnesium sulfate
● Cesarean birth
● Clotting disorders
● DIC
● General anesthesia
● Low implantation of placenta or placenta previa
● Multiparity
● Overdistention of uterus (multifetal pregnancy, hydramnios, large infant)
● Perineal laceration
● Precipitate labor or delivery
● Previous postpartum hemorrhage
● Previous uterine surgery
● Prolonged labor

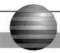

CLINICAL SITUATION

Caring for the client with postpartum hemorrhage

You're assigned to care for a 24-year-old primigravida client who delivered an 8-lb, 9-oz male infant 12 hours ago by spontaneous vaginal delivery over a midline episiotomy. In the client's room 4 hours later, you notice a large amount of blood on her peripad.

What further data collection should be done?
Assess vital signs for signs of shock related to hemorrhage (tachycardia, hypotension), inspect episiotomy incision for signs of a tear, palpate the fundus for uterine atony, and check the bladder for fullness and establish when the client last voided. Assess hemoglobin level and hematocrit if excessive bleeding persists.

Which of the following circumstances is most likely to cause uterine atony, leading to postpartum hemorrhage?
A. Hypertension
B. Cervical and vaginal tears
C. Urine retention
D. Endometritis
Answer: C. Urine retention is most likely to cause uterine atony and subsequent postpartum hemorrhage. Urine retention causes a distended bladder to displace the uterus above the umbilicus and to the side, which prevents the uterus from contracting. The uterus needs to remain contracted if bleeding is to stay within normal limits. Cervical and vaginal tears can cause postpartum hemorrhage, but in the postpartum period, a full bladder is the most common cause of uterine bleeding. Endometritis, an infection of the inner lining of the endometrium, and maternal hypertension don't cause postpartum hemorrhage.

Question for further thought
What nursing action is appropriate if the uterus is boggy (soft) on assessment?

● Retained placental fragments
● Soft, boggy uterus, indicating relaxed uterine tone
● Tocolytic drug use

Data collection findings
- Blood loss greater than 500 ml within the first 24 hours after delivery
- Uterine atony
- Signs of shock (tachycardia, hypotension, oliguria)
- Perineal lacerations
- Retained placental fragments

Diagnostic findings
- Hematology studies show a low fibrinogen level and decreased Hb level, HCT, and PTT.

Nursing diagnoses
- Ineffective tissue perfusion (cardiopulmonary)
- Risk for deficient fluid volume
- Anxiety

Treatment
- Bimanual compression of the uterus and D&C to remove clots
- I.V. replacement of fluids and blood
- Abdominal hysterectomy if other interventions fail to control blood loss

Drug therapy options
- Parenteral administration of methylergonovine (Methergine)
- Rapid I.V. infusion of dilute oxytocin

Patient care goals
- The client will remain hemodynamically stable.
- The client will maintain adequate circulating blood volume.
- The client will verbalize anxiety concerning bleeding.

Nursing interventions
- Monitor vital signs *to assess for complications.*
- Massage the fundus and express clots from the uterus *to increase uterine contraction and tone.*
- Perform a pad count *to assess the amount of vaginal bleeding.*
- Monitor lochia, including amount, color, and odor, *to assess for infection.*
- Monitor the fundus for location *to assess for uterine displacement.*
- Maintain a patent I.V. line for administration of I.V. infusion of dilute oxytocin as ordered *to increase uterine contraction and tone* and methylergonovine as ordered *to increase uterine contraction and tone.*

- Maintain a patent I.V. line for administration of blood products and I.V. fluids as prescribed *to replace volume loss.*
- Provide emotional support *to help alleviate fear and anxiety.*

Evaluation
- The client has stable vital signs.
- The client has blood volume restored as appropriate.
- The client has decreased anxiety over the unexpected complication.

Puerperal infection
Puerperal infection occurs after childbirth in 2% to 5% of all women who have vaginal deliveries and in 15% to 20% of those who have cesarean deliveries. Puerperal infection is one of the leading causes of maternal death.

Possible causes
- Catheterization
- Cesarean delivery
- Colonization of lower genital tract with pathogenic organisms, such as group B streptococcus, *Chlamydia trachomatis, Staphylococcus aureus, Escherichia coli,* and *Gardnerella vaginalis*
- Retained placental fragments

Risk factors
- Excessive number of vaginal examinations
- History of previous infection
- Low socioeconomic status
- Medical conditions such as diabetes mellitus
- Poor general health
- Poor nutrition
- Prolonged labor
- Prolonged rupture of membranes
- Trauma

Data collection findings
- Abdominal pain and tenderness
- Purulent, foul-smelling lochia
- Fever
- Tachycardia
- Chills
- Uterine cramping
- Subinvolution
- Anorexia
- Lethargy

- Malaise

Diagnostic findings
- A catheterized urine specimen may reveal the causative organism.
- A complete blood count may show an elevated WBC count in the upper ranges of normal (more than 30,000/µl) for the postpartum period.
- Cultures of the blood or of the endocervical and uterine cavities may reveal the causative organism.

Nursing diagnoses
- Risk for infection
- Acute pain
- Interrupted family processes

Treatment
- Administration of I.V. fluids (if hydration is needed)
- Appropriate drug therapy, such as broad-spectrum I.V. antibiotics, until a causative organism is identified

Patient care goals
- The client will remain hemodynamically stable.
- The client will have decreased pain.
- The client will improve family interactions as the infection resolves.

Nursing interventions
- Monitor vital signs every 4 hours *to assess for complications.*
- Place the client in Fowler's position *to facilitate lochia drainage.*
- Administer pain medication as ordered *to relieve pain and discomfort.*
- Provide emotional support and reassurance *to ease anxiety.*
- Initiate and maintain I.V. fluid administration as ordered *to replace volume loss.*
- Prepare the client for administration of antibiotics as prescribed *to fight infection.*

Evaluation
- The client has stable vital signs.
- The client reports relief from pain.
- The client has appropriate interaction with family members.

Psychological maladaptation

Psychological maladaptation is depression of a significant depth and duration after childbirth. Many postpartum clients experience some level of mood swings; psychological maladaptation refers to depression that lasts longer than 2 days, indicating a serious problem.

Possible causes
- Hormonal shifts as estrogen and progesterone levels decline
- Stress in the home or work

Risk factors
- History of depression
- Lack of support from family and friends
- Lack of self-esteem
- Troubled childhood

Data collection findings
- Extreme fatigue
- Inability to make decisions
- Inability to stop crying
- Increased anxiety about self and infant's health
- Overall feeling of sadness
- Postpartum psychosis (hallucinations, delusions, potential for suicide or homicide)
- Psychosomatic symptoms (nausea, vomiting, diarrhea)
- Unwillingness to be left alone

Nursing diagnoses
- Fatigue
- Ineffective coping
- Interrupted family processes

Treatment
- Counseling for the at-risk client and family
- Group therapy
- Psychotherapy

Drug therapy options
- Antidepressant: imipramine (Tofranil), nortriptyline (Pamelor)

Patient care goals
- The client will verbalize feelings over life changes and begin to adapt to maternal role.
- The client will demonstrate coping skills to successfully interact with others as well as the infant.

Nursing interventions

● Obtain a health history during the antepartum period *to assess whether the client is at risk for postpartum depression.*

● Assess the client's support systems *to assess the need for additional help.*

● Assess maternal-infant bonding *to assess for signs of depression.*

● Provide emotional support and encouragement *to reduce anxiety.*

● Notify a skilled professional if you observe psychotic symptoms in the client *to promote appropriate care and treatment if these symptoms develop.*

Evaluation

● The client interacts with her infant and family appropriately.

● The client verbalizes decreased anxiety in the maternal role.

● The client demonstrates increased energy in everyday activities.

NEONATAL CARE

A neonate experiences many changes as he adapts to life outside the uterus. Knowledge of these changes and of the normal physiologic characteristics of the neonate provides the basis for normal neonatal care.

Neonatal changes

This is how the neonate's body systems change:

● The cardiovascular system changes from the very first breath, which expands the neonate's lungs and decreases pulmonary vascular resistance. Clamping the umbilical cord increases systemic vascular resistance and left atrial pressure, which functionally closes the foramen ovale (fibrosis may take from several weeks to 1 year).

● The respiratory system also begins to change with the first breath. The neonate's breathing is a reflex triggered in response to noise, light, and temperature and pressure changes. Air immediately replaces the fluid that filled the lungs before birth.

● Renal system function doesn't fully mature until after the 1st year of life; as a result, the neonate has a minimal range of chemical balance and safety. The neonate's limited ability to excrete drugs, coupled with excessive neonatal fluid loss, can rapidly lead to acidosis and fluid imbalances.

FAST FACT

Because the neonate's renal system hasn't fully matured yet, he can easily develop acidosis and fluid imbalances.

● The GI system also isn't fully developed because normal bacteria aren't present in the neonate's GI tract. The lower intestine contains meconium at birth; the first meconium (sterile, greenish black, and viscous) usually passes within 24 hours. Some aspects of GI development include:

– audible bowel sounds 1 hour after birth

– uncoordinated peristaltic activity in the esophagus for the first few days of life

– limited ability to digest fats because amylase and lipase are absent at birth

● frequent regurgitation because of an immature cardiac sphincter.

● Changes in neonatal thermogenesis depend on environment. In an optimal environment, the neonate can produce sufficient heat, but rapid heat loss may occur in a suboptimal thermal environment.

● The neonatal immune system depends largely on three immunoglobulins: immunoglobulin G (IgG), IgM, and IgA. IgG (detected in the fetus at the 3rd month of gestation) is a placentally transferred immunoglobulin, providing antibodies to bacterial and viral agents. The infant synthesizes its own IgG during the first 3 months of life, thus compensating for concurrent catabolism of maternal antibodies. By 20 weeks' gestation, the fetus synthesizes IgM, which is undetectable at birth because it doesn't cross the placenta.

High levels of IgM in the neonate indicate a nonspecific infection. Secretory IgA (which limits bacterial growth in the GI tract) is found in colostrum and breast milk.

In the neonatal hematopoietic system, blood volume accounts for 80 to 85 ml/kg of body weight. The neonate experiences prolonged coagulation time because of decreased levels of vitamin K.

● The full-term neonate's neurologic system should produce equal strength and symmetry in responses and reflexes. Diminished or absent reflexes may indicate a serious neurologic problem, and asymmetrical responses may indicate trauma during birth, including nerve damage, paralysis, or fracture. Some neonatal reflexes gradually weaken and disappear during the early months.

• Jaundice is a major concern in the neonatal hepatic system because of increased serum levels of unconjugated bilirubin from increased RBC lysis, altered bilirubin conjugation, or increased bilirubin reabsorption from the GI tract. Physiologic jaundice appears after the first 24 hours of extrauterine life, pathologic jaundice is evident at birth or within the first 24 hours of extrauterine life, and breast milk jaundice appears after the 1st week of extrauterine life when physiologic jaundice is declining.

Neonatal data collection

Neonatal data collection includes initial and ongoing assessment as well as a thorough physical examination.

Initial assessment

Initial neonatal assessment involves draining secretions, assessing abnormalities, and keeping accurate records.

Nursing interventions

• Suction and administer oxygen as needed *to ensure a proper airway.*
• Dry the neonate under the warmer while keeping the head lower than the trunk *to promote drainage of secretions.*
• Apply a cord clamp and check the number of cord vessels *to assess for abnormal bleeding from the cord.*

• Observe the neonate for voiding and meconium; document the first void and stools.
• Assess the neonate for gross abnormalities and clinical manifestations of suspected abnormalities.
• Prepare the neonate for Apgar scoring even after the 5-minute score is received. (See *Apgar scoring.*)
• Obtain clear footprints and fingerprints (the neonate's footprints are kept on a record that includes the mother's fingerprints), and apply identification bands with matching numbers to the mother (one band) and neonate (two bands) before they leave the delivery room *to provide for proper identification of the neonate.*
• Allow the mother to hold the neonate and to breast-feed *to promote bonding between the mother and neonate.*

Ongoing assessment

Ongoing neonatal physical assessment includes observing and recording vital signs and administering prescribed medications.

Nursing interventions

• Monitor the neonate's vital signs *to assess for cardiovascular and respiratory complications.*
• Take the first temperature by the axillary route (rectal route isn't recommended because of possible rectal mucosa damage).
• Take the apical pulse for 60 seconds (normal rate is 120 to 160 beats/minute).

 NURSING PROCEDURE

Apgar scoring

The Apgar scoring system provides a way to evaluate the neonate's cardiopulmonary and neurologic status. The assessment is performed at 1 and 5 minutes after birth and is repeated every 5 minutes until the infant stabilizes. A score of 8 to 10 indicates that the neonate is in no apparent distress; a score below 8 indicates that resuscitative measures may be needed.

SIGN	0	1	2
Heart rate	Absent	Less than 100 beats/minute	Greater than 100 beats/minute
Respiratory effort	Absent	Slow, irregular	Good crying
Muscle tone	Flaccid	Some flexion of extremities	Active motion
Reflex irritability	None	Grimace	Vigorous cry
Color	Pale, blue	Body pink, blue extremities	Completely pink

- Count respirations with a stethoscope for 60 seconds (normal rate is 30 to 60 breaths/minute).
- Measure and record blood pressure (normal reading ranges from 60/40 mm Hg to 90/45 mm Hg).
- Measure and record the neonate's vital statistics.
- Prepare the neonate for a gestational age assessment.
- Administer prescribed medications such as vitamin K (AquaMEPHYTON), which is a prophylactic against transient deficiency of coagulation factors II, VII, IX, and X.
- Administer erythromycin ointment (Ilotycin), the drug of choice for neonatal eye prophylaxis, *to prevent damage and blindness from conjunctivitis caused by* Neisseria gonorrhoeae *and* Chlamydia; *treatment is required by law.*
- Administer the first hepatitis B vaccine within 12 hours after birth.
- Perform laboratory tests *to assess for abnormalities.*
- Monitor glucose levels and HCT, *which aid in assessing for hypoglycemia and anemia.*

Neonatal physical examination

The neonate should receive a thorough visual and physical examination of each body part. The following is a brief review of normal and abnormal neonatal physiology.

Head

The neonate's head is about one-fourth of its body size. The term molding refers to asymmetry of the cranial sutures due to difficulties during labor and delivery. Cranial abnormalities include:
- cephalhematoma — a collection of blood between a skull bone and the periosteum that doesn't cross suture lines
- caput succedaneum — localized swelling over the presenting part that can cross suture lines.

The neonatal skull has two fontanels: a diamond-shaped anterior fontanel and a triangular-shaped posterior fontanel. The anterior fontanel is located at the juncture of the frontal and parietal bones, measures 1$\frac{1}{8}$" to 1$\frac{5}{8}$" (3 to 4 cm) long and $\frac{3}{4}$" to 1$\frac{1}{8}$" (2 to 3 cm) wide, and closes in about 18 months. The posterior fontanel is located at the juncture of the occipital and parietal bones, measures about $\frac{3}{4}$" across, and closes in 8 to 12 weeks. The fontanels:
- should feel soft to the touch
- shouldn't be depressed — a depressed fontanel indicates dehydration

- shouldn't bulge — bulging fontanels require immediate attention because they may indicate increased intracranial pressure.

Eyes

The neonate's eyes are usually blue or gray because of scleral thinness; permanent eye color is established within 3 to 12 months. Lacrimal glands are immature at birth, resulting in tearless crying for up to 2 months. The neonate may demonstrate transient strabismus. Doll's eye reflex (when the head is rotated laterally, the eyes deviate in the opposite direction) may persist for about 10 days. Subconjunctival hemorrhages may appear from vascular tension changes during birth.

Nose

Because infants are obligatory nose breathers for the first few months of life, nasal passages must be kept clear to ensure adequate respiration. Neonates instinctively sneeze to remove obstructions.

Mouth

The neonate's mouth usually has scant saliva and pink lips. Epstein's pearls may be found on the gums or hard palate, and precocious teeth may also be apparent.

Ears

The neonate's ears are characterized by incurving of the pinna and cartilage deposition. The top of the ear should be above or parallel to an imaginary line from the inner to the outer canthus of the eye. Low-set ears are associated with several syndromes, including chromosomal abnormalities.

Neck

The neonate's neck is typically short and weak with deep folds of skin.

Chest

The neonate's chest is characterized by a cylindrical thorax and flexible ribs. Breast engorgement from maternal hormones may be apparent, and supernumerary nipples may be located below and medially to the true nipples.

Abdomen

The neonatal abdomen is usually cylindrical with some protrusion; a scaphoid appearance indicates diaphragmatic hernia. The umbilical cord is white and gelatinous with two arteries and one vein and begins to dry within 1 to 2 hours after delivery.

Genitalia

Characteristics of a male neonate's genitalia include rugae on the scrotum and testes descended into the scrotum. The urinary meatus is located in one of three places:
- at the penile tip (normal)
- on the dorsal surface (epispadias)
- on the ventral surface (hypospadias).

   In the female neonate, the labia majora cover the labia minora and clitoris, vaginal discharge from maternal hormones appears, and the hymenal tag is present.

Extremities

All neonates are bowlegged and have flat feet. Some neonates may have abnormal extremities. For example, neonates may be polydactyl (more than five digits on an extremity) or syndactyl (two or more digits fused together).

Spine

The neonatal spine should be straight and flat, and the anus should be patent without any fissure. Dimpling at the base of the spine is commonly associated with spina bifida.

Skin

The skin of a neonate can indicate many conditions — some normal and others requiring more serious attention. Assessment findings include:
- acrocyanosis (cyanosis of the hands and feet resulting from adjustments to extrauterine circulation) for the first 24 hours after birth
- milia (clogged sebaceous glands) on the nose or chin
- lanugo (fine, downy hair) appearing after 20 weeks' gestation on the entire body except the palms and soles
- vernix caseosa (a white, cheesy protective coating composed of desquamated epithelial cells and sebum)
- erythema toxicum neonatorum (a transient, maculopapular rash)
- telangiectasia (flat, reddened vascular areas) appearing on the neck, upper eyelid, or upper lip
- port-wine stain (nevus flammeus), a capillary angioma located below the dermis and commonly found on the face
- strawberry hemangioma (nevus vasculosus), a capillary angioma located in the dermal and subdermal skin layers indicated by a rough, raised, sharply demarcated birthmark.

Reflexes

Normal neonates display a number of reflexes, which include:
- Babinski's — when the sole on the side of the small toe is stroked, the neonate's toes fan upward
- grasping — when a finger is placed in each of the neonate's hands, the neonate's fingers grasp tightly enough to be pulled to a sitting position
- Moro's — when lifted above the crib and suddenly lowered, the arms and legs symmetrically extend and then abduct while the fingers spread to form a **C**
- rooting — when the cheek is stroked, the neonate turns his head in the direction of the stroke
- startle — a loud noise such as a hand clap elicits neonatal arm abduction and elbow flexion and the neonate's hands stay clenched
- stepping — when held upright with the feet touching a flat surface, the neonate exhibits dancing or stepping movements
- sucking — sucking motion begins when a nipple is placed in the neonate's mouth
- tonic neck (fencing position) — when the neonate's head is turned while the neonate is lying in a supine position, the extremities on the same side straighten while those on the opposite side flex
- trunk incurvature — when a finger is run laterally down the neonate's spine, the trunk flexes and the pelvis swings toward the stimulated side.

NEONATAL COMPLICATIONS

Common neonatal complications and disorders include drug dependency, fetal alcohol syndrome, human immunodeficiency virus, hypothermia, infections, jaundice, and respiratory distress syndrome.

Drug dependency

Infants born to drug-addicted mothers are at risk for preterm birth, aspiration pneumonia, meconium-stained fluid, and meconium aspiration. Drug-dependent infants may also experience withdrawal from substances, such as heroin and cocaine. Methadone shouldn't be given to neonates because of its addictive nature. (See *Caring for the client with neonatal drug dependency*, page 194.)

Possible causes
- Drug addiction in the mother

CLINICAL SITUATION

Caring for the client with neonatal drug dependency

A client who's 1 day old was born at 28 weeks' gestation to a 16-year-old single mother. You're caring for the client in the neonatal high-risk nursery. She had an Apgar score of 5 at 1 minute after delivery and 8 after 5 minutes. The neonate now demonstrates signs of substance withdrawal, and it's discovered that her mother has a history of cocaine abuse.

What behavior patterns do you expect to see?
The neonate may demonstrate irritability, jitteriness, poor sleep patterns, poor eating pattern, hyperactive reflexes, and vigorous sucking of her hands. She may also have diarrhea, tremors, and frequent yawning. These classic signs and symptoms of drug dependency usually appear within the first 24 hours after birth.

What are appropriate nursing diagnoses for the neonate?
- Ineffective infant feeding pattern
- Deficient fluid volume
- Risk for disorganized infant behavior

Questions for further thought
- What are appropriate goals for the mother and neonate?
- How can you support parenteral adaptation to the neonate?

Data collection findings
- Diarrhea
- Frequent sneezing and yawning
- High-pitched cry
- Hyperactive reflexes
- Increased tendon reflexes
- Irritability
- Jitteriness
- Poor feeding habits
- Poor sleeping pattern
- Tremors
- Vigorous sucking on hands
- Withdrawal symptoms (depend on the length of maternal addiction, the drug ingested, and the time of last ingestion before delivery; usually appear within 24 hours after delivery)

Diagnostic findings
- Drug screen reveals agent abused by mother.

Nursing diagnoses
- Ineffective infant feeding pattern
- Deficient fluid volume
- Risk for disorganized infant behavior

Treatment
- Gavage feedings, if necessary
- I.V. therapy to maintain hydration

Drug therapy options
- Paregoric and phenobarbital (Barbita) to treat withdrawal symptoms

Patient care goals
- The infant will maintain nutrition and demonstrate appropriate weight gain.
- The infant will maintain adequate hydration.
- The infant will develop an improved sleep pattern and more organized behavior.

Nursing interventions
- Monitor cardiovascular status *to detect cardiovascular compromise.*
- Monitor vital signs and fluid intake and output *to assess for complications.*
- Encourage the mother to hold the infant *to promote maternal-infant bonding.*
- Use tight swaddling *for comfort.*
- Place the neonate in a dark, quiet room *to provide a stimulus-free environment.*
- Encourage the use of a pacifier *to meet sucking needs (in cases of heroin withdrawal).*
- Be prepared to administer gavage feeding *because of the neonate's poor sucking reflex (in cases of methadone withdrawal).*
- Maintain fluid and electrolyte balance *to replace fluid loss.*
- Monitor bilirubin levels and assess for jaundice (in cases of methadone withdrawal) *to assess for liver damage.*

Evaluation
- The infant has appropriate weight gain.
- The infant is well hydrated.
- The infant has an established sleep pattern and improved behavior.

Fetal alcohol syndrome

Fetal alcohol syndrome (FAS) results from a mother's chronic or periodic intake of alcohol during pregnancy. The degree of alcohol consumption necessary to cause the syndrome varies. Because alcohol crosses the placenta in the same concentration as is present in the maternal bloodstream, alcohol consumption (particularly binge drinking) is especially dangerous during critical periods of organogenesis. The fetal liver isn't mature enough to detoxify alcohol.

Possible causes
- Risk of teratogenic effects increases proportionally with daily alcohol intake (FAS has been detected in neonates of even moderate drinkers [1 to 2 oz of alcohol daily])

Data collection findings
- Prenatal and postnatal growth retardation
- Facial anomalies (microcephaly, microphthalmia, maxillary hypoplasia, short palpebral fissures)
- Weak sucking reflex
- Sleep disturbances (either always awake or always asleep, depending on the mother's alcohol level close to birth)
- Central nervous system dysfunction (decreased IQ, developmental delays, neurologic abnormalities)

Diagnostic findings
- Chest X-ray may reveal a congenital heart defect.

Nursing diagnoses
- Imbalanced nutrition: Less than body requirements
- Delayed growth and development
- Impaired parenting

Treatment
- Swaddling

Drug therapy options
- I.V. phenobarbital to control hyperactivity and irritability

Patient care goals
- The infant will obtain adequate nutrition.
- The infant will maintain a steady growth pattern.
- The infant will receive adequate care.

Nursing interventions
- Refer the mother to an alcohol treatment center *for ongoing support and rehabilitation.*
- Provide a stimulus-free environment for the neonate. Darken the room, if necessary, *to minimize stimuli.*
- Provide gavage feedings as necessary *to provide adequate nutrition for the infant.*

Evaluation
- The infant maintains a steady growth pattern related to adequate nutrition.
- The infant demonstrates contentment as a result of receiving adequate care.

Hypothermia

A neonate's temperature is about 99° F (37.2° C) at birth. Inside the womb, the fetus was confined in an environment where the temperature was constant. At birth, this temperature can decrease rapidly.

Possible causes
- Cold temperature in delivery environment
- Heat loss due to evaporation, conduction, or convection
- Immature temperature-regulating system
- Inability to conserve heat due to little subcutaneous fat

Data collection findings
- Core body temperature lower than 97.7° F (36.5° C)
- Kicking and crying (a mechanism to increase the metabolic rate to produce body heat)

Diagnostic findings
- Arterial blood gas analysis shows hypoxemia.
- Blood glucose level reveals hypoglycemia.

Nursing diagnoses
- Hypothermia
- Ineffective thermoregulation
- Risk for impaired parent-infant attachment

Treatment
- Radiant warmer

Patient care goals
- The infant will maintain an adequate body temperature.
- The infant will have appropriate interaction with parents.

Nursing interventions

- Dry the neonate immediately *to prevent heat loss.*
- Allow the mother to hold the neonate *to provide warmth.*
- Monitor vital signs every 15 to 30 minutes *to assess temperature fluctuations and complications.*
- Provide a knitted cap for the neonate *to prevent heat loss through the head.*
- Place the neonate in a radiant warmer *to maintain thermoregulation.*

Evaluation

- The infant can maintain a normal body temperature.
- Parent-infant bonding is evident.

Infection

A neonate may contract an infection before, during, or after delivery. Maternal IgM doesn't cross the placenta and IgA requires time to reach optimum levels after birth, limiting the neonate's immune response. Dysmaturity caused by intrauterine growth retardation, preterm birth, or post-term birth can further compromise the neonate's immune system and predispose him to infection.

Sepsis is one of the most significant causes of neonatal morbidity and mortality. Toxoplasmosis, syphilis, rubella, cytomegalovirus, and herpes are common perinatal infections known to affect infants.

Possible causes

- Chorioamnionitis
- Low birth weight or premature birth
- Maternal substance abuse
- Maternal urinary tract infections
- Meconium aspiration
- Nosocomial infection
- Premature labor
- Prolonged maternal rupture of membranes

Data collection findings

- Subtle, nonspecific behavioral changes, such as lethargy or hypotonia
- Feeding pattern changes, such as poor sucking or decreased intake
- Temperature instability
- Sternal retractions
- Apnea
- Abdominal distention
- Vomiting
- Diarrhea
- Pallor
- Petechiae
- Hyperbilirubinemia
- Poor weight gain

Diagnostic findings

- Blood and urine cultures are positive for the causative organism, most commonly gram-positive beta-hemolytic streptococci and gram-negative *Escherichia coli, Aerobacter, Proteus,* and *Klebsiella.*
- Blood chemistry shows increased direct bilirubin levels.
- Complete blood count shows an increased WBC count.
- Lumbar puncture is positive for causative organisms.

Nursing diagnoses

- Hypothermia
- Risk for deficient fluid volume
- Imbalanced nutrition: Less than body requirements

Treatment

- Gastric aspiration
- I.V. therapy to provide adequate hydration
- Temperature regulation

Drug therapy options

- Broad-spectrum antibiotic therapy until the causative organism is identified; then specific antibiotic

Patient care goals

- The infant will have adequate intake to maintain hydration and nutrition.
- The infant will maintain normal temperature.
- The infant will have resolution of infection.

Nursing interventions

- Assess cardiovascular and respiratory status *to assess for complications.*
- Monitor vital signs and assist with transcutaneous blood oxygen tension *to assess for complications.*
- Monitor fluid and electrolyte status *to assess the need for fluid replacement.*
- Initiate and maintain respiratory support as needed *to maintain respiratory filtration.*
- Prepare infant and family for administration of broad-spectrum antibiotics before culture results are received and specific antibiotic therapy after results are received *to treat infection.*

- Provide the family with reassurance and support *to reduce anxiety.*
- Provide the neonate with physiologic supportive care *to maintain a neutral thermal environment.*
- Initiate and maintain I.V. therapy as ordered *to replace fluid loss.*
- Assist with obtaining blood samples and urine specimens *to assess antibiotic therapy efficacy.*

Evaluation
- The infant is hydrated with oral and I.V. fluids.
- The infant maintains a normal temperature.
- The infant is free from infection.

Jaundice
Also called hyperbilirubinemia, neonatal jaundice is characterized by a bilirubin level that:
- exceeds 6 mg/dl within the first 24 hours after delivery
- remains elevated beyond 7 days (in a full-term neonate)
- remains elevated for 10 days (in a premature neonate).

  The neonate's bilirubin levels rise as bilirubin production exceeds the liver's capacity to metabolize it. Unbound, unconjugated bilirubin can easily cross the blood-brain barrier, leading to kernicterus (an encephalopathy).

Possible causes
- Absence of intestinal flora needed for bilirubin passage in the bowel
- Enclosed hemorrhage
- Erythroblastosis fetalis (hemolytic disease of the neonate)
- Hypoglycemia
- Hypothermia
- Impaired hepatic functioning
- Neonatal asphyxia (respiratory failure in the neonate)
- Polycythemia
- Prematurity
- Reduced bowel motility and delayed meconium passage
- Sepsis

Data collection findings
- Jaundice
- Lethargy
- High-pitched crying
- Decreased reflexes
- Opisthotonos
- Seizures

Diagnostic findings
- Bilirubin levels exceed 12 mg/dl in premature or term neonates.
- Conjugated (direct) bilirubin levels exceed 2 mg/dl.
- Bilirubin level rises by more than 5 mg/day.

Nursing diagnoses
- Deficient fluid volume
- Risk for injury
- Risk for impaired parent-infant attachment

Treatment
- Exchange transfusion to remove maternal antibodies and sensitized Hbs if phototherapy fails
- Increased fluid intake
- Phototherapy (preferred treatment)
- Treatment for anemia if jaundice is caused by hemolytic disease

Patient care goals
- The infant will be nurtured by the parents as much as possible.
- The infant will have decreased bilirubin levels.
- The infant will have adequate intake to maintain hydration.

Nursing interventions
- Monitor neurologic status for signs of encephalopathy, *which indicates the potential for permanent damage.*
- Maintain a neutral thermal environment *to prevent hypothermia.*
- Monitor serum bilirubin levels *to assess for reduction of bilirubin.*
- Initiate and maintain phototherapy (provide eye protection while the neonate is under phototherapy lights and remove eye shields promptly when he's removed from the phototherapy lights) *to prevent complications.*
- Allow time for maternal/infant bonding and interaction during phototherapy *to promote bonding.*
- Keep the neonate's anal area clean and dry. *Frequent, greenish stools result from bilirubin excretion and can lead to skin irritations.*
- Provide the parents with support, reassurance, and encouragement *to reduce anxiety.*

Evaluation
- The infant is adequately hydrated.
- The infant has decreased jaundice and bilirubin levels.
- The parents are able to care for the infant.

SPOT CHECK

Which of the following interventions is a preferred treatment for neonatal jaundice?
A. Exchange transfusion
B. Phototherapy
C. Observing and monitoring bilirubin levels
D. Stool softener

Answer: B. The preferred treatment of choice for neonatal jaundice is phototherapy. Exchange transfusion is performed when the bilirubin level rises rapidly despite the use of phototherapy or hydration. Neonates with high bilirubin levels shouldn't just be observed; intervention is necessary. Stool softeners aren't part of medical management for neonatal jaundice.

Respiratory distress syndrome

Respiratory distress syndrome occurs most commonly in preterm infants, infants of diabetic mothers, and infants delivered by cesarean birth. In respiratory distress syndrome, a hyaline-like membrane lines the terminal bronchioles, alveolar ducts, and alveoli, preventing the exchange of oxygen and carbon dioxide.

Possible causes
- Inability to maintain alveolar stability
- Low level or absence of surfactant

Data collection findings
- Nasal flaring
- Expiratory grunting
- Tachypnea (more than 60 breaths/minute)
- Sternal and substernal retractions
- Fine crackles and diminished breath sounds
- Seesaw respirations
- Cyanosis
- Respiratory acidosis
- Hypothermia

Diagnostic findings
- Arterial blood gas analysis reveals respiratory acidosis.
- Chest X-rays reveal bilateral diffuse reticulogranular density.

Nursing diagnoses
- Impaired gas exchange
- Ineffective tissue perfusion (cardiopulmonary)
- Ineffective infant feeding pattern
- Risk for impaired parent-infant attachment

Treatment
- Acid-base balance maintenance
- Endotracheal intubation and mechanical ventilation
- Nutrition supplements (TPN or enteral feedings, if possible)
- Surfactant replacement by way of endotracheal tube
- Temperature regulation with a radiant warmer

Drug therapy options
- indomethacin (Indocin) to promote closure of ductus arteriosus (a fetal blood vessel connecting the left pulmonary artery to the descending aorta)

Patient care goals
- The infant will achieve adequate oxygenation.
- The infant will have adequate nutritional intake.
- The parents will participate in infant care as much as possible.

Nursing interventions
- Monitor cardiovascular, respiratory, and neurologic status *to assess for respiratory distress.*
- Monitor continuous electrocardiography and vital signs *to observe for changes.*
- Maintain ventilatory support status *to maintain air supply.*
- Prepare infant for administration of medications, including endotracheal surfactant, as prescribed *to improve respiratory function.*
- Monitor intake and output *to assess fluid loss.*
- Initiate and maintain I.V. therapy *to maintain fluid levels.*
- Provide adequate nutrition through enteral feedings, if possible, or maintain patency of TPN *to provide adequate nutrition.*
- Maintain thermoregulation *to reduce cold stress.*
- Assist with obtaining blood samples as necessary *to assess for complications.*

Evaluation
- The infant has improved oxygenation and increased lung function.
- The infant demonstrates adequate nutritional intake through appropriate weight gain.
- The parents participate in caring for the infant.

8

Pediatric nursing

Introduction

This chapter focuses on children's health problems from birth through adolescence, especially conditions and disorders that are common to these age-groups:
- infant (birth to age 12 months)
- toddler (ages 1 to 3 years)
- preschooler (ages 4 to 5 years)
- school-age child (ages 6 to 12 years)
- adolescent (ages 13 to 19 years).

The health problems that follow are commonly covered in test questions on the NCLEX-PN examination. The nursing diagnoses specified for each disorder aren't exhaustive; other diagnoses may also be appropriate, depending on the clinical situation. To enhance your understanding, review the section on growth and development in chapter 3, Nursing concepts and skills, pages 25 to 39, and the general information on body systems at the beginning of each adult clinical nursing section.

INFANT DISORDERS

Bronchiolitis

BRONCHIOLITIS, an infection of the lower respiratory tract, produces inflammation and obstruction by thick mucus and edema. In some areas of the lungs, mucus plugs and bronchiolar edema completely obstruct the small bronchioles, resulting in atelectasis. Some of these obstructed bronchioles trap air in the alveoli, producing hyperinflation. Overall, the infant experiences generalized hypoxia and progressive respiratory distress. (See *Pediatric respiratory facts.*)

The infection is viral; RESPIRATORY SYNCYTIAL VIRUS (RSV) is the most common causative agent. Bronchiolitis is most prevalent during winter and spring. It occurs in infants from birth to age 2 years; peak incidence is between

---

Pediatric respiratory facts

A child's respiratory tract differs anatomically from an adult's in ways that predispose the child to many respiratory problems. Here's how a child's respiratory tract differs from an adult's:
- Lungs aren't fully developed at birth.
- Alveoli continue to grow and increase in number through age 8.
- A child's respiratory tract has a narrower lumen than an adult's until age 5; the narrow airway makes the young child prone to airway obstruction and respiratory distress from inflammation, mucus secretion, or a foreign body.
- Elastic connective tissue becomes more abundant with age in the peripheral part of the lung.
- A child's respiratory rate decreases as body size increases.

---

ages 2 and 5 months. Reinfection is common. (See *Pediatric respiratory infections,* pages 200 and 201.)

Possible causes
- RSV
- Other viruses (such as some of the adenoviruses)

Data collection findings
- Air trapping and atelectasis
- Tachypnea
- Dyspnea
- Sternal retractions
- Wheezing, crackles, and rhonchi on auscultation
- Thick mucus
- Signs of a mild upper respiratory infection, such as nasal drainage or pharyngitis
- Low-grade fever for several days
- Sneezing and coughing
- Anorexia
- Signs of otitis media

(Text continues on page 202.)

Pediatric respiratory infections

CONDITION (ETIOLOGY) AND PATHOLOGY	AGE OF PEAK INCIDENCE	MANIFESTATIONS	MANAGEMENT
Acute epiglottiditis (*Haemophilus influenzae,* type B) Infection of epiglottis; can be severe, rapidly progressive, and fatal if untreated	2 to 7 years	• Abrupt onset • Sore throat • Inability to swallow • Tripod positioning (the child remains upright, resting weight on the hands; the chin is thrust out, with the mouth open and drooling) • Froglike sound on inspiration • Marked restlessness and anxiety • High fever	• Don't try to visualize the epiglottis with a tongue blade. • Prepare for intubation or tracheostomy. • Provide high humidity with oxygen and I.V. hydration. • Withhold food and fluids. • Administer antibiotics as ordered. • Encourage Hib vaccine to prevent infection.
Chlamydial pneumonia (bacterial) Acquired as ascending infection before or during birth; nonspecific pathology, but severe disease thought to be responsible for one-third of reported pneumonia cases in infants under age 6 months	Less than 6 months	• Persistent cough • Tachypnea • Normal or mildly elevated temperature • Feeding difficulty • Failure to thrive • Possible accompanying condition: conjunctivitis, chlamydial otitis	• Treat symptomatically. • Administer erythromycin and sulfa drugs, as ordered. (Penicillin isn't effective.)
Pneumococcal pneumonia (bacterial) Involves all or almost all of one or more pulmonary lobes; transmitted by droplet spread	1 to 4 years	• Fever (102° to 105° F [38.9° to 40.6° C]) • Shaking and chills • Headache • Tachycardia • Rapid, shallow respirations • Hacking, nonproductive cough • Pleuritic chest pain • Complications: otitis media, pleural effusion, empyema	• Administer penicillin G and antipyretics, as ordered. • Provide high humidity with oxygen and increased hydration. Suction as needed. • Percuss lung segments with postural drainage. • Use thoracentesis or closed chest drainage (or both) to treat pulmonary complications, if needed.
Staphylococcal pneumonia (bacterial) Bronchopneumonia (begins in bronchioles; exudate consolidates in neighboring lobules)	Infancy (70% of cases) to 2 years	• Mild symptoms of upper respiratory infection, which may progress to tachypnea and anxiety • Fever • Shocklike state • Progressive dyspnea • Complications: empyema, tension pneumothorax, pyopneumothorax	• Treat symptomatically. • Administer semisynthetic penicillins (such as methicillin or nafcillin) because many staphylococcal organisms are penicillin-resistant.
Streptococcal pneumonia (bacterial) Interstitial pneumonitic pneumonia with disseminated infiltration	Not age-specific (usually a complication of strep throat, upper respiratory tract infection, or contagious disease)	• Similar to those of pneumococcal pneumonia in most cases, but sometimes only mild symptoms • Complications: pleural effusion, empyema	• Treat symptomatically. • Administer penicillin G (I.V. or I.M.).

Pediatric respiratory infections *(continued)*

CONDITION (ETIOLOGY) AND PATHOLOGY	AGE OF PEAK INCIDENCE	MANIFESTATIONS	MANAGEMENT
Acute spasmodic laryngitis–spasmodic croup (viral) Inflammation of the larynx, leading to laryngeal muscle spasms and partial obstruction of the upper airway	3 months to 4 years	• Predominantly nighttime attacks that last 1 to 3 hours • Inspiratory stridor with barklike, nonproductive cough • Restlessness • Dyspnea • Anxiety • Slight, if any, temperature elevation	• Provide cool mist. • Help relieve the child's and parents' anxiety.
Acute laryngotracheobronchitis (viral) Inflammation and edema of the larynx, trachea, and bronchi with exudate	1 to 3 years	• Possible marked temperature elevation • Marked dyspnea, tachypnea, bilateral wheezing, diminished breath sounds, prolonged expiration • Tachycardia • Complications: secondary pneumonia, septicemia, cardiac failure	• To maintain an open airway, keep intubation equipment and a tracheostomy set at the bedside, provide cool humidity with oxygen, suction as needed, and administer ordered medication (possibly epinephrine by aerosol or intermittent positive-pressure breathing). • Maintain hydration by giving I.V. fluids. • Take measures to reduce temperature.
Bronchitis (secondary to cystic fibrosis, asthma, or bronchiolitis) Inflammation of the mucous membrane that lines the bronchi	Late infancy and early childhood	• Wheezing if underlying asthma is present • Dry cough, progressing to productive cough with purulent sputum • Moderate emphysema	• Provide high humidity and maintain adequate hydration. • Administer sympathomimetic bronchodilators (subcutaneous epinephrine or oral ephedrine), if ordered.
Atypical primary pneumonia *(Mycoplasma pneumoniae)* Interstitial pneumonitis, bronchitis, bronchiolitis	5 years to adulthood	• Fever • Chills • Headache and malaise • Anorexia • Myalgia • Rhinitis • Sore throat	• Treat symptomatically.
Bronchiolitis (usually respiratory syncytial virus) Inflammation of the lower respiratory tract with obstruction caused by edema and exudate	Infancy and early childhood	• Rapid or insidious onset after upper respiratory tract infection • Mild to marked temperature elevation • Slight to severe cough • Possible signs of obstructive emphysema • Symptoms similar to bronchitis	• Treat symptomatically.

CLINICAL SITUATION

Caring for an infant with RSV

A 5-month-old infant weighing 15.2 lb (6.9 kg) has just been admitted with a diagnosis of respiratory syncytial virus (RSV). His temperature is 101.5° F (38.6° C); respiratory rate, 56 breaths/minute; and apical pulse, 166 beats/minute. His respirations are accompanied by nasal flaring, retractions, and expiratory grunting. The infant is in a high-humidity tent with 30% oxygen and is receiving dextrose 5% in half-normal saline solution I.V. at 25 ml/hour. He may have clear liquids by bottle as tolerated. His parents are present.

What are appropriate nursing diagnoses for this infant?
● Risk for deficient fluid volume *related to increased insensible fluid loss and decreased intake*
● Ineffective airway clearance *related to increased tracheobronchial secretions and bronchial edema*
● Ineffective breathing pattern *related to mucus accumulation and respiratory tract edema*
● Compromised family coping *related to parents' anxiety over infant's illness*

What measures can the nurse take to ease the infant's respirations?
● Suction the nose and mouth as necessary; avoid suctioning the upper respiratory tract if secretions aren't apparent. *Suctioning irritates the mucous membrane, resulting in edema and mucus secretion. This, in turn, can narrow and obstruct the upper airway, further complicating the infant's respiratory problems.*
● Place the infant upright in an infant seat, and closely observe *to ensure that he doesn't slump down. Sitting upright in an infant seat facilitates respirations. If the infant slumps down, his tongue can obstruct the posterior pharynx, interfering with adequate lung expansion.*
● Administer nothing by mouth during an acute phase of dyspnea *to reduce the infant's risk of aspirating secretions and keep him from overtiring.*

Questions for further thought
● Why is adequate hydration required for this infant?
● How can you help relieve the parents' anxiety?

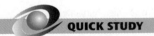

QUICK STUDY

To remember early RSV symptoms, remember the word **WIPERS.**

Wheezing
Intermittent fever
Pharyngitis
Ear infection
Rhinorrhea
Sneezing and coughing

Diagnostic findings
● Diagnostic evaluation of bronchial mucus culture shows RSV.

Nursing diagnoses
● Impaired gas exchange
● Ineffective breathing pattern
● Ineffective airway clearance

Treatment
● Cool mist tent

● Humidified oxygen
● I.V. fluids

Drug therapy options
● Bronchodilator: albuterol (Proventil)
● RSV immune globulin (I.V.)

Patient care goals
● The infant will have a respiratory rate less than 40 breaths/minute and be free from physical signs of respiratory distress within 24 hours.
● The infant will have clear breath sounds and exhibit no accessory muscle use.

Nursing interventions
● Monitor vital signs and pulse oximetry *to determine oxygenation needs and to detect deterioration or improvement in the infant's condition.*
● Assess respiratory and cardiovascular status *to identify signs of respiratory distress or adverse effects of medications. Tachycardia may result from hypoxia or the effects of bronchodilator use.*

FAST FACT

Early signs of respiratory distress include:
- anxiety
- dyspnea
- restlessness
- tachycardia
- tachypnea.

● Use gloves, gowns, and aseptic hand washing as secretion precautions *to prevent the spread of infection.*
● Administer chest physiotherapy after edema has abated *to loosen mucus that may be blocking small airways.*
● Administer humidified oxygen therapy *to liquefy secretions and reduce bronchial edema.*
● Maintain I.V. therapy *to promote hydration and replace electrolytes.*

FAST FACT

The best indicator of fluid balance is found by weighing the client – 2.2 lb (1 kg) of weight loss could indicate 1 L (1.1 qt) of fluid loss.

● Review key teaching topics with family members *to ensure adequate knowledge about the condition and treatments,* including:
– medications, dosages, and adverse reactions
– adequate nutrition and hydration
– importance of humidified environment
– importance of avoiding people with cold symptoms. (See *Caring for an infant with RSV.*)

Evaluation
● The infant has a normal respiratory rate and shows no signs of respiratory distress.
● The infant has clear breath sounds on auscultation.
● The infant doesn't use accessory muscles when breathing.

Cerebral palsy
CEREBRAL PALSY is a neuromuscular disorder resulting from damage to or a defect in the part of the brain that controls motor function. The disorder is most commonly seen in children born prematurely. Although cerebral palsy can't be cured, treatment includes interventions that encourage optimum DEVELOPMENT. Defects are common, including musculoskeletal, neurologic, GI, and nutritional defects as well as other systemic complications (such as abnormal reflexes, fatigue, GROWTH failure, genitourinary complaints, and respiratory infections).

Classifications of cerebral palsy include:
● ataxic type — the least common type; essentially a lack of coordination caused by disturbances in movement and balance
● athetoid type — characterized by involuntary, incoordinate motion with varying degrees of muscle tension (Children with this type of cerebral palsy experience writhing muscle contractions whenever they attempt voluntary movement. Facial grimacing, poor swallowing, and tongue movements cause drooling and poor speech articulation. Despite their abnormal appearance, these children commonly have average or above-average intelligence.)
● spastic type — the most common type, which features hyperactive stretch in associated muscle groups, hyperactive deep tendon reflexes, rapid involuntary muscle contraction and relaxation, contractions affecting extensor muscles, and scissoring (child's legs are crossed and the toes are pointed down, so the child stands on his toes)
● rigid type — an uncommon type that's characterized by rigid postures and lack of active movement
● mixed type — a type that features characteristics of more than one type of cerebral palsy (these children are usually severely disabled).

Possible causes
● Anoxia before, during, or after birth
● Infection
● Trauma (hemorrhage)

Risk factors
● Low birth weight
● Low Apgar scores at 5 minutes
● Metabolic disturbances
● Seizures

Data collection findings
All types
● Abnormal muscle tone and coordination (the most common associated problem)
● Dental anomalies
● Mental retardation of varying degrees in 18% to 50% of cases (most children with cerebral palsy have at least a normal IQ but can't demonstrate it on standardized tests)
● Seizures

- Speech, vision, or hearing disturbances
- Difficulty sucking or keeping the nipple or food in his mouth
- Little voluntarily movement or arm or leg tremors with voluntary movement
- Crossed legs when lifted from behind rather than pulling them up or "bicycling" (normal infant behavior)
- Leg rigidity, making diaper changing difficult
- Persistent use of only one hand or, as he gets older, uses both hands well but not legs

Ataxic cerebral palsy
- Poor balance and muscle coordination
- Unsteady, wide-based gait

Athetoid cerebral palsy
- Slow state of writhing muscle contractions whenever voluntary movement is attempted
- Facial grimacing
- Poor swallowing
- Drooling
- Poor speech articulation

Spastic cerebral palsy
- Hyperactive stretch reflex in associated muscle groups
- Hyperactive deep tendon reflexes
- Rapid involuntary muscle contraction and relaxation
- Contractures affecting the extensor muscles
- Scissoring

Rigid cerebral palsy
- Rigid posture
- Lack of active movement

Mixed cerebral palsy
- Signs of more than one type of cerebral palsy
- Severely disabled

 SPOT CHECK

What are the most common associated problems with cerebral palsy?
Answer: The most common problems are abnormal muscle tone and coordination, which are seen in all types of cerebral palsy.

Diagnostic findings
- Neuroimaging studies determine the site of brain impairment.

- Cytogenic studies (genetic evaluation of the child and other family members) rule out other potential causes.
- Metabolic studies rule out other causes.

Nursing diagnoses
- Impaired physical mobility
- Imbalanced nutrition: Less than body requirements
- Delayed growth and development
- Impaired verbal communication
- Impaired parenting
- Deficient knowledge related to cerebral palsy
- Compromised family coping

Treatment
- High-calorie diet, if appropriate
- Artificial urinary sphincter for the incontinent child who can use hand controls
- Braces or splints and special appliances, such as adapted eating utensils and a low toilet seat with arms, to help the child perform activities independently
- Neurosurgery to decrease spasticity, if appropriate
- Orthopedic surgery to correct contractures
- Range-of-motion (ROM) exercises to minimize contractures (see *Performing passive range-of-motion exercises*)

Drug therapy options
- Muscle relaxant: to decrease spasticity, if appropriate
- Anticonvulsant: phenytoin (Dilantin), phenobarbital (Luminal)

Patient care goals
- The infant will consume adequate daily calories as required.
- The infant will maintain joint mobility and ROM.
- The infant's parents will develop adequate coping mechanisms.
- The infant's parents will demonstrate knowledge of the condition.

Nursing interventions
- Assist with locomotion, communication, and educational opportunities *to enable the child to attain optimal developmental level.*
- Increase caloric intake for the child with increased motor function *to keep up with increased metabolic needs.*
- Make food easy to manage *to decrease stress during mealtimes.*
- Provide a safe environment, for example, by using protective headgear or bed pads *to prevent injury.*

Performing passive range-of-motion exercises

Purpose

Used to move the child's joints through as full a range of motion as possible, passive range-of-motion (ROM) exercises improve or maintain joint mobility and help prevent contractures. Performed by a nurse, a physical therapist, or a caregiver, these exercises are indicated for the child with temporary or permanent loss of mobility, sensation, or consciousness. Passive ROM exercises require recognition of the child's limits of motion and support of all joints during movement.

Implementation

● Determine the joints that need ROM exercises, and consult the physician or physical therapist about limitations or precautions for specific exercises.
● Perform passive ROM at least once each shift, possibly while bathing or turning the child or when the child is in a convenient position. Repeat each exercise at least three times.
● Record which joints were exercised, the presence of edema or pressure areas, any pain resulting from the exercises, any limitation of ROM, and the child's tolerance of the exercises.

Exercising the neck

● Support the child's head with your hands and extend the neck, flex the chin to the chest, and tilt the head laterally toward each shoulder.
● Rotate the head from right to left.

Exercising the shoulders

● Support the child's arm in an extended, neutral position; then extend the forearm and flex it back. Abduct the arm outward from the side of the body, and adduct it back to the side.
● Rotate the shoulder so that the arm crosses the midline, and bend the elbow so that the hand touches the opposite shoulder and then touches the mattress of the bed for complete internal rotation.
● Return the shoulder to a neutral position and, with elbow bent, push the arm backward so that the back of the hand touches the mattress for complete external rotation.

Exercising the elbow

● Place the child's arm at his side with his palm facing up.
● Flex and extend the arm at the elbow.

Exercising the forearm

● Stabilize the child's elbow; then twist the hand to bring the palm up (supination).
● Twist it back again to bring the palm down (pronation).

Exercising the wrist

● Stabilize the forearm, and flex and extend the wrist. Then rock the hand sideways for lateral flexion and rotate the hand in a circular motion.

Exercising the fingers and thumb

● Extend the child's fingers, and then flex the hand into a fist; repeat extension and flexion of each joint of each finger and thumb separately.
● Spread two adjoining fingers apart (abduction), and then bring them together (adduction).
● Oppose each fingertip to the thumb, and rotate the thumb and each finger in a circle.

Exercising the hip and knee

● Fully extend the child's leg, and then bend the hip and knee toward the chest, allowing full joint flexion.
● Next, move the straight leg sideways, out and away from the other leg (abduction), and then back, over, and across it (adduction).
● Rotate the straight leg internally toward the midline and then externally away from the midline.

Exercising the ankle

● Bend the child's foot so that the toes push upward (dorsiflexion); then bend the foot so that the toes push downward (plantar flexion).
● Rotate the ankle in a circular motion.
● Invert the ankle so that the sole of the foot faces the midline, and evert the ankle so that the sole faces away from the midline.

Exercising the toes

● Flex the child's toes toward the sole, and then extend them back toward the top of the foot.
● Spread two adjoining toes apart (abduction), and then bring them back together (adduction).

● Provide rest periods *to promote rest and reduce metabolic needs.*
● Perform ROM exercises if the child is spastic *to maintain proper body alignment and mobility of joints.*
● Promote age-appropriate mental activities and incentives for motor development *to promote growth and development.*
● Divide tasks into small steps *to promote self-care and activity and to increase self-esteem.*
● Refer the child for speech, nutrition, and physical therapy *to maintain or improve functioning.*
● Use assistive communication devices if the child can't speak *to promote a positive self-concept.*

Evaluation
● The infant is maintaining joint mobility and ROM to the best degree possible.
● The infant continues to grow and meet developmental milestones.
● The infant's parents express an understanding of their infant's disorder and associated conditions.
● The infant's parents are providing opportunities for the infant to be stimulated and learn.

Cleft lip and cleft palate

CLEFT LIP and CLEFT PALATE are developmental defects. Cleft lip is a facial malformation resulting from failure of the premaxillary process to merge during gestational weeks 7 and 8. (The malformation may be unilateral or bilateral and may range from a notch in the vermilion border of the lip to a separation extending to the floor of the nose.) Cleft palate results from failure of the palatal process to fuse during the 7th to 12th weeks of gestation.

Long-term problems with cleft palate include impaired speech, malpositioned teeth and maxillary arches, impaired hearing from repeated otitis media, and recurring respiratory infections — all of which can result in impaired growth.

Possible causes
● CONGENITAL defects (in some cases, inheritance plays a role)
● Part of another chromosomal or mendelian abnormality
● Prenatal exposure to TERATOGENS

Data collection findings
● Altered appearance, ranging from a simple notch on the upper lip to complete cleft from the lip edge to the floor of the nostril, on either side of the midline but rarely along the midline itself
● Obvious cleft lip with or without cleft palate at birth (cleft palate without cleft lip may not be detected until a mouth examination is done or until feeding difficulties develop)
● Partial or complete cleft palate
● Difficulty swallowing
● Signs of upper or lower respiratory infections and otitis media, common in infants with cleft palate, resulting from difficulty sucking and swallowing
● Abdominal distention from swallowed air
● Changes in weight and growth pattern since birth
● Altered parent-infant attachment (parents exhibit anxiety and lack of understanding regarding preoperative and postoperative care routines for cleft lip repair)

Diagnostic findings
● Prenatal ultrasonography may indicate severe defects.
● Complete blood count (CBC) shows alterations.
● Serum electrolyte levels are abnormal.
● Urine specific gravity is high due to alterations in oxygenation and nutrition.

Nursing diagnoses
● Impaired swallowing
● Imbalanced nutrition: Less than body requirements
● Risk for aspiration
● Ineffective airway clearance
● Risk for infection
● Risk for impaired parent-infant attachment
● Deficient knowledge related to cleft lip and palate

Treatment
● Cleft lip repair surgery (CHEILOPLASTY) immediately after birth or in early infancy (ages 6 to 12 weeks) to unite the lip and gum edges in anticipation of teeth eruption, providing a route for adequate nutrition and sucking; done after a steady growth rate has been established
● Cleft palate repair surgery (STAPHYLORRHAPHY) usually between ages 1 and 2 years to allow for growth of the palate but before speech patterns develop (infant must be free from ear and respiratory infections and may require several stages of repair over a period of years)

- Long-term, team-oriented care to address speech defects, dental and orthodontic problems, nasal defects, and possible alterations in hearing
- Possible fetal repair if cleft lip is detected on sonogram while the infant is in utero

Patient care goals
- The infant will maintain satisfactory respiratory and nutritional status.
- The infant's suture line will remain intact and free from infection.
- The parents will understand preoperative and postoperative procedures used in the infant's care.
- The parents will participate in the infant's care to the extent they feel comfortable.
- The parents will help plan home care after cheiloplasty and ongoing care of cleft palate.

Nursing interventions
- Monitor vital signs and intake and output *to determine fluid volume status.*
- Assess respiratory status *to detect signs of aspiration.*
- Assess the quality of the infant's suck by determining whether he can form an airtight seal around a finger or nipple placed in his mouth *to determine an effective feeding method.*
- Be alert for respiratory distress when feeding *to avoid aspiration.*
- As the infant grows older, explore his feelings *to assess actual and potential coping problems.*

Preoperative interventions for cleft lip repair
- Feed the infant slowly and in an upright position *to decrease the risk of aspiration.*
- Burp the infant frequently during feeding *to eliminate swallowed air and decrease the risk of emesis.*
- Use gavage feedings if oral feedings are unsuccessful.
- Administer a small amount of water after feedings *to prevent formula from accumulating and becoming a medium for bacterial growth.*

- Give small, frequent feedings *to promote adequate nutrition and prevent tiring the infant.*
- Hold the infant while feeding, and promote sucking between meals. *Sucking is important to speech development.*

Postoperative interventions for cleft lip repair
- Observe for cyanosis as the infant begins to breathe through the nose *to detect signs of respiratory compromise.*
- Keep the infant's hands away from his mouth by using restraints or pinning the sleeves to his shirt; Steri-Strips are used to hold the suture line in place *to prevent tension and maintain an intact suture line.*
- Anticipate the infant's needs *to prevent crying and avoid stress on the suture line;* don't position him prone *to help prevent direct contact with the suture line.*
- Give extra care and support *because the infant can't have his emotional needs met by sucking.*
- Use a syringe with tubing to administer foods at the side of his mouth *to prevent trauma to the suture line.*
- Feed the infant in an upright position, burping after every 1 to 2 oz (29.6 to 59.1 ml) *to decrease the amount of air swallowed and make it easier to manage coughing or gagging.* Rinse his mouth with clear water after formula feeding *to prevent infection of the suture line and decrease the risk of ear infections.* Place the infant in an infant seat after feeding *to decrease the risk of aspiration.*
- When laying the infant down, place him on his right side *to prevent aspiration.*
- Clean the suture line after each feeding by dabbing it with half-strength hydrogen peroxide or saline solution *to prevent crusts and scarring.*
- Encourage the parents to participate in feeding if they feel comfortable doing this. Demonstrate if the parents are hesitant. *These measures can assist the parents if they have fear of traumatizing the suture line.*
- Monitor for pain and administer pain medication as prescribed; note the effectiveness of pain medication *to ensure adequate pain relief.*
- Explain to the parents that cleft palate repair is usually done between ages 1 and 2 years. Ask the parents to explain their understanding of how to care for the infant's cleft palate *to ensure adequate knowledge.*
- Discuss with family members available resources, such as children's medical services, social services, public health associations, and a local cleft palate parent group, *so the parents can receive support and guidance from health care professionals and other parents.*

Preoperative interventions for cleft palate repair

● Feed the infant with a cleft palate nipple or a Teflon implant *to enhance nutritional intake.*
● Wean the infant from the bottle or breast before cleft palate surgery; *the infant must be able to drink from a cup.*

Postoperative interventions for cleft palate repair

● Position the toddler in semi-Fowler's position *to promote a patent airway.*
● Anticipate edema and a decreased airway from the palate closure; this may cause the toddler to appear temporarily dyspneic; assess for signs of altered oxygenation *to promote good respiration.*
● Assess breath sounds and monitor vital signs every 4 hours *to detect signs of respiratory infection from aspiration.*
● Keep hard or pointed objects (such as utensils, straws, and frozen dessert sticks) away from the toddler's mouth *to prevent trauma to the suture line.*
● Use a cup to feed; don't use a nipple or pacifier *to prevent injury to the suture line.*
● Maintain an upright position for 30 minutes after feeding *to prevent aspiration.*
● After each feeding, rinse the toddler's mouth and suture line with at least 1 oz (29.6 ml) of water *to decrease irritation and sloughing of the incision.*
● Use elbow restraints *to keep the toddler's hands out of his mouth.*
● Provide soft toys *to prevent injury.*
● Start the toddler on clear liquids and progress to a soft diet; rinse the suture line by giving the toddler a sip of water after each feeding *to prevent infection.*
● Distract or hold the toddler *to keep his tongue away from the roof of his mouth.*
● Review key teaching topics with family members *to ensure adequate knowledge about the condition and treatment,* including:
– the importance of parental involvement (because it results in facial disfigurement, the condition may cause shock, guilt, and grief for the parents and may block parental bonding with the infant)
– the need for follow-up speech therapy
– understanding of the infant's susceptibility to pathogens and otitis media because of the altered position of the eustachian tubes.

Evaluation

● The infant remains afebrile, has clear breath sounds bilaterally, feeds without aspiration, and maintains admission weight.
● The infant's suture line remains intact and free from inflammation and sloughing.
● The infant has no skin irritation or breakdown under the elbow restraints.
● The infant responds well to cuddling and stops crying quickly after being held.
● The infant's parents participate in feeding the infant and caring for the suture line before discharge.
● The infant's parents verbalize an understanding of long-term cleft palate care and the potential problems with respiratory infection, dentition, and speech development.
● The infant's parents verbalize plans to continue follow-up care with an interdisciplinary cleft lip and cleft palate team.

Clubfoot

CLUBFOOT, also known as talipes, is a congenital disorder in which the foot and ankle are twisted and can't be manipulated into the correct position. Clubfoot occurs in these five forms:
● talipes equinovarus — a combination of positions
● talipes calcaneus — dorsiflexion, as if walking on one's heels
● talipes equinus — plantar flexion, as if pointing one's toes
● talipes valgus — eversion of the ankles, with the feet turning out
● talipes varus — inversion of the ankles, with the soles of the feet facing each other.

 FAST FACT

Nearly all cases of talipes are equinovarus, involving a combination of abnormal positions.

Possible causes

● Arrested development during the 9th and 10th weeks of embryonic life, when the feet are formed
● Deformed talus and shortened Achilles tendon
● Possible genetic predisposition

Data collection findings

● Deformity usually obvious at birth

- Disorder can't be corrected manually (distinguishes true clubfoot from apparent clubfoot)

Diagnostic findings
- X-rays show superimposition of the talus and calcaneus and a ladderlike appearance of the metatarsals.

Nursing diagnoses
- Impaired physical mobility
- Delayed growth and development
- Risk for peripheral neurovascular dysfunction
- Risk for impaired skin integrity
- Risk for impaired parent-infant attachment
- Deficient knowledge related to clubfoot

Treatment
Treatment is administered in three stages:
- correcting the deformity either with a series of casts to gradually stretch and realign the angle of the foot and, after cast removal, application of a Denis Browne splint at night until age 1 or surgical correction
- maintaining the correction until the foot gains normal muscle balance.
- observing the foot closely for several years to prevent the deformity from recurring.

Patient care goals
- The infant will maintain joint mobility and ROM.
- The infant will maintain muscle strength.
- The infant will show no evidence of complications, such as contractures, venous stasis, thrombus formulation, or skin breakdown.
- The infant's parents will verbalize an understanding of the condition and treatment options.

Nursing interventions
- Assess neurovascular status *to ensure circulation to the foot with a cast in place.*
- Ensure that shoes fit correctly *to promote comfort and prevent skin breakdown.*
- Prepare for surgery, if necessary, *to maintain or promote the healing process and decrease anxiety.*

Evaluation
- The infant shows improved joint mobility and ROM.
- The infant shows no sign of circulatory impairment to the legs and maintains skin integrity.

- The infant's parents demonstrate an understanding of care after the infant is home with a clubfoot cast, including cast care and checking for signs of circulatory impairment.
- The infant's parents understand the importance of doing exercises to help maintain the correction.
- The infant's parents exhibit bonding with their infant and appropriate coping skills.

Developmental dysplasia of the hip

DEVELOPMENTAL DYSPLASIA OF THE HIP (DDH), also known as *dislocated hip*, results from an abnormal development of the hip socket. It occurs when the head of the femur is still cartilaginous and the acetabulum (socket) is shallow; as a result, the head of the femur comes out of the hip socket. DDH can affect one or both hips and occurs in varying degrees of dislocation, from partial (subluxation) to complete. (See *Pediatric musculoskeletal facts.*)

DDH is seven times more common in girls than in boys. It's usually diagnosed during the initial pediatric assessment, but screening for DDH should be done at all visits for the 1st year of life. (See *Assessing DDH,* page 210.)

Pediatric musculoskeletal facts

Bones and muscles
- Bones and muscles grow and develop throughout childhood.
- Bone lengthening occurs in the epiphyseal plates at the ends of bones; when the epiphyses close, growth stops.
- Bone healing occurs much faster in a child than in an adult because the child's bones are still growing.
- The younger the child, the faster a bone heals.
- Bone healing takes approximately 1 week for every year of life up to age 10.

Fractures
The most common fractures in children are clavicular fractures and greenstick fractures:
- Clavicular fractures may occur during vaginal birth because the shoulders are the widest part of the body.
- Greenstick fractures of the long bones are related to the increased flexibility of a young child's bones. (The compressed side of the bone bends while the side under tension fractures.)

Assessing DDH

The following illustrations demonstrate signs that would be found in an infant with developmental dysplasia of the hip (DDH).

ASYMMETRIC THIGH AND GLUTEAL FOLDS

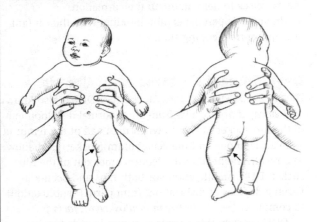

ORTOLANI'S SIGN (HIP CLICK FELT DURING EXTERNAL ROTATION)

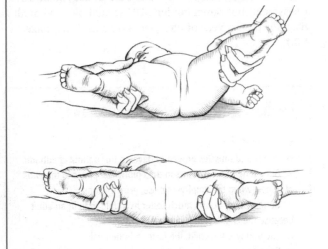

HIP ABDUCTION LIMITED

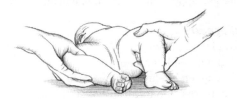

ALLIS' SIGN (ONE KNEE LOWER THAN THE OTHER)

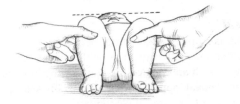

TRENDELENBURG'S SIGN (IN A CHILD OF WEIGHT-BEARING AGE)

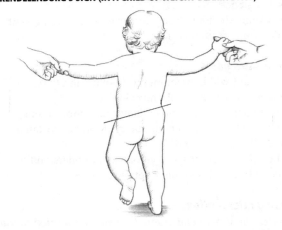

Possible causes
- Breech delivery
- Fetal position in utero
- Genetic predisposition
- Laxity of the ligaments
- Swaddling infants with hip adduction and extension

Data collection findings
- Restricted abduction of the hips
- Appearance of a shortened limb on the affected side
- On the affected side, an increased number of folds on the posterior thigh when the infant is supine with knees bent

Diagnostic findings
- Barlow's sign is present. A click is felt when the infant is placed supine with hips flexed 90 degrees, knees fully flexed, and the hip brought into midabduction.
- Ortolani's sign is present. A click can be felt by the examiner's fingers at the hip area as the femur head snaps out of and back into the acetabulum. It's also palpable

Comparing plaster and synthetic casts

PLASTER CAST	SYNTHETIC CAST
● Heavy	● Lightweight
● Takes 10 to 72 hours to dry	● Takes 5 to 30 minutes to dry
● Molds easily to body parts	● Doesn't mold easily (not useful for small children)
● Smooth exterior	● Rough exterior (can abrade adjacent body parts)
● Inexpensive	● Expensive (three to seven times more costly than a plaster cast)
● Must be protected around water	● Can be immersed in water (observe for macerated skin if dried inadequately)

during examination with the infant's legs flexed and abducted.
● Ultrasonography and magnetic resonance imaging may be used to assess reduction.
● Trendelenburg's test is positive. When the infant or child stands on the affected leg, the opposite pelvis dips to maintain erect posture.
● X-rays show the location of the femur head and a shallow acetabulum. X-rays can also be used to monitor progression of the disorder.

Nursing diagnoses
● Impaired physical mobility
● Risk for peripheral neurovascular dysfunction
● Risk for impaired skin integrity
● Delayed growth and development

Treatment
Treatment varies according to the infant's or child's age. It's most successful when begun before age 2 months, becomes difficult after age 4 years, and is inadvisable after age 6. Regardless of age, the goal of treatment is to maintain abduction and prevent deformity. Treatment may include:
● hip-spica cast or corrective surgery for older children
● Bryant's traction, if the acetabulum doesn't deepen
● triple-cloth diapering, casting, or a Pavlik harness to keep the hips and knees flexed and the hips abducted for at least 3 months; if unsuccessful, corrective surgery. (See *Comparing plaster and synthetic casts.*)

Patient care goals
● The infant will maintain hip abduction.
● The infant will maintain adequate circulation and innervation of the legs while in a cast.
● The infant's skin integrity won't be impaired.

● The parents will demonstrate cast care and be able to provide it at home.

Nursing interventions
● Assess circulation before application of a cast or traction; after application, tickle the infant's feet to get him to wiggle his toes *to detect signs of impaired circulation.* You should be able to place one finger between the skin and the cast. (See *Performing hip-spica cast care,* page 212.)
● Assess for pain that's unrelieved by analgesia *to identify signs of compartment syndrome.*
● Provide skin care *to prevent skin breakdown.*
● Give reassurance that early prompt treatment will probably result in complete correction *to decrease anxiety.*
● Assure the parents that the infant will adjust to restricted movement and return to normal sleeping, eating, and play behaviors in a few days *to ease their anxiety.*
● Inspect the skin, especially around bony prominences, *to detect cast complications and skin breakdown.*
● Review key teaching topics with family members *to ensure adequate knowledge about the condition and treatment,* including:
– correctly splinting or bracing the hips
– receiving frequent checkups
– coping with restricted movement
– removing braces and splints while bathing the infant and replacing them immediately afterward
– stressing good hygiene.

Evaluation
● The infant maintains adequate circulation and innervation of the legs while in the cast.
● The infant is interested in his environment and shows age-appropriate developmental behaviors.

NURSING PROCEDURE

Performing hip-spica cast care

Purpose
A hip-spica cast is applied to maintain hip abduction. Hip-spica cast care is done to:
- protect the cast from urine and feces
- keep the cast dry
- ensure proper blood supply to the legs
- teach the infant's parents how to care for the cast at home.

Implementation
- Check neurovascular status.
- Feel the cast for tightness.
- Blanch toes or toenails every 1 to 2 hours (initially).
- Feel the toes for coldness, and observe for swelling, cyanosis, and pain.
- Feel the cast for warm spots, especially over bony prominences.
- Smell the cast for odors from pressure areas under the cast.
- Observe respirations carefully for signs of impairment.
- Check skin integrity
- Inspect the skin and cast regularly for crumbs.

- Inspect the cast edges.
- Petal the raw cast edges as soon as the cast is dry.
- Keep exposed skin clean and dry.
- Keep small objects and toys away from the infant because they may be put inside the cast.
- Check cast integrity
- Position the infant with the hips lower than the shoulders for toileting. Use a plastic-backed disposable diaper under the cast rim to prevent soiling.
- Turn the infant every 2 hours until the cast is dry; then change the infant's position frequently for comfort.
- Handle a wet cast with the palms. Finger indentation can cause pressure ulcers.
- Check the infant's temperature frequently while the cast is drying.
- Clean the cast with only a damp cloth and a small amount of white cleanser; apply the cleanser only to soiled areas.
- Record the date and time of cast care. Document neurovascular status and skin and cast conditions

- The infant's parents can describe the cast-care procedures they must follow when they bring the infant home from the hospital.

Diarrhea

Diarrhea is an increase in the frequency, volume, and liquidity of stools. Acute diarrhea is the sudden onset of frequent loose or watery stools. Chronic diarrhea begins more slowly, with a gradual increase in the number of stools; consistency becomes loose and unformed.

Diarrhea becomes a problem for infants and children because water and electrolyte loss from the bowel can cause dehydration. Dehydration is classified as isotonic, hypertonic, or hypotonic, based on the relationship of electrolyte loss to fluid loss, and as mild, moderate, or severe, based on the percentage of body weight loss (mild: 2% to 4% weight loss; moderate: 5% to 9% weight loss; severe: 10% or greater weight loss).

Possible causes
- Acute — inflammatory response to an intestinal tract infection

- Chronic — usually results from inflammatory reaction and allergic response or malabsorption syndrome

Data collection findings
Infant
- Stool evaluation
- Stools tinged with blood, mucus, or pus
- Foul-smelling stools
- Change in stool color (light or dark)
- Change in stool consistency or frequency
- Signs of abdominal cramping
- Crying
- Clutching the abdomen
- Flexing the knees to the abdomen
- Signs of dehydration
- Dry mucous membranes
- Sunken anterior fontanel
- Crying without tears
- Decreased number of wet diapers
- Dietary intake (food and fluid) for the 24 hours before the diarrhea started
- Environmental issues, such as source of water, presence of family pets, or travel to another country

Family members

- Similar symptoms in other family members
- Knowledge of illness precautions and how to prevent the spread of infection

Diagnostic findings

- Stool cultures may reveal the presence of bacteria or other infectious agents.
- Microscopic examination of stool may reveal the presence of ova or parasites.
- Stool guaiac test can reveal occult blood.
- Serum electrolytes may reveal signs of dehydration and metabolic acidosis.

Nursing diagnoses

- Risk for infection
- Risk for deficient fluid volume
- Risk for impaired skin integrity
- Delayed growth and development

Treatment

- Replacement of fluids and electrolytes
- Treatment of infection, if present
- Prevention of spread of infection (if applicable)
- Hospitalization, depending on the length of illness, extent of dehydration, serum electrolyte levels, and infant's age

Patient care goals

- The infant's infection won't be transmitted to others.
- The infant will regain fluid and electrolyte balance.
- The infant will have fewer stools per day.
- The infant's skin will remain intact in the perianal area.
- Members of the infant's family will demonstrate understanding of current treatments and the anticipated approach to the diet when oral intake is resumed.
- The infant will maintain or regain his pre-illness developmental level.

Nursing interventions

- Weigh the infant daily using the same scale and at the same time of day *to assist with fluid status evaluation.*
- Maintain hourly intake and output; monitor hydration status (for dehydration and overhydration) every 4 hours *to identify signs of increase or decrease in hydration.*
- Weigh diapers on a gram scale *to help determine fluid loss.* (If stools are watery, apply a pediatric urine collector *to differentiate urine and stool amounts.*)

- Send stools to the laboratory for ordered cultures. Place in double containers *to prevent personnel contamination during the transport.*
- Record amount, consistency, and frequency of stools and perform stool testing for the presence of blood, as ordered, *to determine the infant's elimination patterns and response to therapy.*
- Clean perianal skin thoroughly. Apply protective ointment as needed and report alterations in skin integrity *to help prevent skin irritation and breakdown. (Broken skin can lead to secondary infection.)*
- Administer I.V. fluids at maintenance and greater levels, as ordered, *to provide hydration.*
- Monitor the I.V. administration insertion site and surrounding areas for signs of infiltration *to quickly identify any disruption in the administration of I.V. fluids.*
- Administer oral fluids as ordered when stools decrease in frequency and liquid content. Give food high in sodium content (broth, salted crackers) sparingly *to avoid hypernatremia.*
- Ensure that facility personnel and visitors wash hands carefully and follow facility policies regarding isolation precautions *to prevent the spread of infection to personnel and visitors.*
- Offer the infant a pacifier as desired *to provide for intensified oral needs in response to regression and food and fluid restrictions.*
- Provide age-appropriate sensorimotor stimulation; include auditory (musical toys, verbal conversation), visual (colorful toys, pictures, mobiles), and tactile (stuffed toys, stroking, books) stimuli *to provide appropriate stimulation and activities for maintaining the infant's developmental stage.*
- Encourage parents to remain with the infant as much as possible *to help prevent separation anxiety (fear of abandonment).* The infant needs repeated reassurance of the parents' love and presence.
- Discuss the treatment regimen with family members. Prepare family members for possible follow-up and discharge planning. If the disease is communicable, they should receive written instructions for careful hand washing, disposing of the infant's excretions, and cleaning toilet facilities. Family members should also be taught how to avoid transmitting enteropathologic organisms, with an emphasis on proper hand washing and food handling. If stool specimens are needed from family members, provide written instructions for proper collection and delivery. *These steps help to ensure the planned treatment regimen and prevent the transmission of the infection to others.*

Evaluation

- The infant's body weight is being maintained or is increasing.
- The infant has adequate urine output and a decrease in the number of stools per day.
- The infant has intact skin integrity.
- The infant plays peek-a-boo with parents and staff members.
- The infant's parents express understanding of verbal instructions regarding the hospital treatment regimen and receive, discuss, and express understanding of written discharge instructions.
- Members of the infant's family are free from symptoms and remain so after the infant's discharge from the hospital.

Failure to thrive

FAILURE TO THRIVE is a chronic, potentially life-threatening condition characterized by failure to maintain weight and height above the 5th percentile on age-appropriate growth charts. Most children are diagnosed before age 2. It can result from physical, emotional, or psychological causes.

Possible causes

- Organic — acute or chronic illness (GI reflux, malabsorption syndrome, congenital heart defect, or cystic fibrosis)
- Nonorganic — psychological problem between infant and primary caregiver such as failure to bond
- Mixed — combination of organic and nonorganic causes

Data collection findings

- Altered body posture (infant is stiff or floppy and doesn't cuddle)
- Disparities between chronological age and height and weight
- History of insufficient stimulation and inadequate parental knowledge of child development
- Delayed psychosocial behavior (for example, reluctance to smile or talk)
- History of inadequate feeding techniques, such as bottle propping or insufficient burping
- History of medical problems
- History of sleep disturbances
- Psychosocial family problems
- REGURGITATION of food after almost every feeding, part being vomited and the remainder swallowed (rumination of food)

Diagnostic findings

- Negative nitrogen balance indicates inadequate intake of protein or calories.
- Associated physiologic causes may be detected.
- Reduced creatinine-height index reflects muscle mass and estimates muscle protein depletion.

Nursing diagnoses

- Delayed growth and development
- Imbalanced nutrition: Less than body requirements
- Impaired parenting

Treatment

- High-calorie diet
- Parent counseling
- Respite care for the infant

Drug therapy options

- Vitamin and mineral supplement

Patient care goals

- The infant will have improved growth and development as evidenced by maintaining body weight and meeting age-appropriate milestones.
- The infant's parents will demonstrate improved parenting skills as evidenced by asking appropriate questions about the infant's condition and participating in the infant's care.

Nursing interventions

- Weigh the infant on admission and measure head circumference and length and height *to determine baseline weight.*

 FAST FACT

In general, adequate growth in an infant is considered to be a weight gain of 15 to 30 g per day. With decreased caloric intake, weight will decrease first and then linear growth will slow down, followed by stunted growth of the head. However, the head circumference will be normal in most infants with failure to thrive.

- Assess growth and development using an appropriate tool, such as the Denver Developmental Screening Test, *to determine the infant's developmental level.*
- Properly feed and interact with the infant *to promote nutrition and growth and development.*

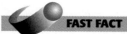
FAST FACT

For a breast-fed infant, the mother should be doing approximately eight feedings (every 3 hours) in a 24-hour period for adequate nutrition. Formula-fed infants typically will have six feedings per day, or about every 4 hours.

- Establish specific times for feeding, bathing, and sleeping *to establish and maintain a structured routine.*
- Provide the infant with visual and auditory stimulation *to promote normal sensory development.*
- Assess parent-infant interaction *to determine whether failure to thrive is due to the parents' inability to form an emotional attachment to the infant.*
- When caring for the infant in the parents' presence, act as a role model for effective parenting skills. Demonstrate comfort measures such as rocking the infant, and show the parents how to hold the infant *to increase the parents' knowledge of routine infant care practices.*
- Teach the parents about normal growth and development, and identify ages at which the infant should be able to master developmental tasks, such as rolling over, crawling, and walking. This will assist the parents in monitoring the infant's growth and development. Also, discuss problem behaviors associated with specific ages, such as colic, temper tantrums, and sleeping difficulties, *to further enhance the parents' understanding of developmental norms.*
- Discuss the infant's need for tactile and sensory stimulation. Demonstrate play activities that promote developmental skills, such as shaking a rattle in front of the infant *to build eye-and-hand coordination* or placing a mobile above the infant *to encourage visual tracking and trunk and head control. Sensory experiences promote* COGNITIVE DEVELOPMENT.

Evaluation
- The infant is maintaining or increasing in body weight and achieving age-appropriate developmental milestones.
- The infant's parents express an understanding of his adequate feeding requirements and of age-appropriate growth and development.
- The infant's parents maintain a loving and supportive relationship with him.

Hirschsprung's disease

In HIRSCHSPRUNG'S DISEASE, also known as *congenital aganglionic megacolon*, a portion of the colon lacks ganglionic cells and the peristaltic waves needed to pass feces through that segment of the colon. The result is chronic constipation as stool accumulates proximal to the aganglionic segment, which is narrowed. However, the infant may pass small ribbonlike stools through the narrow segment despite the internal sphincter's failure to relax. Hirschsprung's disease is four times more common in boys than in girls, and it occurs in 1 out of 5,000 births. (See *Pediatric GI facts.*)

Possible causes
- Lack of ganglionic cells (which normally form along the digestive tract of the fetus between the 5th and 12th week of gestation) beyond a certain point in the intestine. (See *Causes of lower bowel obstruction,* pages 216 and 217.)

Data collection findings
- Absence or delayed passing of meconium stool within 48 hours after birth
- Distended abdomen

Pediatric GI facts

Here are some characteristics of the pediatric GI system:
- Peristalsis occurs within 2½ to 3 hours in the neonate and within 3 to 6 hours in older infants and children.
- Gastric stomach capacity of the neonate is 30 to 60 ml, which gradually increases to 200 to 350 ml by age 12 months and to 1,500 ml as an adolescent.
- The neonatal abdomen is larger than the chest up to ages 4 to 8 weeks, and the musculature is poorly developed.
- The sucking and extrusion reflex persists to ages 3 to 4 months (the extrusion reflex protects the infant from food substances that his system is too immature to digest).
- At age 4 months, saliva production begins and aids in the digestion process.
- Neonates frequently spit up because of the immature muscle tone of the lower esophageal sphincter and the small volume capacity of the stomach.
- Increased myelination of nerves to the anal sphincter allows for physiologic control of bowel function usually around age 2 years.
- The liver's slow development of glycogen storage capacity makes the infant prone to hypoglycemia.
- From ages 1 to 3 years, the composition of intestinal flora becomes more adultlike and stomach acidity increases, reducing the number of GI infections.

Causes of lower bowel obstruction

CONDITION	CHARACTERISTICS	MEDICAL DIAGNOSIS AND TREATMENT	NURSING CARE
Intussusception (telescoping of the intestine into an adjacent portion)	● Incidence: rare in 1st month after birth; most common between ages 3 and 12 months ● Paroxysmal abdominal pain ● Currant-jelly stools (mixture of blood and mucus) ● Vomiting ● Abdominal distention, tenderness, and a palpable mass ● Dehydration and fever progressing to shock	● Air enema (may reduce intussusception; also used in diagnosis) ● Surgery to remove hypoxic bowel section and reconnect remaining healthy bowel sections	● Restore and maintain fluid and electrolyte balance. ● Prevent vomiting and aspiration. ● Carefully assess progression of the infant's stools (normal brown indicates resolved intussusception). ● After surgery, maintain stomach decompression until the infant passes the first stool.
Appendicitis (inflammation of the appendix; the most common cause of abdominal surgery in children)	● Abdominal pain, localized tenderness, and fever ● Initially, generalized pain around the umbilicus, then localized pain in the right lower quadrant ● Changes in behavior, anorexia, or vomiting (common early signs) ● White blood cell (WBC) count of 15,000 to 20,000/μl ● Constipation or diarrhea ● Possible perforation (indicated by sudden pain relief) or peritonitis (indicated by increased pain, rigid abdomen, obvious guarding of the abdomen, high fever, and elevated WBC count) if untreated	● Surgical removal of the appendix ● Management of peritonitis, shock, dehydration, and infection ● Chest X-ray to differentiate appendicitis from pneumonia (pneumonia may cause referred pain in the right lower quadrant and thus may be misdiagnosed as appendicitis) ● Barium GI series and ultrasonography to differentiate appendicitis from other abdominal problems	● Don't administer enemas or laxatives or apply heat to the abdomen. ● When the appendix isn't perforated, perform the same postoperative care as for any abdominal surgery. ● When the appendix is perforated (and Penrose drains are in place), place the child in semi-Fowler's position or on his right side after surgery. ● Change dressings frequently, and provide meticulous skin care at the operative site.
Imperforate anus (absent anal opening or opening obliterated by thin, translucent membrane)	● One of the most common congenital anomalies caused by abnormal development ● Absence of anus noted when taking the first rectal temperature in the neonatal unit ● Absence of meconium ● Possible meconium in urine, indicating an associated rectourethral fistula	● Digital and endoscopic examination ● Abdominal X-ray with opaque marker at the anal dimple and with the infant in the inverted position (the air outlines a blind rectal pouch) ● Surgery to reconstruct the anus and perform a colon pull-through or sigmoid colostomy with anastomosis and pull-through 1 year later	● After anorectal repair, place the infant in a side-lying or prone position, with the hips elevated to keep pressure off the sutures. ● Feed the infant when peristalsis returns. ● Help the parents adjust to the infant's congenital disorder. ● Conduct a thorough assessment and history taking particularly concerning diet and bowel habits. ● Preoperatively, teach parents colostomy care and what to expect postoperatively. ● Monitor abdominal distention: Measure girth every 8 hours. ● Provide resources for parents going home.

Causes of lower bowel obstruction *(continued)*

CONDITION	CHARACTERISTICS	MEDICAL DIAGNOSIS AND TREATMENT	NURSING CARE
Hirschsprung's disease (congenital aganglionic megacolon)	● Four times more common in boys than in girls ● Incidence: 1 in 5,000 births ● Failure to pass meconium within 48 hours after birth ● Food refusal, vomiting, and abdominal distention ● Inadequate weight gain, constipation, abdominal distention, episodes of vomiting, and diarrhea in older infant ● Chronic symptoms of constipation, ribbon-like foul stools, abdominal distention, and impaction in older child	● Diagnosis in early infancy based on signs of intestinal obstruction ● Dilated proximal colon and aganglionic segment indicated by barium enema ● Diagnosis confirmed by rectal biopsy ● Anorectal manometry may be used: pressure-sensitive catheter and balloon placed in the rectum and pressures of the internal and external sphincters recorded ● Two-stage bowel resection performed surgically, with a temporary colostomy for 4 to 6 weeks	● Observe for signs of complications, such as fever, bloody diarrhea, and vomiting, and notify the physician if these occur. ● Keep the infant in an upright position, for example, in an infant seat. ● After colostomy, keep the area around the stoma clean and dry and cover with dressings or a colostomy or ileostomy appliance to absorb drainage. Watch for prolapse, discoloration, or excessive bleeding (slight bleeding is common). ● After the final corrective surgery, keep the wound clean and dry. Don't use a rectal thermometer. The infant will have a bowel movement in 3 to 4 days, which may create discomfort. Watch for signs of anastomic leaks (sudden development of abdominal distention, temperature spike, or extreme irritability). ● Because an infant with Hirschsprung's disease needs surgery and hospitalization so early in life, provide emotional support to family members.

● Lack of stool in the rectum
● Episodes of vomiting and diarrhea
● Foul-smelling stool
● Presence of ribbonlike or pellet-shaped stools
● Constipation
● Anemia
● Refusal of food; inadequate weight gain
● Thin, undernourished appearance

Diagnostic findings
● Rectal examination reveals absence of stool in the rectum.

● Barium enema films show a dilated colon segment proximal to the narrowed aganglionic segment of colon.
● Rectal biopsy confirms the diagnosis.

Nursing diagnoses
● Imbalanced nutrition: Less than body requirements
● Risk for deficient fluid volume
● Risk for infection
● Deficient knowledge related to Hirschsprung's disease
● Disturbed sleep pattern

Treatment

● Surgery (two-stage bowel resection with a temporary colostomy for 4 to 6 weeks)

Patient care goals

● The child's bowel will be emptied preoperatively and prepared for a colostomy.
● The child's parents will understand the procedures involved in preoperative bowel preparation, the surgical procedure and desired outcome, and changes in body function.
● The child will regain and maintain fluid and electrolyte balance.
● The child will heal without infection postoperatively.
● The child will have adequate nutrition to provide for growth and weight gain.
● The child will participate in appropriate age-related activities.
● The child's colostomy will function normally.
● The child's parents will understand and participate in colostomy care.
● The child and parents will return home able to cope with the child's altered body functions.

Nursing interventions

Before surgery

● Prepare the child's bowel for surgery by administering antibiotics and saline colonic enemas until the bowel is clear *to reduce bacterial flora.* This preparation isn't necessary in the neonate, whose bowel is sterile.
● Teach the child's parents about the surgical procedure (temporary colostomy with or without pull-through anastomosis to anus) and about required preoperative care *to reduce anxiety.* Space the explanations *to prevent anxiety and confusion from too much information.*

After surgery

● Weigh the child at the same time each day, using the same scale, to obtain accurate weight measurements, *which can help in monitoring the child's fluid balance and nutritional state.*
● Monitor and record abdominal circumference at least once every shift *to evaluate for abdominal distention, which can crowd the diaphragm and interfere with respirations.* Use a pen to mark where the measurement is taken.
● Withhold food and fluids until bowel sounds return, the nasogastric (NG) tube is removed, and the colostomy or anastomosed bowel can tolerate feedings; begin with small, frequent meals. *Bowel decompression continues postoperatively until bowel sounds return.*

● Change the child's diaper frequently, especially immediately after each bowel movement, *to prevent contamination of the surgical site and promote healing.* The stoma typically is placed low on the abdomen *so that the child may not need stoma bags and the skin surrounding the stoma won't be abraded.*
● If stoma bags are necessary, change stomal dressings with each bowel movement. Keep the diaper below the stoma. Use appropriate-sized ostomy supplies. *Changing dressings prevents contamination of the surgical site and promotes healing. Keeping the diaper below the stoma avoids contaminating the stoma with urine. Appropriate-sized ostomy supplies can help prevent skin breakdown.*
● Involve the parents early in dressing changes and irrigations, if ordered, *to help them gradually accept their child's altered body functions.*
● Evaluate the child's pain level; include the parents' assessment of the child's behavior *because parents know their child's behavior and commonly can assess their child's pain level.* Provide pain relief measures, such as medications, distraction, and relaxation techniques, *to relieve pain.*

Evaluation

● The child returns home free from stomal infection.
● The child's discomfort is relieved by nonnarcotic analgesia.
● The child has an average of at least one bowel movement each day and is free from abdominal distention.
● The child begins to enjoy mealtimes and eats without discomfort.
● The child gains weight and continues to develop at the appropriate developmental rate.
● The child's parents are performing stoma care and irrigations as instructed.

Myelomeningocele

MYELOMENINGOCELE, the most severe SPINA BIFIDA defect, is a protruding, saclike cyst, usually in the lumbosacral area, that contains meninges, spinal fluid, and a portion of the spinal cord with its nerves. This congenital neural tube defect is readily apparent at birth. The myelomeningocele is commonly encased in a thin membrane that's prone to tears and leakage of cerebrospinal fluid (CSF). The extent of neurologic dysfunction depends on the level of the vertebral column at which the defect occurs. Lumbosacral lesions tend to be associated with flaccid paralysis of the legs; NEUROGENIC BLADDER and fecal incontinence; musculoskeletal deformities, including flexion or extension contractures; talipes varus or valgus; and hip dislocation or subluxation.

HYDROCEPHALUS associated with Arnold-Chiari malformation (downward displacement of the cerebellar tonsils through the foramen magnum into the cervical spinal canal) occurs in approximately 90% of those with lumbosacral myelomeningocele.

Possible causes
- Combination of genetic and environmental factors
- Exposure to a teratogen
- Part of a multiple-malformation syndrome (for example, chromosomal abnormalities, such as trisomy 13 or 18 syndrome)

Data collection findings
- Saclike structure protruding over the spine with evidence of solid matter on TRANSILLUMINATION (light passed through the side of the sac); translucent sac may indicate MENINGOCELE rather than myelomeningocele
- Permanent neurologic dysfunction (paralysis)
- Increased head circumference or unusual disproportion between the head and chest circumferences, which may indicate hydrocephalus before other neurologic symptoms appear (a neonate's head circumference is normally about 1″ [2.5 cm] larger than the chest circumference)
- Hydrocephalus
- Increased intracranial pressure (ICP)
- Arnold-Chiari syndrome
- Curvature of the spine
- Clubfoot
- Possible mental retardation
- Knee contractures

Diagnostic findings
- Amniocentesis reveals a neural tube defect.
- Elevated alpha-fetoprotein levels in the mother's blood may indicate a neural tube defect.
- Acetylcholinesterase measurement can be used to confirm the diagnosis.
- After birth, spinal X-ray can be used to show the bone defect.
- Chromosomal abnormalities associated with neural tube defects may be revealed by fetal karyotype and biochemical test results.
- Myelography can be used to differentiate spina bifida from other spinal abnormalities, particularly spinal cord tumors.
- Ultrasound may be used to identify the open neural tube or ventral wall defect.

Nursing diagnoses
- Impaired physical mobility
- Risk for infection
- Impaired skin integrity
- Delayed growth and development
- Risk for impaired parent-infant attachment

Treatment
- Surgical closure of the sac by skin grafts 24 to 48 hours after birth or after the infant can more easily tolerate the procedure (doesn't reverse neurologic deficits)
- Supportive measures to promote independence and prevent further complications
- Placement of VENTRICULOPERITONEAL SHUNT to treat hydrocephalus (see *Ventriculoperitoneal shunt*, page 220)

Patient care goals
- During hospitalization, the infant will:
– maintain an intact myelomeningocele sac before surgery
– maintain stable vital signs and neurologic status
– show no symptoms of increased ICP (indicating shunt malfunction or infection)
– maintain ROM and corrective positioning
– maintain skin integrity
– maintain urinary elimination without bladder distention and no sign of urinary tract infection (UTI) due to catheterization.
- The infant's parents will:
– demonstrate at least three positive signs of attachment within 72 hours
– verbalize an understanding of operative procedures, the need to report signs of increased ICP and infection promptly, and the need for long-term follow-up of problems related to myelomeningocele and hydrocephalus
– demonstrate appropriate care techniques (for example, monitoring neurologic status for increased ICP, monitoring for infection, and performing intermittent catheterization and ROM exercises), which they will continue after discharge.

Nursing interventions
Before surgery
- Hold and cuddle the infant on your lap, and position him on his abdomen; handle the infant carefully and don't apply pressure to the defect *to prevent injury at the site of the defect.*
- Clean the defect, inspect it often, and cover it with sterile dressings moistened with sterile normal saline solution *to prevent infection.*

Ventriculoperitoneal shunt

This illustration shows the placement of the ventriculoperitoneal shunt. Note that the end in the peritoneal cavity is coiled to allow room for growth of the infant.

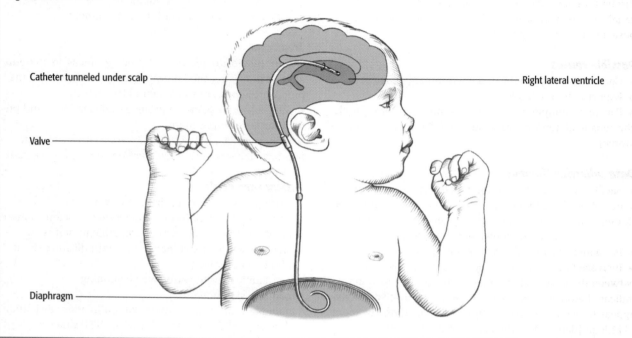

Catheter tunneled under scalp

Valve

Diaphragm

Right lateral ventricle

● In most cases, the infant can't wear a diaper or a shirt until after surgical correction *because it will irritate the sac,* so keep him warm in an infant Isolette *to prevent hypothermia.*
● Watch for signs of hydrocephalus. Measure head circumference daily. Be sure to mark the spot where the measurement was made *to ensure accurate readings.*
● Watch for signs of meningeal irritation, such as fever and nuchal rigidity, *to detect signs of meningitis.*
● Contractures can be minimized by passive ROM exercises and casting. Moderately abduct the hips with a pad between the knees or with sandbags and ankle rolls *to prevent hip dislocation.*
● Monitor intake and output. Watch for decreased skin turgor and dryness *to detect dehydration.*
● Provide a diet high in calories and protein *to ensure adequate nutrition.*

After surgery to correct myelomeningocele
● Watch for hydrocephalus, which follows surgery in many cases. Measure the infant's head circumference, as

ordered, *to detect signs of hydrocephalus and to prevent associated complications.*
● Monitor vital signs often *to detect early signs of shock, infection, and increased ICP.* (See *Signs of increased intracranial pressure.*)
● Change the dressing regularly, as ordered, and check for and report signs of drainage, wound rupture, and infection *to promote early treatment and prevent complications.*
● Place the infant in the prone position *to protect and assess the site.*
● If leg casts have been applied to treat deformities, watch for signs that the infant is outgrowing the cast. Regularly check distal pulses *to ensure adequate circulation.*

After placement of ventriculoperitoneal shunt to treat hydrocephalus
● Place the infant flat, with hips abducted or on the nonsurgical side; change his position every hour *to help prevent too-rapid decompression of the intracranial fluid.* Hip abduction continues to be necessary because of the neurologic deficit to the lower body. A side-lying position must be on the nonsurgical side *to avoid putting pressure on the*

shunt valve. Changing the infant's position reduces the risk of hypostatic pneumonia and pressure ulcers.

● Document head circumference every shift; assess and document vital signs and neurologic status (anterior fontanelle and pupils, blood pressure, level of irritability, sucking reflex, listlessness, and seizure activity) every 4 hours *to identify complications.* The valve opens at a certain intraventricular pressure and closes when the pressure is sufficiently reduced by fluid drainage. A depressed fontanelle may indicate a successful shunt if unaccompanied by other signs of dehydration (such as increased heart rate or respirations, decreased urine output, and irritability). A tense, bulging fontanelle indicates a nonfunctioning shunt and increased ICP. Signs of increased ICP may indicate infection or shunt malfunction, the greatest postoperative hazards.

● Pump the shunt, if ordered, by depressing the valve firmly and quickly with the index finger; leave the finger lightly in place to check for refill. Teach the parents this procedure. Although not performed routinely, *shunt pumping may be needed to maintain valve patency or assess valve function.* The physician orders the desired pumping frequency.

● Maintain strict intake and output records, monitoring I.V. fluid intake every hour, *to reduce the risk of cerebral edema and increased ICP.* The physician may restrict fluids for the first 24 to 48 hours.

● Observe for abdominal distention to assess for signs of an ileus or peritonitis, which can be caused by CSF drainage.

● Have the parents assume more responsibility for the infant's care, including feeding, passive ROM exercises, skin care, and hygiene. Provide positive reinforcement and guidance. *Active participation and feedback enhance learning. The parents must become more involved with the infant's care during hospitalization if they're to provide adequate care after the infant is discharged.*

● Give the parents a list of signs of infection and increased ICP; include the physician's telephone number. *A written list reminds the parents of signs that require medical treatment.*

● Have the parents demonstrate their understanding of long-term follow-up care that the infant will need, including continuous medical evaluation of hydrocephalus and myelomeningocele, orthopedic evaluation and possible appliance, and urologic evaluation to maintain bowel and bladder control and prevent UTI. The shunt will require periodic readjustment *to compensate for growth or malfunction.*

Signs of increased intracranial pressure

Infant
● Refusal of feedings or difficulty feeding
● Irritability, altered level of consciousness (LOC)
● Vomiting
● Bulging fontanel
● Increased frontal occipital circumference
● High-pitched cry
● Setting-sun sign (eyes are rotated downward, and the sclera are visible above the pupil)
● Cries when picked up but settles when lying still

Child
● Headache in the morning (with or without vomiting)
● Altered LOC
● Ataxia
● Irritability
● Lethargy

● Tell the parents what to expect regarding the infant's future development and refer them to an early childhood development program and support group *so they have a general idea of what to expect and how best to help the infant at each stage of development.*

● When spina bifida is diagnosed prenatally, refer the parents to a genetic counselor, *who can provide information and support the couple's decisions on how to manage the pregnancy.*

● Review key teaching topics with the parents *to ensure adequate knowledge about the condition and treatment,* including:
– handling the infant without applying pressure to the defect
– coping with the infant's physical problems
– recognizing early signs of complications, such as hydrocephalus, pressure ulcers, and UTIs
– recognizing signs of shunt blockage, such as morning headache, vomiting, or irritability
– maintaining a positive attitude and working through feelings of guilt, anger, and helplessness
– conducting intermittent catheterization and conduit hygiene
– emptying the child's bowel by administering a glycerin suppository as needed

– recognizing developmental lags (a possible result of hydrocephalus)
– ensuring maximum mental development
– planning activities appropriate to the infant's age and abilities.

Evaluation

● The infant's vital signs remain stable, his fontanel remains soft to slightly depressed, and he's alert with a lusty cry.
● The infant is free from infection.
● The infant's skin remains intact.
● The infant's parents assume more responsibility for his care; they demonstrate an understanding of procedures, complication signs, and the need for long-term follow-up evaluation and treatment.

Pyloric stenosis

In PYLORIC STENOSIS, hyperplasia and hypertrophy of the circular muscle at the pylorus narrow the pyloric canal, thereby preventing the stomach from emptying normally. The defect is most common in male infants younger than age 4 months.

Infants with pyloric stenosis are usually well for the first few weeks after birth. As the hypertrophy and hyperplasia progress, pyloric obstruction becomes apparent. Typically, the infant initially regurgitates occasionally after feeding; later, he begins to regurgitate after every feeding. Vomiting quickly progresses (usually within 1 to 2 weeks) to projectile vomiting. Moderate to severe dehydration occurs as vomiting increases.

Possible causes

● Exact cause unknown

Data collection findings

● Projectile emesis during or shortly after feedings, preceded by reverse peristaltic waves (going left to right) but not by nausea; resumption of eating after vomiting
● Olive-sized bulge palpated below the right costal margin
● Poor weight gain
● Tetany
● Symptoms of malnutrition and dehydration despite the infant's apparent adequate intake of food
● Symptoms appearing at about 4 weeks in formula-fed infants and at about 6 weeks in breast-fed infants

Diagnostic findings

● Arterial blood gas (ABG) analysis reveals metabolic alkalosis.
● Blood chemistry tests may reveal hypocalcemia, hypokalemia, and hypochloremia.
● Hematest reveals blood in emesis.
● Ultrasound shows hypertrophied sphincter.
● Endoscopy reveals hypertrophied sphincter.

Nursing diagnoses

● Risk for deficient fluid volume
● Imbalanced nutrition: Less than body requirements
● Risk for infection

Treatment

● Nothing-by-mouth status maintained before surgery
● I.V. therapy to correct fluid and electrolyte imbalances
● Possible insertion of an NG tube for gastric decompression
● Surgical intervention (pyloromyotomy performed by laparoscopy)

Drug therapy options

● Potassium supplements (only after proper kidney function is confirmed)
● I.V. calcium

Patient care goals

Before surgery, the infant will:
● regain fluid and electrolyte balance
● not vomit after feeding
● be free from infection
● gain depleted body fat and protein stores
● develop at the appropriate level.
  After surgery, the infant will:
● regain fluid and electrolyte balance
● not vomit after feeding
● be free from infection
● gain depleted body fat and protein stores
● develop at the appropriate level
● gain weight.
  The infant's parents will understand care to be continued at home, including:
● feeding and positioning techniques
● incision care
● behaviors to expect and which behaviors to report
● importance of providing warm, loving care.

Nursing interventions

- Weigh the infant daily *to assess growth.*
- Monitor vital signs and intake and output *to assess renal function and to check for signs of dehydration.*
- Assess for metabolic alkalosis and dehydration from frequent emesis *to detect early complications.*
- Assess abdominal and cardiovascular status *to detect early signs of compromise.*
- Provide small, frequent, thickened feedings and burp the infant frequently (preoperatively) *to promote nutrition and prevent aspiration.*
- Position the infant on his right side with the head of the bed elevated *to prevent the aspiration of vomitus.*

After surgery

- Feed the infant small amounts of oral electrolyte solution at first and then increase the amount and concentration of food until normal feeding is achieved *to meet nutritional needs and prevent vomiting.*
- Provide a pacifier *to meet nonnutritive sucking needs and maintain comfort.*
- Provide routine postoperative care *to maintain and improve the infant's condition and to detect early complications.* Position the infant on his right side with the head of the bed elevated *so if vomiting occurs there's little chance of aspiration. Positioning the infant on his right side possibly aids the flow of fluid through the pyloric valve by gravity.*
- Keep the incision area clean. *The infant is at an increased risk for infection because the incision is near the diaper area.*
- Review key teaching topics with family members *to ensure adequate knowledge about the condition and treatment,* including:
– feeding the infant, including specific formula, volume, and technique
– preventing infection.

Evaluation

- The infant ingests appropriate amounts of formula without regurgitating or vomiting and shows appropriate weight gain.
- The infant's parents can:
– explain feeding and positioning techniques
– describe incision care
– list signs and symptoms of incision infection.
- The parents demonstrate a warm, caring relationship with the infant.

Sudden infant death syndrome

SUDDEN INFANT DEATH SYNDROME (SIDS) is the sudden death of an infant in which a postmortem examination fails to confirm the cause of death. The peak age is 3 months; 90% of cases occur before age 6 months, especially during the winter and early spring months.

Infants who are diagnosed with SIDS are typically described as healthy with no previous medical problems. Death commonly occurs sometime after the infant has been put down to sleep.

Possible causes

- Possibly an abnormality in the control of ventilation, causing prolonged apneic periods with profound hypoxia and cardiac arrhythmias
- Undetected abnormalities, such as an immature respiratory system and respiratory dysfunction (see *Recommendations for decreasing SIDS*)

Data collection findings

- Death that occurs during sleep without noise or struggle
- History of low birth weight
- History of siblings with SIDS

Diagnostic findings

- Autopsy is the only way to diagnose SIDS. Autopsy findings indicate pulmonary edema, intrathoracic petechiae, and other minor changes suggesting chronic hypoxia.

Recommendations for decreasing SIDS

Research is being done to investigate the causes that may lead to sudden infant death syndrome (SIDS). For instance, there's a decreased incidence of SIDS in infants maintained in the supine position for sleep. The American Academy of Pediatrics has set forth the following recommendations to decrease the incidence of SIDS:

- Place the infant on his back to sleep.
- Don't place the infant on a waterbed, sofa, soft mattress, or other soft surface to sleep.
- Avoid soft materials in the infant's sleeping area, such as pillows, stuffed toys, loose blankets, and quilts and comforters.
- Make sure that the infant's crib meets the safety standards of the Consumer Product Safety Commission and the ASTM (formerly the American Society for Testing and Materials).

Nursing diagnoses
- Ineffective coping
- Dysfunctional grieving
- Fear
- Hopelessness
- Deficient knowledge related to SIDS
- Spiritual distress

Treatment
- If the parents bring the infant to the emergency department, the physician decides whether to attempt resuscitation.
- If successfully resuscitated, the infant is temporarily placed on mechanical ventilation. After he's extubated, the infant is tested for infantile apnea and the parents are given a home apnea monitor.

Drug therapy options
- Epinephrine, atropine and, after ABG analysis, sodium bicarbonate, if appropriate (according to Pediatric Advanced Life Support protocols)

Patient care goals
- Family members will use available support systems to assist in coping with fear.
- Family members will share feelings about the event.
- Family members will identify feelings of hopelessness regarding the current situation.
- Family members will use effective coping strategies to ease spiritual discomfort.
- Family members will seek appropriate support persons for assistance.

Nursing interventions
- Because most infants with SIDS can't be resuscitated, focus your interventions on providing emotional support for the family. Keep in mind that grief may be coupled with guilt. Also, the parents may express anger at emergency department personnel, each other, or anyone involved with the infant's care. Stay calm and let them express their feelings. The parents need to express these feelings *to prevent dysfunctional grieving.*
- Let the parents touch, hold, and rock the infant, if desired, and allow them to say goodbye to the infant *to facilitate the grieving process.*
- Provide literature on SIDS and support groups and suggest psychological support for the surviving children *to help prevent maladaptive emotional responses to loss, to promote a realistic perspective on the tragedy, and to promote coping.*

Evaluation
- Family members cope with their grief, as demonstrated by sharing their feelings, utilizing support systems, and having realistic perspectives about the tragedy.
- Family members cope with their feelings of hopelessness, fear, and guilt.

Tracheoesophageal fistula and esophageal atresia

Tracheoesophageal FISTULA is an abnormal passage between the esophagus and the trachea. A reflux of gastric juice after feeding can allow acidic stomach contents to cross the fistula, irritating the trachea.

Esophageal ATRESIA occurs when the proximal end of the esophagus ends in a blind pouch; food from the esophagus can't enter the stomach.

Esophageal atresia and tracheoesophageal fistula occur in many combinations and may be associated with other defects. Esophageal atresia with tracheoesophageal fistula is the most common of these conditions. Esophageal atresia alone is the second most common of these conditions. (See *Common types of tracheoesophageal fistulas and esophageal atresia.*)

Esophageal atresia with tracheoesophageal fistula occurs when:
- the distal end of the esophagus ends in a blind pouch and the proximal end of the esophagus is linked to the trachea by a fistula.
- the proximal end of the esophagus ends in a blind pouch and the distal portion of the esophagus is connected to the trachea by a fistula.

Possible causes
- Prematurity (contributing factor)

Data collection findings
Esophageal atresia
- Excessive salivation and drooling due to an inability to pass food through the esophagus
- Regurgitation of undigested formula immediately after feeding; possible respiratory distress and cyanosis if secretions are aspirated
- Inability to insert an NG tube

Tracheoesophageal fistula
- Excessive drooling of saliva (possibly the first symptom)

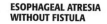

Common types of tracheoesophageal fistulas and esophageal atresia

These illustrations depict two common types of tracheoesophageal fistulas and esophageal atresia.

ESOPHAGEAL ATRESIA WITH FISTULA TO THE DISTAL SEGMENT

(Occurrence: approximately 85% to 88%)

ESOPHAGEAL ATRESIA WITHOUT FISTULA

(Occurrence: approximately 6% to 8%)

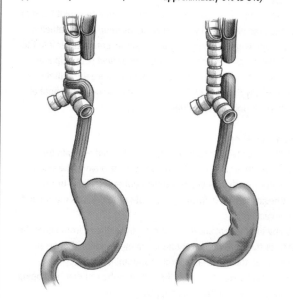

● Choking, coughing, and intermittent cyanosis during feeding due to food going into the trachea through the fistula
● Tracheal irritation from gastric acids that reflux across the fistula
● Abdominal distention from air going into the stomach through the fistula

Esophageal atresia with tracheoesophageal fistula
● Excessive salivation and drooling due to an inability to pass food through the esophagus
● Regurgitation of undigested formula immediately after feeding; possible respiratory distress and cyanosis if secretions are aspirated
● Signs of respiratory distress (coughing, choking, and intermittent cyanosis) because the infant has difficulty tolerating oral foods and handling oral secretions or refluxed gastric contents
● Inability to insert an NG tube

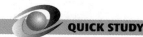

QUICK STUDY

Remember the 3 C's when assessing for tracheoesophageal fistula.
1. Coughing
2. Choking
3. Cyanosis

Diagnostic findings
● Neonates are fed first with a few sips of sterile water to detect anomalies and to avoid aspiration of formula or breast milk into the lungs.
● Abdominal X-rays reveal air in the stomach.
● Fluoroscopy, using radiopaque fluid carefully introduced into the esophagus, reveals atresia.
● Bronchoscopy shows a blind pouch.

Nursing diagnoses
● Imbalanced nutrition: Less than body requirements
● Risk for infection
● Risk for impaired parent-infant attachment

Treatment
● Percutaneous endoscopic gastrostomy (PEG) tube insertion (infant not fed orally)
● Surgical correction by ligating the tracheoesophageal fistula and reanastomosing the esophageal ends (in many cases, repair is done in stages)

Patient care goals
● The infant will have adequate nutritional intake.
● The infant will be afebrile and demonstrate no symptoms of infection.
● The parents will participate in the infant's care.

Nursing interventions
● Monitor vital signs *to detect tachycardia and tachypnea, which could indicate hypoxemia.*
● Assess respiratory status *to detect poor respiratory status, which may result in hypoxemia.*
● Position the infant with his head elevated 30 degrees *to decrease reflux at the distal esophagus.*
● Suction as needed *to stimulate coughing and clear airways.* (See *Performing oronasopharyngeal suction,* page 226.)

NURSING PROCEDURE

Performing oronasopharyngeal suction

Purpose

Oronasopharyngeal suction removes secretions from the pharynx by a suction catheter inserted through the mouth or nostril. Used to maintain a patent airway, this procedure helps the client who can't clear his airway effectively with coughing and expectoration, such as the unconscious or severely debilitated client. The procedure should be done as often as necessary, depending on the client's condition.

Because the catheter may inadvertently slip into the lower airway or esophagus, oronasopharyngeal suction is an aseptic procedure that requires sterile equipment. Apply suction for only 10 to 15 seconds at a time to minimize tissue trauma and prevent hypoxia.

After suctioning, record the date; time; reason for suctioning; technique used; amount, color, consistency, and odor (if any) of the secretions; the client's respiratory status before and after the procedure; any complications and the nursing action taken; and the client's tolerance of the procedure.

Implementation

- Check for a physician's order if one is required by your facility.
- Check vital signs. Evaluate the client's ability to cough and deep-breathe.
- Explain the procedure to the client or his parents, including that it may cause coughing or gagging. Provide reassurance throughout the procedure.
- Position the client in semi-Fowler's or high Fowler's position, if tolerated.
- Turn on the suction from the wall or portable unit, and set the pressure (usually between 80 and 120 mm Hg). Occlude the end of the connecting tubing to check suction pressure.
- Using strict aseptic technique, open the suction catheter kit or the packages containing the sterile catheter, disposable container, and gloves. Put on the gloves; consider your dominant hand sterile and your nondominant hand nonsterile. Using your nondominant hand, pour saline solution into the sterile container.
- With your nondominant hand, place a small amount of water-soluble lubricant on the sterile area.

- Pick up the catheter with your dominant (sterile) hand, and attach it to the connecting tubing. Use your nondominant hand to control the suction valve while your dominant hand manipulates the catheter.

For nasal insertion

- Raise the tip of the client's nose with your nondominant hand to straighten the passageway and facilitate insertion of the catheter. Without applying suction, gently insert the suction catheter into the client's naris. Roll the catheter between your fingers to help it advance through the turbinates. Continue to advance the catheter approximately 5″ to 6″ (12.5 to 15 cm) until you reach the pool of secretions or until the client begins to cough.

For oral insertion

- Without applying suction, gently insert the catheter into the client's mouth. Advance it 3″ to 4″ (7.5 to 10 cm) along the side of the client's mouth until you reach the pool of secretions or the client begins to cough. Suction both sides of the client's mouth and pharyngeal area.
- Using intermittent suction, withdraw the catheter from either the mouth or the nose with a continuous rotating motion. Between passes, wrap the catheter around your dominant hand
- If secretions are thick, clear the lumen of the catheter by dipping it in normal saline solution and applying suction.
- Repeat the procedure until gurgling or bubbling sounds stop and respirations are quiet.
- After completing suctioning, pull your sterile glove off over the coiled catheter and then remove your nonsterile glove. Discard both gloves as well as the container of water.
- Flush the connecting tubing with normal saline solution.
- Let the client rest after suctioning while you continue to observe him. The frequency and duration of suctioning depends on the client's tolerance for the procedure and any complications.

- Keep the PEG tube open and suspended above the infant *to release gas.*
- If feeding the infant through a PEG tube after surgery, anticipate abdominal distention from air; keep the infant upright during feedings *to reduce the chance of refluxed* *stomach contents and aspiration pneumonia,* and keep the tube open and elevated before and after feedings.
- Administer gastrostomy feedings only by gravity flow — not a feeding pump — *to help meet nutritional and meta-*

CLINICAL SITUATION

Caring for an infant with tracheoesophageal fistula

An infant has been in the newborn nursery for about 3½ hours when he suddenly becomes cyanotic and begins coughing and choking. The nurse notices that he has excessive mucus in his mouth and that he has been drooling. The infant is scheduled to be fed the first bottle of glucose water in about 2 hours. A diagnosis of a tracheoesophageal fistula with esophageal atresia has been made. The infant receives an esophagostomy, and a gastrostomy (PEG) tube is placed.

What are appropriate interventions following surgery?
● Observe and care for wounds, and apply and change sterile dressings as needed. If the infant has undergone a cervical esophagostomy, perform special skin care *to prevent breakdown from continuous moisture. Carefully observe all incision sites for signs of infection and take appropriate measures to prevent it.*
● Maintain adequate respiratory exchange and prevent pneumonia, as follows:
– Maintain a patent airway by carefully suctioning the infant's trachea, nose, and mouth as needed. Use the specially marked suction catheter as a guide *to prevent trauma to the anastomosis site.* During surgery, the surgeon measures and marks a suction catheter at a distance slightly above the anastomosis site; the catheter's length is communicated to all caregivers.
– Keep a laryngoscope and endotracheal tube at bedside *in case extreme edema causes obstruction.*
– Periodically check the chest tubes by auscultating both lungs for breath sounds, checking for loose connections and kinking, and checking the drainage system for proper functioning every 4 to 8 hours based on the infant's condition *to ensure that the infant's lungs are fully expanded.*
– Place the infant in an Isolette with humidity and oxygen *to reduce tracheal drying and irritation.*
– Keep the infant on his back or left side and elevate the head of the bed 30 degrees *to help prevent aspiration of secretions and make breathing easier.*
● On the 2nd or 3rd postoperative day, begin PEG tube feedings. Continue the feedings, if tolerated, for 10 to 14 days. *This delay helps avoid postoperative vomiting.* Tube feedings maintain the infant's nutrition while bypassing the operative site *to promote heal-*

ing. Within 10 to 14 days, the anastomosis should heal completely; the surgeon may order an upper GI series to confirm healing.
● Begin oral feedings with sterile water or expressed breast milk, observing the infant carefully *to ensure that he can swallow without choking.* Progress to small, frequent formula feedings; supplement these with PEG tube feedings if the infant can't consume enough orally to meet nutritional needs. *Sterile water or expressed breast milk is given initially because it causes fewer problems than other solutions if the infant aspirates it or can't swallow.* Small, frequent formula feedings are gradually increased until they're sufficient to meet the infant's needs. The stomach will expand as the amount of food increases.

How can the nurse prepare the parents for home care?
● Teach proper care of the PEG tube and an esophagostomy if the infant has had a staged palliative procedure. If a staged repair is performed and anastomosis is delayed until age 18 to 24 months, the infant will be sent home with a PEG tube and an esophagostomy.
● Teach the parents to recognize signs of wound infection, including swelling, redness, foul or oozing drainage, and elevated temperature. *The infant typically is discharged 2 or 3 weeks after surgery; infection is possible even after discharge.*
● Teach the parents to recognize signs of esophageal stenosis: choking or coughing with feeding, refusal to eat, and painful swallowing. *Recurring esophageal stenosis and dysphagia are common complications of scarring, which may develop at the anastomosis site.*
● Teach correct positioning of the infant after feeding (on his back or right side, with the head of the bed slightly elevated), *which helps prevent regurgitation into the esophagus.*
● Teach the parents *to* recognize signs of respiratory distress, including nasal flaring, retractions, and grunting. *Respiratory distress may accompany dysphagia, or a fistula may develop at the operative site where the esophagus is separated from the trachea.*

Question for further thought
● How could the nurse provide mild sensorimotor stimulation to the infant?

bolic requirements. (See *Caring for an infant with tracheo-esophageal fistula.*)

After surgery
● Maintain patency of chest tube and respiratory support *to prevent respiratory compromise.*

● Keep a suction catheter ready *to eliminate secretions and prevent aspiration.*
● Mark the catheter to indicate the distance from the infant's nose to the point just above the anastomosis *to avoid causing trauma to the anastomosis site.*
● Make sure the NG tube is secure and handle it with extreme caution *to avoid displacement.*
● Administer antibiotics as prescribed *to prevent infection.*
● Monitor intake and output, including total parenteral nutrition, *to maintain nutritional support.*
● Review key teaching topics with the parents, such as proper care of the infant at home (for example, feeding and bathing techniques), *to ensure adequate knowledge about the condition and treatment.*

Evaluation
● The infant receives enough nutrition — either in formula or breast milk — to maintain growth without choking, coughing, or aspirating.
● The parents demonstrate the ability to provide care without anxiety.
● The parents can list the signs of wound infection and esophageal STENOSIS.
● The parents demonstrate caring behaviors toward the infant.

TODDLER DISORDERS

Acute acetaminophen poisoning

Because toddlers and preschoolers are mobile, active, and curious, they're especially vulnerable to accidental ingestion. Among drugs that children ingest most frequently, acetaminophen (Tylenol) ranks number one. Although aspirin poisoning has decreased, it still occurs in young children. Like acetaminophen, aspirin is readily available in most homes and is taken freely by adults, whom children imitate. Also, children's aspirin and acetaminophen are brightly colored and have appealing flavors.

In acetaminophen poisoning, hepatic damage results from a metabolite of acetaminophen. Usually, the liver enzyme glutathione combines with and neutralizes the metabolite, which is then excreted in the urine. With ingestion of large acetaminophen doses, the metabolite overwhelms glutathione, causing hepatic necrosis. (Administration of acetylcysteine [Mucomyst] provides a substitute for glutathione.) Hepatotoxicity occurs at plasma levels greater than 200 mg/ml at 4 hours after ingestion and greater than 50 mg/ml by 12 hours after ingestion.

Possible causes
Acetaminophen poisoning is caused by acetaminophen overdose. Other substances children commonly ingest include soap, plants, cleaning agents, detergents, vitamins, and other drugs. (See *Common poisoning agents.*)

Data collection findings
● Anorexia
● Nausea
● Diaphoresis
● Liver dysfunction
● Right upper quadrant tenderness and jaundice evident 72 to 96 hours after ingestion
● Shock
● Oliguria
● Pallor
● Hypothermia
● Severe hypoglycemia
● Encephalopathy
● Hepatic failure, death, or resolution of symptoms 7 to 8 days after ingestion

Diagnostic findings
● Blood glucose levels are decreased.
● Serum aspartate aminotransferase (AST) and serum alanine aminotransferase (ALT) levels become elevated soon after ingestion.
● Prothrombin time (PT) is prolonged.

Nursing diagnoses
● Risk for poisoning
● Risk for imbalanced fluid volume
● Deficient knowledge related to poisoning
● Activity intolerance

Treatment
● Gastric lavage or emesis induction with ipecac syrup
● Hyperthermia blanket
● I.V. fluid
● Oxygen therapy (intubation and mechanical ventilation may be required)

Drug therapy options
● Acetylcysteine (Mucomyst) in 1 loading dose and 17 maintenance doses
● Emetic: ipecac syrup

Patient care goals
● The child will maintain or regain normal liver function.
● The child will regain fluid and electrolyte balance.

Common poisoning agents

SUBSTANCE INGESTED	ASSESSMENT	TREATMENT
Salicylates (such as aspirin)	● Determine whether ingestion is acute or chronic. ● Assess for signs and symptoms of salicylate poisoning, including deep respirations, decreased level of consciousness, dehydration, metabolic acidosis, blood loss, and tinnitus. ● Assess the parents' knowledge of proper aspirin administration. ● Assess the child's serum salicylate levels; peak levels may vary with enteric-coated aspirin.	● Remove aspirin from the child's stomach by giving ipecac syrup or administering gastric lavage, as ordered. ● Administer activated charcoal as ordered to absorb the drug in the stomach. ● Administer electrolyte solutions and sodium bicarbonate as ordered to correct metabolic acidosis. ● Administer diazepam for seizure control. ● Offer adequate calories and fluids to meet the child's increased metabolic demands. ● Administer vitamin K for bleeding
Lead	● Identify high-risk groups by screening for pica (an abnormal desire to eat substances not normally eaten, such as lead paint or hair) and an environment high in lead. (Universal blood screening is recommended for infants and children ages 6 months to 6 years.) ● Observe for signs of encephalopathy: hyperactivity, aggression, impulsiveness, lethargy, irritability, clumsiness, learning difficulties, short attention span, convulsions, mental retardation, and coma. ● Observe for signs of anemia: fatigability, irritability, decreased hemoglobin level, and exercise intolerance. ● Observe for signs of renal damage: excretion of glucose, protein, amino acids, and phosphate.	● Administer chelating agents, such as EDTA and dimercaprol, which cause lead to be removed from blood and soft tissues, deposited in bone, and excreted in urine. ● EDTA and dimercaprol are given in a series of deep I.M. injections, in rotating sites; multiple injections may result in painful fibrotic tissues. ● Adverse reactions to EDTA include hypocalcemia (resulting in tetany and seizures) and nephrotoxicity (resulting in decreased urine output). ● Eliminate lead from the environment; a few chips of paint the size of a thumbnail contain 100 mg of lead (200 times the safe daily dose). Other sources of lead are unglazed pottery, colored newsprint, and painted food wrappers.
Hydrocarbons (petroleum distillates, such as kerosene, gasoline, turpentine, lighter fluid, furniture polish, metal polish, cleaning fluid, and insecticides)	● Recognize early signs of toxicity: gagging, choking, coughing, nausea, vomiting, lethargy, drowsiness, weakness, and respiratory symptoms (from inhalation of vapors), including cyanosis, retractions, grunting, and tachypnea.	● Maintain a patent airway. ● Give nothing by mouth. ● Don't give emetics. ● Call the poison control center.
Corrosives (oven and drain cleaners, dishwasher detergents, and other strong detergents and cleaning agents)	● Observe for signs of toxicity: severe, burning pain of the mouth, lips, tongue, throat, and stomach; white, swollen oral mucous membranes; swollen tongue and pharynx; violent vomiting with blood; shock; anxiety; and agitation.	● Maintain a patent airway. ● Administer steroids as ordered. ● Give nothing by mouth except as ordered. ● Give analgesics as needed. ● Don't give emetics; vomiting will redamage tissue. ● Call the poison control center.

- The child will regain a normal energy level.
- The child's parents will learn about emergency measures to take for a child with acute acetaminophen poisoning.
- The child's parents will learn how to childproof their home.

Nursing interventions

- Monitor liver function studies immediately and 3 and 6 months after the incident *to detect signs of liver damage and to monitor the treatment's effectiveness.*
- Monitor vital signs and intake and output every 1 to 4 hours. *Tachycardia and decreased urine output may signify dehydration.*
- Assess cardiovascular and GI status *to detect the treatment's effectiveness.*
- Administer hyperthermia therapy by using a warming blanket, limiting exposure during routine nursing care, and covering the child with warm blankets *to help the child become normothermic.*
- Administer acetylcysteine in a juice. *Acetylcysteine has an offensive odor and taste. Administering this drug in juice will help the child swallow it.* For small children, administer it directly into an NG tube to avoid this difficulty.

 SPOT CHECK

What's the best way to administer acetylcysteine?
Answer: Acetylcysteine has an offensive odor and taste, so administering it in juice helps a child swallow it. For a small child, you may need to use an NG tube.

- Record fluid intake and output. *Monitoring the child's fluid balance helps to evaluate for signs of fluid retention and decreased urine output, which can be caused by hepatic failure. Vomiting and anorexia also may decrease urine output, further complicating fluid balance assessment.*
- Monitor the child's activity level and level of consciousness (LOC) *to assess for signs of hepatic coma (the most severe stage of hepatic toxicity), which is indicated by reduced activity level and altered LOC.*
- Allow the parents to express their feelings about circumstances surrounding the poisoning *to help them resolve feelings of guilt and to refocus their attention on promoting the child's recovery and health.*
- Teach the child's parents about poison control measures, such as keeping ipecac syrup in the home, placing the telephone number for the poison control center near the telephone, and viewing the home from a toddler's eye level to find hazards. *Poisoning is an emergency. Advance preparation can lead to earlier intervention, resulting in milder toxicity.*
- Tell the parents to store all medications and drugs out of the child's reach and sight. List several examples of over-the-counter medications, such as aspirin and cold remedies, because many people don't realize these contain potent drugs.
- Caution the parents not to store drugs in containers without safety caps if small children are part of the household.
- Have the parents teach their children not to take non-food items without supervision.
- Instruct the parents to read the labels of cold remedies for ingredients, recommended dosages, and contraindications.
- Explain all procedures and treatments to the parents *to reduce anxiety.*

Evaluation

- The child regains fluid and electrolyte balance and normal liver function and returns home free from complications.
- The child's parents don't feel guilty about the poisoning.
- The child's parents have made their home childproof.

Anemia, iron deficiency

ANEMIA is a reduction either in the volume of red blood cells (RBCs) or in hemoglobin (Hb) concentration. These reductions diminish the blood's capacity to carry oxygen and therefore reduce the amount of oxygen available to tissue. Anemia is the most common hematologic disorder in infants and children. Symptoms of anemia result from tissue hypoxia and the body's compensatory response.

Iron deficiency anemia, the most prevalent nutritional disorder in the United States, occurs most commonly in children between ages 6 months and 2 years (iron stores are depleted between the 5th and 6th month) and again during adolescence. Iron deficiency anemia is characterized by poor RBC production. Insufficient body stores of iron lead to:

- depleted RBC mass
- decreased Hb concentration (hypochromia)
- decreased oxygen-carrying capacity of the blood.

In the early stages of iron deficiency anemia, the child may be asymptomatic. Compensatory mechanisms effectively prevent most overt symptoms at that point. Blood viscosity is reduced because the number of RBCs is reduced. Such hemodilution results in decreased peripheral resistance, which increases the volume of blood returned to the heart. The cardiac workload increases as the heart pumps faster to circulate the thinned blood. If the condition persists, the heart may enlarge and have a functional systolic murmur. Increased cardiac output (from tachycardia and cardiac dilatation) compensates for the decreased number of RBCs. However, with exercise, infection, emotional stress, or circulatory overload, cardiac failure may occur.

QUICK STUDY

Think **PLATE** to remember key blood components.

Plasma
Leukocytes
AB antigens
Thrombocytes
Erythrocytes

Possible causes

● Blood loss secondary to drug-induced GI bleeding (from anticoagulants, aspirin, or steroids) or due to heavy menses, hemorrhage from trauma, GI ulcers, or cancer
● Inadequate dietary intake of iron, which may occur following prolonged nonsupplemented breast-feeding or bottle-feeding of infants or during periods of stress such as rapid growth in children and adolescents
● Iron malabsorption, as in chronic diarrhea, partial or total gastrectomy, and malabsorption syndromes, such as celiac disease and pernicious anemia
● Intravascular hemolysis-induced hemoglobinuria or paroxysmal nocturnal hemoglobinuria
● Mechanical erythrocyte trauma caused by a prosthetic heart valve or vena cava filters

Data collection findings

Anemia progresses gradually, and many children are initially asymptomatic, except for symptoms of an underlying condition. Symptoms can be vague and insidious. Children with advanced anemia display:
● pallor
● irritability
● fatigue
● dyspnea on exertion
● inability to concentrate
● listlessness
● headache
● susceptibility to infection

● tachycardia
● growth retardation
● edema.
   With chronic iron deficiency anemia, children may also display:
● numbness and tingling of the extremities
● vasomotor disturbances
● neuralgic pain
● cracks in corners of the mouth
● smooth tongue
● spoon-shaped, brittle nails
● dysphagia
● signs of infection, such as tugging at the ear (otitis media), runny nose, reluctance to swallow (sore throat), coughing, sneezing, and elevated temperature.

Diagnostic findings

● Bone marrow studies reveal depleted or absent iron stores and normoblastic hyperplasia.
● Hb level, hematocrit, and serum ferritin level are low.
● Mean corpuscular Hb level is decreased in severe anemia.
● RBC count is low, with microcytic and hypochromic cells. In early stages, RBC count may be normal, except in infants and children.
● Serum iron levels are low, with high binding capacity.
● Positive fecal occult blood test (Hemoccult) results can indicate chronic hidden blood loss, which is a cause of anemia.

Nursing diagnoses

● Imbalanced nutrition: Less than body requirements
● Impaired gas exchange
● Risk for infection
● Delayed growth and development
● Activity intolerance

Treatment

● Increased iron intake by adding foods rich in iron to diet (iron supplements may be added)

Drug therapy options

● Oral iron preparation or a combination of iron and ascorbic acid (which enhances iron absorption); iron dextran (InFeD), if additional therapy is needed
● Vitamin B_{12} (cyanocobalamin), if intrinsic factor is lacking

Infant iron needs

An infant should receive only breast milk or commercial formula with iron until age 6 months. From age 6 months to 1 year, the infant should receive breast milk or iron-fortified formula and cereal with a gradual introduction of other baby foods. As a rule, an infant should receive no more than 32 oz of milk per day. One quart of milk provides only 0.5 mg of iron, whereas 1 tbs of fortified baby cereal provides 2.5 to 5 mg of iron. Infants with iron deficiency anemia should receive no more than 16 oz of milk per day, because it's deficient in iron, zinc, and vitamin C and has a high renal solute load.

Patient care goals

● The child won't develop cardiac complications from the anemia.
● The child's iron intake will increase sufficiently to replace depleted stores and to maintain RBC production.
● The child will remain free from infection.
● The child's parents will provide a nutritionally balanced diet that has enough iron.
● The child will return to physical activity levels appropriate to developmental age.

Nursing interventions

● Carefully assess a child's drug history. *Certain drugs, such as pancreatic enzymes and vitamin E, may interfere with iron metabolism and absorption; other drugs, such as aspirin and steroids, can cause GI bleeding.*
● Provide passive stimulation; allow frequent rest; give small, frequent feedings; and elevate the head of the bed *to decrease oxygen demands.*
● Implement proper hand washing *to decrease the risk of infection.*
● Provide foods high in iron (liver, whole grains, and dark, leafy vegetables) *to replenish iron stores.* (See *Infant iron needs.*)
● Monitor the infant for signs of infection *to identify complications from inadequate nutrition.*
● Administer iron before meals with citrus juice. *Iron is best absorbed in an acidic environment.*
● Give liquid iron through a straw *to prevent staining the child's skin and teeth.* For infants, administer by oral syringe toward the back of the mouth.
● Don't give iron with milk products. *Milk products may interfere with iron absorption.*

● Monitor the child's cardiac function *to identify signs of increased cardiac workload, such as tachycardia or tachypnea, which may lead to cardiac failure.*
● Monitor reticulocyte count *to evaluate the child's response to treatment.* The reticulocyte count should begin to increase approximately 1 week after beginning iron supplements.
● Be supportive of family members and keep them informed of the child's status *to decrease anxiety.*
● Review key teaching topics with family members *to ensure adequate knowledge about the condition and treatment,* including:
– keeping iron supplements safely stored out of the child's reach at home
– brushing teeth after iron administration
– reporting reactions to iron supplementation, such as nausea, vomiting, diarrhea, constipation, fever, or severe stomach pain, which may require a dosage adjustment
– providing a nutritionally balanced diet with adequate amounts of iron.

Evaluation

● The child doesn't develop cardiac decompensation.
● The child's reticulocyte count indicates rapid RBC proliferation; RBC and Hb levels are within normal range.
● The child demonstrates appropriate physical and emotional development for his age.
● The child's parents understand that they must provide a balanced, iron-rich diet.
● The child is free from infection at discharge.

Congenital heart disease, acyanotic

Congenital heart disease occurs in approximately 8 to 10 of every 1,000 live births and — like prematurity — is a major cause of death in the 1st year. Congenital heart defects are of two types (based on alteration in blood flow): acyanotic, in which deoxygenated blood isn't mixed in the systemic circulation (the child doesn't appear blue), and cyanotic, in which deoxygenated blood is mixed in the systemic circulation (the child usually appears blue or dusky). Congenital heart defects may be further categorized by normal, decreased, or increased pulmonary blood flow. (See *Common congenital heart defects.*)

In an acyanotic defect, blood is usually shunted from the left (oxygenated) side of the heart to the right (unoxygenated) side. Acyanotic defects include:
● AORTIC STENOSIS — a narrowing or fusion of the aortic valves, interfering with left ventricular outflow

Common congenital heart defects

Major acyanotic defects

Atrial septal defect

An abnormal opening between the right and left atria

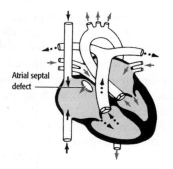

Atrial septal defect

Coarctation of the aorta

A narrowing of the aortic lumen that results in a preductal or postductal obstruction

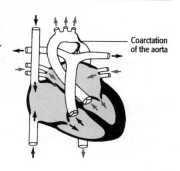

Coarctation of the aorta

Patent ductus arteriosus

A defect resulting from the failure of the ductus to close, causing shunting of blood to the pulmonary artery

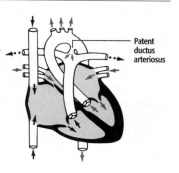

Patent ductus arteriosus

Ventricular septal defect

An abnormal opening between the right and left ventricles

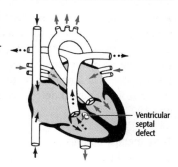

Ventricular septal defect

Major cyanotic defects

Complete transposition of great vessels

A defect in which the aorta arises from the right ventricle and the pulmonary artery arises from the left ventricle

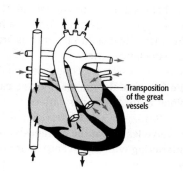

Transposition of the great vessels

Tetralogy of Fallot

A combination of four defects: pulmonic stenosis, ventricular septal defect, overriding aorta, and hypertrophy of the right ventricle

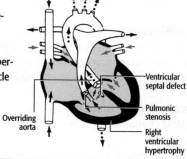

Ventricular septal defect

Pulmonic stenosis

Overriding aorta

Right ventricular hypertrophy

Tricuspid atresia

Characterized by absence of tricuspid valve and no blood flow between the right atrium and right ventricle, a small right ventricle, a large left ventricle, an atrial septal defect, a small ventricular septal defect and, usually, diminished pulmonary circulation

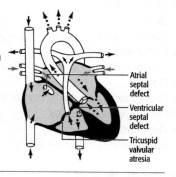

Atrial septal defect

Ventricular septal defect

Tricuspid valvular atresia

Truncus arteriosus

A defect in which normal septation of the embryologic bulbar trunk into an aorta and pulmonary artery doesn't occur (a single arterial trunk overrides the ventricles and receives blood from them through a ventricular septal defect)

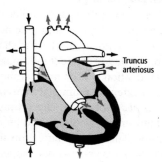

Truncus arteriosus

● ATRIAL SEPTAL DEFECT — a defect stemming from a patent foramen ovale or the failure of a septum to develop completely between the atria (there's an abnormal opening between the right and left atria)

● COARCTATION OF THE AORTA — a narrowing of the aortic arch, usually distal to the ductus arteriosus beyond the left subclavian artery

● PATENT DUCTUS ARTERIOSUS — a defect resulting from the failure of the ductus to close, causing shunting of blood to the pulmonary artery

● PULMONARY ARTERY STENOSIS — a narrowing or fusing of valve leaflets at the entrance of the pulmonary artery, interfering with right ventricular outflow

● VENTRICULAR SEPTAL DEFECT — a defect occurring when the ventricular septum fails to complete its formation between the ventricles, resulting in a left-to-right shunt.

Possible causes

● Defects between structures that inhibit blood flow to the system or alter pulmonary resistance
● Defects in the septa that lead to left-to-right shunt

Data collection findings

● Mild cyanosis (if the condition leads to right-sided heart failure)
● Respiratory distress
● Tachycardia
● Tachypnea
● Machinelike heart murmur (in patent ductus arteriosus)
● Congested cough
● Diaphoresis
● Fatigue
● Poor growth and development due to increased energy expenditure for breathing
● Hepatomegaly
● Frequent respiratory infections

Diagnostic findings

● Chest X-ray results and cardiac catheterization are used to confirm the type of acyanotic heart defect:

– In *aortic stenosis*, chest X-ray shows left ventricular hypertrophy and prominent pulmonary vasculature. Cardiac catheterization is used to determine the degree of shunting and extent of pulmonary vascular disease.

– In *atrial septal defect*, chest X-ray shows an enlarged right atrium and ventricle and prominent pulmonary vasculature. Cardiac catheterization shows right atrial blood that's more oxygenated than superior vena cava blood. It's also used to determine the degree of shunting and the extent of pulmonary vascular disease.

– In *coarctation of the aorta*, chest X-ray shows left ventricular hypertrophy, wide ascending and descending aorta, and prominent collateral circulation. Cardiac catheterization shows affected collateral circulation and pressures in the right and left ventricles.

– In *patent ductus arteriosus*, chest X-ray shows prominent pulmonary vasculature and enlargement of the left ventricle and aorta. Cardiac catheterization is used to determine the extent of pulmonary vascular disease and shows an oxygen content higher in the pulmonary artery than in the right ventricle.

– In *pulmonary artery stenosis*, chest X-ray shows right ventricular hypertrophy. Cardiac catheterization is used to gather evidence about the degree of shunting.

– In *ventricular septal defect*, chest X-ray may be normal for small defects or show cardiomegaly with a large left atrium and ventricle. In a large defect, chest X-ray may show prominent pulmonary vasculature. Cardiac catheterization is used to determine the size and exact location of the ventricular septal defect and the degree of shunting.

Nursing diagnoses

● Decreased cardiac output
● Impaired gas exchange
● Risk for infection
● Anxiety
● Deficient knowledge related to heart disease

Treatment

● For *aortic stenosis:* surgery (valvulotomy or commissurotomy)
● For *atrial septal defect:* surgery to patch the hole (mild defects may close spontaneously)
● For *coarctation of the aorta:* inoperable if coarctation is proximal to the ductus arteriosus; closed heart resection if coarctation is distal to the ductus arteriosus
● For *patent ductus arteriosus:* ligation of the patent ductus arteriosus in closed-heart operation
● For *pulmonary artery stenosis:* open-heart surgery to separate the pulmonary valve leaflets
● For *ventricular septal defect:* pulmonary artery banding to prevent heart failure and permanent correction with a patch, later, when heart is larger (spontaneous closure of the ventricular septal defect occurs in some children by age 3)

Drug therapy options

● Digoxin (Lanoxin)
● Diuretic: furosemide (Lasix)

- Indomethacin (Indocin) to achieve pharmacologic closure in patent ductus arteriosus
- Prophylactic antibiotics to prevent endocarditis

Patient care goals
- The child will exhibit signs of improved gas exchange and cardiac output.
- The child and family members will exhibit decreased anxiety.
- Members of the child's family will verbalize knowledge about the disorder, treatment, care at home, and how to contact appropriate community resources.

Nursing interventions
- Explain the heart defect and answer questions *to prepare the child for cardiac catheterization.*
- Monitor vital signs, pulse oximetry, and intake and output *to assess renal function and detect change.*
- Assess cardiovascular and respiratory status *to detect early signs of decompensation.*
- Take apical pulse for 1 minute before giving digoxin and hold the drug if the heart rate is less than 100 beats/minute (which indicates bradycardia in an infant) *to prevent toxicity.*
- Monitor fluid status, enforcing fluid restrictions as appropriate *to prevent fluid overload.*
- Weigh the child daily *to determine fluid overload or deficit.*
- Organize physical care and anticipate the child's needs *to reduce the child's oxygen demands.*
- Give the child high-calorie, easy-to-chew, and easy-to-digest foods *to maintain adequate nutrition and decrease oxygen demands.*
- Maintain normal body temperature *to prevent cold stress.*
- Raise the head of the bed or place the child in an infant car seat *to ease breathing.*
- Prepare the child and parents for the sights and sounds of the intensive care unit (ICU) *to reduce anxiety.*

Evaluation
- The child's incision site remains free from infection.
- The child remains free from respiratory infections and endocarditis.
- The child exhibits normal respirations and adequate oxygen saturation.
- The child exhibits no signs of heart failure, no evidence of severe skin mottling, adequate urine output, and a normal liver on palpation.

- The child and family members exhibit decreased anxiety. The child takes part in age-appropriate activities. Family members express concerns, ask appropriate questions about the child's condition, and participate in the child's care.

Congenital heart disease, cyanotic

The skin of a child with a cyanotic heart disease usually appears blue or dusky because unoxygenated blood or a mixture of oxygenated and unoxygenated blood is shunted through the cardiovascular system. This shunting can lead to left-sided heart failure, decreased oxygen supply to the body, and the development of collateral circulation. (For more information, review *Common congenital heart defects,* page 233.)

Cyanotic heart defects include:
- TRANSPOSITION OF THE GREAT VESSELS or arteries — a defect in which the aorta arises from the right ventricle and the pulmonary artery arises from the left ventricle
- TETRALOGY OF FALLOT — a defect consisting of pulmonary artery stenosis, ventricular septal defect, hypertrophy of the right ventricle, and an overriding aorta
- hypoplastic left heart syndrome (HLHS) — a defect consisting of aortic valve atresia, mitral atresia or stenosis, diminutive or absent left ventricle, and severe hypoplasia of the ascending aorta and aortic arch
- TRICUSPID VALVULAR ATRESIA — a defect characterized by absence of the tricuspid valve, lack of blood flow between the right atrium and the right ventricle, a small right ventricle, a large left ventricle, an atrial septal defect, a small ventricular septal defect and, usually, diminished pulmonary circulation.

Possible causes
- Any condition that increases pulmonary vascular resistance
- Structural defects

Data collection findings
- Cyanosis
- Crouching position assumed frequently
- History of inadequate feeding
- Clubbing
- Increasing cyanosis as the foramen ovale or ductus arteriosus closes (in transposition of the great vessels), leading to loss of consciousness, also known as a tet spell (in tetralogy of Fallot)

● Increasing dyspnea, cyanosis, and tachypnea during the first few days after birth; without treatment, heart failure after closure of the ductus (in HLHS)
● Irritability
● Tachycardia
● Tachypnea

Diagnostic findings
● ABG analysis shows diminished arterial oxygen saturation.
● Cardiac catheterization results confirm the diagnosis by allowing visualization of defects and measurement of oxygen saturation level.
● CBC shows polycythemia. (Hypoxia stimulates the body to increase RBC production.)

Nursing diagnoses
● Decreased cardiac output
● Impaired gas exchange
● Risk for infection
● Anxiety
● Deficient knowledge related to heart disease

Treatment
For transposition of the great vessels or arteries
● Corrective surgery to redirect blood flow by switching the position of the major blood vessels (performed around age 1)
● Palliative surgery to provide communication between the chambers

For tetralogy of Fallot
● Complete repair or palliative treatment during the 1st year to increase blood flow to the lungs by bypassing pulmonic stenosis (Blalock-Taussig shunt to connect the right pulmonary artery to the right subclavian artery)
● Oxygen therapy
● Repair of ventricular septal defect and stenosis (may be done in stages)

For HLHS
● Heart transplant
● Three-stage procedure that involves restructuring the heart (without surgery, death occurs in early infancy)
– Stage I (Norwood procedure) — the pulmonary artery is divided; one end is sewn shut and the other is connected to the aorta and patched to create a new aorta; a shunt is placed to connect the aorta to the pulmonary artery

– Stage II (Hemi-Fontan procedure) — the superior vena cava and right pulmonary artery are joined; the shunt placed in stage I is removed
– Stage III (Fontan procedure) — a conduit is used to bypass the right ventricle, thus diverting systemic venous blood to the main pulmonary artery

For tricuspid valvular atresia
● Systemic to pulmonary shunt or pulmonary artery banding

Drug therapy options
● Morphine during tet spell
● Propranolol (Inderal) as prophylactic
● Prostaglandin E to keep the ductus arteriosus patent

Patient care goals
● The child will exhibit signs of improved gas exchange and cardiac output.
● The child and family members will exhibit decreased anxiety.
● Members of the child's family will verbalize knowledge about the disorder, treatment, care at home, and how to contact appropriate community resources.

Nursing interventions
● Assess cardiovascular and respiratory status *to detect early signs of compromise.*
● Monitor vital signs and pulse oximetry *to detect hypoxia.*
● Monitor intake and output *to assess renal status.*
● Provide oxygen when necessary *to compensate for impaired oxygen exchange.*
● Anticipate needs and prevent distress *to decrease oxygen demands on the child.*
● Use a nipple designed for premature infants *to decrease the energy needed for sucking.*
● Provide adequate hydration *to prevent sequelae of polycythemia.*
● Administer prophylactic antibiotics *to prevent endocarditis.*
● Provide thorough skin care *to prevent skin breakdown.*
● Prepare the child for cardiac catheterization *to decrease anxiety.*
● Prepare the child and parents for the sights and sounds of the ICU *to decrease anxiety.*
● Explain the difference between palliative and corrective procedures to the child's parents *to improve knowledge regarding diagnosis and treatment.*

Evaluation

- The child's incision site remains free from infection.
- The child remains free from respiratory infections and endocarditis.
- The child exhibits normal respirations and adequate oxygen saturation.
- The child exhibits no signs of heart failure, no evidence of severe skin mottling, adequate urine output, and a normal liver on palpation.
- The child and family members exhibit decreased anxiety. The child takes part in age-appropriate activities. Family members express concerns, ask appropriate questions about the child's condition, and participate in the child's care.

Croup

CROUP is a group of related upper airway respiratory conditions that commonly affect toddlers. It includes acute spasmodic laryngitis, acute obstructive laryngitis, and acute laryngotracheobronchitis.

Possible causes

- Virus-induced edema around the larynx

Data collection findings

- Barking, brassy cough or hoarseness, sometimes described as a "seal bark" cough
- Inspiratory stridor with varying degrees of respiratory distress
- Condition usually begins at night and during cold weather and frequently recurs
- Crackles and decreased breath sounds (indicate the condition has progressed to bronchi)
- Increased dyspnea and lower accessory muscle use
- Either gradual or sudden onset

Diagnostic findings

- If bacterial infection is the cause, throat cultures may identify the organisms and their sensitivity to antibiotics as well as rule out diphtheria.
- Laryngoscopy may reveal inflammation and obstruction in epiglottal and laryngeal areas.
- Neck X-ray shows areas of upper airway narrowing and edema in subglottic folds and rules out the possibility of foreign body obstruction as well as masses and cysts.

Nursing diagnoses

- Impaired gas exchange

- Ineffective breathing pattern
- Ineffective airway clearance
- Risk for imbalanced fluid volume
- Anxiety

Treatment

- Clear liquid diet to keep mucus thin
- Cool humidification during sleep with a cool mist tent or room humidifier
- Rest from activity
- Tracheostomy and oxygen administration

Drug therapy options

- Antipyretic: acetaminophen (Tylenol)
- Inhaled racemic epinephrine (AsthmaNefrin)
- Corticosteroid: methylprednisolone sodium succinate (Solu-Medrol) to alleviate respiratory distress

Patient care goals

- The child will maintain adequate ventilation as evidenced by relief of respiratory distress.
- The child's temperature will be within normal range.
- The child will maintain a patent airway.
- The child's parents will demonstrate an understanding of the illness and treatment.
- The child's parents will use available support systems to assist with coping.

Nursing interventions

- Assess respiratory and cardiovascular status *to detect indications that obstruction is worsening.*
- Monitor vital signs and pulse oximetry *to detect early signs of respiratory compromise.*
- Administer oxygen therapy and maintain the child in a cool mist tent, if needed. *Cool mist helps liquefy secretions.* (See *Mist tent therapy,* page 238.)
- Administer medications, as ordered, and note their effectiveness *to maintain or improve the child's condition.*
- Provide emotional support for the parents *to decrease anxiety.*
- Provide age-appropriate activities for the child confined to the mist tent *to ease anxiety.*
- Monitor for rebound obstruction if the child is receiving racemic epinephrine; *the drug's effects are short term and may result in rebound obstruction.*

Evaluation

- The child's respirations return to normal with no further signs of respiratory distress.

NURSING PROCEDURE

Mist tent therapy

Purpose
Also known as a croupette for infants or a cool-humidity tent for children, a mist tent houses a nebulizer that transforms distilled water into mist. Mist tent therapy benefits the child by providing a cool, moist environment. This atmosphere eases breathing and helps to decrease respiratory tract edema, liquefy secretions, and reduce fever. Oxygen may also be administered along with the mist.

Implementation
Setup
● If you're required to set up the mist tent, place the tent frame and the plastic tenting at the head of the crib or bed. Then cover the mattress with a bed sheet, cover the bed sheet with a plastic sheet or linen-saver pad (tucked under the mattress), and cover these layers with a bath blanket.
● Next, fill the reservoir of the nebulizer with sterile distilled water and make sure that the inlet for air contains a clean filter. If the child will have oxygen in the tent, make sure that the oxygen flowmeter connects to the tent. Then turn the flowmeter to the desired setting. Be sure to analyze the percentage of oxygen being delivered. Wait 2 minutes after mist begins filling the tent before placing the child in it.
● Carefully explain the mist tent's purpose to the child and his parents.
● Elevate the head of the bed to a position that enhances comfort. Consider placing an infant in an infant seat. If the child will be in the room alone, position him on his side.

● Use a stockinette cap, booties, and bath blanket, as needed, to keep the child from becoming chilled as the mist condenses inside the tent.
● Change the child's bed sheets and clothing as they dampen, and check his temperature frequently.
● Monitor the child frequently for a change in condition, keeping in mind that the mist may make observation difficult. Because the tent alone won't stop an infant or a small child from falling out of bed, raise the side rails all the way.
● If secretions coat the inside of the tent, wipe the tent down with a facility-approved cleaner such as soap and water. Also clean the reservoir with sterile water to prevent bacterial growth.
● To prevent a fire, forbid toys or games that may spark or trigger an electric shock, such as battery-operated toys. Also, remove the electric call light and give older children a handbell instead. If oxygen is being administered, check the percentage of oxygen delivered at least once every 4 hours.
● For bathing, remove the child from the tent to prevent hypothermia.
● Record the date and time the child was placed in the tent and removed from the tent. Describe the child's respiratory status, including breath sounds, sputum production, and perfusion. Record the percentage of oxygen being delivered, the date and time of all analyses, and the oxygen saturation.

● The child's vital signs are within normal range.
● The child's parents verbalize an understanding of methods to decrease laryngeal spasm, such as taking the child into the bathroom, turning on the shower, and letting the room fill with steam.
● The child's parents demonstrate appropriate coping.

Down syndrome
The first disorder researchers attributed to a chromosomal aberration, DOWN SYNDROME is characterized by:
● mental retardation
● dysmorphic facial features
● other distinctive physical abnormalities (60% of clients have congenital heart defects, respiratory infections,

chronic myelogenous leukemia, and a weak immune response to infection).

Possible causes
● Genetic nondisjunction, with three chromosomes on the 21st pair (total of 47 chromosomes)

 SPOT CHECK

What is the most probable cause of Down syndrome?
Answer: Down syndrome usually results from trisomy 21, in which chromosome 21 has three copies instead of the normal two, resulting in a karyotype of 47 chromosomes instead of the normal 46.

Risk factors
● Maternal age (the older the age of the mother, the greater the risk of genetic nondisjunction)

Data collection findings
● Brushfield's spots (marbling and speckling of the iris)
● Flat nose and low-set ears
● Hypotonia
● Mild to moderate retardation
● Protruding tongue (because of a small oral cavity)
● Short stature with pudgy hands
● Simian crease (a single crease across the palm)
● Small head with slow brain growth
● Upward slanting eyes

Diagnostic findings
● Amniocentesis allows prenatal diagnosis. It's recommended for women older than age 34 regardless of a negative family history or for a woman of any age if she or the father carries a translocated chromosome.
● Karyotype shows the specific chromosomal abnormality.

Nursing diagnoses
● Delayed growth and development
● Risk for injury
● Risk for aspiration
● Ineffective coping

Treatment
● Treatment for coexisting conditions — congenital heart problems, visual defects, or hypothyroidism
● Skeletal, immunologic, metabolic, biochemical, and oncologic problems treated as per specific problem

Drug therapy options
● Megavitamin therapy (controversial): promotes growth and development potential

 FAST FACT

Special education programs, available in most communities, permit a child with Down syndrome to maximize his potential and promote self-esteem. His physical condition and self-image can also benefit from special athletic programs.

Patient care goals
● The child will demonstrate age-appropriate skills and behaviors to the extent possible.

● The child will participate in developmental stimulation programs to increase skill levels.
● The child's parents will express an understanding of norms for growth and development.
● The child's parents will express an understanding of the condition and demonstrate appropriate coping skills.

Nursing interventions
● Provide activities appropriate for the child *to support optimal development of the child.*
● Set realistic, reachable, short-term goals; break tasks into small steps *to encourage their successful accomplishment.*
● Use behavior modification, if applicable, *to promote safety and prevent injury to the child and others.*
● Provide stimulation and communicate at a level appropriate to the child's mental age rather than chronological age *to promote a healthy emotional environment.*
● Provide a safe environment *to prevent injury.*
● Mainstream daily routines *to promote normalcy.*

Evaluation
● The child's potential is maximized through stimulation and learning.
● The child's parents express knowledge of the condition and seek treatment for any coexisting conditions.
● The child's parents demonstrate appropriate coping, such as utilizing support groups and contacting early intervention programs.

Duchenne's muscular dystrophy
A genetic disorder that occurs only in males, DUCHENNE'S MUSCULAR DYSTROPHY (also called *pseudohypertrophic dystrophy*) is marked by muscular deterioration that progresses throughout childhood. It generally results in death from cardiac or respiratory failure in the late teens or early 20s due to a defect on the X chromosome, resulting in a lack of production of dystrophin. The absence of dystrophin results in the breakdown of muscle fibers. Muscle fibers are replaced with fatty deposits and collagen in muscles. There's no known cure.

Possible causes
● Sex-linked recessive trait

Data collection findings
● Begins with pelvic girdle weakness, indicated by waddling gait and falling
● Gowers' sign (use of hands to push self up from floor)

- Eventual muscle weakness and wasting
- Cardiac or pulmonary failure
- Decreased ability to perform self-care activities
- Delayed motor development
- Eventual contractures and muscle hypertrophy

Diagnostic findings

- Electromyography typically demonstrates short, weak bursts of electrical activity in affected muscles.
- Muscle biopsy shows variations in the size of muscle fibers and, in later stages, shows fat and connective tissue deposits, with no dystrophin.

Nursing diagnoses

- Impaired physical mobility
- Impaired walking
- Impaired gas exchange
- Compromised family coping

Treatment

- Gene therapy (under investigation to prevent muscle degeneration)
- High-fiber, high-protein, low-calorie diet
- Physical therapy
- Surgery to correct contractures
- Use of devices, such as splints, braces, trapeze bars, overhead slings, and a wheelchair, to help preserve mobility

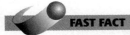

FAST FACT

The primary focus of treatment in Duchenne's muscular dystrophy is to help the child remain as active and independent as possible.

Patient care goals

- The child will maintain muscle strength.
- The child will maintain joint mobility and ROM.
- The child will show no evidence of complications.
- The child will achieve the highest level of mobility possible within the confines of the disease.
- The child will maintain normal cardiorespiratory status for as long as possible.
- The child's parents will recognize the early signs of respiratory complications, such as tachypnea and use of accessory muscles to breathe.

Nursing interventions

- Perform ROM exercises *to promote joint mobility.*

- Provide emotional support to the child and parents *to decrease anxiety and promote coping mechanisms.*
- Assist with genetic counseling *to inform the child and family about passing the disorder on to future children.*
- If respiratory involvement occurs, encourage coughing, deep-breathing exercises, and diaphragmatic breathing *to maintain a patent airway and mobilize secretions to prevent complications associated with retained secretions.*
- Encourage use of a footboard or high-topped sneakers and a foot cradle *to increase comfort and prevent footdrop.*
- Encourage adequate fluid intake, increase dietary fiber, and obtain an order for a stool softener *to prevent constipation associated with inactivity.*

Evaluation

- The child maintains muscle strength, joint mobility, and ROM to the fullest degree possible.
- The child's parents verbalize an understanding of the disease and keep the child as active and involved as possible.
- The child's parents verbalize an understanding of possible respiratory complications and how to handle a respiratory infection. Urge the parents to report signs of infection to the physician immediately.

Nephrotic syndrome

NEPHROTIC SYNDROME (also known as idiopathic nephrotic syndrome or minimal change nephrotic syndrome) develops when large amounts of plasma protein are lost in urine because of increased glomerular permeability. The syndrome occurs most commonly in preschool-age children. About 80% of those affected display no other signs of systemic or renal disease; about 60% are boys. The pathogenesis of nephrotic syndrome isn't clearly understood. The increased glomerular permeability to plasma protein results in massive proteinuria, hypoproteinemia, hypovolemia, edema, and hyperlipidemia. (See *Pediatric genitourinary facts.*)

Possible causes

- Unknown

Data collection findings

- Generalized edema, starting as facial puffiness and progressing over a period of weeks to abdominal swelling, respiratory difficulty, and labial or scrotal swelling
- Diminished urine volume; urine dark in color, opalescent, and frothy; urine specific gravity greatly increased; high protein level; and low RBC level

- Lethargy, irritability, decreased activity tolerance, and fatigability
- Ascites
- Anorexia
- Regression in developmental level in response to illness and hospitalization

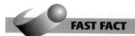

FAST FACT

The nephrotic syndrome symptom triad includes:
- proteinuria
- hypoalbuminemia
- edema.

Diagnostic findings
- Urinalysis reveals an increased number of hyaline, granular, and waxy, fatty casts as well as oval fat bodies and consistent, heavy proteinuria.
- Blood values reveal increased levels of cholesterol, phospholipids, and triglycerides and decreased albumin levels.
- Renal biopsy provides a histologic identification.

Nursing diagnoses
- Risk for imbalanced fluid volume
- Imbalanced nutrition: Less than body requirements
- Impaired skin integrity
- Risk for infection

Treatment
- Usually symptomatic and supportive (may consist of providing a regular diet with no added salt)

Drug therapy options
- Immunosuppressant therapy, including cyclophosphamide (Cytoxan) for 2 to 3 months
- Loop diuretics if edema alters respiratory status
- Steroid therapy until urine is free from protein

Patient care goals
- The child will remain free from secondary infection.
- The child will have increased urine output, decreased proteinuria, decreased body weight, decreased edema, decreased respiratory effort, and increased appetite within 7 to 21 days.
- The child will maintain or regain age-appropriate development.

Pediatric genitourinary facts

- An infant has a much greater percentage of total body water in extracellular fluid (42% to 45%) than an adult does (20%).
- Because of the increased percentage of water in a child's extracellular fluid, the child's water turnover rate is two to three times greater than an adult's. Every day, 50% of an infant's extracellular fluid is exchanged, compared with only 20% of an adult's; a child is therefore more susceptible than an adult to dehydration.
- A neonate also has a greater ratio of body surface area to body weight than an adult; this results in greater fluid loss through the skin.
- A neonate's kidneys attain the adult number of nephrons (about 1 million in each kidney) shortly after birth. The nephrons, which form urine, continue to mature throughout early childhood.
- A neonate's renal system can maintain a healthy fluid and electrolyte status. However, it doesn't function as efficiently during stress as an adult's renal system.
- An infant's kidneys don't concentrate urine at an adult level (average specific gravity is less than 1.010 for an infant, compared with 1.010 to 1.030 for an adult).
- An infant usually voids 5 to 10 ml/hour, a 10-year-old child usually voids 10 to 25 ml/hour, and an adult usually voids 35 ml/hour.
- A child has a short urethra; therefore, organisms can be easily transmitted into the bladder, increasing the risk of bladder infection.

Nursing interventions
- Monitor the child's vital signs (including blood pressure) every 4 hours *to identify increased blood pressure which, although rare, may indicate renal failure. Increased temperature and pulse rate could be related to a secondary infection.*
- Prevent visitors and staff members with respiratory symptoms or other infections from coming in close contact with the child. *Children with nephrotic syndrome are susceptible to secondary infection because the plasma proteins lost in the urine are immunoglobulins.*
- Maintain the child on complete bed rest in semi-Fowler's position until edema subsides. *Bed rest decreases tissue oxygen demands. Semi-Fowler's position decreases upward pressure of the ascitic abdomen on the diaphragm.*
- Turn the child every 2 hours and provide support (sheepskin pad, special skin care) to extremely edematous

areas, such as the scrotum, *to help prevent infection.* Taut, edematous skin breaks down quickly. Skin surfaces should be cleaned and separated by clothing or padding.
● Keep strict intake and output records. Document voiding times and the volume, color, and specific gravity of urine. Test urine with a dipstick after each voiding, and document the presence or absence of proteins and RBCs. Corticosteroids are used in the primary treatment of a client with nephrosis. Within 7 to 21 days of starting treatment, urine excretion should increase and proteinuria should disappear. *Careful monitoring helps to evaluate the child's response to therapy.*
● Assess and document edema status at least every shift. Accurately measure body weight and abdominal girth daily and assess the periorbital area, abdomen, sacrum, pretibial area, and extremities *to identify the degree of fluid accumulation or fluid shift.*
● Offer the child small amounts of a no-salt-added regular diet at frequent intervals *to promote adequate nutrition.* Severe salt and fluid restrictions are usually unnecessary unless the child shows signs of renal failure. Although increased protein may be desirable, children with nephrotic syndrome are anorexic and don't usually accept a high-protein diet.
● As the child's energy level permits, offer toys that are age-appropriate, such as large blocks, crayons and coloring books, illustrated books, music boxes, and large puzzles *to enhance normal growth and development and prevent boredom.*
● Before discharge, prepare the parents for providing home care, as follows, *to promote careful monitoring* because the syndrome is marked by remissions and exacerbations:
– Tell the parents to report weight gain, headaches, nausea, fever, and other signs of infection, which may signal a relapse.
– Teach the parents how to test urine for protein to identify early signs of an exacerbation. (Parents should participate in urine testing in the hospital and continue testing at least twice weekly at home.) The child should receive medical attention before extensive edema occurs.
– Inform the parents of adverse reactions to corticosteroids, including cushingoid response and masking of usual infection signs. Warn them not to stop therapy suddenly; if the drug is stopped suddenly, the child will develop signs of shock and vascular collapse, requiring emergency care.
– Tell the parents what kind of behaviors to expect in response to illness and hospitalization. Regressive behaviors, especially increased dependence and clinging behav-

iors, may persist for several weeks. Discuss limit setting to maintain normalcy for the child.

Evaluation
● The child remains free from secondary infection.
● The child responds positively to steroid therapy.
● The child shows more interest in his surroundings and participates willingly in age-appropriate activities before discharge.

Otitis media

OTITIS MEDIA is inflammation of the middle ear that may or may not be accompanied by infection. Fluid presses on the tympanic membrane, causing pain and leading to possible rupture or perforation. This condition may be acute or chronic and secretory or suppurative.

Acute otitis media is common in children. Its incidence increases during the winter months, paralleling the seasonal increase in nonbacterial respiratory tract infections. With prompt treatment, the prognosis for a client with acute otitis media is excellent; however, prolonged accumulation of fluid in the middle ear cavity causes chronic otitis media and, possibly, perforation of the tympanic membrane.

Possible causes
All types
● Obstructed eustachian tube
● Wider, shorter, more horizontal eustachian tubes and increased lymphoid tissue in children as well as other anatomic anomalies

Acute secretory otitis media
● Barotrauma (pressure injury caused by inability to equalize pressure between the environment and the middle ear), as occurs during rapid aircraft descent in a person with upper respiratory tract infection or during rapid underwater ascent in scuba diving (barotitis media)
● Obstruction of the eustachian tube secondary to eustachian tube dysfunction from viral infection or allergy, which causes a buildup of negative pressure in the middle ear that promotes transudation of sterile serous fluid from blood vessels in the membrane of the middle ear

Acute suppurative otitis media
● Bacterial infection with pneumococci, *Haemophilus influenzae* (the most common cause in children under age 6), *Moraxella (Branhamella) catarrhalis,* beta-hemolytic

group A streptococci, staphylococci (most common cause in children age 6 or older), or gram-negative bacteria
- Respiratory tract infection, allergic reaction, nasotracheal intubation, or position changes that allow nasopharyngeal flora to reflux through the eustachian tube and colonize the middle ear

Chronic secretory otitis media
- Persistent eustachian tube dysfunction from mechanical obstruction (adenoidal tissue overgrowth or tumors), edema (allergic rhinitis or chronic sinus infection), or inadequate treatment of acute suppurative otitis media

Chronic suppurative otitis media
- Inadequate treatment of acute otitis episodes
- Infection by resistant strains of bacteria
- Tuberculosis (rarely)

Data collection findings
Acute secretory otitis media
- Echo heard by child when speaking; vague feeling of top-heaviness (caused by accumulation of fluid)
- Popping, crackling, or clicking sounds on swallowing or with jaw movement
- Sensation of fullness in the ear
- Severe conductive hearing loss

Acute suppurative otitis media
- Bulging and erythema of tympanic membrane
- Dizziness
- Fever (mild to very high)
- Hearing loss (usually mild and conductive)
- Nausea and vomiting
- Pain pattern (pulling the pinna doesn't exacerbate pain)
- Pain that suddenly stops (occurs if tympanic membrane ruptures)
- Purulent drainage in the ear canal from tympanic membrane rupture
- Severe, deep, throbbing pain (from pressure behind the tympanic membrane)
- Signs of upper respiratory tract infection (sneezing and coughing)
- Tinnitus

Chronic otitis media
- Cholesteatoma (cystlike mass in the middle ear)
- Decreased or absent tympanic membrane mobility
- Painless, purulent discharge in chronic suppurative otitis media
- Thickening and scarring of the tympanic membrane

Diagnostic findings
Acute secretory otitis media
- Otoscopy reveals clear or amber fluid behind the tympanic membrane and tympanic membrane retraction, which causes the bony landmarks to appear more prominent. If hemorrhage into the middle ear has occurred, as in barotrauma, the tympanic membrane appears blue-black.

Acute suppurative otitis media
- Culture of the ear drainage identifies the causative organism.
- Otoscopy reveals obscured or distorted bony landmarks of the tympanic membrane.
- Pneumatoscopy may show decreased tympanic membrane mobility, but this procedure is painful with an obviously bulging, erythematous tympanic membrane.

Chronic otitis media
- Otoscopy shows thickening, sometimes scarring, and decreased mobility of the tympanic membrane.
- Pneumatoscopy shows decreased or absent tympanic membrane movement.

Nursing diagnoses
- Acute pain
- Ineffective thermoregulation
- Deficient knowledge related to otitis media

Treatment
Acute secretory otitis media
- Concomitant treatment of the underlying cause, such as elimination of allergens or adenoidectomy for hypertrophied adenoids
- Inflation of the eustachian tube by performing Valsalva's maneuver several times per day (may be the only treatment required)
- Myringotomy and aspiration of middle ear fluid if decongestant therapy fails, followed by insertion of a polyethylene tube into the tympanic membrane for immediate and prolonged equalization of pressure (the tube falls out spontaneously after 9 to 12 months)

Acute suppurative otitis media
- Myringotomy for children with severe, painful bulging of the tympanic membrane

Chronic otitis media
- Elimination of eustachian tube obstruction
- Excision for cholesteatoma

● Mastoidectomy
● Treatment of otitis externa; myringoplasty and tympanoplasty to reconstruct middle ear structures when thickening and scarring are present

Drug therapy options
Acute secretory otitis media
● Nasopharyngeal decongestant therapy for at least 2 weeks; sometimes used indefinitely with periodic evaluation (current research questions the benefits of this practice but it's still done)

Acute suppurative otitis media
● Amoxicillin-clavulanate potassium (Augmentin) in areas with a high incidence of beta-lactamase-producing *H. influenzae* and in children who aren't responding to amoxicillin
● Antibiotic therapy, usually amoxicillin (Amoxil) (must be used with discretion to prevent development of resistant strains of bacteria in children with recurring otitis); for prevention, broad-spectrum antibiotics, such as cefuroxime (Ceftin) or amoxicillin-clavulanate potassium in high-risk children
● Cefaclor (Ceclor) or co-trimoxazole (Bactrim) for children who are allergic to penicillin derivatives

Chronic otitis media
● Broad-spectrum antibiotics, such as cefuroxime or amoxicillin-clavulanate potassium, for exacerbations of otitis media

Patient care goals
● The child will be afebrile and demonstrate no signs of secondary infection.
● The child will receive pain relief.
● The parents will verbalize knowledge about the condition, treatment, postoperative care (if applicable), and preventive measures.

Nursing interventions
● Monitor vital signs *to determine baseline values and detect early signs of worsening infection.*
● Watch for and report headache, fever, severe pain, or disorientation *to detect early signs of complications.*
● Administer analgesics, as needed, or recommend applying heat to the external ear *to relieve pain.*
● Identify and treat allergies *to prevent recurrences of otitis media.*

● Encourage the child and parents to complete the prescribed course of antibiotic treatment *to prevent reinfection.*
● For children with acute secretory otitis media, watch for and immediately report pain and fever *to detect early signs of secondary infection.*
● Tell the parents to avoid feeding an infant in a supine position or putting him to bed with a bottle *to prevent reflux of nasopharyngeal flora.*
● Encourage the child to perform Valsalva's maneuver several times daily *to promote eustachian tube patency.*
● After myringotomy, maintain drainage flow; place sterile cotton loosely in the external ear *to absorb drainage,* and change the cotton frequently *to prevent infection.*
● After tympanoplasty, reinforce dressings and observe for excessive bleeding from the ear canal *to assess for fluid volume deficit.*
● Review key teaching topics with the child and family members *to ensure adequate knowledge about the condition and treatment,* including:
– avoiding blowing the nose or getting the ear wet when bathing
– instilling nasopharyngeal decongestants properly, if prescribed
– recognizing upper respiratory tract infections and getting treatment early
– reporting complications, such as increasing fever, severe pain, or altered LOC.

Evaluation
● The child demonstrates a body temperature within normal range.
● The child experiences pain relief from analgesics.
● The parents express an understanding of discharge instructions if a surgical procedure has been performed.
● The parents state interventions appropriate to preventing future infections.

PRESCHOOL CHILD DISORDERS

Asthma
ASTHMA is a reversible respiratory disorder of bronchial obstruction and irritation after exposure to stimuli. It's the leading cause of acute and chronic illness in children. Attacks may be triggered by many different stimuli, including:
● allergens, such as wool, animals, and foods

- environmental pollutants
- exercise
- weather change
- infections
- medications
- emotions.

Most clients with asthma have extrinsic (immunoglobulin E [IgE]–mediated) disease, although exercise- or infection-induced (non-IgE-mediated) disease isn't uncommon. Most asthmatic clients experience a first attack before age 4. Asthma produces:

- inflammation of the mucous membranes
- smooth-muscle bronchospasm
- increased mucus secretion leading to airway obstruction and air trapping.

Possible causes
- Hyperresponsiveness of the lower airway (may be an idiopathic or intrinsic hyperresponsive reaction to an allergen, exercise, or environmental change)

Data collection findings
- Prolonged expiration with an expiratory wheeze (in severe distress, possibly an inspiratory wheeze)
- Unequal or decreased breath sounds
- Diaphoresis
- Dyspnea
- Alteration in chest contour from chronic air trapping
- Altered cerebral function
- Exercise intolerance
- Fatigue, apprehension, and restlessness
- Recent exposure to attack triggers
- Parents' lack of knowledge of asthma, its causes, diagnostic workup, and management
- Use of accessory muscles

 FAST FACT

Stay observant. Decreased wheezing – caused by decreased air movement in the airways – can indicate deterioration in a child's condition.

Diagnostic findings
- Oxygen saturation levels measured by pulse oximetry may show decreased oxygen saturation.
- ABG measurement may show increased partial pressure of arterial carbon dioxide ($PaCO_2$) from respiratory acidosis.

- Skin test is used to identify the source of the allergy.
- Sputum analysis is used to rule out respiratory infection.
- Chest X-rays may demonstrate hyperinflation, pulmonary infiltrates, and atelectasis.

Nursing diagnoses
- Impaired gas exchange
- Ineffective airway clearance
- Anxiety
- Risk for deficient fluid volume
- Caregiver role strain

Treatment
- Chest physiotherapy (after edema has abated)
- Hyposensitization through the use of allergy shots, if appropriate
- Parenteral fluids to thin mucus secretions
- Oxygen therapy as tolerated

Drug therapy options
- Bronchodilator: albuterol (Proventil)
- Chromone derivative: cromolyn (Intal) to prevent the release of mast cell products after an antigen-antibody union has taken place
- Corticosteroids (inhaled) to decrease edema of the mucous membranes; for chronic asthma, daily doses to control chronic inflammation

Patient care goals
- The child's respiratory rate will be within the age-appropriate normal range and normal breath sounds will be present throughout all lung fields by discharge.
- The child will maintain adequate hydration.
- The child will attain normal respiratory oxygenation on room air.
- The child will respond positively to the nursing staff in nonthreatening situations and receive comfort and support from the parents during invasive procedures.
- The child's parents will express understanding of the current treatment and the planned diagnostic workup.
- The child's parents will discuss concerns about caring for a child with asthma and demonstrate understanding of how to allergy-proof their home.

Nursing interventions
- Assess respiratory and cardiovascular status. *Tachycardia, tachypnea, and quiet breath sounds signal worsening respiratory status.*

● Monitor vital signs *to detect changes and prevent complications.*

● Assess the nature of the child's cough (hacking, unproductive progressing to productive), especially at night, in the absence of infection. *Early detection and treatment reduce respiratory distress.*

● Modify the environment to avoid an allergic reaction; remove the offending allergen. *Allergens can trigger an asthma attack.*

● Rinse the child's mouth after he inhales medication *to promote comfort and prevent irritation to the oral mucosa.*

● For exercise-induced asthma, give prophylactic treatments of cromolyn or beta-adrenergic blockers 10 to 15 minutes before the child exercises. *Premedication before exercise may prevent an asthma attack.*

● Position the child upright *to assist with breathing.*

● Assist the child with the use of inhaled medications. Monitor the child's respiratory status *to evaluate the response to medications,* as follows:
– Auscultate the lungs for rate, depth, and adventitious sounds.
– Assess for changes in the amount and quality of cough and sputum.
– Assess the use of accessory muscles and energy expended on breathing.

● Monitor the child's level of oxygenation through oxygen saturation *to evaluate for stable oxygen saturation levels.*

● Offer the child small sips of fluids, but avoid cold beverages. Record intake and output. *Promoting adequate fluid intake is important, but cold beverages should be avoided because they can trigger bronchospasm. Recording intake and output helps in evaluating the effectiveness of treatment.*

● Have the parents stay with the child during invasive procedures *to reduce anxiety.* Family-centered care should be maintained. Offer simple explanations of all procedures to be done.

● Teach parents the purpose and use of a peak expiratory flow meter (PEFM). *The PEFM has color zones that aid in guiding the treatment of asthma at home and aid in early identification of respiratory infections.*

● Teach allergen control measures in the home. Specific allergens identified by skin tests need to be removed, if possible, or minimized. Humidity should be kept below 50% to remove dust mites. Exposure to animals should be limited.

● Help parents plan activities *to encourage normal child development.* Asthmatic children should be encouraged to participate in all age-appropriate activities, including sports, particularly those that require an even-level expenditure of energy, such as distance running or swimming.

SPOT CHECK

What prophylactic action can be taken for a child who has exercise-induced asthma?

Answer: Prophylactic treatments of cromolyn or beta-adrenergic blockers taken 10 to 15 minutes before exercise may prevent an asthma attack.

● Forbid smoking in the child's environment. *Secondhand smoke can trigger an asthma attack.*

● Review key teaching topics with family members *to ensure adequate knowledge about the condition and treatment,* including:
– use of breathing exercises to increase ventilatory capacity
– proper use of inhalers
– ways to avoid allergens.
  During an acute attack:

● Provide moist oxygen, if necessary, *to promote mobilization of secretions.*

● Allow the child to sit upright *to ease breathing. This position promotes chest expansion.*

● Monitor for alterations in vital signs (especially cardiac stimulation and hypotension) *to detect signs of impending respiratory arrest and cardiac decompensation.*

● Monitor urine for glucose if the child is receiving corticosteroids *to detect early signs of hyperglycemia.*

● Administer inhaled medications by metered-dose inhaler, and monitor peak flow rates. *Peak flow rates indicate the degree of lung impairment.*

● Maintain a calm environment; provide emotional support and reassurance *to decrease anxiety and decrease oxygen demands.*

● Monitor the effectiveness of drug therapy. *Failure to respond to drugs during an acute attack can result in status asthmaticus.*

Evaluation

● The child breathes easily and with normal breath sounds.

● The child breathes room air and has normal oxygen saturation levels.

● The child takes fluids freely and has a normal hydration status.

● The child's parents outline a plan for coping with upcoming tests and measures to decrease the child's exposure to allergens.
● The child's parents correctly describe asthma and the treatment the child needs.

Hemophilia

HEMOPHILIA results from a deficiency in one of the coagulation factors. Hemophilia affects 1 in 5,000 males. The types of hemophilia are:
● hemophilia A (also called factor VIII deficiency or classic hemophilia), the most common type (75% of all cases)
● hemophilia B (also called factor IX deficiency or Christmas disease)
● hemophilia C (factor XI deficiency).
   Hemophilia is an X-linked recessive disorder. The inheritance pattern is described below:
● If the father has the disorder and the mother doesn't, all daughters will be carriers but sons won't have the disease.
● If the mother is a carrier and the father doesn't have hemophilia, each son has a 50% chance of getting hemophilia and each daughter has a 50% chance of being a carrier.

Possible causes
● Genetic inheritance

Data collection findings
● Multiple bruises without petechiae
● Prolonged bleeding after circumcision, immunizations, or minor injuries
● Bleeding into the throat, mouth, and thorax
● Hemarthrosis
● Peripheral neuropathies from bleeding near peripheral nerves

Diagnostic findings
● Partial thromboplastin time (PTT) is prolonged.

SPOT CHECK

What is a classic sign of hemophilia?
Answer: A classic sign of hemophilia is prolonged bleeding after minor injuries.

Nursing diagnoses
● Risk for deficient fluid volume
● Risk for injury
● Acute pain
● Anxiety
● Powerlessness

Treatment
● Avoidance of aspirin, sutures, and cauterization, which may aggravate bleeding
● Blood transfusion, if necessary
● Cryoprecipitate to maintain an acceptable serum level of the clotting factor; usually done by the family at home
● Assessment of human immunodeficiency virus (HIV) status (child is at increased risk for acquiring HIV through blood product transfusions)
● Administration of fresh frozen plasma to restore deficient coagulation factors
● Promotion of vasoconstriction during bleeding episodes by applying ice, pressure, and hemostatic agents

Drug therapy options
● Desmopressin acetate to promote the release of factor VIII in individuals with mild or moderate hemophilia A

Patient care goals
● The child will show evidence of hemodynamic stability.
● The child's fluid volume will remain within a normal range.
● The child will express feelings of comfort and decreased pain.
● The child's parents will demonstrate adequate coping skills.

Nursing interventions
● Monitor vital signs and intake and output *to assess renal status and monitor for fluid overload or dehydration.*
● Assess cardiovascular status and check for signs of bleeding; *fever, tachycardia, or hypotension may indicate hypovolemia.*
● Measure the joint's circumference and compare it to that of the unaffected joint *to assess for bleeding into the joint, which may lead to hypovolemia.*
● Note swelling, pain, or limited joint mobility. *Changes may indicate progressive decline in function.*
● Assess for joint degeneration from repeated hemarthroses *to detect the extent of damage.*
● Pad toys and other objects in the child's environment *to promote child safety and prevent bleeding.*

- Recommend protective headgear, soft foam Toothettes (instead of bristle toothbrushes), and stool softeners as appropriate *to prevent bleeding.*
- Discourage abnormal weight gain, *which increases the load on joints.*

When bleeding occurs
- Elevate the affected extremity above the heart *to decrease circulation to the affected area and promote venous return.*
- Immobilize the site *to prevent clots from dislodging.*
- Decrease anxiety *to lower the child's heart rate.*

Treating hemarthrosis
- Immobilize the affected extremity; elevate it in a slightly flexed position *to prevent further injury.*
- Decrease pain and anxiety *to lower the child's heart rate and minimize blood loss.*
- Avoid excessive handling or weight bearing for 48 hours *to prevent bleeding and to rest the site.*
- Begin mild ROM exercises after 48 hours *to facilitate absorption and prevent contractures.*

Evaluation
- The child is hemodynamically stable, with minimal complications.
- The child's parents understand how to respond during a bleeding episode.
- The child's parents can recognize signs of further bleeding, such as increased pain and swelling, fever, and symptoms of shock.
- The child's parents verbalize an understanding of the need to protect their child from injury while avoiding unnecessary restrictions that impair his normal development. For instance, the knees and elbows of a child's clothing can be padded to protect these joints during falls.

Leukemia
Leukemia is the most common form of cancer in children, with peak onset between ages 3 and 5. The 5-year survival rate varies from 50% to 90%, depending on the type of leukemia. Leukemia's main feature is a rapid increase in the number of immature white blood cells (WBCs).

Leukemic cells have the same properties as malignant cells of solid tumors, including:
- high metabolic rate
- infiltration of surrounding tissue
- migration to other body parts.

Because leukemic cells proliferate rapidly in the bone marrow, other blood components are deprived of nutrients and crowded out. The result is progressive anemia from decreased erythrocyte levels and bleeding problems from decreased thrombocyte levels. Though increased in number, the leukemic WBCs can't fight infection.

The leukemic cells tend to migrate first to the highly vascular organs of the reticuloendothelial system (the spleen, liver, and lymph glands). Infiltration of the central nervous system (CNS) results in signs of increased ICP and meningeal irritation. Finally, all organs are involved, and the child is deprived of metabolic nutrients, resulting in generalized wasting.

In children, the most common type of leukemia is ACUTE LYMPHOCYTIC LEUKEMIA (ALL). This type of leukemia is marked by extreme proliferation of immature lymphocytes (blast cells). In adolescents, acute myelogenous leukemia is more common and is believed to result from a malignant transformation of a single stem cell.

Clinical findings for leukemia may appear with surprising abruptness in children, with few, if any warning signs. (See *Signs and symptoms of leukemia.*)

Possible causes
- Chemical exposure and viruses
- Chromosomal disorders
- Down syndrome
- Ionizing radiation

Data collection findings
- Low-grade fever
- Petechiae and ecchymosis
- Lassitude
- History of infections
- Pallor
- Bone and joint pain
- Lymphadenopathy
- Decrease in all blood cells when bone marrow undergoes atrophy (leads to anemia, bleeding disorders, and immunosuppression)
- Blood in urine, stool, or emesis
- Pathologic fractures (when bone marrow undergoes hypertrophy)
- Poor wound healing and oral lesions.
- Enlarged spleen, liver, and lymph nodes
- Leukemic meningitis

Diagnostic findings
- Blast cells appear in the peripheral blood (where they normally don't appear).

Signs and symptoms of leukemia

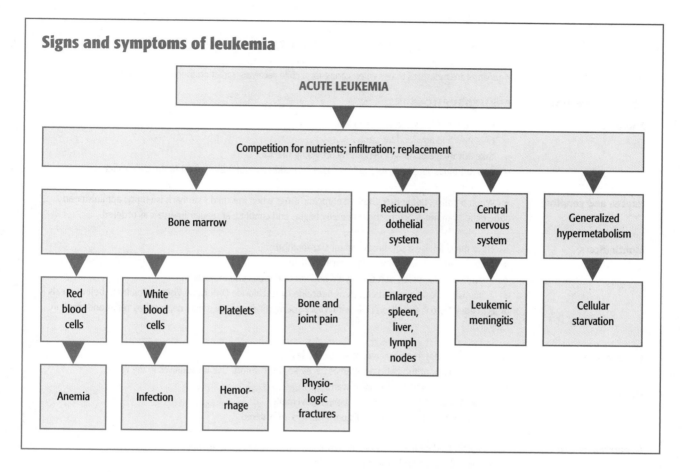

● Blast cells may be as high as 95% in the bone marrow (they're normally less than 5%) as measured by marrow aspiration in the posterior iliac crest (the sternum can't be used in children).

● Initial WBC count may be less than 10,000/µl at the time of diagnosis in a child with ALL between ages 3 and 7. (This child has the best prognosis.)

● Lumbar puncture indicates whether leukemic cells have crossed the blood-brain barrier.

Nursing diagnoses

● Risk for infection
● Acute pain
● Chronic pain
● Interrupted family processes
● Ineffective protection

Treatment

● Bone marrow transplantation (marrow from a twin or another donor with identical human leukocyte antigen,

usually a sibling, is transfused to repopulate the recipient's bone marrow with normal cells)

● High-protein, high-calorie, bland diet
● I.V. fluids as necessary
● Oxygen therapy, if needed
● Radiation therapy
● Transfusion therapy as needed

Drug therapy options

● Analgesic: acetaminophen (Tylenol), acetaminophen with codeine, ibuprofen (Motrin), morphine sulfate for pain relief
● Antiemetic: hydroxyzine (Atarax), ondansetron (Zofran)
● Chemotherapy with agents: cytarabine (Cytosar-U); intrathecal chemotherapy usually with methotrexate (Folex)
● Corticosteroid: prednisone (Deltasone)

Patient care goals

● The child will have a normal temperature and be free from signs of infection at the time of discharge.

Implementation for adverse reactions to radiation therapy and chemotherapy

The following table describes key nursing care measures to use when caring for a child receiving radiation therapy and chemotherapy.

ADVERSE REACTION	NURSING IMPLICATIONS
Anorexia	● Allow the child to select his own food. ● Give the child any food he wants. ● Take advantage of hungry periods by providing snacks. ● Add nutritious supplements (such as custards, puddings, and milk shakes) to the child's diet.
Nausea and vomiting	● When possible, administer chemotherapeutic drugs when the child's stomach is empty; administer an antiemetic 20 minutes before chemotherapy begins and continue at regular intervals as ordered.
Mouth ulcers	● Have the child use a soft-bristle, infant-size toothbrush. ● Provide frequent mouthwash with normal saline. ● Provide a bland, moist, soft diet; avoid hot and cold foods and beverages. ● Administer a local anesthetic, such as lidocaine hydrochloride (Xylocaine Viscous Solution), before meals or as needed for comfort. (Don't use with a very young child because it may depress gag reflex and result in aspiration.)
Rectal ulcers	● Don't use rectal thermometers or suppositories. ● Give sitz baths or tub baths as often as necessary for comfort. Use no additives in the water. ● Expose the affected area to air or warm heat. ● Apply A and D Ointment before a bowel movement. ● Provide dietary fiber, fluids, and stool softeners, as ordered.
Hemorrhagic cystitis	● Maintain fluid intake above maintenance level, usually 3,000 ml/m²/day. ● Monitor the child for burning pain on urination. ● Encourage frequent voiding; arouse the child at night to void. An empty bladder reduces the amount of time that the bladder is exposed to the alkylating agent in urine.
Alopecia	● Keep the scalp clean and dry to prevent infection. ● Obtain a baseball cap or favorite hat for the child to wear. ● Tell the child's parents to keep his head covered when exposed to the sun, wind, or cold.

● The child will experience pain control through medication and alternative comfort measures.
● The child and family members will demonstrate appropriate coping skills to deal with the problems of the disease.

Nursing interventions

● Monitor vital signs and intake and output *to determine fluid volume deficit and renal status.*
● Give special attention to mouth care *to prevent infection and bleeding.*

● Inspect the skin frequently *to assess for skin breakdown.*
● Give increased amounts of fluids *to flush chemotherapeutic drugs through the kidneys.*
● Provide a high-protein, high-calorie, bland diet with no raw fruits or vegetables. *Eliminating raw fruits and vegetables helps prevent infection. A diet meeting the child's caloric requirements helps ensure that the child's maintenance and growth needs are met.*

Caring for a child with acute lymphocytic leukemia

The nurse is reviewing discharge instructions with the parents of a 4-year-old boy diagnosed with acute lymphocytic leukemia (ALL) during this admission. The child has a recent history of a bad cold and several sore throats, bruises and petechiae over his body without a history of injuries, anorexia, weight loss, and fatigue.

What key points should be included in the discharge instructions?

● Teach the parents how to assess and care for the child, including how to observe for signs of chronic and acute blood loss (see "Shock," in chapter 4, pages 61 to 69). Tell them to take necessary measures to prevent hemorrhage, such as padding the child's sleeping and living area and keeping sharp objects out of the child's reach.

● Instruct the parents to monitor the child for infection and to take measures to prevent it, such as:
– removing broken toys and other sharp objects from the child's environment
– screening visitors for signs of infection
– advising visitors to use good hand-washing technique.

● Instruct the parents to ensure the child maintains a well-balanced diet.

● Advise the parents to schedule analgesia *to get maximum pain relief and optimal mental functioning.*

● Support the child and his parents through the grief process (see "Grieving," in chapter 3, page 43). The child and his parents will experience differing levels of anticipatory grief and loss. *They'll profit from support during this time.*

● Inform the parents of expected adverse effects of medication, as follows:
– Give the parents specific instructions on which adverse effects need medical attention: mouth and rectal ulcers, hemorrhagic cystitis, peripheral neuropathy, infection, and dehydration.
– Inform the parents that adverse effects of drugs don't indicate a return of leukemia.

Questions for further thought

● How can the nurse evaluate the parents' understanding of the instructions provided?
● What response or action indicates a need for further instructions?

● Provide pain relief as ordered, and document effectiveness and adverse effects. *Analgesics depress the CNS, thereby reducing pain.*

● Monitor the CNS *to assess for changes such as confusion that may result from cerebral damage.*

● Provide nursing measures to ease adverse reactions to radiation and chemotherapy *to promote comfort and encourage adequate nutritional intake.* (See *Implementation for adverse reactions to radiation therapy and chemotherapy.*)

● Review key teaching topics with the child and family *to ensure adequate knowledge about the condition and treatment,* including:
– avoiding infection
– adjusting to changes in body image
– contacting support groups
– recognizing signs and symptoms of infection and the need to seek immediate medical attention. (See *Caring for a child with acute lymphocytic leukemia.*)

Evaluation

● The child is free from infection at the time of discharge.
● The child verbalizes pain relief with the measures being used.
● The child and parents verbalize understanding of the disease, treatment measures, and when to seek medical attention.
● The child and parents express understanding of various coping strategies.

Reye's syndrome

REYE'S SYNDROME is an acute illness that causes fatty infiltration of the liver, kidneys, brain, and myocardium. It can lead to hyperammonemia, encephalopathy, and increased ICP.

Possible causes

● Acute viral infection, such as upper respiratory tract, type B influenza, or varicella (Reye's syndrome almost always follows within 1 to 3 days of infection)
● Concurrent aspirin use (high incidence)

FAST FACT

To prevent Reye's syndrome, use nonsalicylate analgesics and antipyretics.

Data collection findings

Reye's syndrome develops in five stages. The severity of signs and symptoms varies with the degree of encephalopathy and cerebral edema:

● stage 1 — vomiting, lethargy, hepatic dysfunction
● stage 2 — hyperventilation, delirium, hyperactive reflexes, hepatic dysfunction
● stage 3 — coma, hyperventilation, decorticate rigidity, hepatic dysfunction
● stage 4 — deepening coma, decerebrate rigidity, large fixed pupils, minimal hepatic dysfunction
● stage 5 — seizures, loss of deep tendon reflexes, flaccidity, respiratory arrest (death is usually a result of cerebral edema or cardiac arrest).

Diagnostic findings

● Blood test results show elevated serum ammonia levels; serum fatty acid and lactate levels are also increased.
● CSF shows a WBC count less than 10/µl; with coma, there's increased CSF pressure.
● Coagulation studies reveal prolonged PT and PTT.
● Liver biopsy shows fatty droplets uniformly distributed throughout cells.
● Liver function studies show that AST and ALT are elevated to twice their normal levels.

Nursing diagnoses

● Decreased intracranial adaptive capacity
● Ineffective thermoregulation
● Impaired gas exchange
● Risk for deficient fluid volume
● Impaired physical mobility
● Risk for impaired skin integrity

Treatment

● Decompressive craniotomy
● Endotracheal intubation and mechanical ventilation to control $PaCO_2$ levels
● Enteral or parenteral nutrition as needed
● Exchange transfusion
● Induced hypothermia
● Transfusion of fresh frozen plasma

Drug therapy options

● Osmotic diuretic: mannitol (Osmitrol)
● Vitamin: phytonadione (AquaMEPHYTON)

Patient care goals

● The child will maintain a normal respiratory status, as evidenced by a normal respiratory rate.

● The child will maintain adequate ventilation.
● The child will maintain orientation to his environment without evidence of deficit.
● The child will maintain joint mobility and ROM.
● The child will maintain skin integrity.

Nursing interventions

● Assist with maintenance of ICP monitoring with a subarachnoid screw or other invasive device *to closely assess for increased ICP.*
● Monitor vital signs and pulse oximetry *to determine oxygenation status.*
● Assess cardiac, respiratory, and neurologic status *to evaluate the effectiveness of interventions and monitor for complications such as seizures.*
● Monitor fluid intake and output *to prevent fluid overload.*
● Monitor blood glucose levels *to detect hyperglycemia or hypoglycemia and to prevent complications.*
● Maintain seizure precautions *to prevent injury.*
● Keep the head of the bed at a 30-degree angle *to decrease ICP and promote venous return.*
● Prevent dislodgement of the pulmonary artery catheter used to assess pulmonary artery pressures *to assess cardiopulmonary status.*
● Maintain oxygen therapy, which may include intubation and mechanical ventilation, *to promote oxygenation and maintain thermoregulation.*
● Maintain I.V. lines for administration of blood products as necessary *to increase oxygen-carrying capacity of the blood and prevent hypovolemia.*
● Administer medications, as ordered, and monitor for adverse effects *to detect complications.*
● Provide a hypothermia blanket as needed and monitor the client's temperature every 15 to 30 minutes while the blanket is in use *to prevent injury and maintain thermoregulation.*
● Check for loss of reflexes and signs of flaccidity *to determine the degree of neurologic involvement.*
● Provide good skin and mouth care and perform ROM exercises *to prevent alteration in skin integrity and promote joint motility.*
● Provide postoperative craniotomy care if necessary *to promote wound healing and prevent complications.*
● Be supportive of the family and keep them informed of the child's status *to decrease anxiety.*

Evaluation

● The child returns to a normal respiratory state without signs of respiratory distress.

- The child has minimal neurologic complications as ICP decreases, as evidenced by reflexes, LOC, and orientation.
- The child maintains joint mobility and ROM and skin integrity during his recuperation.
- The parents verbalize an understanding of avoiding Reye's syndrome by using nonsalicylate analgesics and antipyretics.

SCHOOL-AGE CHILD DISORDERS

Hypothyroidism

HYPOTHYROIDISM occurs when the body doesn't produce enough thyroid gland hormone, the hormone necessary for normal growth and development. (See *Understanding thyroid gland hormones.*)

Two types of hypothyroidism exist. Congenital hypothyroidism is present at birth. Acquired hypothyroidism is commonly due to thyroiditis, an inflammation of the thyroid gland that results in injury or damage to thyroid tissue. Hypothyroidism is three times more common in girls than in boys.

Early diagnosis and treatment offer the best hope. Infants treated before age 3 months usually grow and develop normally. Children who remain untreated beyond age 3 months and children with acquired hypothyroidism who remain untreated beyond age 2 suffer irreversible cognitive impairment. Skeletal abnormalities, however, may be reversible with treatment.

Possible causes
- Antithyroid drugs taken during pregnancy (in infants)
- Chromosomal abnormalities
- Chronic autoimmune thyroiditis (in children older than age 2)
- Defective embryonic development that causes congenital absence or underdevelopment of the thyroid gland (most common cause in infants)
- Inherited enzymatic defect in the synthesis of thyroxine (T_4) caused by an autosomal recessive gene (in infants)

Data collection findings
General findings
- Delayed dentition
- Enlarged tongue
- Hypotonia
- Legs shorter in relation to trunk size
- Cognitive impairment (develops as the disorder progresses)

> ## Understanding thyroid gland hormones
>
> The thyroid gland secretes the iodinated hormones thyroxine and triiodothyronine. These hormones:
> - act on many tissues to increase metabolic activity and protein synthesis
> - are necessary for normal growth and development
> - may lead to varying degrees of hypothyroidism (from a mild, clinically insignificant form to life-threatening myxedema coma) if deficient.

- Short stature with the persistence of infant proportions
- Short, thick neck

Slow basal metabolic rate
- Cool body and skin temperature
- Decreased perspiration
- Dry, scaly skin
- Easy weight gain
- Slow pulse

Untreated hypothyroidism in infants
- Hoarse crying
- Persistent jaundice
- Respiratory difficulties

Untreated hypothyroidism in older children
- Bone and muscle dystrophy
- Cognitive impairment
- Stunted growth (dwarfism)

Diagnostic findings
- Electrocardiogram shows bradycardia and flat or inverted T waves in untreated infants.
- Hip, knee, and thigh X-rays reveal the absence of the femoral or tibial epiphyseal line and delayed skeletal development that's markedly inappropriate for the child's chronological age.
- In myxedema coma, laboratory tests may also show low serum sodium levels, decreased pH, and increased $Paco_2$, indicating respiratory acidosis.
- Increased gonadotropin levels accompany sexual precocity in older children and may coexist with hypothyroidism.

● Serum cholesterol, alkaline phosphatase, and triglyceride levels are elevated.
● Normocytic normochromic anemia is present.
● Radioimmunoassay confirms hypothyroidism with low triiodothyronine and T_4 levels.
● Thyroid scan and ^{131}I uptake tests show decreased uptake levels and confirm the absence of thyroid tissue in athyroid children.
● Thyroid-stimulating hormone (TSH) level is decreased when hypothyroidism is due to hypothalamic or pituitary insufficiency.
● TSH level is increased when hypothyroidism is due to thyroid insufficiency.

FAST FACT

Newborn screens are blood tests performed on every neonate to determine the presence of certain congenital disorders. Hypothyroidism and phenylketonuria are the only two disorders screened for in every state of the United States. However, a positive result should always be confirmed with further testing, such as the radioimmunoassay for T_4, TSH, or both.

Nursing diagnoses
● Delayed growth and development
● Disturbed body image
● Constipation
● Compromised family coping
● Deficient knowledge

Treatment
● Routine monitoring of T_4 and TSH levels
● Periodic evaluation of growth to ensure thyroid replacement is adequate

Drug therapy options
● Oral thyroid hormone: levothyroxine (Synthroid)
● Supplemental vitamin D (to prevent rickets resulting from rapid bone growth)

Patient care goals
● The child will suffer minimally from the disease as evidenced by maintaining normal T_4 and TSH levels and meeting age-appropriate developmental milestones.
● The child and parents will demonstrate an understanding of the disease and its long-term effects.
● The child and parents will understand and comply with the treatment regimen.

● The child and parents will state adverse effects of thyroid replacement medication.
● The child and parents will cope with this chronic illness.

Nursing interventions
● Monitor blood pressure and pulse rate; report hypertension and tachycardia. *These signs of hyperthyroidism indicate that the dose of thyroid replacement medication is too high.*
● Check rectal temperature every 2 to 4 hours. Keep the child normothermic *to reduce metabolic demands.*
● Provide parents with support, referrals, and counseling as necessary *to help them cope with the possibility of caring for a physically and cognitively impaired child.*
● Adolescent girls require future-oriented counseling that stresses the importance of adequate thyroid replacement during pregnancy. Ideally, females should have excellent control before conception *to prevent congenital hypothyroidism in their child.*

Evaluation
● The child maintains normal thyroid hormone levels, thus experiencing minimal effects of the disease.
● The child and parents comply with thyroid replacement therapy and return for appropriate thyroid hormone level monitoring
● The child's parents engage the child in stimulating activities to help him reach maximum potential.

Pediculosis
HEAD LICE (*Pediculosis capitis*) is a contagious infestation of lice eggs, which look like white flecks, that firmly attach to hair shafts near the base. The cause of this disorder isn't related to the hygiene of a child or family members; however, head lice is easily transmitted among children and family members.

Possible causes
● Sharing of clothing and combs; close physical contact with peers (for example, in gym class [common in school-age children])

Data collection findings
● Pruritus of the scalp
● White flecks attached to the hair shafts

Diagnostic findings
- Examination reveals lice eggs firmly attached near the base of hair shafts.

Nursing diagnoses
- Impaired skin integrity
- Disturbed body image
- Social isolation

Treatment
- Removal of lice and eggs using a fine-toothed comb

Drug therapy options
- Pyrethrins (RID) or permethrin (Nix) shampoos (should be used for other family members and classmates as well)
- Lindane (Kwell) in resistant cases

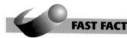 **FAST FACT**

When applying insecticidal treatments, carefully follow the manufacturer's directions to avoid neurotoxicity.

Patient care goals
- The child will exhibit improved or healing wounds, if any.
- The child will report feelings of increased comfort.
- The child will verbalize feelings about changed body image or social isolation.
- The child and his parents will demonstrate appropriate treatment application.

Nursing interventions
- Carefully follow the manufacturer's directions when applying medicated shampoo *to avoid neurotoxicity.*
- Confine the child to home for 24 hours *to reduce the risk of transmission.*
- Repeat treatment in 7 to 12 days *to ensure that all the eggs have been killed.*

Evaluation
- The child is free from infestation.
- The child and his parents demonstrate an understanding of methods to avoid reinfestation, including washing bed linens, hats, combs, and brushes, and refraining from exchanging combs, brushes, headgear, or clothing with other children.

Sickle cell anemia

SICKLE CELL ANEMIA, also called sickle cell disease, occurs in about 1 out of 400 blacks; it's rare in whites. In sickle cell anemia, Hb, in the presence of low oxygen tension (caused by hypoxia, acidosis, dehydration, or fever), crystallizes quickly, causing RBCs to bend into a crescent (or sickle) shape. The sickle cells accumulate, obstructing capillary flow throughout the body. The thickened blood results in capillary stasis, obstructed blood flow, and thrombosis. Ischemia occurs distal to the thrombosis, causing further oxygen depletion and sickling, which can lead to necrosis. The body hemolyzes the fragile sickle cells, quickly producing severe anemia (sickle cell crisis). (See *Sickling phenomenon,* page 256.)

Possible causes
- Genetic inheritance (sickle cell anemia is an autosomal recessive trait; the child inherits the gene that produces Hb S from two healthy parents who carry the defective gene)

Data collection findings
- Vary with the child's age
- Rare before age 4 months (fetal Hb prevents excessive sickling)

Infants
- Colic from pain caused by an abdominal infarction
- Dactylitis or hand-foot syndrome from infarction of the small bones of the hands and feet
- Splenomegaly from sequestered RBCs

Toddlers and preschoolers
- Pain at site of vaso-occlusive crisis
- Hypovolemia and shock from sequestration of large amounts of blood in the spleen

School-age children and adolescents
- Extreme pain at crisis site
- Poor healing of leg wounds from inadequate peripheral circulation of oxygenated blood
- History of pneumococcal pneumonia and other infections due to atrophied spleen
- Enuresis
- Priapism
- Delayed growth and development and delayed sexual maturity

Sickling phenomenon

This diagram shows the cycle of sickling phenomenon in sickle cell anemia.

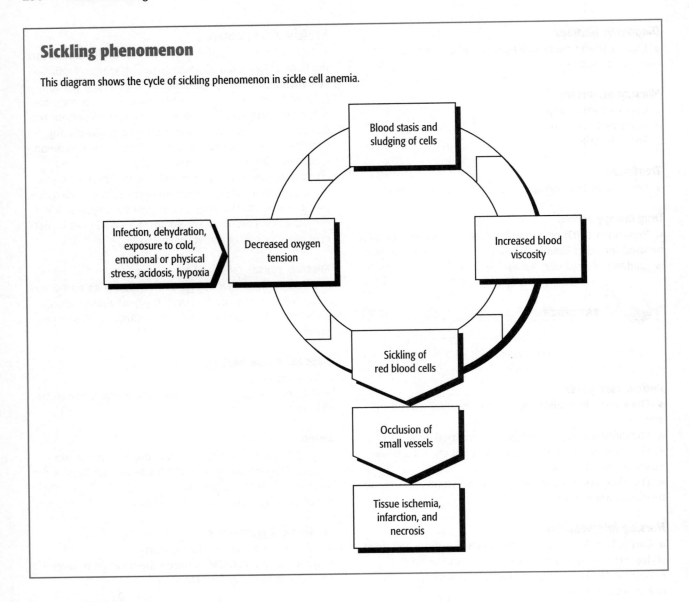

Diagnostic findings
● Laboratory studies show Hb level is 6 to 9 g/dl (in a toddler).
● More than 50% Hb S indicates sickle cell disease; a lower level of Hb S indicates sickle cell trait.
● RBCs are crescent-shaped and prone to agglutination.

Nursing diagnoses
● Ineffective tissue perfusion (peripheral)
● Acute pain
● Risk for infection
● Ineffective coping
● Compromised family coping
● Deficient knowledge related to sickle cell anemia

Treatment
● Bed rest
● Hydration with I.V. fluid (may be increased to 3 L [3.2 qt] per day during crisis)
● Short-term oxygen therapy (long-term oxygen decreases bone marrow activity, further aggravating anemia)
● Transfusion therapy as necessary
● Treatment of acidosis as necessary

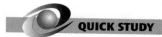

Drug therapy options

- Analgesic: morphine
- Antineoplastic: hydroxyurea (Droxia)
- Pneumococcal vaccine

Patient care goals

- The child's progressive sickling process will be halted.
- The child will maintain adequate levels of blood oxygen concentration.
- The child will be free from infection.
- The child will receive pain relief.
- The parents and child will verbalize knowledge about the condition, treatment, and options for genetic counseling.

Nursing interventions

- Administer sufficient pain medication (concerns about addiction are clinically unfounded) *to promote comfort.* A narcotic may be administered using a client-controlled analgesia pump at a continuous base rate with periodic rescue boluses available. *Lack of pain relief can cause further sickling.*

- Assess cardiovascular, respiratory, and neurologic status. *Tachycardia, dyspnea, or hypotension may indicate fluid volume deficit or electrolyte imbalance. Change in LOC may signal neurologic involvement.*
- Assess for symptoms of acute chest syndrome from a pulmonary infarction *to identify early complications.*
- Assess vision *to monitor for retinal infarction.*
- Encourage the child to receive the pneumococcal vaccine *to prevent infection.*
- Give large amounts of oral or I.V. fluids *to prevent fluid volume deficit, induce hemodilution, and prevent further sickling and additional complications.*

- Teach the child relaxation techniques *to decrease the child's stress level.*
- Maintain the child's normal body temperature *to prevent stress and maintain adequate metabolic state.*
- Monitor vital signs and intake and output *to assess renal function and hydration status.*
- Provide proper skin care *to prevent skin breakdown.*
- Reduce the child's energy expenditure *to improve oxygenation.*
- Remove tight clothing *to prevent inadequate circulation.*
- Suggest family screening and initiate genetic counseling *to identify possible carriers of the disease.*
- Review key teaching topics with the child and family members *to ensure adequate knowledge about the condition and treatment,* including:
  – avoiding activities that promote a crisis, such as excessive exercise, mountain climbing, or deep-sea diving
  – avoiding high altitudes
  – recognizing signs of infection and actions to take to help prevent infection
  – seeking early treatment of illness to prevent dehydration
  – avoiding aspirin use, which enhances acidosis and promotes sickling.

Evaluation

- The child returns home with an improved Hb level and without signs and symptoms of sickle cell crisis.
- The child continues to perform age-appropriate developmental tasks.
- The child's parents monitor his health status, avoid situations that precipitate a crisis, and seek early aggressive medical care for infections or signs of crisis.
- The child is infection-free at discharge.
- The parents relate an awareness of the child's condition, the importance of early treatment, and options for genetic counseling.

Type 1 diabetes mellitus

DIABETES is a disorder of carbohydrate metabolism characterized by insufficient insulin to allow glucose to cross the cell membrane. Type 1 diabetes (formerly called juvenile diabetes or insulin-dependent diabetes) most commonly occurs in childhood. Children with this type of diabetes must take insulin to replace what their pancreas can no longer produce.

Type 1 diabetes is most commonly diagnosed during childhood or adolescence but can occur at any time from infancy to about age 30. The psychological and emotional demands of growth and development and the generally increased but unpredictable activity levels of children com-

Age-related concerns with type 1 diabetes

Infants
● Careful monitoring of insulin needs secondary to rapid metabolism and growth and an infant's potential for acute illnesses
● Frequent infections and, in late infancy, food preferences that make management difficult
● Difficulty of recognizing hypoglycemia and ketoacidosis in infants

Toddlers
● Erratic activity patterns, decreased growth rate, and finicky eating behaviors that affect insulin needs
● Toddlers who have difficulty understanding why their parents purposely hurt them with fingersticks and injections
● Difficulty of recognizing hypoglycemia and ketoacidosis in toddlers

Preschoolers
● Readiness to learn about the disease and participate in care
● Resistance to daily injections (management of resistant behavior may be more difficult at this age than any other)

School-age children
● Adequate cognitive and motor ability for participating actively in managing diabetes (that is, injecting insulin, planning diet and exercise, and blood testing)
● Use of disease to achieve secondary gain such as pretending to be ill to stay home from school
● Increased participation in active sports (can present problems in balancing diet, insulin, and activity)

Adolescents
● Should be capable of self-management (however, rapid growth and metabolic changes make management complex)
● Effect of chronic disease on identity formation
● Need to express grief and anger at burden (group discussions, health clinics for diabetic adolescents, and juvenile diabetes camps are effective)

---

plicate management. (See *Age-related concerns with type 1 diabetes*.)

Possible causes
● Autoimmune mechanisms
● Genetic predisposition
● Viral infection

Hyperglycemia
● Cortisone use
● Decreased exercise with no decrease in food intake
● Decreased use of insulin
● Increased sugar intake
● Increased stressors
● Infection

Hypoglycemia
● Excessive exercise
● Failure to eat
● Increased insulin use

Data collection findings
● Polydipsia
● Polyphagia
● Polyuria

Hyperglycemia
● Nausea
● Vomiting
● Fruity breath odor
● Headache
● Dry, flushed skin
● Fatigue
● Weakness
● Abdominal cramping
● Thin appearance and possible malnourishment

Hypoglycemia
● Diaphoresis
● Tremors
● Palpitations
● Tachycardia
● Behavior changes (belligerence, confusion, slurred speech)

Diagnostic findings
● Fasting plasma glucose level (no caloric intake for at least 8 hours) is greater than or equal to 126 mg/dl.
● Plasma glucose value in the 2-hour sample of the oral glucose tolerance test is greater than or equal to 200 mg/

dl. This test should be performed after a loading dose of 75 g (2.6 oz) of anhydrous glucose.

● A random plasma glucose value (obtained without regard to the time of the child's last food intake) greater than or equal to 200 mg/dl and accompanied by symptoms of diabetes indicates diabetes mellitus.

● Test for glycosuria and ketonuria using dipstick, Clinitest, Acetest, Keto-Diastix, or glucose enzymatic test strip is positive.

 SPOT CHECK

True or false? Fruity breath odor, dry flushed skin, and vomiting are signs and symptoms of hypoglycemia.

Answer: False. These are signs and symptoms of hyperglycemia.

Nursing diagnoses
● Imbalanced nutrition: Less than body requirements
● Risk for deficient fluid volume
● Disturbed body image

Treatment
● Exercise
● Strict diet planned to meet nutritional needs, control blood glucose levels, and reach and maintain appropriate body weight

Drug therapy options
● Insulin replacement

Patient care goals
Outcomes relate to the school-age child. Age-appropriate modifications — such as increased parental involvement with insulin administration — should be made, depending on the child's age.

● The child and parents will state the onset, peak, and duration of action for the insulin form being taken.
● The child will accurately and safely draw up and administer insulin daily during the hospital stay.
● The child and parents will demonstrate an understanding of appropriate body sites for insulin administration and rotation scheduling.
● The child and parents will accurately test the child's blood for glucose at least four times per day.
● The child and parents will state appropriate actions to take in case of illness or a change in the normal activity schedule.
● The child and parents will state at least three signs or symptoms of hyperglycemia and hypoglycemia.

● The child and parents will describe appropriate action to take during an insulin reaction.
● The child and parents will be able to discuss the principles and rationales of the required diet.

Nursing interventions
● Monitor vital signs and fluid intake and output. *High urine output may signify hyperglycemia. Weak, thready pulse may indicate hypoglycemia.*
● Monitor blood glucose level and electrolytes *to detect early signs of electrolyte imbalance.*
● If you're unsure whether the child is hypoglycemic or hyperglycemic and the child is stuporous or unconscious, treat him for hypoglycemia. *If he's hypoglycemic, he'll respond quickly; if he's hyperglycemic, this action won't significantly worsen his condition.*
● Evaluate the child's understanding of type 1 diabetes and his attitude about the need to manage it. *This will help you to plan teaching.*
● Correct any misconception the child or adolescent has regarding type 1 diabetes and the therapeutic regimen. Use age-appropriate teaching materials *to increase knowledge of the condition and instill confidence for the child's ability to manage it.*
● Provide an opportunity for the child to interact with peers who have experienced diabetes *to decrease feelings of isolation and sense of being different from others.*
● Discuss issues surrounding peer pressure. Ask the adolescent whether he feels that social pressure causes him to ignore his diet or avoid self-administering insulin. Ask whether he feels embarrassed by his disorder. Explore ways of dealing with peer pressure. *Peer pressure is a reality that each adolescent must learn to deal with.*

Hyperglycemia
● Administer regular insulin for fast action *to promote euglycemia and prevent complications.*
● Administer I.V. fluids without dextrose *to flush out acetone and maintain hydration.*
● Monitor electrolytes and ABG levels and maintain I.V. line for possible administration of bicarbonate as needed *to combat acidosis.*
● Monitor blood glucose level *to detect early changes and prevent complications such as diabetic ketoacidosis.*

Hypoglycemia
● Give a fast-acting carbohydrate, such as honey, orange juice, or sugar cubes, followed later by a protein source *to establish normal glucose levels, thereby preventing complications of hypoglycemia.*

Teaching about insulin administration

Here are some important elements to teach children, adolescents, and parents about insulin administration:
● When both types of insulin are used, clear insulin should be drawn up first to prevent contamination.
● The vial shouldn't be shaken; intermediate forms are suspensions and should be gently rotated to prevent air bubbles.
● Injection sites should be rotated to prevent lipodystrophy.
● The infant, child, or adolescent should eat when the insulin peaks (for example, at midafternoon and bedtime)
● Insulin requirements may be altered with illness, stress, growth, food intake, and exercise; blood glucose measurements are the best way to determine insulin adjustments.

● If the child is stuporous or unconscious, maintain the patency of the I.V. line for administration of glucagon (subcutaneously, I.V., or I.M.) or dextrose I.V. *to prevent complications of hypoglycemia.*
● Review key teaching topics with the child and family members *to ensure adequate knowledge about the condition and treatment,* including:
– complying with the prescribed treatment program (see *Teaching about insulin administration*)
– monitoring blood glucose levels
– understanding the importance of good hygiene
– preventing, recognizing, and treating hypoglycemia and hyperglycemia
– understanding the effect of blood glucose control on long-term health
– managing diabetes during minor illness, such as a cold, flu, or an upset stomach, including testing urine for ketones
– providing the child or adolescent with written materials that cover the teaching topic
– providing the child or adolescent with information about the Juvenile Diabetes Foundation.

Evaluation
● The child and family members accurately monitor blood glucose levels.
● The child and family members verbalize knowledge about the disease, required treatment, and dietary needs.
● The child and family members can state the signs of hyperglycemia and hypoglycemia and know how to intervene appropriately.

● The child verbalizes strategies to cope with peer pressure and shows verbal evidence of a positive self-image.

Urinary tract infection
UTI is a microbial invasion of the kidneys, ureters, bladder, or urethra. The risk of UTIs varies depending on the child's age and the presence of obstructive uropathy or voiding dysfunction. In the neonatal period, UTIs occur most frequently in males, possibly because of the higher incidence of congenital abnormalities in male neonates. By age 4 months, UTIs are much more common in girls than in boys. The increased incidence in girls continues throughout childhood.

After infancy, nearly all UTIs occur when bacteria enter the urethra and ascend the urinary tract. Females are especially at risk for infection because the female urethra is much shorter than the male urethra. The female urethra is more subject to direct contamination because of its proximity to the anal opening. *Escherichia coli* causes approximately 75% to 90% of all UTIs in females.

Possible causes
● Incomplete bladder emptying
● Irritation by bubble baths
● Poor hygiene
● Reflux

Data collection findings
● Frequent urges to void with pain or burning on urination
● Urine that's cloudy and foul-smelling
● Low-grade fever
● Lethargy
● Hematuria
● Abdominal pain
● Enuresis
● Poor feeding patterns

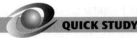 **QUICK STUDY**

To remember the clinical findings associated with UTI, think, "The urinary tract is **FULL** of infection."

    Frequent urges to void
    Urine that's foul-smelling and cloudy
    Low-grade fever
    Lethargy

Diagnostic findings
- Clean-catch urine culture yields large amounts of bacteria.
- Urine pH is increased.

Nursing diagnoses
- Impaired urinary elimination
- Acute pain
- Risk for infection
- Deficient knowledge related to UTI

Treatment
- Cranberry juice (acidifies urine)
- Forced fluids (flushes infection from the urinary tract)

Drug therapy options
- Antibiotic: co-trimoxazole (Bactrim) or ampicillin (to prevent glomerulonephritis)

Patient care goals
- The child will report increased comfort.
- The child will have minimal complications.
- The child and her parents will verbalize an understanding of the condition.

Nursing interventions
- Monitor input and output *to determine whether fluid replacement therapy is adequate.*
- Assess toileting habits for proper front-to-back wiping and proper hand washing *to prevent recurrent infection.*
- Encourage increased intake of fluids and cranberry juice *to flush the infection from the urinary tract and acidify the urine.*
- Assist the child when necessary to ensure that the perineal area is clean after elimination. *Cleaning the perineal area by wiping from the area of least contamination (urinary meatus) to the area of greatest contamination (anus) helps prevent UTIs.*

Evaluation
- The child expresses relief from symptoms, such as pain, urinary frequency, and burning on urination.
- The child has no complications resulting from the infection.
- The child and her parents demonstrate the need to complete the full course of antibiotics.
- The child and her parents demonstrate an understanding of the methods to avoid a UTI, such as avoiding bubble baths, using the toilet every 2 hours, and performing proper toilet hygiene (wiping from front to back).

ADOLESCENT DISORDERS

Acne vulgaris
An inflammatory disease of the sebaceous follicles, ACNE VULGARIS primarily affects adolescents, although lesions can appear as early as age 8. Although acne strikes boys more commonly and more severely, it usually occurs in girls at an earlier age and tends to last longer, sometimes into adulthood. The prognosis is good with treatment.

Possible causes
- Androgen-stimulated sebum production
- Follicular occlusion
- No longer attributed to dietary influences (such theories appear to be groundless)
- *Propionibacterium acnes,* a normal skin flora

Risk factors
- Androgen stimulation
- Certain drugs, including corticosteroids, corticotropin, androgens, iodides, bromides, trimethadione, phenytoin, isoniazid, lithium, and halothane; cobalt irradiation; or total parenteral nutrition
- Cosmetics
- Emotional stress
- Exposure to heavy oils, greases, or tars
- Heredity
- Oral contraceptives (many females experience an acne flare-up during their first few menses after starting or discontinuing oral contraceptives)
- Trauma or rubbing from tight clothing
- Unfavorable climate

Data collection findings
- Closed comedo, or whitehead (acne plug not protruding from the follicle and covered by the epidermis)
- Open comedo, or blackhead (acne plug protruding and not covered by the epidermis)
- Inflammation and characteristic acne pustules, papules or, in severe forms, acne cysts or abscesses (caused by rupture or leakage of an enlarged plug into the dermis)
- Acne scars from chronic, recurring lesions

Diagnostic findings

Diagnostic testing isn't necessary. The appearance of characteristic acne lesions, especially in an adolescent, confirms the presence of acne vulgaris.

Nursing diagnoses

- Impaired skin integrity
- Disturbed body image
- Risk for infection
- Risk for situational low self-esteem

Treatment

- Acne surgery (in severe cases)
- Cryotherapy
- Exposure to ultraviolet light (but never when a photosensitizing agent such as tretinoin is being used)

Drug therapy options

- Intralesional corticosteroid injection
- Oral isotretinoin (Accutane) (limited to those with severe papulopustular or cystic acne who don't respond to conventional therapy)
- Systemic therapy: usually tetracycline (Achromycin) (decreases bacterial growth; alternatively, erythromycin [tetracycline is contraindicated during pregnancy and childhood because it discolors developing teeth])
- Topical medication: benzoyl peroxide (Benzac), clindamycin (Cleocin), or erythromycin (Benzamycin)
- Antibacterial agent alone or in combination with tretinoin (retinoic acid, Retin-A) or a keratolytic
- Antiandrogenic agent: estrogens or spironolactone (Aldactazide)

Patient care goals

- The adolescent will exhibit improved or healed wounds or lesions.
- The adolescent and parents will demonstrate an understanding of skin-care regimen.
- The adolescent will voice his feelings about his changed body image.

Nursing interventions

- Try to identify predisposing factors *to determine whether any may be eliminated or modified.*
- Explain the causes of acne to the adolescent and family. Make sure they understand that the prescribed treatment is more likely to improve acne than a strict diet and fanatic scrubbing with soap and water. Provide written instructions regarding treatment *to eliminate misconceptions.*

- Instruct the adolescent receiving tretinoin to apply it at least 30 minutes after washing the face and at least 1 hour before bedtime. Warn against using it around the eyes or lips *to prevent damage.* After treatments, the skin should look pink and dry. If it appears red or starts to peel, the preparation may have to be weakened or applied less often.
- Advise the adolescent to avoid exposure to sunlight or to use a sunscreen *to prevent photosensitivity reaction.* If the prescribed regimen includes tretinoin and benzoyl peroxide, tell the adolescent to use one preparation in the morning and the other at night *to avoid skin irritation.*
- Instruct the adolescent to take tetracycline on an empty stomach and not to take it with antacids or milk *because it interacts with their metallic ions and is then poorly absorbed.*
- Tell the adolescent who is taking isotretinoin to avoid vitamin A supplements, which can worsen adverse effects. Also, discuss how to deal with the dry skin and mucous membranes that usually occur during treatment. Warn the female adolescent about the severe risk of teratogenesis, and recommend effective contraception during treatment if she's sexually active. Monitor liver function and lipid levels *to avoid toxicity.*
- Inform the adolescent that acne may take a long time to clear — even years for complete resolution. Encourage continued local skin care even after acne clears. Explain the adverse effects of all drugs *to promote compliance.*
- Pay special attention to the adolescent's perception of his physical appearance and offer emotional support *to help the adolescent cope with the effects of his illness.*

Evaluation

- The adolescent has improved skin integrity and acne diminishes.
- The adolescent expresses positive feelings about his body image.
- The adolescent and his parents understand predisposing factors for acne, such as cosmetic use or emotional stress.

Cystic fibrosis

CYSTIC FIBROSIS of the pancreas (also known as fibrocystic disease of the pancreas and mucoviscidosis) is a generalized dysfunction of the exocrine glands characterized by thickened and tenacious secretions that occlude glandular ducts, causing dysfunction in many organ systems. It's a chronic, life-shortening disease that occurs in 1 out of every 2,500 to 3,000 live births and primarily affects white children.

Possible causes
- Genetic inheritance (research suggests that there may be as many as 300 genes that code for cystic fibrosis)

Data collection findings
Overall
- Failure to thrive
- Malnutrition

Respiratory
- Excess inspissated mucus plugs in the airways leading to chronic obstructive pulmonary disease
- History of chronic, productive cough and recurrent respiratory infections, typically due to Pseudomonas infections

GI
- Thickened bile, which obstructs the ducts and results in eventual liver cirrhosis
- Bulky, greasy, foul-smelling stools that contain undigested food
- Distal intestinal obstruction syndrome (a partial or complete intestinal obstruction due to thick intestinal secretions)
- Increased appetite from undigested food lost in stools
- Meconium ileus at birth (the earliest symptom)
- Obstruction of pancreatic ducts preventing digestive enzymes from being released, resulting in decreased absorption of nutrients, especially fat-soluble vitamins (A, D, E, and K)
- Rectal prolapse due to large, bulky stools

Reproductive
- Blockage of the vas deferens by secretions, resulting in sterility in males
- Delayed puberty
- Viscous cervical secretions, which can lead to decreased fertility in females

Integumentary
- Channel defect in sweat glands, preventing sodium and chloride reabsorption, which places the child or adolescent at risk for abnormal salt loss and dehydration
- Salty taste of skin

Diagnostic findings
- Chest X-ray indicates early signs of obstructive lung disease.
- Sweat test using pilocarpine iontophoresis is positive.
- Stool specimen analysis indicates the absence of trypsin.

Nursing diagnoses
- Ineffective airway clearance
- Risk for infection
- Imbalanced nutrition: Less than body requirements
- Activity intolerance

Treatment
- Chest physiotherapy
- Multivitamins twice per day, especially fat-soluble vitamins
- High-protein formula and high-calorie supplement such as PediaSure

Drug therapy options
- Antibiotics (I.V.) for Pseudomonas infection when infection interferes with daily functioning
- Mucolytic (dornase alfa [Pulmozyme]), bronchodilator, or antibiotic nebulizer inhalation treatment before chest physiotherapy
- Pancrelipase (Pancrease) for oral pancreatic enzyme replacement

Patient care goals
- The child will maintain adequate ventilation.
- The child will be free from acute respiratory infection.
- The child's nutrition will be adequate to meet his needs.
- The child will continue to achieve age-appropriate developmental tasks.
- The child and parents will cope with chronic cystic fibrosis.

Nursing interventions
- Assess respiratory and cardiovascular status *for early detection of hypoxia.*
- Monitor vital signs and intake and output *to detect dehydration, which may worsen respiratory status. Dehydration can cause even thicker mucus secretions in the respiratory tract as well as constipation in children with cystic fibrosis.*
- Monitor pulse oximetry *to detect early signs of hypoxia.*
- Administer pancreatic enzymes with meals and snacks *to aid digestion and absorption of nutrients.*

NURSING PROCEDURE

Performing chest physiotherapy

Purpose
Chest physiotherapy (PT) includes postural drainage, chest percussion and vibration, and coughing and deep-breathing exercises. Together, these techniques mobilize and eliminate secretions, reexpand lung tissue, and promote efficient use of respiratory muscles. Chest PT helps prevent or treat atelectasis and may also help prevent pneumonia.

Postural drainage performed in conjunction with percussion and vibration encourages peripheral pulmonary secretions to empty by gravity into the major bronchi or trachea and is accomplished by sequential repositioning of the client. Usually, secretions drain best with the client positioned so that the bronchi are perpendicular to the floor. Lower and middle lobe bronchi usually empty best with the client in the head-down position; upper lobe bronchi, in the head-up position.

Percussing the chest with cupped hands mechanically dislodges thick, tenacious secretions from the bronchial walls. Vibration can be used with percussion or as an alternative when percussion can't be tolerated.

Implementation
- Explain the procedure to the child and provide privacy.
- Wash your hands.
- Auscultate the child's lungs to determine baseline respiratory status.

Postural drainage
- Position the child as ordered. In generalized disease, drainage usually begins with the lower lobes, continues with the middle lobes, and ends with the upper lobes. In localized disease, drainage begins with the affected lobes and then proceeds to the other lobes to avoid spreading the disease to uninvolved areas.
- Instruct the child to remain in each position for 10 to 15 minutes. During this time, perform percussion and vibration as ordered.

Percussion
- Instruct the child to breathe slowly and deeply, using the diaphragm, to promote relaxation. Hold your hands in a cupped shape, with fingers flexed and thumbs pressed tightly against your index fingers. Percuss each segment for 1 to 2 minutes by alternating your hands against the child in a rhythmic manner. Listen for a hollow sound on percussion to verify correct performance of the technique.

Vibration
- Ask the child to inhale deeply and then exhale slowly through pursed lips. During exhalation, firmly press your fingers and the palms of your hands against the chest wall. Tense the muscles of your arms and shoulders in an isometric contraction to send fine vibrations through the chest wall. Vibrate during five exhalations over each chest segment.
- After postural drainage, percussion, or vibration, instruct the child to inhale deeply through his nose and then exhale in three short huffs. Then have him inhale deeply again and cough through a slightly open mouth. Three consecutive coughs are highly effective. An effective cough sounds deep, low, and hollow; an ineffective one, high-pitched. Have the child perform exercises for about 1 minute and then rest for 2 minutes. Gradually progress to a 10-minute exercise period four times daily.
- Auscultate the child's lungs to evaluate the effectiveness of therapy.
- Record the date and time of chest PT; positions for secretion drainage and length of time each is maintained; chest segments percussed or vibrated; color, amount, odor, and viscosity of secretions produced and the presence of any blood; any complications and nursing actions taken; and the child's tolerance of treatment.

FAST FACT

When administering pancreatic enzymes, open the capsule and add the powder to a small amount of cold applesauce if the child can't swallow the capsule.

- Provide high-calorie, high-protein foods with added salt *to replace sodium loss and promote normal growth.*
- Encourage breathing exercises, verify that the child receives ordered respiratory treatments, and perform chest physiotherapy two to four times per day *to mobilize secretions, maintain lung capacity, and increase oxygenation.* (See *Performing chest physiotherapy.*)

CLINICAL SITUATION

Caring for an adolescent with cystic fibrosis

A 16-year-old boy was diagnosed with cystic fibrosis at age 16 months and has been hospitalized many times for the condition. This time, he's in acute respiratory distress with an upper and lower respiratory tract infection. He has a fever of 101.8° F (38.8° C), a respiratory rate of 38 breaths/minute, and a pulse rate of 128 beats/minute. His skin is dusky, and his nail beds are cyanotic. He has a barrel chest and supraclavicular and intercostal retractions. He's orthopneic, highly anxious, and restless. The adolescent appears small for his age, thin and wasted, with little, if any, subcutaneous fat. He has a distended abdomen, a voracious appetite, and pale, transparent skin and is easily fatigued, displaying malaise, irritability, and lethargy. The adolescent is receiving oxygen by face mask.

What are appropriate steps to take when assessing the adolescent?

● Assess the level of the adolescent's respiratory distress and infection, noting respiratory rate and depth; skin color; breath sounds; amount, color, and consistency of sputum; temperature; and clubbing of fingers and toes. *Clubbing of fingers and toes stems from chronic hypoxia.*

● Assess the adolescent's cardiac status, noting blood pressure and apical pulse rate, rhythm, and quality. *Chronic obstructive pulmonary disease can progress to cor pulmonale (right-sided heart failure), which can be a cause of death in cystic fibrosis.*

● Assess the adolescent's nutritional status, estimating the thickness of subcutaneous tissue and comparing his weight and height with growth chart measurements. *Diminished amounts of pancreatic enzymes result in malnutrition and malabsorption.*

● Assess the adolescent's fluid and electrolyte balance. *Prevention of dehydration is important because dehydration thickens mucoid secretions.*

● Assess the family's ability to cope with the acute episode and their continuing ability to cope with chronic cystic fibrosis. *This clarifies their need for support or counseling.*

● Assess the adolescent's developmental level (see the section on Growth and development, pages 25 to 39). *This assessment helps the nurse to determine whether the adolescent is meeting age-appropriate developmental expectations.*

How can the nurse assist the adolescent in maintaining an age-appropriate developmental level?

● The adolescent is different from his peers and needs guidance in identifying ways in which he's the same, *to help him through the teen years, when peer relationships are most important.*

● Encourage independence within the limits imposed by his condition. *This promotes a feeling of control over his situation and helps him regain and maintain self-esteem.*

● Allow the adolescent to participate in decisions about care. Explain procedures, treatments, and routines directly and candidly. Approach him as an adult; don't condescend to or berate him. *This will help him regain a sense of control.*

Questions for further thought

● What referrals are appropriate for the adolescent and his family members?

● What adverse reactions would occur if the adolescent became dehydrated?

● Encourage physical activity *to promote normal development.*

● Review key teaching topics with the child and family members *to ensure adequate knowledge about the condition and treatment,* including:

– avoiding cough suppressants and antihistamines because the child must be able to cough and expectorate

– genetic counseling for the family

– promoting as normal a life as possible for the child. (See *Caring for an adolescent with cystic fibrosis.*)

Evaluation

● The child is afebrile and doesn't exhibit signs of respiratory infection.

● The child's nutritional intake results in slow, steady weight gain and meets his growth needs.

● The child and family members perform aerosol therapy (if ordered) and chest physical therapy accurately and as frequently as necessary to prevent respiratory infection.

● The parents state that they will seek medical care for respiratory infections or weight loss and have the child see the physician routinely for preventive care.

● The child engages in age-appropriate behaviors.

Meningitis

MENINGITIS is an inflammation of the brain and spinal cord meninges. It's most common in infants and toddlers. The incidence of meningitis is greatly reduced with routine *Haemophilus influenzae* type B vaccine.

Possible causes

● Viral or bacterial agents, transmitted by the spread of droplets (organisms enter the blood from the nasopharynx or middle ear)

Data collection findings

● Nuchal rigidity that may progress to opisthotonus (arching of the back)
● Positive Brudzinski's sign (the child flexes the knees and hips in response to passive neck flexion)
● Positive Kernig's sign (inability to extend leg when hip and knee are flexed)
● Coma
● Delirium
● Fever
● Headache
● High-pitched cry
● Irritability
● Onset gradual or abrupt following an upper respiratory infection
● Petechial or purpuric lesions possibly present in bacterial meningitis
● Projectile vomiting
● Seizures

 SPOT CHECK

Positive responses to which tests help establish a diagnosis of meningitis?
Answer: A positive Brudzinski's sign and positive Kernig's sign help to establish a diagnosis of meningitis.

Diagnostic findings

● Lumbar puncture shows increased CSF pressure, cloudy color, increased WBC count and protein level, and a decreased glucose level if the meningitis is caused by bacteria.

Nursing diagnoses

● Decreased intracranial adaptive capacity
● Ineffective breathing pattern
● Risk for injury
● Hyperthermia
● Anxiety

Treatment

● Burr holes to evacuate subdural effusion, if present
● Droplet precautions; should be maintained until at least 24 hours of effective antibiotic therapy have elapsed; continued precautions recommended for meningitis caused by *H. influenzae* or *Neisseria meningitidis*
● Hypothermia blanket
● Oxygen therapy may require intubation and mechanical ventilation to induce hyperventilation to decrease ICP
● Seizure precautions
● Treatment for coexisting conditions

Drug therapy options

● Analgesic (treats pain of meningeal irritation)
● Corticosteroid: dexamethasone (Decadron)
● Parenteral antibiotic: ceftazidime (Fortaz), ceftriaxone (Rocephin); possibly intraventricular administration of antibiotics

Patient care goals

● The child will maintain normal vital signs, including adequate ventilation and temperature within the normal range.
● The child will express feelings of comfort and relief from pain.
● The child will maintain fluid volume within the normal range.
● The child and his parents will verbalize an understanding of the condition and its treatment.

Nursing interventions

● Monitor vital signs and intake and output *to assess for fluid volume excess.*
● Assess the child's neurologic status frequently *to monitor for signs of increased ICP.*
● Provide a dark and quiet environment. *Environmental stimuli can increase ICP or stimulate seizure activity.*
● Maintain seizure precautions *to prevent injury.*
● Administer medications as ordered *to combat infection and decrease ICP.*
● Move the child gently *to prevent a rise in ICP.*
● Maintain isolation precautions, as ordered, *to prevent the spread of infection.*
● Provide emotional support for the family *to decrease anxiety.*
● Examine the infant for bulging fontanels and measure head circumference; *hydrocephalus is a complication that can result from meningitis.*

Evaluation
- The child expresses relief from symptoms and has no complications.
- The child's vital signs are normal.
- The child and his parents express an understanding of methods to prevent meningitis, including seeking proper medical treatment for chronic sinusitis or other chronic infections.

Scoliosis

SCOLIOSIS, a lateral curvature of the spine, occurs more commonly in girls than in boys. About 10% of preadolescent children have some degree of scoliosis. The curvature progresses insidiously and may be prominent before the condition is diagnosed. It becomes more obvious at prepuberty, a time of rapid growth. The curve progression stops when bone growth stops. (See *Defects of the spinal column,* page 268.)

Possible causes
- Nonstructural, functional, or postural scoliosis — a nonprogressive **C** curve from some other condition, such as poor posture, unequal leg length, and poor vision
- Structural or progressive scoliosis — a progressive **S** curve with a primary and compensatory curvature resulting in spinal and rib changes

Data collection findings
Nonstructural scoliosis
- Disappearing curve in the spinal column when the child bends at the waist to touch the toes

Structural scoliosis
- Failure of the spinal curve to straighten when the child bends forward with the knees straight and the arms hanging down toward the feet (the hips, ribs, shoulders, and shoulder blades are asymmetrical)

Diagnostic findings
- X-rays may aid the diagnosis.

Nursing diagnoses
- Chronic pain
- Disturbed body image
- Delayed growth and development
- Powerlessness

Treatment
Nonstructural scoliosis
- Postural exercises
- Shoe lifts

Structural scoliosis
- Harrington, Luque, Wisconsin segmental spine instrumentation, Texas Scottish Rite, or Cotrel-Dubousset rods for curves greater than 40 degrees (to realign the spine or when curves fail to respond to orthotic treatment) along with spinal fusion with a bone graft from the iliac crest
- Possible prolonged bracing (Milwaukee, thoracolumbosacral orthoses, or Boston brace) to slow progression of condition

Patient care goals
- The adolescent's scoliosis will be arrested.
- The adolescent and her parents will comply with bracing and traction recommendations.
- The adolescent will accept the brace and activity restrictions.
- The adolescent will physically adjust to the brace and help to select clothing to wear with it.
- The adolescent will develop a positive self-image and continue with developmental tasks of adolescence.
- The parents will demonstrate understanding and support of the adolescent's independence.

Nursing interventions
- Review key teaching topics with the adolescent and parents *to ensure adequate knowledge about the condition and treatment,* including:
– performing stretching exercises for the spine
– taking steps to help the adolescent maintain self-esteem.

Adolescent with bracing
- Instruct the adolescent and parents that the brace must be worn 16 to 23 hours each day *to slow progression of the condition.*
- Advise the adolescent to wear a cotton T-shirt under the brace *to protect the skin.*
- Examine the skin, especially over bony prominences, daily *to evaluate for signs of skin breakdown.*

After spinal fusion and insertion of rods
- Monitor vital signs and intake and output *to prevent fluid volume deficit.*
- Turn the child only by logrolling for the first 24 to 48 hours, depending on the type of instrumentation used, *to prevent injury.*

Defects of the spinal column

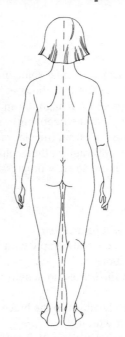

The normal spine in the upright position is vertically aligned, not twisted.

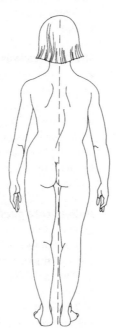

A child with mild to moderate spinal curvature (the upright spine has a marked serpentine twist) may benefit from corrective bracing or surgery.

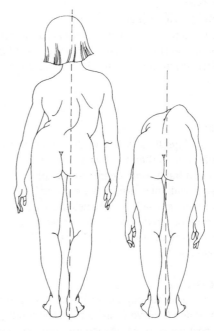

The rib hump, a hallmark of severe scoliosis, is accentuated when the child bends forward. A child with severe curvature is generally treated with surgery.

● Maintain correct body alignment *to promote joint mobility and prevent injury.*
● Maintain the bed in a flat position *to prevent injury and complications.*
● Help the child adjust to the increase in height and altered self-perception *to promote self-esteem and decrease anxiety.*
● Perform neurologic assessment of lower extremities and report any abnormalities to the physician immediately *to detect any change in condition.*

Evaluation
● The adolescent and her parents comply with the bracing regimen, and the scoliosis doesn't progress.
● The adolescent has a positive self-image.
● The adolescent continues to develop independence.
● The parents support the need for independence while allowing the adolescent to be dependent when appropriate.

● The adolescent maintains her friendships with peers, who accept her in a brace.
● The adolescent returns for scheduled follow-up visits.

9 Adult nursing

Introduction

This section reviews nursing care of adult clients with physiologic health problems, which are organized by body system for easy reference. As in other sections of this book, the text follows the nursing process format to help you solve the nursing problems presented. Selected clinical situations (case studies) represent their high incidence among hospitalized clients or demonstrate principles essential to safe practice.

Before you begin reading this section, consider reviewing the entries on the nursing process, acid-base balance, fluid and electrolyte balance, shock, immobility, and perioperative nursing.

CARDIOVASCULAR SYSTEM

The cardiovascular system is made up of the heart and a network of arteries, veins, and smaller blood vessels that transport blood to and from all body organs and tissues.

Cardiovascular structure and function

The cardiovascular system serves several vital functions, including:
- transporting life-supporting oxygen and nutrients to cells
- removing metabolic waste products
- carrying hormones from one part of the body to another.

Heart

The central organ of the cardiovascular system is the heart, which propels blood through the body by continuous rhythmic contractions. Review these other characteristics of the heart:
- It's a muscular organ composed of two atria (left and right) and two ventricles (left and right).

- The heart is surrounded by a pericardial sac that consists of two layers:
  - visceral (inner) layer
  - parietal (outer) layer.
- The heart wall has three layers:
  - epicardium (visceral pericardium) — the outer layer
  - myocardium — the thick, muscular middle layer
  - endocardium — the inner layer.
- Inside the heart are four valves:
  - The *tricuspid valve* and *mitral valve* lie between the atria and ventricles; because of their location, they're also called atrioventricular (AV) valves. These valves prevent backflow of blood during systole.
  - The *pulmonic semilunar valve* lies between the right ventricle and the pulmonary artery. The *aortic semilunar valve* lies between the left ventricle and the aorta. These valves prevent backflow of blood during diastole.

Coronary arteries

The heart is nourished by blood from two main arteries, the left coronary artery and the right coronary artery (RCA):
- As the left coronary artery branches off the aorta, it branches into the left anterior descending (LAD) artery and the circumflex artery. The LAD artery then supplies blood to the anterior wall of the left ventricle, the anterior ventricular septum, and the apex of the left ventricle. The circumflex artery supplies blood to the left atrium, the lateral and posterior portions of the left ventricle.
- The RCA fills the groove between the atria and the ventricles and gives rise to the acute marginal artery, which becomes the posterior descending artery. The RCA sends blood to the sinoatrial (SA) and AV nodes and to the right atrium. The posterior descending artery supplies the posterior and inferior walls of the left ventricle and the posterior portion of the right ventricle.

Cardiac circulation

Blood circulates through the heart along the following pathway:
- from the inferior and superior venae cavae to the right atrium
- through the tricuspid valve to the right ventricle
- through the pulmonic valve to the pulmonary artery
- to the lungs, where blood is oxygenated
- through the pulmonary veins to the left atrium
- through the mitral valve to the left ventricle
- through the aortic valve to the aorta and throughout the body.

Conduction

The system that conducts electrical impulses and coordinates the heart's contractions consists of the SA node, internodal tracts, AV node, bundle of His, right and left bundle branches, and Purkinje fibers.

A normal electrical impulse is initiated at the SA node, the heart's intrinsic pacemaker, which results in the following chain of events:
- atrial depolarization
- atrial contraction
- impulse transmission to the AV node
- impulse transmission to the bundle of His, bundle branches, and Purkinje fibers
- ventricular depolarization
- ventricular contraction
- ventricular repolarization.

Cardiac function

Cardiac function is assessed by measuring these parameters:
- Cardiac output is the total amount of blood ejected from a ventricle per minute. Cardiac output equals stroke volume multiplied by heart rate ($CO = SV \times HR$).
- Stroke volume is the amount of blood ejected from a ventricle with each beat.
- Ejection fraction is the percent of left ventricular end-diastolic volume ejected during systole (normally 60% to 70%).

Systemic circulation

Blood is carried throughout the body in arteries and veins and through smaller vessels, such as arterioles, capillaries, and venules. Think of them as a series of large and small canals forming an interlocking system of blood flow:

- Arteries carry oxygenated blood from the heart to the tissues. They consist of three layers — the intima, media, and adventitia.
- Arterioles are small-resistance vessels that feed into capillaries.
- Capillaries join arterioles to venules (larger, lower-pressured vessels than arterioles), where nutrients and wastes are exchanged.
- Venules join capillaries to veins.
- Veins are large-capacity, low-pressure vessels that return unoxygenated blood to the heart.

CARDIOVASCULAR DISORDERS

Major cardiovascular disorders include angina; aortic aneurysm (abdominal and thoracic); arrhythmias; arterial occlusive disease; cardiac tamponade; cardiomyopathy; coronary artery disease (CAD); endocarditis, infective; heart failure; hypertension; myocardial infarction (MI); pericarditis; pulmonary edema; Raynaud's disease; rheumatic fever and rheumatic heart disease; thrombophlebitis; valvular heart disease; and venous insufficiency (chronic).

For all major cardiovascular disorders, the goal of nursing management is to decrease cardiac workload and increase myocardial blood supply so that tissue oxygenation increases and overall damage to the heart is reduced.

Angina

ANGINA — chest pain that results from myocardial ischemia — is the most common symptom of CAD, the term for cardiac conditions that result from myocardial ischemia, usually secondary to atherosclerosis. Angina is an imbalance between myocardial oxygen supply and demand.

Angina is generally categorized as one of three main forms:
- With *stable angina*, symptoms are consistent and pain is relieved by rest.
- With *unstable angina*, pain is marked by increasing severity, duration, and frequency. Pain from unstable angina responds slowly to nitroglycerin.
- With *variant angina*, pain is unpredictable and may occur at rest.

Possible causes
- Activity or disease that increases metabolic demands

Ischemic pain patterns

Ischemic pain experienced during a myocardial infarction radiates in various directions, as illustrated here.

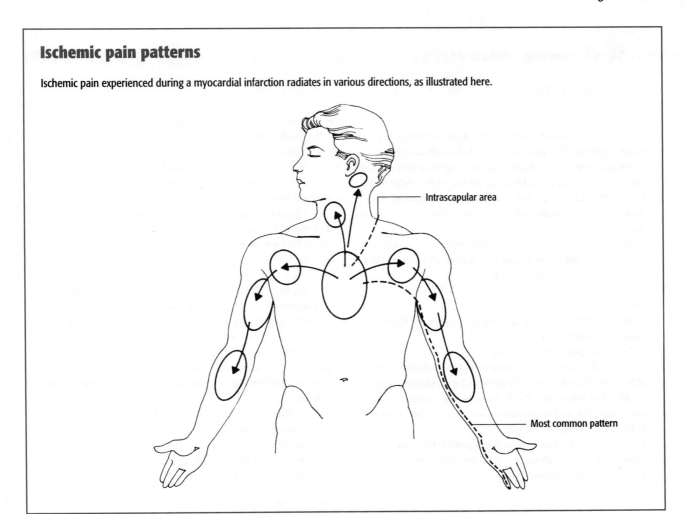

Intrascapular area

Most common pattern

- Aortic stenosis
- Atherosclerosis
- Pulmonary stenosis
- Small-vessel disease (associated with rheumatoid arthritis, radiation injury, or lupus erythematosus)
- Thromboembolism
- Vasospasm

Data collection findings

- Pain that may be substernal, crushing, or compressing; may radiate to the arms, jaw, or back; usually lasts 3 to 5 minutes and usually occurs after exertion, emotional excitement, or exposure to cold but can also develop when the client is at rest (see *Ischemic pain patterns*)
- Anxiety
- Diaphoresis
- Dyspnea
- Tachycardia
- Palpitations
- Epigastric distress

Diagnostic findings

- Blood chemistry test results may show increased cholesterol and low-density lipoprotein levels (LDL), low high-density lipoprotein (HDL) levels, and elevated triglycerides.
- Cardiac enzyme levels are within normal limits.
- Coronary arteriography shows narrowing of the coronary arteries.
- Electrocardiogram (ECG) may show ST-segment depression and T-wave inversion during angina.

NURSING PROCEDURE

Obtaining an ECG

Purpose

One of the most valuable and frequently used diagnostic tools, electrocardiography (ECG) measures the heart's electrical activity as waveforms. Impulses moving through the heart's conduction system create electric currents that can be monitored on the body's surface. Electrodes attached to the skin detect these electric currents and transmit them to an instrument that produces a record (ECG) of cardiac activity.

ECG can be used to identify myocardial ischemia and infarction, rhythm and conduction disturbances, chamber enlargement, electrolyte imbalances, and drug toxicity.

Implementation

● Place the ECG machine close to the client's bed, and plug the power cord into the wall outlet.

● Explain the procedure to the client.

● Position the client supine in the center of the bed with his arms at his sides. You may raise the head of the bed to promote comfort.

● Place the electrodes on flat, fleshy areas. Avoid muscular and bony areas. If an area is excessively hairy, shave it. Clean excess oil or other substances from the skin.

● Apply electrode paste or gel or the disposable electrodes to the client's wrists and the medial aspects of his ankles. Position chest gel or electrodes as follows:

– V_1: Fourth intercostal space at right sternal border

– V_2: Fourth intercostal space at left sternal border

– V_3: Halfway between V_2 and V_4

– V_4: Fifth intercostal space at midclavicular line

– V_5: Fifth intercostal space at anterior axillary line (halfway between V_4 and V_6)

– V_6: Fifth intercostal space at midaxillary line, level with V_4.

● Connect the leadwires to the electrodes as indicated by the coding on the tip of each leadwire.

● Enter the appropriate information as prompted by the ECG machine.

● Check to see that the paper speed selector is set to the standard 25 mm/second and that the machine is set to full voltage.

● Ask the client to breathe normally, lie still, and not talk. Press the AUTO button. Observe the tracing quality of all 12 leads.

● When the machine finishes recording the 12-lead ECG, remove the electrodes and clean the client's skin. After disconnecting the leadwires from the electrodes, dispose of or clean the electrodes as indicated.

● Label the ECG recording with the client's name, room number, and facility identification number. Document in your notes the test's date and time as well as significant responses by the client. Record the date, time, and client's name and room number on the ECG itself. Note any appropriate clinical information on the ECG.

● Holter monitoring may reveal ST-segment depression and T-wave inversion during angina.

● Stress test results include abnormal ECG results and chest pain.

Nursing diagnoses

● Acute pain

● Anxiety

● Activity intolerance

● Deficient knowledge related to cardiovascular disease

Treatment

● Low-fat, low-cholesterol (and low-calorie, if necessary) diet

● Coronary artery bypass grafting

● Oxygen therapy

● Percutaneous coronary intervention

● Semi-Fowler's position

Drug therapy options

● Anticoagulant: heparin

● Aspirin

● Beta-adrenergic blocker: atenolol (Tenormin), metoprolol (Lopressor), nadolol (Corgard), propranolol (Inderal)

● Calcium channel blocker: diltiazem (Cardizem), nicardipine (Cardene), nifedipine (Procardia), verapamil (Calan)

● Nitrate: isosorbide dinitrate (Isordil), nitroglycerin (Nitrostat), topical nitroglycerin (Nitrol), transdermal nitroglycerin (Transderm-Nitro)

Patient care goals

● The client will reduce cardiovascular events by modifying risk factors.

● The client will increase activity tolerance through appropriate treatment.

● The client will decrease anxiety by increasing his knowledge of cardiovascular status and decreasing the number of episodes of ischemic pain.

Nursing interventions

● Assess cardiovascular status, hemodynamic variables, and vital signs *to detect evidence of cardiac compromise and response to treatment.*
● Monitor and record intake and output *to monitor fluid status.*
● Administer medications, as prescribed, *to increase oxygenation and to reduce cardiac workload.* If systolic blood pressure is less than 90 mm Hg, hold the nitrate and beta-adrenergic blocker and notify the physician. If heart rate is less than 60 beats/minute, hold the beta-adrenergic blocker and notify the physician *to prevent complications that can occur as a result of therapy.*
● Assess the client for chest pain, and evaluate its characteristics. *Assessment allows for the care plan to be modified as necessary.*
● Advise the client to rest if pain begins *to reduce cardiac workload.*
● Obtain a 12-lead ECG during an acute attack *to check for ischemic changes.* (See *Obtaining an ECG.*)
● Keep the client in semi-Fowler's position *to promote chest expansion and ventilation.*
● Maintain the client's prescribed diet (low fat, low cholesterol and, if necessary, low calorie) *to reduce the risk of CAD.*
● Encourage weight reduction and smoking cessation, if necessary, *to reduce the risk of CAD.*
● Encourage the client to express anxiety, fears, or concerns *because anxiety can increase oxygen demands.*
● Administer oxygen *to increase oxygen supply during anginal attack.*

Evaluation

● The client describes appropriate lifestyle changes to help prevent anginal episodes.
● The client understands and complies with the prescribed treatment plan.
● The client has fewer anginal episodes.
● The client demonstrates increased activity tolerance.

Aortic aneurysm, abdominal

An ABDOMINAL AORTIC ANEURYSM results from damage to the medial layer of the abdominal portion of the aorta. Aneurysm commonly results from atherosclerosis which, over time, causes weakening in the medial layer of the artery. Continued weakening from the force of blood flow results in outpouching of the artery and formation of the aneurysm. The aneurysm may then rupture, leading to hemorrhage, hypovolemic shock, and even death.

An abdominal aneurysm can be one of four types:
● dissecting (the vessel wall ruptures, and a blood clot is retained in an outpouching of tissue)
● false (bilateral outpouching in which layers of the vessel wall separate from creating a cavity)
● fusiform (bilateral outpouching)
● saccular (unilateral outpouching).

Possible causes

● Atherosclerosis
● Congenital defect
● Hypertension
● Infection
● Marfan syndrome
● Syphilis
● Trauma

Data collection findings

● Commonly asymptomatic
● Diminished femoral pulses
● Lower abdominal pain and lower back pain
● Systolic blood pressure in the legs lower than that in the arms
● Abdominal pulsations
● Abdominal mass to the left of the midline
● Bruits over the site of the aneurysm
● Severe back or abdominal pain with hypotension (indicates rupture)

Diagnostic findings

● Abdominal computed tomography (CT) scan shows aneurysm.
● Abdominal ultrasound shows aneurysm.
● Arteriography shows aneurysm.
● ECG differentiates an aneurysm from MI.

Nursing diagnoses

● Ineffective tissue perfusion (peripheral)
● Acute pain
● Death anxiety
● Risk for deficient fluid volume

Treatment

● Abdominal aortic aneurysm resection
● Bed rest

Drug therapy options
- Analgesic: oxycodone (OxyContin)
- Antihypertensive: hydralazine (Apresoline), nitroprusside (Nitropress), nitroglycerin
- Beta-adrenergic blocker: propranolol (Inderal), metoprolol (Lopressor)

Patient care goals
- The client will be hemodynamically stable.
- The client will have pain relief.
- The client will maintain adequate peripheral tissue perfusion.

Nursing interventions
- Assess cardiovascular status, and monitor and record vital signs. *Tachycardia, dyspnea, or hypotension may indicate fluid volume deficit caused by rupture of the aneurysm.*
- Monitor intake and output and the results of laboratory studies. *Low urine output and high specific gravity indicate hypovolemia.*
- Observe the client for signs and symptoms of hypovolemic shock from aneurysm rupture, such as anxiety, restlessness, severe back pain, decreased pulse pressure, increased thready pulse, and pale, cool, moist, clammy skin.
- Gently palpate the abdomen to check for distention. *Increasing distention may signify impending rupture.*
- Check peripheral circulation — including pulses, temperature, color, and any sites where the client is experiencing abnormal sensations — *to detect poor arterial blood flow.*
- Assess pain *to detect enlarging aneurysm or rupture.*
- Administer medications, as prescribed, *to reduce hypertension and control pain.*
- Encourage the client to express his feelings, such as a fear of dying, *to reduce anxiety.*
- Maintain a quiet environment *to control blood pressure and reduce the risk of rupture.*

Evaluation
- The client maintains stable vital signs and doesn't exhibit signs of bleeding.
- The client verbalizes pain relief.
- The client verbalizes decreased fear after treatment.
- The client has palpable peripheral pulses.

SPOT CHECK

A client comes into the emergency department with a dissecting aortic aneurysm. Is he at greatest risk for septic shock, anaphylactic shock, cardiogenic shock, or hypovolemic shock?

Answer: A dissecting aortic aneurysm is a precursor to aortic rupture, which leads to hemorrhage and hypovolemic shock.

Aortic aneurysm, thoracic

THORACIC AORTIC ANEURYSM is characterized by an abnormal widening of the ascending, transverse, or descending part of the aorta. Aneurysm of the ascending aorta is most common and most commonly fatal.

The aneurysm may be *dissecting,* a hemorrhagic separation in the aortic wall, usually within the medial layer; *saccular,* an outpouching of the arterial wall, with a narrow neck; or *fusiform,* a spindle-shaped enlargement encompassing the entire circumference of the aorta.

Some aneurysms progress to serious and eventually lethal complications, such as rupture of an untreated thoracic dissecting aneurysm into the pericardium, with resulting tamponade.

Possible causes
- Atherosclerosis
- Congenital disorders such as coarctation of the aorta
- Fungal infection (infected aneurysm) of the aortic arch and descending segments
- Hypertension
- Syphilis, usually of the ascending aorta (uncommon because of antibiotics)
- Trauma, usually of the descending thoracic aorta, from an accident that shears the aorta transversely (acceleration-deceleration injuries)

Data collection findings
Ascending aneurysm
- Pain (described as severe, boring, and ripping and extending to the neck, shoulders, lower back, or abdomen)
- Unequal intensities of the right carotid and left radial pulses
- Bradycardia
- Pericardial friction rub caused by a hemopericardium

Descending aneurysm
- Pain (described as sharp and tearing, usually starting suddenly between the shoulder blades and possibly radiating to the chest)

Transverse aneurysm
- Pain (described as sharp and tearing and radiating to the shoulders)
- Dyspnea
- Dry cough
- Dysphagia
- Hoarseness

Diagnostic findings
- Aortography, the definitive test, shows the lumen of the aneurysm, its size and location, and the false lumen in a dissecting aneurysm.
- Blood chemistry test results may show low hemoglobin (Hb) level because of blood loss from a leaking aneurysm.
- Chest X-ray shows widening of the aorta.
- CT scan can be used to confirm and locate the aneurysm and may be used to monitor its progression.
- Echocardiography may be used to identify a dissecting aneurysm of the aortic root.
- ECG is used to distinguish a thoracic aneurysm from an MI.
- Transesophageal echocardiography can be used to detect and measure the aneurysm in the ascending or descending aorta.

Nursing diagnoses
- Acute pain
- Anxiety
- Decreased cardiac output

Treatment
- Surgery (resection of aneurysm through a Dacron or Teflon graft replacement and, possibly, replacement of the aortic valve)

Drug therapy options
- Analgesic
- Antihypertensive: nitroprusside (Nitropress)
- Negative inotropic: propranolol (Inderal), metoprolol (Lopressor)

Patient care goals
- The client will remain hemodynamically stable.
- The client will have pain relief.
- The client will verbalize understanding of the illness and its treatment.

Nursing interventions
- Monitor the client's blood pressure *to detect fluid volume deficit*. Also, maintain safety of lines and devices for pulmonary artery wedge pressure (PAWP) and central venous pressure (CVP).
- Evaluate pain, breathing, and carotid, radial, and femoral pulses *to detect early signs of aneurysm rupture.*
- Review laboratory test results, which must include a complete blood count (CBC) with differential, electrolyte levels, typing and crossmatching for whole blood, arterial blood gas (ABG) analysis, and urinalysis, *to note Hb levels and ensure that the client can tolerate surgery.*
- Insert an indwelling urinary catheter *to closely monitor urine output.*
- Maintain an I.V. line for administration of dextrose 5% in water or lactated Ringer's solution and an antibiotic, if needed.
- Assist with monitoring blood pressure every 5 minutes until it stabilizes *to note the effectiveness of treatment and to prevent hypotension caused by a large dose of nitroprusside.*
- With suspected bleeding from an aneurysm, maintain the safety of the I.V. line for whole-blood transfusion *to adequately replace fluid volume deficit.*
- Explain diagnostic tests. If surgery is scheduled, explain the procedure and expected postoperative care (I.V. lines, endotracheal [ET] and drainage tubes, cardiac monitoring, ventilation) *to alleviate the client's anxiety.*

After thoracic aneurysm repair
- Evaluate the client's level of consciousness (LOC). Monitor vital signs, pulse rate, urine output, and pain, and maintain safety of devices for monitoring of pulmonary artery pressure (PAP), PAWP, and CVP *to guide the treatment regimen and evaluate its effectiveness.*
- Carefully observe respiratory function, record the type and amount of chest tube drainage, and frequently assess heart and breath sounds *to detect early signs of compromise.*
- Monitor I.V. therapy *to prevent fluid excess, which may occur with rapid fluid replacement.*
- Give medications as appropriate *to improve the client's condition.*
- Watch for signs of infection, especially fever, and excessive wound drainage *to initiate treatment promptly and prevent complications such as sepsis.*
- Assist with range-of-motion (ROM) exercises of legs *to prevent thromboembolism due to venostasis during prolonged bed rest.*
- After the client's vital signs and respiration have stabilized, encourage him to turn, cough, and deep-breathe; assist, if needed. If necessary, provide intermittent positive pressure breathing *to promote lung expansion.*

- Help the client walk as soon as he's able *to prevent complications of immobility, such as pneumonia and thromboembolism formation.*
- Before discharge, ensure adherence to antihypertensive therapy by explaining the need for such drugs and the expected adverse reactions. Teach the client how to monitor his blood pressure *to prevent complications associated with ineffective blood pressure management such as stroke.*
- Throughout hospitalization, offer the client and family members psychological support *to relieve anxiety and feelings of helplessness.*

Evaluation
- The client has stable vital signs.
- The client verbalizes pain relief.
- The client cooperates with the treatment regimen and states understanding of the illness.

Arrhythmias
With cardiac ARRHYTHMIAS, abnormal electrical conduction or automaticity changes heart rate and rhythm. Arrhythmias vary in severity, from mild and asymptomatic ones that require no treatment (such as sinus arrhythmia, in which heart rate increases and decreases with respirations) to catastrophic ventricular fibrillation (VF), which necessitates immediate resuscitation.

Arrhythmias are generally classified according to origin (atrial or ventricular). The effect on cardiac output and blood pressure, partially influenced by the site of origin, determines the clinical significance. The most common arrhythmias include atrial fibrillation (AF), asystole, VF, and ventricular tachycardia (VT).

Possible causes
- Congenital
- Degeneration of conductive tissue
- Drug toxicity
- Electrolyte imbalance
- Heart disease
- MI
- Myocardial ischemia

Data collection findings
AF
- Complaints of feeling faint
- Irregular pulse with no pattern to the irregularity
- Palpitations
- Possibly asymptomatic

Asystole
- No pulse
- No palpable blood pressure
- Apnea
- Cyanosis

VF
- No pulse
- No palpable blood pressure
- Apnea

VT
- Chest pain
- Diaphoresis
- Dizziness
- Hypotension
- Possible loss of consciousness
- Weak pulse

Diagnostic findings
AF
- ECG shows irregular atrial rhythm, atrial rate greater than 400 beats/minute, irregular ventricular rhythm, QRS complexes of uniform configuration and duration, indiscernible PR interval, and no P waves or P waves that appear as erratic, irregular baseline fibrillation waves.

Asystole
- ECG shows no atrial or ventricular rate or rhythm and no discernible P waves, QRS complexes, or T waves.

VF
- ECG shows rapid and chaotic ventricular rhythm, wide and irregular QRS complexes, and no visible P waves.

VT
- ECG shows ventricular rate 140 to 220 beats/minute, wide and bizarre QRS complexes, and no discernible P waves. VT may start or stop suddenly.

Nursing diagnoses
- Decreased cardiac output
- Ineffective tissue perfusion (cardiopulmonary)
- Impaired gas exchange

Treatment
AF
- Radiofrequency catheter ablation
- Synchronized cardioversion

Asystole

- Advanced cardiac life support (ACLS) protocol for endotracheal intubation and possible transcutaneous pacing
- Cardiopulmonary resuscitation (CPR)

VF

- ACLS protocol for endotracheal intubation
- CPR
- Defibrillation
- Implantable cardioverter-defibrillator

VT

- ACLS protocol for endotracheal intubation, if pulseless
- CPR, if pulseless
- Implantable cardioverter-defibrillator
- Synchronized cardioversion, if symptomatic

Drug therapy options
AF

- Antiarrhythmic (if client's condition is stable): amiodarone (Cordarone), digoxin (Lanoxin), diltiazem (Cardizem), procainamide (Pronestyl), verapamil (Calan)

Asystole

- Antiarrhythmic: atropine or epinephrine (Adrenalin) per ACLS protocol

VF

- Antiarrhythmic: amiodarone, epinephrine, lidocaine (Xylocaine), magnesium sulfate, procainamide, vasopressin (Pitressin) per ACLS protocol

VT

- Antiarrhythmic: amiodarone, epinephrine, lidocaine, magnesium sulfate, procainamide, or vasopressin per ACLS protocol if pulseless
- Antiarrhythmic: amiodarone, lidocaine, procainamide, or sotalol (Betapace) per ACLS protocol if stable monomorphic VT with normal cardiac function
- Antiarrhythmic: amiodarone or lidocaine per ACLS protocol if stable monomorphic VT with poor ejection fraction
- Antiarrhythmic: beta-adrenergic blockers, lidocaine, amiodarone, procainamide, or sotalol per ACLS protocol if polymorphic VT with normal baseline QT interval
- Antiarrhythmic: isoproterenol (Isuprel), lidocaine, magnesium, or phenytoin (Dilantin) per ACLS protocol if polymorphic VT with prolonged baseline QT interval

Patient care goals

- The client will have improved cardiac circulation.

- The client will have adequate cardiac output.
- The client will have adequate oxygenation.

Nursing interventions

- Assess an unmonitored client for rhythm disturbances *to promptly identify and treat life-threatening arrhythmias.*
- If the client's pulse is abnormally rapid, slow, or irregular, watch for signs of hypoperfusion, such as hypotension and diminished urine output, *to prevent such complications as renal failure and cerebral anoxia.*
- Document any arrhythmias in a monitored client *to create a record of their occurrence.* Assess the client for possible causes and effects *so that proper treatment can be instituted.*
- When life-threatening arrhythmias develop, rapidly assess LOC, respirations, and pulse *to avoid crises.*
- Initiate CPR, if indicated, *to maintain cerebral perfusion until other ACLS measures are successful.*
- Evaluate the client for altered cardiac output resulting from arrhythmias. *Decreased cardiac output may cause inadequate perfusion of major organs, leading to irreversible damage.*
- If trained, perform defibrillation early for VT and VF. *Studies show that early intervention with defibrillation improves the client's chance of survival.*
- Prepare the client for medication administration, as needed, and for medical procedures (for example, cardioversion) if indicated *to ensure prompt treatment of life-threatening arrhythmias.*
- Monitor the client for predisposing factors — such as fluid and electrolyte imbalance — and for signs of toxic reaction to his drug therapy, especially if he's taking digoxin. If he has such a reaction, his next dose may need to be withheld. *Alleviating predisposing factors decreases the risk of arrhythmias.*
- Provide adequate oxygen and reduce the heart's workload, while carefully maintaining metabolic, neurologic, respiratory, and hemodynamic status, *to prevent arrhythmias in a cardiac client.*
- Restrict the client's activity after permanent pacemaker insertion. Monitor the pulse rate regularly, and watch for signs of decreased cardiac output. *These measures avert permanent pacemaker malfunction.*
- If the client has a permanent pacemaker, warn him about environmental hazards, as indicated by the pacemaker manufacturer, *to avoid pacemaker malfunction.*

Evaluation

- The client has stable vital signs and a controlled cardiac rhythm.
- The client maintains optimal oxygenation.

Arterial occlusive disease

With ARTERIAL OCCLUSIVE DISEASE, the obstruction or narrowing of the lumen of the aorta and its major branches causes an interruption of blood flow, usually to the legs and feet. Arterial occlusive disease may affect the carotid, vertebral, innominate, subclavian, mesenteric, and celiac arteries. Occlusions may be acute or chronic and commonly cause severe ischemia, skin ulceration, and gangrene.

Arterial occlusive disease is more common in males than in females. The prognosis depends on the location of the occlusion, the development of collateral circulation to counteract reduced blood flow and, in acute disease, the time elapsed between occlusion and its removal.

Possible causes
- Atherosclerosis
- Emboli formation
- Thrombosis
- Trauma or fracture

Risk factors
- Age
- Diabetes
- Family history of vascular disorders, an MI, or stroke
- Hyperlipemia
- Hypertension
- Smoking

Data collection findings
Femoral, popliteal, or innominate arteries
- Mottling of the extremity
- Pallor
- Paralysis and paresthesia in the affected arm or leg
- Pulselessness distal to the occlusion
- Sudden and localized pain in the affected arm or leg (most common symptom)
- Temperature change that occurs distal to the occlusion

Internal and external carotid arteries
- Diminished pulses with an auscultatory bruit over affected vessels
- Transient ischemic attacks (TIAs), which produce transient monocular blindness, dysarthria, hemiparesis, possible aphasia, confusion, decreased mentation, and headache
- Stroke

Subclavian artery
- Subclavian steal syndrome (characterized by the backflow of blood from the brain through the vertebral artery on the same side as the occlusion into the subclavian artery distal to the occlusion; clinical effects of vertebrobasilar occlusion and exercise-induced arm claudication)

Vertebral and basilar arteries
- TIAs, which produce binocular vision disturbances, vertigo, dysarthria, and falling down without loss of consciousness

Diagnostic findings
- Arteriography shows collateral circulation and the type (thrombus or embolus), location, and degree of obstruction.
- Doppler ultrasonography shows decreased blood flow distal to the occlusion.
- EEG and a CT scan may be necessary to rule out brain lesions.
- Ophthalmodynamometry helps to determine the degree of obstruction in the internal carotid artery by comparing ophthalmic artery pressure to brachial artery pressure on the affected side. A more- than-20% difference between pressures suggests insufficiency.

Nursing diagnoses
- Ineffective tissue perfusion (type depends on the location of the occlusion)
- Acute pain
- Fear

Treatment
- Exercise such as walking
- Smoking cessation
- Surgery (for acute arterial occlusive disease), including atherectomy, balloon angioplasty, bypass graft, embolectomy, laser angioplasty, patch grafting, stent placement, thromboendarterectomy, or amputation

Drug therapy options
- Anticoagulant: heparin, warfarin (Coumadin)
- Antiplatelet drug: aspirin, pentoxifylline (Trental), cilostazol (Pletal)
- Thrombolytic: alteplase (Activase), streptokinase (Streptase), urokinase (Abbokinase)

Patient care goals
- The client will have increased perfusion to the affected area.

- The client will report decreased pain in the affected area.
- The client will verbalize less fear regarding occlusion and treatment.

Nursing interventions

- Advise the client to stop smoking and to follow the prescribed medical regimen *to modify risk factors and promote adherence.*

Preoperative (during an acute episode)

- Check for the most distal pulses and inspect skin color and temperature *to assess the client's circulatory status.* Decreased tissue perfusion causes mottling; skin also becomes cooler, and skin texture changes.
- Provide pain relief as needed *to help decrease ischemic pain.*
- Prepare the client for administration of heparin by continuous I.V. drip as needed to prevent thrombi. Use an infusion monitor or pump *to ensure the proper flow rate.*
- Wrap the client's affected foot in soft cotton batting and reposition it frequently *to prevent pressure on any one area.* Strictly avoid elevating or applying heat to the affected leg. *Directly heating extremities causes increased tissue metabolism; if arteries don't dilate normally, tissue perfusion decreases and ischemia may occur.*
- Watch for signs of fluid and electrolyte imbalance, and monitor intake and output for signs of renal failure (urine output less than 30 ml/hour). *Electrolyte imbalances and renal failure are complications that may occur as a result of arterial occlusion and tissue damage.*
- If the client has a carotid, innominate, vertebral, or subclavian artery occlusion, monitor him for signs of CVA, such as numbness in an arm or a leg and intermittent blindness, *to detect early signs of decreased cerebral perfusion.*

Postoperative

- Monitor the client's vital signs *to assess for changes in his condition.* Continuously assess circulatory function by inspecting skin color and temperature and by checking for distal pulses. In charting, compare earlier assessments and observations. Watch closely for signs of hemorrhage (such as tachycardia and hypotension) and check dressings for excessive bleeding *to prevent or detect postoperative complications.*
- If the client has a carotid, innominate, vertebral, or subclavian artery occlusion, assess neurologic status frequently for changes in LOC, muscle strength, and pupil size *to ensure prompt treatment of deteriorating neurologic status.*
- If the client has mesenteric artery occlusion, connect a nasogastric tube (NG) to low intermittent suction. Monitor

intake and output. *(Low urine output may indicate damage to renal arteries during surgery.)* Assess abdominal status. *Increasing abdominal distention and tenderness may indicate extension of bowel ischemia with resulting gangrene, necessitating further excision, or peritonitis.*
- If the client has saddle block occlusion, check distal pulses *to assess for adequate circulation.* Watch for signs of renal failure and mesenteric artery occlusion (such as severe abdominal pain) and cardiac arrhythmias, which may precipitate embolus formation, *to ensure prompt recognition and treatment of complications.*
- If the client has iliac artery occlusion, monitor urine output *to assess for signs of renal failure from decreased perfusion to the kidneys as a result of surgery.* Provide meticulous catheter care *to prevent complications.*
- If the client has femoral or popliteal artery occlusion, assist with early ambulation and discourage prolonged sitting *to encourage circulation to the extremities.*
- After amputation, check the client's stump carefully for drainage and record its color and amount and the time *to detect hemorrhage.* Elevate the stump and administer analgesics *to treat edema and pain.* Because phantom limb pain is common, explain this phenomenon to the client *to reduce his anxiety.*
- When preparing the client for discharge, instruct him to watch for signs of recurrence (pain, pallor, numbness, paralysis, absence of pulse) that can result from graft occlusion or occlusion at another site. Warn him against wearing constrictive clothing. *These measures enable the client to participate in his care and allow him to make more informed decisions about his health status.*

Evaluation

- The client discusses lifestyle adjustments to reduce the risk of occlusion.
- The client expresses a decreased level of pain.
- The client demonstrates decreased fear after being treated for occlusion.

 QUICK STUDY

Remember the signs and symptoms of acute occlusion by the six P's.

1. Pain
2. Pallor
3. Paralysis
4. Paresthesia
5. Polar (coldness)
6. Pulselessness

Cardiac tamponade

In CARDIAC TAMPONADE, a rapid, unchecked rise in intrapericardial pressure impairs diastolic filling of the heart. The rise in pressure usually results from blood or fluid accumulation in the pericardial sac.

If fluid rapidly accumulates, this condition is commonly fatal and necessitates emergency lifesaving measures. (See *Caring for the client with cardiac tamponade.*) Slow accumulation and rise in pressure, as in pericardial effusion associated with cancer, may not produce immediate symptoms because the fibrous wall of the pericardial sac can gradually stretch to accommodate as much as 1 to 2 L (1 to 2 qt) of fluid.

Possible causes

- Dressler's syndrome
- Effusion (in cancer, bacterial infections, tuberculosis [TB] and, rarely, acute rheumatic fever)
- Hemorrhage from nontraumatic causes (such as rupture of the heart or great vessels or anticoagulant therapy in a client with pericarditis)
- Hemorrhage from trauma (such as gunshot or stab wounds of the chest and perforation by a catheter during cardiac or central venous catheterization or after cardiac surgery)
- MI
- Uremia

Data collection findings

- Anxiety
- Diaphoresis
- Dyspnea
- Reduced arterial blood pressure
- Restlessness
- Tachycardia
- Muffled heart sounds on auscultation
- Narrow pulse pressure
- Neck vein distention
- Pallor or cyanosis
- Hepatomegaly
- Increased venous pressure
- Pulsus paradoxus (an abnormal inspiratory drop in systemic blood pressure greater than 15 mm Hg)
- Upright, leaning forward posture

Diagnostic findings

- Chest X-ray shows a slightly widened mediastinum and cardiomegaly.
- Echocardiography records pericardial effusion with collapse of the cardiac chambers during diastole.

- ECG may reveal changes produced by acute pericarditis. This test is useful to rule out other cardiac disorders.
- Pulmonary artery catheterization detects increased right atrial pressure, right ventricular diastolic pressure, and CVP.

Nursing diagnoses

- Decreased cardiac output
- Ineffective tissue perfusion (cardiopulmonary)
- Anxiety

Treatment

- Pericardiocentesis (needle aspiration of the pericardial cavity), surgical creation of an opening to drain fluid, or thoracotomy

Drug therapy options

- Heparin antagonist: protamine sulfate in heparin-induced tamponade
- Inotropic agent: dopamine (Intropin), isoproterenol (Isuprel)
- Vitamin: vitamin K (AquaMEPHYTON) in warfarin-induced cardiac tamponade

Patient care goals

- The client will maintain hemodynamic stability.
- The client will have adequate tissue perfusion.
- The client will have decreased anxiety after appropriate treatment.

Nursing interventions
If the client needs pericardiocentesis

- Explain the procedure to the client *to alleviate anxiety.*
- Keep a pericardial aspiration needle attached to a 50-ml syringe by a three-way stopcock, an ECG machine, and an emergency cart with a defibrillator at the bedside. Make sure the equipment is turned on and ready for immediate use *to avoid treatment delay.*
- Position the client at a 45- to 60-degree angle. Connect the precordial ECG lead to the hub of the aspiration needle with an alligator clamp and connecting wire. When the needle touches the myocardium during fluid aspiration, an ST-segment elevation or premature ventricular contractions will be seen. *Monitoring the client's ECG ensures the accuracy of the procedure and helps prevent complications*
- Monitor blood pressure during and after pericardiocentesis to monitor for complications, such as hypotension, *which may indicate cardiac chamber puncture.*

CLINICAL SITUATION

Caring for the client with cardiac tamponade

A 40-year-old male client is admitted to the telemetry unit after being involved in a motor vehicle accident during which he forcefully struck the steering wheel. Slight bruising is evident over the sternal area. On admission, the client's electrocardiogram (ECG) is normal and he denies chest discomfort. Six hours after admission, the client suddenly complains of chest discomfort and difficulty breathing. He's diaphoretic and anxious.

What emergency measures should be instituted?
A. Notify the physician, administer oxygen, assess vital signs, obtain an ECG, and have an emergency cart nearby containing a pericardiocentesis needle.
B. Assess vital signs, obtain an ECG, and administer nitroglycerin and morphine.
C. Notify the family, make the client comfortable, and administer a sedative.
D. Notify the physician, obtain blood work, administer oxygen, and obtain an ECG.
Answer: A. Trauma to the chest can result in cardiac tamponade. Because this is a life-threatening situation, notify the physician immediately, administer oxygen to improve cardiac perfusion, assess vital signs to evaluate hemodynamic status, obtain an ECG to detect arrhythmias or ischemia, and have emergency equipment available in case the client's condition deteriorates and pericardiocentesis becomes necessary.

Questions for further thought
● What further measures, other than pericardiocentesis, could be taken to relieve cardiac tamponade?
● What nursing diagnoses apply to the client complaining of chest discomfort and exhibiting signs of anxiety?

● Maintain the I.V. infusion *to maintain blood pressure.* Watch for a rise in blood pressure, *which indicates relief of cardiac compression.*
● Watch for complications of pericardiocentesis, such as VF, vasovagal response, and coronary artery or cardiac chamber puncture, *to prevent crisis.*
● Closely monitor ECG changes, blood pressure, pulse rate, LOC, and urinary output *to detect signs of decreased cardiac output.*

If the client needs thoracotomy
● Explain the procedure to him. Tell him what to expect postoperatively (chest tubes, drainage bottles, administration of oxygen). Teach him how to turn, deep-breathe, and cough *to prevent postoperative complications and to relieve the client's anxiety.*
● Prepare the client for administration of antibiotics *to prevent or treat infection* and protamine sulfate or vitamin K as needed *to prevent hemorrhage.*
● Postoperatively, monitor critical parameters, such as vital signs and ABG levels, and assess heart and breath sounds *to detect early signs of complications such as reaccumulation of fluid.*
● Give pain medication as needed *to alleviate pain and promote comfort.*
● Maintain the chest drainage system and be alert for complications, such as hemorrhage and arrhythmias, *to prevent further decompensation.*

Evaluation
● The client has stable vital signs and adequate oxygenation.
● The client verbalizes an understanding of his condition and its treatment.

Cardiomyopathy

In CARDIOMYOPATHY, the myocardium (middle muscular layer) around the left ventricle becomes flabby, altering cardiac function and resulting in decreased cardiac output. Increased heart rate and increased muscle mass compensate in early stages; in later stages, however, heart failure develops.

The three types of cardiomyopathy are:
● dilated (congestive) — the most common form, in which dilated heart chambers contract poorly, causing blood to pool and reducing cardiac output
● hypertrophic (obstructive) — in which a hypertrophied left ventricle can't relax and fill properly
● restrictive (obliterative) — a rare form, characterized by stiff ventricles resistant to ventricular filling.

Possible causes
Dilated cardiomyopathy
● Chronic alcoholism
● Infection
● Metabolic and immunologic disorders
● Pregnancy and postpartum disorders

Hypertrophic cardiomyopathy
- Congenital
- Chronic hypertension

Restrictive cardiomyopathy
- Amyloidosis
- Cancer and other infiltrative diseases
- Postradiation treatment
- Diabetes mellitus

Data collection findings
- Chest pain
- Cough
- Crackles on lung auscultation
- Enlarged heart
- Dependent pitting edema
- Dyspnea; paroxysmal nocturnal dyspnea
- Enlarged liver
- Fatigue
- Jugular vein distention
- Murmur; third (S_3) or fourth (S_4) heart sounds
- Syncope

Diagnostic findings
- Cardiac catheterization excludes the diagnosis of CAD.
- Chest X-ray shows cardiomegaly and pulmonary congestion.
- ECG findings indicate left ventricular hypertrophy, nonspecific changes, or low voltage.
- Echocardiogram shows decreased myocardial function and enlarged chamber sizes.

Nursing diagnoses
- Decreased cardiac output
- Impaired gas exchange
- Activity intolerance

Treatment
- Dietary changes: establishing a low-sodium diet with vitamin supplements
- Dual-chamber pacing (for hypertrophic cardiomyopathy)
- Surgery (when medication fails): heart transplantation or cardiomyoplasty (for dilated cardiomyopathy); ventricular myotomy (for hypertrophic cardiomyopathy)

Drug therapy options
- Beta-adrenergic blocker: propranolol (Inderal), nadolol (Corgard), metoprolol (Lopressor) for hypertrophic cardiomyopathy
- Calcium channel blocker: particularly, verapamil (Calan) and diltiazem (Cardizem) for hypertrophic cardiomyopathy
- Diuretic: furosemide (Lasix), bumetanide (Bumex), metolazone (Zaroxolyn) for dilated cardiomyopathy
- Inotropic drug: dobutamine (Dobutrex), milrinone (Primacor), digoxin (Lanoxin) for dilated cardiomyopathy
- Oral anticoagulant: warfarin (Coumadin) for dilated cardiomyopathy

Patient care goals
- The client will remain hemodynamically stable.
- The client will have adequate oxygenation.
- The client will have increased activity tolerance.

Nursing interventions
- Monitor the client's heart beat for irregularity.
- Monitor laboratory results *to detect abnormalities, such as hypokalemia, from the use of diuretics.*
- Monitor respiratory status *to detect evidence of heart failure, such as dyspnea and crackles.*
- Assess cardiovascular status, vital signs, and hemodynamic variables *to detect heart failure.*
- Monitor and record intake and output *to detect fluid volume overload.*
- Keep the client in semi-Fowler's position *to enhance gas exchange.*
- Maintain bed rest *to reduce oxygen demands on the heart.*
- Administer oxygen and medications, as prescribed, *to improve oxygenation and cardiac output.*
- Maintain the client's prescribed diet. *A low-sodium diet reduces fluid retention.*

Evaluation
- The client has stable vital signs.
- The client has stable respiratory status.
- The client has safely increased his activity level.

Coronary artery disease
CORONARY ARTERY DISEASE (CAD) results from the buildup of atherosclerotic plaque in the arteries of the heart. This causes a narrowing of the arterial lumen and reduces blood flow to the myocardium.

Possible causes
- Arteriosclerosis
- Atherosclerosis

Risk factors

- Aging
- Depletion of estrogen after menopause
- Diabetes
- Genetics
- High-fat, high-cholesterol diet
- Hyperlipidemia
- Hypertension
- Obesity
- Sedentary lifestyle
- Smoking
- Stress

Data collection findings

- Angina (substernal, compressing, or pressure) that may radiate to the arms, jaw, or back; usually lasts 3 to 5 minutes; and usually occurs after exertion, emotional excitement, or exposure to cold but can also develop at rest

Diagnostic findings

- Blood chemistry test results may show increased cholesterol levels; specifically, decreased HDL levels and increased LDL levels.
- Coronary arteriography shows narrowing of the coronary arteries.
- ECG or Holter monitoring shows ST-segment depression and T-wave inversion during anginal episode.
- Stress test reveals ST-segment changes and provokes chest discomfort.

Nursing diagnoses

- Acute pain
- Impaired gas exchange
- Activity intolerance

Treatment

- Activity changes, including weight loss (if necessary)
- Percutaneous coronary intervention, such as atherectomy, percutaneous transluminal coronary angioplasty, or coronary artery stent
- Coronary artery bypass surgery
- Low-cholesterol, low-fat and, if appropriate, low-calorie and low-sodium diet with more dietary fiber

Drug therapy options

- Analgesic: morphine sulfate (I.V.)
- Anticoagulant: heparin
- Antilipemic: atorvastatin (Lipitor), cerivastatin (Baycol), gemfibrozil (Lopid), lovastatin (Mevacor), nicotinic acid (Niaspan), pravastatin (Pravachol), simvastatin (Zocor)

- Aspirin
- Beta-adrenergic blocker: metoprolol (Lopressor), nadolol (Corgard), propranolol (Inderal)
- Calcium channel blocker: nifedipine (Procardia), diltiazem (Cardizem), verapamil (Calan)
- Nitrate: isosorbide dinitrate (Isordil), nitroglycerin (Nitro-Bid)

Patient care goals

- The client will demonstrate increased activity tolerance.
- The client will have adequate oxygenation.
- The client will report pain relief.

Nursing interventions

- Obtain an ECG during anginal episodes *to detect evidence of ischemia.*
- Monitor laboratory studies. Monitor cardiac enzyme levels *to rule out MI.*
- Assess cardiovascular status, vital signs, and hemodynamic variables *to detect evidence of compromise.*
- Monitor intake and output *to detect changes in fluid status.*
- Encourage the client to express anxiety, fears, or concerns *to help cope with illness.*
- Administer nitroglycerin sublingually *to provide pain relief from anginal episodes.*

Evaluation

- The client demonstrates increased activity tolerance.
- The client maintains stable respiratory status.
- The client remains free from pain.

Endocarditis, infective

INFECTIVE ENDOCARDITIS (IE) is a bacterial or fungal infection of the endocardium, the heart valves, or a cardiac prosthesis. This invasion produces vegetative growths on the heart valves, the endocardial lining of a heart chamber, or the endothelium of a blood vessel that may embolize to the spleen, kidneys, central nervous system (CNS), and lungs. This disorder is also called *endocarditis* or *bacterial endocarditis.*

In IE, fibrin and platelets aggregate on the valve tissue and engulf circulating bacteria or fungi that flourish and produce friable verrucous vegetations. Such vegetations may cover the valve surfaces, causing ulceration and necrosis; they may also extend to the chordae tendineae, leading to their rupture and subsequent valvular insufficiency.

Untreated IE is usually fatal but, with proper treatment, about 70% of clients recover. The prognosis is worse when IE causes severe valvular damage, leading to insufficiency and heart failure, or when it involves a prosthetic valve.

Possible causes
- Enterococci
- I.V. drug abuse
- Staphylococci (especially *Staphylococcus aureus*)
- Streptococci (especially *Streptococcus viridans*)

Risk factors
- Coarctation of the aorta
- Degenerative heart disease
- Marfan syndrome
- Patent ductus arteriosus
- Pulmonary stenosis
- Subaortic and valvular aortic stenosis
- Tetralogy of Fallot
- Ventricular septal defects

Data collection findings
- Intermittent, recurring fever
- Night sweats
- Malaise
- Arthralgia
- Chills
- Fatigue
- Weakness
- Anorexia
- Weight loss
- Petechiae
- Roth's spots
- Osler's nodes
- Janeway's lesions
- Signs of cerebral, pulmonary, renal, or splenic infarction
- Valvular insufficiency
- Heart murmur
- Sublingual splinter hemorrhage
- Splenomegaly

Diagnostic findings
- Blood chemistry test results may include normal or elevated white blood cell (WBC) count, abnormal histiocytes (macrophages), elevated erythrocyte sedimentation rate (ESR), normocytic normochromic anemia (in 70% to 90% of endocarditis cases), and positive serum rheumatoid factor (RF) (in about one-half of clients with endocarditis after the disease is present for 3 to 6 weeks).
- Echocardiography may reveal valvular damage.

- ECG may show AF and other arrhythmias that accompany valvular disease.
- Three blood cultures taken at 1-hour intervals enable identification of the causative organism in up to 90% of clients.

Nursing diagnoses
- Decreased cardiac output
- Activity intolerance
- Risk for injury

Treatment
- Bed rest
- Sufficient fluid intake
- Surgery (in cases of severe valvular damage) to replace the defective valve

Drug therapy options
- Antibiotic (infecting organism determines which drug is used)
- Aspirin

Patient care goals
- The client will have increased activity tolerance as the infection is resolved.
- The client will remain hemodynamically stable.
- The client will remain free from complications of IE.

Nursing interventions
- Before giving an antibiotic, obtain a client history of allergies *to prevent anaphylaxis.*
- Observe the client for signs of infiltration and inflammation, both possible complications of long-term I.V. drug administration, at the venipuncture site. Rotate venous access sites *to reduce the risk of these complications.*
- Watch for signs and symptoms of embolization (petechiae, hematuria, pleuritic chest pain, left upper quadrant pain, paresis), a common occurrence during the first 3 months of treatment. *These signs and symptoms may indicate impending peripheral vascular occlusion or splenic, renal, cerebral, or pulmonary infarction.*
- Monitor the client's renal status (blood urea nitrogen [BUN] levels, creatinine clearance, and urine output) *to check for signs of renal emboli or evidence of toxic reaction to the drug therapy.*
- Observe the client for signs of heart failure, such as dyspnea, tachypnea, tachycardia, crackles, neck vein distention, edema, and weight gain. *Detecting heart failure early ensures prompt intervention and treatment and decreases the risk of heart failure progressing to pulmonary edema.*

- Provide reassurance by teaching the client and family members about IE and the need for prolonged treatment. Tell them to watch closely for fever, anorexia, and other signs and symptoms of relapse about 2 weeks after treatment stops. Suggest quiet diversionary activities to prevent excessive physical exertion. *Having the client and family members involved in care gives them a feeling of control and promotes adherence with long-term therapy.*
- Make sure a susceptible client understands the need for prophylactic antibiotics before, during, and after dental work, childbirth, and genitourinary, GI, or gynecologic procedures *to prevent further episodes of endocarditis.*

Evaluation
- The client demonstrates increased activity tolerance.
- The client has stable vital signs.
- The client is free from infection and without complications.

Heart failure

HEART FAILURE occurs when the heart can't pump enough blood to meet the body's metabolic needs. It can occur on the left side or right side of the heart:
- Left-sided heart failure causes mostly pulmonary signs and symptoms, such as shortness of breath, dyspnea on exertion, and a moist cough.
- Right-sided heart failure causes systemic signs, such as edema and swelling, jugular vein distention, and hepatomegaly.

Possible causes
- Atherosclerosis
- Cardiac conduction defects
- Chronic obstructive pulmonary disease (COPD)
- Fluid overload
- Hypertension
- MI
- Pulmonary hypertension
- Valvular insufficiency
- Valvular stenosis

Data collection findings
Left-sided heart failure
- Dyspnea
- Crackles
- Orthopnea
- Paroxysmal nocturnal dyspnea
- Tachypnea
- Tachycardia

- Gallop rhythm, S_3 or S_4 heart sound
- Fatigue
- Anxiety
- Arrhythmias
- Cough

Right-sided heart failure
- Dependent edema
- Weight gain
- Fatigue
- Jugular vein distention
- Tachycardia
- Gallop rhythm, S_3 or S_4
- Nausea
- Anorexia
- Hepatomegaly
- Ascites

FAST FACT

Left-sided heart failure causes pulmonary symptoms. Right-sided heart failure causes systemic symptoms.

Diagnostic findings
Left-sided heart failure
- ABG levels indicate hypoxemia and hypercapnia.
- Blood chemistry test results reveal decreased potassium and sodium levels and increased BUN and creatinine levels.
- Chest X-ray shows increased pulmonary congestion and left ventricular hypertrophy.
- ECG may show left ventricular hypertrophy or acute ST-T wave changes.
- Echocardiography shows increased size of cardiac chambers and decreased wall motion.
- Hemodynamic monitoring reveals increased PAP and PAWP and decreased cardiac output.

Right-sided heart failure
- ABG levels indicate hypoxemia.
- Blood chemistry test results show decreased sodium and potassium levels and increased BUN and creatinine levels.
- Chest X-ray reveals pulmonary congestion, cardiomegaly, and pleural effusions.
- ECG may show left and right ventricular hypertrophy or acute ST-T wave changes.
- Echocardiogram shows increased size of chambers and decrease in wall motion.

● Hemodynamic monitoring shows increased right atrial pressure, CVP, and right ventricular pressure and decreased cardiac output.

Nursing diagnoses
● Excess fluid volume
● Activity intolerance
● Ineffective health maintenance

Treatment
● Low-sodium diet and limited intake of fluids
● Intra-aortic balloon pump (IABP)
● Oxygen therapy (possibly intubation and mechanical ventilation)
● Left ventricular assist device (for left-sided heart failure)
● Paracentesis (for right-sided heart failure)
● Thoracentesis (for right-sided heart failure)

Drug therapy options
● Analgesic: morphine sulfate (I.V.)
● Angiotensin-converting enzyme (ACE) inhibitor: captopril (Capoten), enalapril (Vasotec), lisinopril (Prinivil)
● Beta-adrenergic blocker: carvedilol (Coreg), metoprolol (Lopressor)
● Cardiac glycoside: digoxin (Lanoxin)
● Diuretic: bumetanide (Bumex), furosemide (Lasix), metolazone (Zaroxolyn), spironolactone (Aldactone)
● Inotropic agent: inamrinone (Inocor), dobutamine (Dobutrex), dopamine (Intropin)
● Nitrate: isosorbide dinitrate (Isordil), nitroglycerin (Nitro-Bid)
● Vasodilator: nitroprusside (Nitropress)

Patient care goals
● The client will understand how to cope with necessary lifestyle changes.
● The client won't develop preventable complications.
● The client will understand how to continue therapy at home.

Nursing interventions
● Assess cardiovascular status, vital signs, and hemodynamic variables *to detect signs of reduced cardiac output.*
● Assess respiratory status *to detect increasing fluid in the lungs and respiratory failure.*
● Keep the client in semi-Fowler's position *to increase chest expansion and improve ventilation.*
● Administer medications, as prescribed, *to enhance cardiac performance and reduce excess fluids.*

Low-salt diet

Many medical conditions, such as heart failure and high blood pressure, necessitate decreased salt intake. Reduced salt intake can also reduce the risk of high blood pressure. Include the following tips when instructing your client about a low-salt diet:
● Avoid salty foods.
● Look for sodium content on the labels of medicines and foods. Pay close attention to the amount of sodium per serving.
● Use reduced-sodium or no-salt-added products.
● Use herbs and spices instead of salt. Be aware that some seasonings, such as horseradish, and additives, such as monosodium glutamate, are high in sodium.
● Prepare food by baking, broiling, steaming, roasting, or poaching without salt. Order food prepared this way in restaurants. Skip gravies, soups, and salad dressings, unless low-salt varieties are available.
● Eat fresh fruits and vegetables. If canned foods must be used, get low-salt types and rinse them.
● Get permission before using a salt substitute. Many contain potassium or ammonium, which can cause harm if the client has kidney, liver, or heart disease.

● Administer oxygen *to enhance arterial oxygenation.*
● Measure and record intake and output. *Intake greater than output may indicate fluid retention.*
● Monitor laboratory test results *to detect electrolyte imbalances, renal failure, and impaired cardiac circulation.*
● Provide suctioning, if necessary, assist with turning, and encourage coughing and deep breathing *to prevent pulmonary complications.*
● Restrict oral fluids *to avoid worsening the client's condition.*
● Weigh the client daily *to detect fluid retention.* A weight gain of 2 lb (0.9 kg) in 1 day or 5 lb (2.3 kg) in 1 week indicates fluid gain.
● Measure and record the client's abdominal girth. *An increase in abdominal girth suggests worsening fluid retention and right-sided heart failure.*
● Make sure the client maintains a low-sodium diet *to reduce fluid accumulation.* (See *Low-salt diet.*)
● Encourage the client to express his feelings, such as a fear of dying, *to reduce anxiety.*

Evaluation
● The client accurately describes recommended dietary restrictions and medication regimens.
● The client hasn't experienced complications.

- The client verbalizes important signs and symptoms to report.

Hypertension

Persistent elevation of systolic or diastolic blood pressure (systolic pressure greater than 140 mm Hg, diastolic pressure greater than 90 mm Hg) indicates HYPERTENSION. Hypertension results from a narrowing of the arterioles, which increases peripheral resistance, necessitating increased force to circulate blood through the body.

There are two major types of hypertension:
- Essential hypertension, the most common type, has no known cause, but many factors play a role in its development.
- Secondary hypertension is caused by renal disease or other systemic disease.

Hypertension is classified according to three stages:
- stage 1 — systolic pressure 140 to 159 mm Hg, diastolic pressure 90 to 99 mm Hg
- stage 2 — systolic pressure 160 to 179 mm Hg, diastolic pressure 100 to 109 mm Hg
- stage 3 — systolic pressure greater than 180 mm Hg or diastolic pressure greater than 110 mm Hg.

Possible causes
- Coarctation of the aorta
- Cushing's disease
- Neurologic disorders
- No known cause (essential hypertension)
- Oral contraceptive use
- Pheochromocytoma
- Pregnancy
- Primary hyperaldosteronism
- Renovascular disease
- Thyroid, pituitary, or parathyroid disease
- Use of such drugs as cocaine, epoetin alfa, and cyclosporine

Risk factors
- Aging
- Atherosclerosis
- Diet (sodium and caffeine)
- Family history
- Obesity
- Race (incidence is higher in blacks)
- Sex (incidence is higher in males older than age 40)
- Smoking
- Stress

Data collection findings
- Asymptomatic
- Elevated blood pressure
- Dizziness
- Headache
- Left ventricular hypertrophy
- Heart failure
- Cerebral ischemia
- Renal failure
- Papilledema
- Vision disturbances, including blindness

Diagnostic findings
- Blood chemistry test results may show elevated sodium, BUN, creatinine, and cholesterol levels.
- Blood pressure measurements result in sustained readings higher than 140/90 mm Hg.
- Chest X-ray reveals cardiomegaly.
- ECG shows left ventricular hypertrophy.
- Echocardiogram may show left ventricular hypertrophy.
- Ophthalmoscopic examination shows retinal changes, such as severe arteriolar narrowing, papilledema, and hemorrhage.
- Urinalysis discloses proteinuria, red blood cells (RBCs), and WBCs.

Nursing diagnoses
- Ineffective health maintenance
- Imbalanced nutrition: More than body requirements

Treatment
- Regular exercise to reduce weight, if appropriate
- Low-sodium diet and limitation of alcohol intake (see *Stepped-care approach to antihypertensive therapy*)

Drug therapy options
- ACE inhibitor: captopril (Capoten), enalapril (Vasotec), lisinopril (Prinivil)
- Angiotensin receptor blocker: candesartan (Atacand), irbesartan (Avapro), losartan (Cozaar)
- Antihypertensive: doxazosin (Cardura), methyldopa (Aldomet), hydralazine (Apresoline), prazosin (Minipress)
- Beta-adrenergic blocker: carteolol (Cartrol), metoprolol (Lopressor), penbutolol (Levatol), propranolol (Inderal)
- Calcium channel blocker: diltiazem (Cardizem), nicardipine (Cardene), nifedipine (Procardia), verapamil (Calan)

Stepped-care approach to antihypertensive therapy

The diagram below illustrates the four-step approach to antihypertensive therapy that's recommended by the National Institutes of Health. The progression of therapy is based on the client's response, which is defined two ways: The client has achieved the target blood pressure set by the physician, or the client is making considerable progress toward this goal.

Step 1

Begin lifestyle modifications, including:
- weight reduction
- moderation of alcohol intake
- regular physical activity
- reduction of sodium intake
- smoking cessation.

If the client fails to achieve the desired blood pressure or make significant progress

Step 2

Continue lifestyle modifications and begin drug regimen, including:
- beta-adrenergic blocker or angiotensin-converting enzyme inhibitor (initially)
- diuretic , calcium antagonist, $alpha_1$-receptor-adrenergic antagonist, or mixed alpha- and beta-adrenergic antagonist (if initial drug regimen is ineffective or unacceptable).

If the client fails to achieve the desired blood pressure or make significant progress

Step 3

Increase drug dosage.
    OR
Substitute another drug in the same class.
    OR
Add a second antihypertensive from a different class.

If the client fails to achieve the desired blood pressure or make significant progress

Step 4

Add a second or third antihypertensive or a diuretic if not already prescribed. These agents may include direct-acting vasodilators, $alpha_1$-receptor antagonists, and peripherally acting adrenergic neuron antagonists.

Source: U.S. Department of Health and Human Services, National Institutes of Health. *Sixth Report of the Joint National Committee on Prevention, Detection, Evaluation, and Treatment of High Blood Pressure.* Washington, D.C.: Government Printing Office, 1997.

- Diuretic: bumetanide (Bumex), furosemide (Lasix), spironolactone (Aldactone), hydrochlorothiazide (HydroDIURIL)
- Vasodilator: nitroprusside (Nitropress)

Patient care goals

- The client will exhibit a reduction in blood pressure.
- The client will express understanding and acceptance of necessary lifestyle changes.

Nursing interventions

- Assess cardiovascular status, including vital signs, *to detect cardiac compromise.*
- Take an average of two or more blood pressure readings *to establish hypertension.*
- Check the client's blood pressure in lying, sitting, and standing positions *to determine whether orthostatic hypotension is present.* Also check for pallor, diaphoresis, and vertigo.
- Assess neurologic status, and observe the client for changes that may indicate an alteration in cerebral perfusion (stroke or hemorrhage).
- Monitor and record intake and output and daily weight *to detect fluid volume overload.*
- Administer medications as prescribed *to lower blood pressure.*
- Make sure the client maintains a low-sodium, low-cholesterol diet *to help minimize hypertension.*
- Encourage the client to express his feelings about daily stress *to reduce anxiety.*
- Maintain a quiet environment *to reduce stress.*

Evaluation

- The client maintains reduced blood pressure.
- The client expresses understanding of the need for a low-calorie, low-sodium diet.
- The client has made necessary lifestyle changes.
- The client describes the medication regimen.

Myocardial infarction

With MYOCARDIAL INFARCTION (MI), reduced blood flow in one of the coronary arteries leads to myocardial ischemia, injury, and necrosis. With a Q-wave MI, tissue damage extends through all myocardial layers. With a non-Q-wave MI, usually only the innermost layer is damaged.

Possible causes

- Coronary artery occlusion
- Coronary artery spasm

- Coronary artery stenosis

Risk factors

- Aging
- Decreased serum HDL levels
- Diabetes mellitus
- Drug use, specifically use of amphetamines or cocaine
- Elevated serum triglyceride, LDL, and cholesterol levels
- Excessive intake of saturated fats, carbohydrates, or salt
- Family history of CAD
- Hypertension
- Obesity
- Postmenopausal woman
- Sedentary lifestyle
- Smoking
- Stress

Data collection findings

- Crushing substernal chest pain that may radiate to the jaw, back, and arms; may wax and wane (angina is a crescendo pain); and is unrelieved by rest or nitroglycerin (may not be present in clients with silent MI)
- Dyspnea
- Diaphoresis
- Arrhythmias
- Tachycardia
- Anxiety
- Pallor
- Hypotension
- Nausea and vomiting
- Elevated temperature

Diagnostic findings

- ECG shows deep, widened Q wave, elevated or depressed ST segment, and T-wave inversion or cardiac arrhythmias.
- Blood chemistry test results show increased creatine kinase (CK), lactate dehydrogenase (LD), lipid, and troponin T levels; increased WBC count; positive CK-MB fraction; and flipped LD1 (LD1 levels exceed LD2 levels, the reversal of their normal patterns).

Nursing diagnoses

- Acute pain
- Anxiety
- Activity intolerance

Treatment

- Bed rest with bedside commode

Diet to lower cholesterol

A client can significantly reduce elevated cholesterol levels by following sound nutritional guidelines. As with any sensible diet, total caloric intake varies widely among individuals but shouldn't exceed the amount needed to achieve and maintain a desirable weight. Nutritionists generally recommend the following percentages of total caloric intake (with primary sources in parentheses):

- Carbohydrates (fruits, vegetables, legumes, whole grains), 50% to 60%
- Protein (dairy products, eggs, meats, fish), approximately 15%
- Fat (total fat intake should be less than 25% to 35%)
- Saturated fat (beef, bacon, cheese, coconut oil), less than 7%
- Polyunsaturated fat (corn, cottonseed, and safflower oils), up to 10%
- Monounsaturated fat (peanut, olive, and canola oils), up to 20%.

   The client with a high cholesterol level should limit fat intake to less than 200 mg/day; he can accomplish this by including plenty of low-cholesterol foods in his diet and avoiding such high-cholesterol foods as organ meats, eggs, and shellfish — all of which contain significant amounts.

LOW-CHOLESTEROL FOODS	HIGH-CHOLESTEROL FOODS
• Fish (except shellfish), skinless chicken and turkey, lean meats • Dry peas, beans • Tofu • Egg whites (2 whites = 1 whole egg in recipes), cholesterol-free egg substitutes • Skim or low-fat (1% fat) milk and buttermilk (liquid, powdered, or evaporated); nonfat or low-fat yogurt and cottage cheese (1% fat); low-fat or nonfat farmer, pot, and hard cheese (2 to 6 g fat per ounce); low-fat or light cream cheese and sour cream; sherbet and sorbet • Fresh, frozen, canned, and dried fruits and vegetables • Whole-grain breads and cereals (oatmeal, whole wheat, rye, bran, multigrain), rice, pasta, angel food cake, low-fat crackers and cookies, homemade baked goods using unsaturated oils sparingly • Baking cocoa; unsaturated vegetable oil; olive, canola, safflower, sesame, soybean, and sunflower oils; margarine, shortening, mayonnaise, and salad dressing made with unsaturated oil	• Shellfish, fatty cuts of beef, lamb, pork, spareribs, organ meats, cold cuts, sausage, hot dogs, bacon, sardines, roe • Egg yolks • Whole milk (4% fat; regular, evaporated, or condensed), cream, half-and-half, imitation milk products, most nondairy creamers, whipped toppings; whole-milk yogurt and cottage cheese (4% fat); all natural cheeses (blue, Roquefort, Camembert, cheddar, Swiss), cream cheeses, sour cream; ice cream • Vegetables prepared in butter, cream, and other sauces • Homemade breads in which eggs are a major ingredient; egg noodles; commercially baked goods (pies, cakes, doughnuts, croissants, pastries, muffins, biscuits, crackers, cookies) • Chocolate; butter; coconut, palm, or palm kernel oil; lard; bacon fat; dressings made with egg yolk; coconut

Source: Recommendations for total caloric intake, National Cholesterol Education Program; National Heart, Lung, and Blood Institute; National Institutes of Health (NIH Publication No. 01-3670, May 2001). *Therapeutic Lifestyle Changes Diet Tip Sheet Daily Food Guide Food Groups.* Cholesterol Education Program. *www.nhlbi.nih.gov/chd/TIPSHEETS/FOODGROUP.HTM.*

- Bleeding precautions (if thrombolytic therapy was administered)
- Coronary artery bypass graft
- IABP
- Left ventricular assist device
- Low-calorie, low-cholesterol, low-fat diet
- Monitoring of vital signs, urine output, ECG results, and hemodynamic status
- Ongoing laboratory studies (ABG, CK with isoenzymes, electrolyte, and cardiac troponin levels)
- Oxygen therapy

- Percutaneous coronary intervention
- Possibly a pacemaker for symptomatic bradycardia or heart block
- Pulmonary artery catheterization (to detect left- or right-sided heart failure)

Drug therapy options
- Analgesic: morphine sulfate (I.V.)
- ACE inhibitor: captopril (Capoten), enalapril (Vasotec)
- Antiarrhythmic: lidocaine (Xylocaine), procainamide (Pronestyl)

- Anticoagulant: heparin I.V. after thrombolytic therapy
- Antihypertensive: hydralazine (Apresoline)
- Aspirin
- Atropine I.V. for symptomatic bradycardia or heart block
- Beta-adrenergic blocker (contraindicated if client also has hypotension or bronchospasm): metoprolol (Lopressor), nadolol (Corgard), propranolol (Inderal)
- Calcium channel blocker: diltiazem (Cardizem), nifedipine (Procardia), verapamil (Calan)
- Nitrate: nitroglycerin I.V. (Nitro-Bid)
- Platelet GP IIb-IIIa receptor antagonist (for non–Q-wave MI): abciximab (ReoPro), tirofiban (Aggrastat)
- Thrombolytic (for ST-segment elevation or MI): anistreplase (Eminase), streptokinase (Streptase), tissue plasminogen activator (Activase) (given within 6 hours of onset of symptoms but most effective when started within 3 hours)

Patient care goals
- The client won't develop preventable complications.
- The client will understand the necessary treatment and lifestyle changes.

Nursing interventions
- Monitor and record vital signs and hemodynamic variables *to monitor response to therapy and detect complications.*
- Monitor and record intake and output *to assess renal perfusion and possible fluid retention.*
- Monitor laboratory values *to detect myocardial damage, abnormal electrolyte levels, drug levels, renal function, and coagulation.*
- Assess cardiovascular and respiratory status *to watch for signs of heart failure, such as an S_3 or S_4 gallop, crackles, cough, tachypnea, and edema.*
- Make sure the client maintains bed rest *to reduce oxygen demands on the heart.*
- Administer oxygen, as prescribed, *to improve oxygen supply to the heart.*
- Obtain an ECG reading during acute pain *to detect myocardial ischemia, injury, or infarction.*
- Maintain the client's prescribed diet *to reduce fluid retention and cholesterol levels.* (See *Diet to lower cholesterol.*)
- Provide postoperative care, if necessary, *to avoid postoperative complications and to help the client achieve a full recovery.*
- Allay the client's anxiety *because anxiety increases oxygen demands.*

Evaluation
- The client explains how and when to take his medication and states reportable adverse reactions.
- The client describes appropriate lifestyle changes to reduce the risk of a future cardiac event.
- The client experiences no complications.

Pericarditis

PERICARDITIS is an inflammation of the pericardium, the fibroserous sac that envelops, supports, and protects the heart. It occurs in acute and chronic forms. Acute pericarditis can be fibrinous or effusive, with purulent, serous, or hemorrhagic exudate; chronic constrictive pericarditis is characterized by dense fibrous pericardial thickening. The prognosis depends on the underlying cause but is generally good in acute pericarditis, unless constriction occurs.

Possible causes
- Bacterial, fungal, or viral infection (infectious pericarditis)
- Drugs, such as hydralazine or procainamide
- High-dose radiation to the chest
- Hypersensitivity or autoimmune disease, such as acute rheumatic fever (most common cause of pericarditis in children), systemic lupus erythematosus (SLE), and rheumatoid arthritis
- Idiopathic factors (most common in acute pericarditis)
- Neoplasms (primary, or metastasis from lungs, breasts, or other organs)
- Postcardiac injury, such as MI (which later causes an autoimmune reaction [Dressler's syndrome] in the pericardium), trauma, or surgery that leaves the pericardium intact but causes blood to leak into the pericardial cavity
- Uremia

Data collection findings
Acute pericarditis
- Sharp sudden pain that usually starts over the sternum and radiates to the neck, shoulders, back, and arms (unlike the pain of MI, pericardial pain is commonly pleuritic, increasing with deep inspiration and decreasing when the client sits up and leans forward, pulling the heart away from the diaphragmatic pleurae of the lungs)
- Pericardial friction rub (grating sound heard as the heart moves)
- Symptoms of cardiac tamponade (pallor, clammy skin, hypotension, pulsus paradoxus, neck vein distention)

- Symptoms of heart failure (dyspnea, orthopnea, tachycardia, ill-defined substernal chest pain, feeling of fullness in the chest)

Chronic pericarditis
- Pericardial friction rub
- Symptoms similar to those of chronic right-sided heart failure (fluid retention, ascites, hepatomegaly)
- Gradual increase in systemic venous pressure

Diagnostic findings
- Blood tests reflect inflammation and may show normal or elevated WBC count, especially in infectious pericarditis; elevated ESR; and slightly elevated cardiac enzyme levels with associated myocarditis.
- Culture of pericardial fluid obtained by open surgical drainage or cardiocentesis sometimes identifies a causative organism in bacterial or fungal pericarditis.
- Echocardiography confirms the diagnosis when it shows an echo-free space between the ventricular wall and the pericardium (in cases of pleural effusion).
- ECG shows the following changes in acute pericarditis:
– elevation of ST segments in the standard limb leads and most precordial leads without significant changes in QRS morphology that occur with MI
– atrial ectopic rhythms such as AF
– diminished QRS voltage in pericardial effusion.

Nursing diagnoses
- Acute pain
- Decreased cardiac output
- Deficient knowledge related to pericarditis

Treatment
- Bed rest
- Pericardiocentesis (in cases of cardiac tamponade), partial pericardectomy (for recurrent pericarditis), total pericardectomy (for constrictive pericarditis)

Drug therapy options
- Antibiotic: according to sensitivity of infecting organism
- Corticosteroid: methylprednisolone (Solu-Medrol)
- Nonsteroidal anti-inflammatory drug (NSAID): aspirin, indomethacin (Indocin)

Patient care goals
- The client will have relief from pain.
- The client will maintain hemodynamic stability.
- The client will understand the information provided about his current illness and its treatment.

Nursing interventions
- Provide complete bed rest *to decrease oxygen demands on the heart.*
- Assess pain in relation to respiration and body position *to distinguish pericardial pain from myocardial ischemic pain.*
- Place the client in an upright position *to relieve dyspnea and chest pain.*
- Provide analgesics and oxygen and reassure the client with acute pericarditis that his condition is temporary and treatable *to promote client comfort and allay anxiety.*
- Assist with monitoring the client for signs of cardiac compression or cardiac tamponade, possible complications of pericardial effusion. Signs include decreased blood pressure, increased CVP, and pulsus paradoxus. Keep a pericardiocentesis set handy whenever pericardial effusion is suspected *because cardiac tamponade requires immediate treatment.*
- Explain tests and treatments to the client. If surgery is necessary, he should learn deep-breathing and coughing exercises beforehand *to alleviate fear and anxiety and promote adherence with the postoperative treatment regimen.* Postoperative care is similar to that given after cardiothoracic surgery.

Evaluation
- The client verbalizes relief from pain.
- The client states an understanding of current illness and necessary treatment.
- The client has stable vital signs.

Pulmonary edema

PULMONARY EDEMA is a complication of left-sided heart failure. It occurs when pulmonary capillary pressure exceeds intravascular osmotic pressure, resulting in increased pressure in the capillaries of the lungs and acute transudation of fluid. Such increased pressure and fluid accumulation lead to impaired oxygenation and hypoxia.

Possible causes
- Adult respiratory distress syndrome
- Atherosclerosis
- Drug overdose (heroin, barbiturates, morphine sulfate)
- Heart failure
- Hypertension
- MI
- Myocarditis
- Overload of I.V. fluids
- Smoke inhalation

- Valvular disease

Data collection findings
- Agitation, restlessness, intense fear
- Blood-tinged, frothy sputum and paroxysmal cough
- Cold, clammy skin
- Crackles auscultated over lung fields
- Dyspnea
- Orthopnea
- Tachypnea
- Jugular vein distention
- Syncope
- Tachycardia
- S_3 and S_4
- Chest pain

Diagnostic findings
- ABG levels show respiratory alkalosis or acidosis and hypoxemia.
- ECG reveals tachycardia and ventricular enlargement.
- Hemodynamic monitoring shows increases in PAP, PAWP, and CVP as well as decreased cardiac output.
- Pulse oximetry reveals hypoxia.

Nursing diagnoses
- Impaired gas exchange
- Excess fluid volume
- Anxiety

Treatment
- Bed rest and ROM isometric exercises
- Low-sodium diet and limited intake of oral fluids
- Oxygen therapy with possible intubation and mechanical ventilation
- Hemodialysis and ultrafiltration, if available

Drug therapy options
- Analgesic: morphine sulfate I.V.
- ACE inhibitor: captopril (Capoten), enalapril (Vasotec), lisinopril (Prinivil)
- Beta-adrenergic blocker: carvedilol (Coreg), metoprolol (Lopressor)
- Cardiac glycoside: digoxin (Lanoxin)
- Diuretic: bumetanide (Bumex), furosemide (Lasix), metolazone (Zaroxolyn)
- Inotropic agent: inamrinone (Inocor), dobutamine (Dobutrex), milrinone (Primacor)
- Nitrate: isosorbide dinitrate (Isordil), nitroglycerin (Nitro-Bid)
- Vasodilator: nitroprusside sodium (Nitropress)

Patient care goals
- The client will have decreased pulmonary congestion and fluid volume.
- The client will experience no preventable complications.
- The client will demonstrate improvement in physiologic and psychological comfort.

Nursing interventions
- Assist with assessment of cardiovascular status, hemodynamic variables, and respiratory status *to detect changes in fluid balance.* Tachycardia, S_3, hypotension, increased respiratory rate, and crackles indicate increased fluid volume.
- Monitor and record intake and output. *Intake greater than output and elevated specific gravity suggest fluid retention.*
- Weigh the client daily *to detect fluid retention. A weight gain of 2 lb (0.9 kg) in 1 day or 5 lb (2.3 kg) in 1 week indicates fluid gain.*
- Monitor laboratory values. *BUN and creatinine levels indicate renal function; electrolyte and Hb levels and hematocrit (HCT) indicate fluid status.*
- Keep the client in high Fowler's position if his blood pressure tolerates; if he's hypotensive, keep him in semi-Fowler's position if tolerated. *Elevating the head of the bed reduces venous return to the heart and promotes chest expansion.*
- Administer oxygen, as prescribed, *to increase alveolar oxygen concentration and enhance arterial blood oxygenation.*
- Administer medications *to improve gas exchange, improve myocardial function, and reduce anxiety.*
- Note the color, amount, and consistency of sputum. *Sputum amount and consistency may indicate hydration status. A change in color or foul-smelling sputum may indicate a respiratory tract infection.*
- Withhold food and fluids, as directed, *to prevent aspiration.*
- Encourage the client to express his feelings, such as a fear of suffocation, *to reduce anxiety and lessen oxygen demands.*

Evaluation
- The client demonstrates a decrease in pulmonary congestion and fluid volume as evidenced by improved respiratory effort and oxygenation.
- The client doesn't develop complications.

Raynaud's disease

RAYNAUD'S DISEASE is characterized by episodic vasospasm in the small peripheral arteries and arterioles, precipitated by exposure to cold or stress. This condition occurs bilaterally and usually affects the hands or, less commonly, the feet.

Raynaud's disease is most prevalent in women, particularly between puberty and age 40. A benign condition, it requires no specific treatment and has no serious sequelae.

Raynaud's phenomenon, however, a condition commonly associated with several connective tissue disorders — such as scleroderma, SLE, and polymyositis — has a progressive course, leading to ischemia, gangrene, and amputation. Differentiating the two disorders is difficult because some clients who experience mild symptoms of Raynaud's disease for several years may later develop overt connective tissue disease — most commonly scleroderma.

Possible causes
- Unknown (most probable theory involves an antigen-antibody immune response)

Data collection findings
- Typically, blanching of the skin on the fingers, which then becomes cyanotic before changing to red (after exposure to cold or stress)
- Numbness and tingling relieved by warmth
- Sclerodactyly, ulcerations, or chronic paronychia (in longstanding disease)

Diagnostic findings
- Arteriography reveals vasospasm.
- Plethysmography reveals intermittent vessel occlusion.

Nursing diagnoses
- Ineffective tissue perfusion (peripheral)
- Risk for injury
- Acute pain

Treatment
- Avoidance of cold
- Smoking cessation (if appropriate)
- Sympathectomy (used in fewer than one-quarter of clients)

Drug therapy options
- Calcium channel blocker: diltiazem (Cardizem), nifedipine (Procardia)
- Vasodilator: phenoxybenzamine (Dibenzyline), reserpine (Serpalan)

Patient care goals
- The client will have improved peripheral circulation.
- The client won't develop complications from repeated peripheral vasospasm.
- The client will have relief from pain.

Nursing interventions
- Warn against exposure to the cold. Tell the client to wear mittens or gloves in cold weather or when handling cold items or defrosting the freezer *to prevent vasospasm, which causes onset of symptoms.*
- Advise the client to avoid stressful situations and to stop smoking *to prevent exacerbation of symptoms.*
- Instruct the client to inspect the skin frequently and to seek immediate care for signs of skin breakdown or infection *to prevent complications.*
- Teach the client about drugs, their use, and their adverse effects *to prevent further complications.*
- Provide psychological support and reassurance *to allay the client's fear of amputation and disfigurement.*

Evaluation
- The client reports decreased incidents of peripheral vasoconstriction.
- The client doesn't develop complications of illness.
- The client verbalizes pain relief.

Rheumatic fever and rheumatic heart disease

Commonly recurrent, acute RHEUMATIC FEVER is a systemic inflammatory disease of childhood that follows a group A beta-hemolytic streptococcal infection. RHEUMATIC HEART DISEASE refers to the cardiac manifestations of rheumatic fever and includes pancarditis (myocarditis, pericarditis, and endocarditis) during the early acute phase and later chronic valvular disease.

Long-term antibiotic therapy can minimize recurrence of rheumatic fever, reducing the risk of permanent cardiac damage and eventual valvular deformity. However, severe pancarditis occasionally produces fatal heart failure during the acute phase. Of the clients who survive this complication, about 20% die within 10 years.

This disease strikes most commonly during cool, damp weather in the winter and early spring. In the United States, it's most common in the northern states.

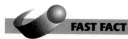

Rheumatic fever follows a group A beta-hemolytic streptococcal infection. Rheumatic heart disease refers to the cardiac manifestations of rheumatic fever.

Possible causes
● Hypersensitivity reaction to a group A beta-hemolytic streptococcal infection

Data collection findings
● Signs and symptoms of carditis
● Temperature of at least 100.4° F (38° C)
● Migratory joint pain or polyarthritis
● Skin lesions such as erythema marginatum (in only 5% of clients)
● Transient chorea (can develop up to 6 months after the original streptococcal infection)

Diagnostic findings
● Blood tests show elevated WBC count and ESR and slight anemia during periods of inflammation.
● Cardiac catheterization evaluates valvular damage and left ventricular function in severe cardiac dysfunction.
● Cardiac enzyme levels may be increased in severe carditis.
● Chest X-rays show normal heart size (except with myocarditis, heart failure, or pericardial effusion).
● C-reactive protein is positive (especially during the acute phase).
● Echocardiography helps evaluate valvular damage, chamber size, and ventricular function.
● ECG shows a prolonged PR interval in 20% of clients.

Nursing diagnoses
● Decreased cardiac output
● Activity intolerance
● Chronic pain

Treatment
● Strict bed rest until temperature returns to normal without medication, ESR is normal, and ECG returns to baseline
● Corrective valvular surgery (in cases of persistent heart failure)

Drug therapy options
● Antibiotic: erythromycin (Erythrocin), penicillin (Pfizerpen)
● NSAID: aspirin, indomethacin (Indocin)

Patient care goals
● The client will maintain hemodynamic stability and adequate cardiac output and will exhibit no arrhythmias.
● The client will increase his activity as infection subsides.
● The client will obtain relief from pain.

Nursing interventions
● Before giving penicillin, ask the client whether he has ever had a hypersensitivity reaction to it. Even if the client has never had a reaction to penicillin, warn that such a reaction is possible *to adequately inform the client about possible treatment complications.*
● Tell the client to stop taking the drug and immediately report the development of a rash, fever, chills, or other signs of allergy at any time during penicillin therapy *to prevent anaphylaxis.*
● Instruct the client to watch for and report early signs of heart failure, such as dyspnea and a hacking, nonproductive cough, *to prevent further cardiac decompensation.*
● Stress the need for bed rest during the acute phase, and suggest appropriate, physically undemanding diversions. *These measures decrease oxygen demands of the heart.*
● After the acute phase, encourage family and friends to spend as much time as possible with the client *to minimize boredom.*
● If the client has severe carditis, help him prepare for permanent changes in his lifestyle *to promote positive coping strategies.*
● Warn the client to watch for and immediately report signs of recurrent streptococcal infection — sudden sore throat, diffuse throat redness and oropharyngeal exudate, swollen and tender cervical lymph glands, pain on swallowing, a temperature of 101° to 104° F (38.3° to 40° C), headache, and nausea — *to prevent complications associated with delayed treatment such as heart valve damage.* Urge the client to avoid people with respiratory tract infections *to prevent reinfection.*
● Make sure the client understands the need to comply with prolonged antibiotic therapy and follow-up care and the need for additional antibiotics during dental surgery *to prevent reinfection.*
● Arrange for a visiting nurse to oversee home care if necessary *to promote adherence.*

Evaluation
● The client reports decreased pain.
● The client has stable vital signs.

- The client tolerates increased activity.

Thrombophlebitis

THROMBOPHLEBITIS is marked by inflammation of the venous wall and thrombus formation. It may affect deep veins or superficial veins. The thrombus may occlude a vein or detach and embolize to the lungs.

Possible causes

- Hypercoagulability (from cancer, blood dyscrasias, oral contraceptives)
- Injury to the venous wall (from I.V. injections, fractures, antibiotics)
- Venous stasis (from varicose veins, pregnancy, heart failure, prolonged bed rest)

Data collection findings

Deep vein thrombophlebitis
- Tenderness to touch in calf or thigh
- Positive Homans' sign
- Edema
- Cramping pain

Superficial vein thrombophlebitis
- Induration and redness along a superficial vein
- Warmth and tenderness along a superficial vein

Diagnostic findings

Deep vein thrombophlebitis
- Hematology reveals increased WBC count.
- Photo-plethysmography shows venous-filling defects.
- Ultrasound reveals decreased blood flow.
- Venography shows venous-filling defects.

Nursing diagnoses

- Acute pain
- Ineffective tissue perfusion (peripheral)
- Impaired skin integrity

Treatment

Deep vein thrombophlebitis
- Bed rest and elevation of the affected extremity
- Embolectomy and insertion of a vena cava umbrella or filter
- Antiembolism stockings
- Warm, moist compresses

Superficial vein thrombophlebitis
- Warm, moist compresses

Drug therapy options

- Anticoagulant: heparin (Liquaemin), warfarin (Coumadin) for deep vein thrombophlebitis
- Anti-inflammatory: aspirin, NSAID

Patient care goals

- The client will report pain relief.
- The client will exhibit healing of the injured site.
- The client will have improved circulation to the affected area.

Nursing interventions

Deep vein thrombophlebitis
- Assess pulmonary status. *Crackles, dyspnea, tachypnea, hemoptysis, and chest pain suggest pulmonary embolism.*
- Assess cardiovascular status. *Tachycardia and chest pain may indicate pulmonary embolism.*
- Check for Homans' sign. *Although it suggests deep vein thrombosis, it may be unreliable because it isn't specific to this condition.*
- Assess the client for bleeding *due to anticoagulant therapy.*
- Monitor and record vital signs, such as hypotension, tachycardia, tachypnea, and restlessness. Observe the client for bruising, epistaxis, blood in stool, bleeding gums, and painful joints. *Tachypnea and tachycardia may suggest pulmonary embolism or hemorrhage.*
- Perform neurovascular checks *to detect nerve or vascular damage.*
- Obtain blood samples for laboratory tests. *Partial thromboplastin time (PTT) and platelet count in a client on heparin and prothrombin time (PT) in a client receiving warfarin should be $1\frac{1}{2}$ to 2 times the control. International normalized ratio (INR) should be 2 to 3 times the control if the client is receiving warfarin. A decreasing Hb level and HCT indicate blood loss.*
- Keep the client in bed and elevate the affected extremity *to promote venous return and reduce swelling.*
- Assist with administration of medications, as prescribed, *to control or dissolve blood clots.*
- Apply warm, moist compresses *to improve circulation to the affected area and relieve pain and inflammation.*
- Measure and record the circumference of the client's thighs and calves. Compare measurement to the unaffected leg *to assess for worsening inflammation.*

Superficial vein thrombophlebitis
- Apply warm moist compresses to improve circulation to the area and relieve pain and inflammation.

- Monitor the site for increased redness and drainage, which may indicate infection.

Evaluation

- The client verbalizes pain relief.
- The client exhibits complete healing at the injury site.
- The client has improved circulation to the affected area.

SPOT CHECK

The nurse administers warfarin (Coumadin) to a client with deep vein thrombophlebitis. Which laboratory value indicates that the client has a therapeutic level of warfarin: PTT 1¼ to 2 times the control, PT 1¼ to 2 times the control, INR 3 to 4, or HCT 32%?
Answer: Warfarin is at a therapeutic level when the PT is 1¼ to 2 times the control. Values greater than this increase the risk of bleeding and hemorrhage; lower values increase the risk of blood clot formation. Heparin, not warfarin, prolongs the PTT. The INR may also be used to determine whether warfarin is at a therapeutic level; an INR of 2 to 3 is considered therapeutic. HCT doesn't provide information on the effectiveness of warfarin; however, decreasing HCT in a client taking warfarin may be a sign of hemorrhage.

Valvular heart disease

With VALVULAR HEART DISEASE, three types of mechanical disruption can occur: stenosis, or narrowing, of the valve opening; incomplete closure of the valve; or prolapse of the valve. These conditions can result from such disorders as endocarditis (most common), congenital defects, and inflammation, and they can lead to heart failure.

Valvular heart disease occurs in several forms. The most common include:

- AORTIC INSUFFICIENCY, in which blood flows back into the left ventricle during diastole, causing fluid overload in the ventricle, which dilates and hypertrophies (the excess volume causes fluid overload in the left atrium and, finally, the pulmonary system; left-sided heart failure and pulmonary edema eventually result)
- MITRAL INSUFFICIENCY, in which blood from the left ventricle flows back into the left atrium during systole, causing the atrium to enlarge to accommodate the backflow (as a result, the left ventricle also dilates to accommodate the increased volume of blood from the atrium and to compensate for diminishing cardiac output)
- MITRAL STENOSIS, in which narrowing of the valve by valvular abnormalities, fibrosis, or calcification obstructs blood flow from the left atrium to the left ventricle (conse-

quently, left atrial volume and pressure rise and the chamber dilates)

- MITRAL VALVE PROLAPSE (MVP), in which one or both valve leaflets protrude into the left atrium (*MVP syndrome* is the term used when the anatomic prolapse is accompanied by assessment findings unrelated to the valvular abnormality)
- TRICUSPID INSUFFICIENCY, in which blood flows back into the right atrium during systole, decreasing blood flow to the lungs and left side of the heart (cardiac output also lessens; fluid overload in the right side of the heart can eventually lead to right-sided heart failure).

QUICK STUDY

Remember the word **SIP** to distinguish the types of mechanical disruption that occur in heart valves.

Stenosis
Incomplete closure
Prolapse

Possible causes
Aortic insufficiency

- Endocarditis
- Hypertension
- Idiopathic origin
- Rheumatic fever
- Syphilis

Mitral insufficiency

- Hypertrophic cardiomyopathy
- Left-sided heart failure
- MVP
- Rheumatic fever

Mitral stenosis

- Rheumatic fever

MVP

- Neuroendocrine and metabolic abnormalities

Tricuspid insufficiency

- Endocarditis
- Rheumatic fever
- Right-sided heart failure
- Trauma

Data collection findings
Aortic insufficiency
- Dyspnea
- Palpitations
- Angina
- Fatigue
- Cough
- Pulmonary vein congestion
- Rapidly rising and collapsing pulses

Mitral insufficiency
- Angina
- Dyspnea
- Fatigue
- Orthopnea
- Peripheral edema

Mitral stenosis
- Dyspnea on exertion
- Palpitations
- Fatigue
- Orthopnea
- Weakness
- Peripheral edema

MVP
- Possibly asymptomatic
- Dizziness
- Chest pain
- Fatigue
- Palpitations
- Headache

Tricuspid insufficiency
- Dyspnea
- Fatigue
- Peripheral edema

Diagnostic findings
Aortic insufficiency
- Cardiac catheterization shows reduction in arterial diastolic pressures.
- Echocardiography shows left ventricular enlargement.
- ECG shows sinus tachycardia and left ventricular hypertrophy.
- X-ray shows left ventricular enlargement and pulmonary vein congestion.

Mitral insufficiency
- Cardiac catheterization shows mitral insufficiency and elevated atrial and PAWPs.
- Echocardiography shows abnormal valve leaflet motion.
- ECG may show left atrial and ventricular hypertrophy.
- X-ray shows left atrial and ventricular enlargement.

Mitral stenosis
- Cardiac catheterization shows diastolic pressure gradient across the valve and elevated left atrial pressure and PAWP.
- Echocardiography shows thickened mitral valve leaflets.
- ECG shows left atrial hypertrophy.
- X-ray shows left atrial and ventricular enlargement.

MVP
- Color-flow Doppler studies show mitral insufficiency.
- ECG shows prolapse of the mitral valve into the left atrium.

Tricuspid insufficiency
- Echocardiography shows systolic prolapse of the tricuspid valve.
- ECG shows right atrial or right ventricular hypertrophy.
- X-ray shows right atrial dilation and right ventricular enlargement.

Nursing diagnoses
- Decreased cardiac output
- Activity intolerance
- Anxiety

Treatment
- Sodium restrictions (in cases of heart failure)
- Open-heart surgery using cardiopulmonary bypass for valve replacement (in severe cases)

Drug therapy options
- Anticoagulant: warfarin (Coumadin) to prevent thrombus formation if the client is in atrial fibrillation and after valve replacement surgery

Patient care goals
- The client will remain hemodynamically stable.
- The client will have decreased anxiety over illness after appropriate education.
- The client will tolerate increased activity.

Nursing interventions

- Watch closely for signs of heart failure or pulmonary edema and for adverse effects of drug therapy *to prevent cardiac decompensation.*
- Place the client in an upright position *to relieve dyspnea.*
- Make sure the client maintains bed rest and provide assistance with bathing, if necessary, *to decrease oxygen demands on the heart.*
- If the client undergoes surgery, watch for hypotension, arrhythmias, and thrombus formation. Assist with monitoring of vital signs, ABG levels, intake and output, daily weight, blood chemistry test results, chest X-rays, and pulmonary artery catheter readings *to detect early signs of postoperative complications and ensure early intervention and treatment.*
- Allow the client to verbalize concerns over being unable to meet life demands because of activity restrictions *to reduce anxiety.*

Evaluation

- The client has stable vital signs and a controlled cardiac rhythm.
- The client verbalizes a decreased level of anxiety about the medical condition, discusses treatment, and states an understanding of the illness.
- The client demonstrates improved activity tolerance as the medical condition permits, such as taking part in activities of daily living (ADLs) with no significant change in heart rate or vital signs.

Venous insufficiency, chronic

CHRONIC VENOUS INSUFFICIENCY generally results from physiologic changes secondary to deep vein thrombophlebitis. It's a reverse flow of blood in the lower extremities caused by incompetent vessels and resulting in increased pressure in the vessels during ambulation.

Possible causes

- Leg trauma
- Superficial venous insufficiency secondary to congenital or acquired arteriovenous fistula
- Tumor (causing obstruction in the pelvic veins)

Data collection findings

- Progressive edema of the leg (particularly the lower leg)
- Itching of the skin
- Dull discomfort of the lower legs worsened by periods of standing
- Pain (if ulceration is present)

- Thin, shiny, atrophic and cyanotic skin on legs
- Brownish pigmentation of legs
- Eczema, with superficial weeping dermatitis

Diagnostic findings

- Duplex Doppler ultrasonography and impedence plethysmography rule out phlebitis.

Nursing diagnoses

- Risk for injury
- Ineffective tissue perfusion (peripheral)

Patient care goals

- The client will maintain skin integrity.
- The client will have improved circulation to the lower extremities.

Nursing interventions

- Instruct the client initially to maintain bed rest with legs elevated *to diminish chronic edema.*
- Suggest intermittent elevation of the legs during the day and elevation of the legs at night (above the level of the heart) *to promote circulation.*
- Advise the client to avoid long periods of sitting or standing *to decrease venous stasis.*
- Make sure to use properly fitted graduated compression stockings *to avoid venous compression.*
- Administer wet compresses to weeping dermatitis four times daily *to facilitate drainage.*
- Apply an Unna's boot to the affected extremity *to promote healing.*

Drug therapy options

- Antibiotic (if active infection is present)
- Anticoagulant (if recurrent thrombophlebitis): warfarin (Coumadin)

Evaluation

- The client has stable vital signs.
- The client states an understanding of his illness and its treatment and demonstrates decreased anxiety.
- The client has increased activity tolerance.

NEUROLOGIC SYSTEM

The neurologic system serves as the body's communication network. It processes information from the outside world (through the sensory portion) and coordinates and organizes the functions of all other body systems.

Neurologic system structure and function

Major parts of the neurologic system include the brain, spinal cord, and peripheral nerves. The complex tissues that make up the neurologic system include billions of neurons (nerve cells).

Neurons

A neuron is a highly specialized conductor cell that receives and transmits electrochemical nerve impulses. Delicate, threadlike nerve fibers called *axons* and *dendrites* extend from the neuron cell body and transmit signals. Axons carry impulses away from the cell body; dendrites carry impulses toward the cell body. A covering called a *myelin sheath* protects the entire neuron. Neurotransmitters — including the substances acetylcholine (ACh), serotonin, dopamine, endorphins, gamma-aminobutyric acid, and norepinephrine — conduct impulses across a synapse and into the next neuron.

QUICK STUDY

To help you remember the cranial nerves (and their order) think of the mnemonic "**O**n **O**ld **O**lympus' **T**owering **T**ops, **A** **F**inn **A**nd **G**erman **V**iewed **S**ome **H**ops."

  Olfactory (CN I)
  Optic (CN II)
  Oculomotor (CN III)
  Trochlear (CN IV)
  Trigeminal (CN V)
  Abducens (CN VI)
  Facial (CN VII)
  Acoustic (CN VIII)
  Glossopharyngeal (CN IX)
  Vagus (CN X)
  Spinal accessory (CN XI)
  Hypoglossal (CN XII)

Central nervous system

The central nervous system (CNS) includes the brain and spinal cord. These fragile structures are protected by the skull and vertebrae, cerebrospinal fluid (CSF), and three membranes: the dura mater, the pia mater, and the arachnoid membrane.

Brain

The brain is a mass of neural tissue that includes the lobed cerebrum and other related structures.

Cerebrum

The cerebrum, the largest part of the brain, houses the nerve center that controls motor and sensory functions and intelligence. It's divided into hemispheres. Because motor impulses descending from the brain cross in the medulla, the right hemisphere controls the left side of the body and the left hemisphere controls the right side of the body. Several fissures divide the cerebrum into four lobes:
- frontal lobe — the site of personality, memory, reasoning, concentration, and motor control of speech
- parietal lobe — the site of sensation, integration of sensory information, and spatial relationships
- temporal lobe — the site of hearing, speech, memory, and emotion
- occipital lobe — the site of vision and involuntary eye movements.

Other structures

Other parts of the brain include the thalamus, hypothalamus, cerebellum, and brain stem:
- The thalamus is a structure located deep in the brain that consists of two oval-shaped parts, one located in each hemisphere. The thalamus is referred to as "the relay station of the brain" because it receives input from all of the senses except olfaction (smell), analyzes that input, and then transmits that information to other parts of the brain.
- The hypothalamus, located beneath the thalamus, controls sleep and wakefulness, temperature, respiration, blood pressure, sexual arousal, fluid balance, and emotional response.
- The cerebellum, at the brain's base, coordinates muscle movements, maintains balance, and controls posture.
- The brain stem provides the connection between the spinal cord and the brain. It contains three sections:
– The midbrain mediates pupillary reflexes and eye movements; it's also the reflex center for the third and fourth cranial nerves.
– The pons helps regulate respiration; it's also the reflex center for the fifth through eighth cranial nerves and mediates chewing, tasting, saliva secretion, and equilibrium.
– The medulla oblongata contains the vomiting, vasomotor, respiratory, and cardiac centers.

Spinal cord

The spinal cord functions as a two-way conductor pathway between the brain stem and the peripheral nervous system. It consists of gray matter and white matter:

● Gray matter is made up of cell bodies and dendrites and axons.

● White matter contains ascending (sensory) and descending (motor) tracts, sending signals up to the brain and motor signals out to the muscles.

Peripheral nervous system

The peripheral nervous system delivers messages from the spinal cord to the body's outlying areas. The system's main nerves are grouped into:

● 31 pairs of spinal nerves, which carry mixed impulses (motor and sensory) to and from the spinal cord

● 12 pairs of cranial nerves, including olfactory, optic, oculomotor, trochlear, trigeminal, abducent, facial, acoustic, glossopharyngeal, vagus, spinal accessory, and hypoglossal.

Autonomic nervous system. The autonomic nervous system, a subdivision of the peripheral nervous system, controls involuntary body functions, such as digestion, respiration, and cardiovascular function. It's divided into two cooperating systems to maintain homeostasis — the sympathetic nervous system and the parasympathetic nervous system:

● The sympathetic nervous system coordinates activities that handle stress (the flight or fight response).

● The parasympathetic nervous system conserves and restores energy stores.

NEUROLOGIC DISORDERS

Major neurologic disorders include acute head injury, amyotrophic lateral sclerosis (ALS), Bell's palsy, brain tumor, cerebral aneurysm, encephalitis, Guillain-Barré syndrome, increased intracranial pressure (ICP), meningitis, multiple sclerosis (MS), myasthenia gravis (MG), Parkinson's disease, SEIZURE DISORDERS such as epilepsy, spinal cord injury, stroke, and trigeminal neuralgia.

Acute head injury

ACUTE HEAD INJURY results from a trauma to the head, leading to brain injury or bleeding within the brain. Effects of injury may include edema and hypoxia. Manifestations of the injury can vary greatly from a mild cognitive effect to severe functional deficits.

A head injury is classified by brain injury type: fracture, hemorrhage, or trauma. Fractures can be depressed, comminuted, or linear. Hemorrhages are classified as epidural, subdural, intracerebral, or subarachnoid.

Possible causes

● Assault
● Automobile accident
● Blunt trauma
● Fall
● Penetrating trauma

Data collection findings

● Disorientation to time, place, or person
● Unequal pupil size, loss of pupillary reaction (if edema is present) (see *Using the Glasgow Coma Scale*, page 302)
● Decreased LOC
● Paresthesia
● Otorrhea, rhinorrhea, and frequent swallowing (if a CSF leak occurs)

Diagnostic findings

● CT scan shows hemorrhage, cerebral edema, or shift of midline structures.
● EEG may reveal seizure activity.
● ICP monitoring shows increased ICP.
● Magnetic resonance imaging (MRI) shows hemorrhage, cerebral edema, or shift of midline structures.
● Skull X-ray may show skull fracture.

Nursing diagnoses

● Ineffective tissue perfusion (cerebral)
● Decreased intracranial adaptive capacity
● Risk for injury

Treatment

● Cervical collar (until neck injury is ruled out)
● Craniotomy: surgical incision into the cranium (may be necessary to evacuate a hematoma or evacuate contents to make room for swelling to prevent herniation)
● Oxygen therapy: intubation and mechanical ventilation (to provide controlled hyperventilation to decrease elevated ICP)
● Restricted oral intake for 24 to 48 hours
● Ventriculostomy: insertion of a drain into the ventricles (to drain CSF in the presence of hydrocephalus, which may occur as a result of head injury; can also be used to monitor ICP)

Using the Glasgow Coma Scale

To quickly assess a client's level of consciousness and to uncover baseline changes, use the Glasgow Coma Scale. This assessment tool grades consciousness in relation to eye opening and motor and verbal responses. A decreased reaction score in one or more categories warns of impending neurologic crisis. A client who scores 7 or less is comatose and probably has severe neurologic damage.

If the client has an endotracheal tube or a tracheostomy tube and can't respond verbally, use the abbreviation "T" to score him. For example, if the client scores a 5 for best verbal response but he has a tracheostomy tube in place, this score is noted as 5T.

TEST	CLIENT'S REACTION	SCORE
Eye-opening response	Opens spontaneously	4
	Opens to verbal command	3
	Opens to pain	2
	No response	1
Best motor response	Obeys verbal command	6
	Localizes painful stimuli	5
	Flexion-withdrawal	4
	Flexion-abnormal (decorticate rigidity)	3
	Extension (decerebrate rigidity)	2
	No response	1
Best verbal response	Oriented and converses	5
	Disoriented and converses	4
	Inappropriate words	3
	Incomprehensible sounds	2
	No response	1
Total		**3 to 15**

Drug therapy options
- Analgesic: codeine phosphate
- Anesthetic: lidocaine (Xylocaine)
- Anticonvulsant: phenytoin (Dilantin)
- Barbiturate: pentobarbital (Nembutal), if unable to control ICP with diuresis
- Diuretic: mannitol (Osmitrol), furosemide (Lasix) to combat cerebral edema
- Dopamine (Intropin) to maintain cerebral perfusion pressure above 50 mm Hg (if blood pressure is low and ICP is elevated)
- Glucocorticoid: dexamethasone (Decadron) to reduce cerebral edema
- Histamine-2 (H_2) receptor antagonist: cimetidine (Tagamet), ranitidine (Zantac), famotidine (Pepcid), nizatidine (Axid)
- Mucosal barrier fortifier: sucralfate (Carafate)
- Posterior pituitary hormone: vasopressin (Pitressin) if the client develops diabetes insipidus

Patient care goals
- The client will have improved cerebral perfusion.
- The client will have decreased ICP.
- The client will remain free from injury.

Nursing interventions
- Assess neurologic and respiratory status *to monitor for signs of increased ICP and respiratory distress.*
- Observe for signs of increasing ICP (including ICP greater than 20 mm Hg for more than 10 minutes) *to avoid treatment delay and prevent neurologic compromise.*
- Assist with monitoring and recording vital signs and intake and output, specific gravity, laboratory studies, and pulse oximetry *to detect early signs of compromise.*

Implementing seizure precautions

Purpose

By taking appropriate precautions, you can help protect a client from injury, aspiration, and airway obstruction in the event that he has a seizure. Plan your precautions using information obtained from the client's history. What kind of seizure has the client previously had? Is he aware of exacerbating factors? Sleep deprivation, missed doses of anticonvulsants, and even upper respiratory infections can increase seizure frequency in some people who have had seizures. Was his previous seizure an acute episode, or did it result from a chronic condition?

Remember that a client with preexisting seizures who is being admitted for a change in medication, treatment of an infection, or detoxification may be at greater risk for seizures.

Implementation

- Explain the reasons for the precautions to the client.
- *To protect the client's limbs, head, and feet from injury if he has a seizure while in bed,* cover the side rails, headboard, and footboard with side rail pads or bath blankets. If you use blankets, keep them in place with adhesive tape.
- Be sure to keep the side rails raised while the client is in bed *to prevent falls.* Keep the bed in a low position *to minimize injuries that may occur if the client climbs over the rails.*
- Place an airway at the client's bedside, or tape it to the wall above the bed according to your facility's protocol. Keep suction equipment nearby in case you need to establish a patent airway. Explain to the client how the airway will be used.
- If the client has frequent or prolonged seizures, prepare an I.V. heparin lock *to facilitate administration of emergency medications.*
- Document that seizure precautions have been implemented.

- Assess for CSF leak as evidenced by otorrhea or rhinorrhea. *A CSF leak could leave the client at risk for infection.*
- Assess pain. *Pain may cause anxiety and increase ICP.*
- Check cough and gag reflex *to prevent aspiration.*
- Check for signs of diabetes insipidus (low urine specific gravity, high urine output) *to maintain hydration.*
- Monitor I.V. fluids *to maintain hydration.*
- Administer oxygen and maintain position and patency of ET tube, if present, *to maintain airway and hyperventilate the client to lower ICP.*

- Provide suctioning; if the client is able, assist with turning, coughing, and deep breathing *to prevent pooling of secretions.*
- Maintain position, patency, and low suction of the NG tube *to prevent vomiting.*
- Maintain seizure precautions *to uphold client safety.* (See *Implementing seizure precautions.*)
- Assist with administration of medications as prescribed *to decrease ICP and pain.*
- Allow a rest period between nursing activities *to avoid an increase in ICP.*
- Encourage the client to express feelings about changes in his body image *to allay anxiety.*
- Provide appropriate sensory input and stimuli with frequent reorientation *to foster awareness of the environment.*
- Provide a means of communication, such as a communication board, *to prevent anxiety.*
- Provide eye, skin, and mouth care *to prevent tissue damage.*
- Turn the client every 2 hours or maintain him in a rotating bed if his condition allows *to prevent skin breakdown.*

Evaluation

- The client has an improved LOC.
- The client doesn't exhibit signs of increased ICP.
- The client remains free from injury.

Amyotrophic lateral sclerosis

AMYOTROPHIC LATERAL SCLEROSIS (ALS), commonly known as Lou Gehrig disease, is a progressive, degenerative disorder that leads to decreased motor function in the upper and lower motor neuron systems. In ALS, myelin sheaths are destroyed and replaced with scar tissue, resulting in distorted or blocked nerve impulses. Nerve cells die and muscle fibers have atrophic changes resulting in progressive motor dysfunction. The disease affects males three times more commonly than females.

Possible causes

- Genetic predisposition
- Nutritional deficiency related to a disturbance in enzyme metabolism
- Slow-acting virus
- Unknown

Data collection findings

- Muscle weakness
- Fasciculations
- Dysphagia

- Awkwardness of fine finger movements
- Fatigue
- Atrophy of tongue
- Dyspnea
- Nasal quality of speech
- Spasticity

Diagnostic findings
- CK level is elevated.
- Electromyogram (EMG) shows decreased amplitude of evoked potentials.

Nursing diagnoses
- Ineffective airway clearance
- Impaired physical mobility
- Ineffective health maintenance

Treatment
- Symptomatic relief

Drug therapy options
- Anticholinergic: dicyclomine (Bentyl)
- Anticonvulsant: gabapentin (Neurontin)
- Antispasmodic: baclofen (Lioresal), lorazepam (Ativan)
- Investigational: thyrotropin-releasing hormone, interferon
- Neuroprotective agent: riluzole (Rilutek)

Patient care goals
- The client will maintain a patent airway and adequate ventilation.
- The client will maintain joint mobility and ROM.
- The client will maintain care of himself and his environment without evidence of deficit.

Nursing interventions
- Assess neurologic and respiratory status *to detect decreases in neurologic functioning.*
- Assess swallow and gag reflexes *to decrease the risk of aspiration.*
- Monitor and record vital signs and intake and output *to determine baseline assessment and detect changes from baseline.*
- Administer medications as prescribed *to help the client achieve maximum potential.*
- Devise an alternate method of communication, when necessary, *to help the client communicate and to decrease the client's anxiety and frustration.*

- Encourage the client to verbalize his feelings and maintain his independence for as long as possible *to decrease anxiety and promote self-esteem.*
- Suction oral pharynx as necessary *to stimulate cough and clear airways.*
- Maintain the client's diet *to improve his nutritional status.*

Evaluation
- The client has adequate gas exchange.
- The client demonstrates the ability to use muscles and joints effectively.
- The client demonstrates the ability to perform self-care.

Bell's palsy

BELL'S PALSY affects the seventh cranial (facial) nerve and produces unilateral facial weakness or paralysis. Onset is rapid. Although the disorder affects all age-groups, it's most common in people younger than age 60. In 80% to 90% of clients, it subsides spontaneously, with complete recovery in 1 to 8 weeks; however, recovery may be delayed in older adults. If recovery is partial, contractures may develop on the paralyzed side of the face. Bell's palsy may recur on the same or opposite side of the face.

FAST FACT

There are two facial nerves, one on each side. Bell's palsy occurs when one of those nerves becomes swollen and pinched.

Possible causes
- Blockage of the seventh cranial nerve resulting from infection, hemorrhage, tumor, meningitis, or local trauma

Data collection findings
- Inability to completely close the eye on the affected side
- Pain around the jaw or ear
- Unilateral facial weakness
- Eye rolls upward and tears excessively when the client attempts to close it
- Ringing in the ears
- Taste distortion on the affected anterior portion of the tongue

Diagnostic findings
- EMG helps predict the level of expected recovery by distinguishing temporary conduction defects from a pathologic interruption of nerve fibers.

NURSING PROCEDURE

Performing mouth care

Purpose

Given in the morning, at bedtime, or after meals, mouth care entails brushing and flossing the teeth and inspecting the mouth. Proper mouth care results in removal of soft plaque deposits and calculus from the teeth and gum cleaning and massage. These practices reduce mouth odor and also help prevent infection. By freshening the client's mouth, mouth care also enhances appreciation of food, thereby aiding appetite and nutrition.

Although the ambulatory client can usually perform mouth care alone, the bedridden client may require partial or full assistance. The comatose client requires use of suction equipment to prevent aspiration during oral care.

Implementation

● Wash your hands thoroughly and put on gloves.
● Explain the procedure to the client.
● Provide privacy.

Supervising mouth care for a bedridden client
● Encourage the client to perform his own mouth care if possible.
● Place the client in Fowler's position. Arrange the equipment on the overbed table in front of the client and position a mirror if available.
● Drape a towel over the client's chest. Tell him to floss his teeth while looking into the mirror.
● Then instruct the client to brush his teeth and gums while looking into the mirror. Encourage him to rinse frequently during brushing, using a mix of mouthwash and water. Provide facial tissues for him to wipe his mouth.

Performing mouth care
● Perform mouth care for the comatose client or the conscious client incapable of self-care. If the client wears dentures, clean them thoroughly.

● Position the client on his side, with his face extended over the edge of the pillow.
● Arrange the equipment on the overbed table or bedside stand, including the oral suction equipment if necessary. Place a linen-saver pad under the client's chin and an emesis basin near his cheek.
● Lubricate the client's lips with petroleum jelly. If necessary, insert a bite-block to hold the client's mouth open during oral care.
● If possible, use a dental floss holder and direct it as close to the gum as possible without injuring the sensitive tissues around the tooth.
● Then, using a toothbrush with toothpaste, brush the client's lower teeth from the gum line up; the upper teeth, from the gum line down. Place the brush at a 45-degree angle to the gum line, and press the bristles gently into the gingival sulcus. Using short, gentle strokes *to prevent gum damage,* brush the buccal surfaces (toward the cheek) and the lingual surfaces (toward the tongue) of the bottom teeth. Use just the tip of the brush for the lingual surfaces of the front teeth. Then, using the same technique, brush the buccal and lingual surfaces of the top teeth. Next, brush the biting surfaces of the bottom and top teeth, using a back-and-forth motion. Hold the emesis basin steady under the client's cheek, and wipe his mouth and cheeks with facial tissues as needed.
● After brushing the client's teeth, take a sponge-tipped mouth swab dipped in mouthwash solution and gently stroke the gums, buccal surfaces, palate, and tongue to clean the mucosa and stimulate circulation.
● Record the date and time of mouth care in your notes. Also note any unusual conditions, such as bleeding, edema, mouth odor, excessive secretions, or plaque on the tongue.

Nursing diagnoses

● Acute pain
● Disturbed sensory perception (gustatory)
● Disturbed body image

Treatment

● Electrotherapy after the 14th day of prednisone therapy to help prevent facial muscle atrophy

● Moist heat
● Facial sling

Drug therapy options

● Corticosteroid: prednisone (Deltasone) to reduce facial nerve edema and improve nerve conduction and blood flow

Patient care goals
● The client will experience increased comfort and relief from pain.
● The client will report improved sensation and function in the affected area.
● The client will state positive feelings about himself.

Nursing interventions
● During treatment with prednisone, watch for adverse reactions, especially GI distress and fluid retention. If GI distress is troublesome, a concomitant antacid usually provides relief and prevents further complications.
● If the client has diabetes, prednisone must be used with caution and necessitates frequent monitoring of serum glucose levels. *Hyperglycemia is an adverse reaction to prednisone therapy.*
● Apply moist heat to the affected side of the face, taking care not to burn the skin.
● Teach the client to massage his face using a gentle upward motion two to three times daily for 5 to 10 minutes. When he's ready for active exercises, teach him to exercise by grimacing in front of a mirror. *These practices help maintain muscle tone.*
● Arrange for privacy at mealtimes *to reduce embarrassment.*
● Apply a facial sling *to improve lip alignment.*
● Give the client frequent and complete mouth care, being careful to remove residual food that collects between the cheeks and gums *to prevent breakdown of the oral mucosa.* (See *Performing mouth care,* page 305.)
● Offer psychological support. Give reassurance that recovery is likely within 1 to 8 weeks *to allay the client's anxiety.*

Evaluation
● The client reports adequate pain control.
● The client has improved sensation and function in the affected area.
● The client makes positive statements regarding his facial appearance and functional ability.

Brain tumor

A BRAIN TUMOR is an abnormal mass found in the brain resulting from unregulated cell growth and division. These tumors can either infiltrate and destroy surrounding tissue or be encapsulated and displace brain tissue. The lesion's presence causes compression of blood vessels, producing ischemia, edema, and increased ICP.

Symptoms and manifestations vary depending on the location of the tumor in the brain. The tumor can be primary (originating in the brain tissue) or secondary (metastasizing from another area of the body). Tumors are classified according to the tissue of origin, such as gliomas (composed of neuroglial cells), meningiomas (originating in the meninges), and astrocytomas (composed of astrocytes).

Possible causes
● Environmental
● Genetic

Data collection findings
Tumor in any area
● Deficits in cerebral function
● Headache

Tumor in the frontal lobe
● Aphasia
● Memory loss
● Personality changes

Tumor in the temporal lobe
● Aphasia
● Seizures

Tumor in the parietal lobe
● Motor seizures
● Sensory impairment

Tumor in the occipital lobe
● Homonymous hemianopsia (defective vision or blindness affecting the right halves or the left halves of the visual field of the two eyes)
● Visual hallucinations
● Visual impairment

Tumor in the cerebellum
● Impaired coordination
● Impaired equilibrium

Diagnostic findings
● CT scan shows location and size of tumor.
● MRI also shows location and size of tumor.

Nursing diagnoses
- Disturbed sensory perception (kinesthetic)
- Anxiety
- Risk for injury

Treatment
- Craniotomy
- High-calorie diet
- Radiation therapy

Drug therapy options
- Anticonvulsant: phenytoin (Dilantin)
- Antineoplastic: vincristine (Oncovin), lomustine (CeeNU), carmustine (BiCNU)
- Diuretic: mannitol (Osmitrol), furosemide (Lasix) if increased ICP
- Glucocorticoid: dexamethasone (Decadron)
- H_2-receptor antagonist: cimetidine (Tagamet), ranitidine (Zantac), famotidine (Pepcid), nizatidine (Axid)
- Mucosal barrier fortifier: sucralfate (Carafate)

Patient care goals
- The client will recognize limitations imposed by his illness and will express his feelings about these limitations.
- The client will express feelings about his diminished capacity to perform his usual roles.
- The client will remain free from injury.

Nursing interventions
- Assess neurologic and respiratory status *to determine baseline and deviations from baseline assessment.*
- Assess pain. *Continuous assessment correlates the client's subjective complaints and behavior with organic pathology.*
- Assess for increased ICP *to facilitate early intervention and prevent neurologic complications.*
- Monitor and record vital signs, intake and output, and laboratory studies *to determine baseline and detect early deviations from baseline assessment.*
- Monitor for signs and symptoms of syndrome of inappropriate antidiuretic hormone (edema, weight gain, positive fluid balance, high urine specific gravity) *to facilitate early intervention and prevent increased ICP through fluid restriction and I.V. infusion of normal saline solution.*
- Turn and reposition the client every 2 hours *to maintain skin integrity.*
- Maintain the client's diet *to promote healing.*

- Encourage the client to drink fluids, or monitor I.V. fluids if the client can't drink adequate amounts, *to maintain hydration.*
- Administer oxygen *to prevent ischemia.*
- Administer enteral nutrition or ensure safety of central line for total parenteral nutrition (TPN), as indicated, *to meet nutritional needs.*
- Limit environmental noise. *Auditory stimuli can contribute to increased ICP.*
- Encourage the client to express his feelings about changes in his body image and fear of dying *to decrease anxiety.*
- Assist with monitoring ABG levels. *Hypercapnia results in vasodilation, increased cerebral blood volume, and increased ICP.*
- Maintain normothermia and control shivering. *Shivering causes isometric muscle contraction, which can increase ICP.*
- Provide rest periods. *Cerebral blood flow increases during rapid eye-movement sleep.*
- Maintain seizure precautions and administer anticonvulsants, as ordered. *Seizures increase intrathoracic pressure, decrease cerebral venous outflow, and increase cerebral blood volume, thereby increasing ICP.*

Evaluation
- The client demonstrates ability to function despite sensory or motor deficits.
- The client demonstrates effective coping mechanisms in dealing with limitations of illness.
- The client remains free from injury.

Cerebral aneurysm
A CEREBRAL ANEURYSM is an outpouching of a cerebral artery that results from weakness of the middle layer of an artery. It usually results from a congenital weakness in the structure of the artery and remains asymptomatic until it ruptures.

Cerebral aneurysms are classified by type: saccular (berry), fusiform, and giant. Saccular aneurysms, the most common, occur at the base of the brain at the juncture where the large arteries bifurcate.

Possible causes
- Atherosclerosis
- Congenital weakness
- Head trauma

Data collection findings

- Asymptomatic until aneurysm ruptures
- Headache (commonly described by the client as the worst he has ever had)
- Decreased LOC
- Diplopia, ptosis, blurred vision
- Fever
- Hemiparesis
- Nuchal rigidity
- Seizure activity

Diagnostic findings

- Cerebral angiogram identifies the aneurysm.
- CT scan shows a shift of intracranial midline structures and blood in subarachnoid space.
- Lumbar puncture (contraindicated with increased ICP) shows increased CSF pressure, protein level, and WBC count and grossly bloody and xanthochromic CSF.
- MRI shows shift of intracranial midline structures and blood in subarachnoid space.

Nursing diagnoses

- Ineffective tissue perfusion (cerebral)
- Decreased intracranial adaptive capacity
- Anxiety

Treatment

- Aneurysm and seizure precautions
- Aneurysm clipping
- Bed rest
- Head of bed elevated 30 degrees
- I.V. therapy
- Oxygen therapy (intubation and mechanical ventilation with hyperventilation, if increased ICP)

Drug therapy options

- Analgesic: codeine sulfate
- Anticonvulsant: phenytoin (Dilantin)
- Antihypertensive: hydralazine (Apresoline), nitroprusside (Nitropress), labetalol (Trandate), metoprolol (Lopresor), esmolol (Brevibloc)
- Calcium channel blocker: nimodipine (Nimotop) preferred drug to prevent cerebral vasospasm
- Glucocorticoid: dexamethasone (Decadron)
- H_2-receptor antagonist: cimetidine (Tagamet), ranitidine (Zantac), famotidine (Pepcid)
- Vasopressor: dopamine (Intropin) to maintain systolic blood pressure at 140 to 160 mm Hg
- Mucosal barrier fortifier: sucralfate (Carafate)
- Stool softener: docusate sodium (Colace)

Patient care goals

- The client will maintain adequate ventilation and oxygenation.
- The client will have stable cerebral perfusion.
- The client will express feelings of calmness.

Nursing interventions

- Assess neurologic status *to screen for changes in the client's condition.*
- Maintain a quiet environment and assist the client with relaxation using sedatives and pain medication as appropriate *to reduce ICP.*
- Maintain patency of the I.V. site for administration of diuretics *to prevent or treat increased ICP.*
- Assist with administration of crystalloid solutions after aneurysm clipping *to induce hypervolemia and increase cerebral perfusion, thus decreasing the risk of vasospasm.*
- Administer oxygen (may require intubation and mechanical ventilation with hyperventilation). *Hypercapnia results in vasodilation, increased cerebral blood volume, and increased ICP.*
- Keep the head of the bed elevated to 30 degrees *to reduce increased ICP.*
- Monitor for Cushing's triad (bradycardia, systolic hypertension, and wide pulse pressure), *which is a sign of impending hemorrhage.*
- Take vital signs every 1 to 2 hours initially, then every 4 hours when the client becomes stable *to detect early signs of decreased cerebral perfusion pressure or increased ICP.*
- Allow a rest period between nursing activities *to reduce increased ICP.*
- Maintain seizure precautions and administer anticonvulsants, as ordered. *Seizures increase intrathoracic pressure, decrease cerebral venous outflow, and increase cerebral blood volume, thereby increasing ICP.*
- Provide skin care and turn the client every 2 hours *to prevent pressure ulcers.*
- Maintain adequate nutrition *to facilitate tissue healing and meet metabolic needs.*
- Minimize constipation and straining at defecation *to prevent increased ICP.*
- If the client has a potentially compromised airway, use antiemetics or NG suction *to prevent nausea and vomiting, which may increase ICP.*

SPOT CHECK

A client undergoes a surgical clipping of a cerebral aneurysm. To prevent vasospasm, postsurgical care focuses on maintaining an optimal cerebral perfusion pressure. This is best accomplished by administering:

A. diuretics such as furosemide (Lasix).
B. blood products such as cryoprecipitate.
C. the calcium channel blocker nifedipine (Procardia).
D. volume expanders such as crystalloids.

Answer: D. To prevent vasospasm following repair of a cerebral aneurysm, treatment focuses on increasing cerebral perfusion. This can be accomplished by giving volume expanders such as crystalloids. Diuretics would decrease cerebral perfusion by reducing volume. Cryoprecipitate isn't used as a volume expander. Nimodipine (Nimotop), not nifedipine (Procardia), is the calcium channel blocker indicated for use in cerebral vasospasm treatment and prevention.

Evaluation
- The client has adequate ventilation and oxygenation.
- The client is alert and oriented.
- The client demonstrates calm behavior.

Encephalitis

ENCEPHALITIS is a severe inflammation and swelling of the brain, usually caused by a mosquito-borne or, in some areas, a tick-borne virus. Transmission also may occur through ingestion of infected goat's milk and accidental injection or inhalation of the virus. Eastern equine encephalitis may produce permanent neurologic damage and is commonly fatal.

In encephalitis, intense lymphocytic infiltration of brain tissues and the leptomeninges causes cerebral edema, degeneration of the brain's ganglion cells, and diffuse nerve cell destruction.

Possible causes
- Exposure to virus

Data collection findings
- Sudden onset of fever
- Headache
- Meningeal irritation (stiff neck and back) and neuronal damage (drowsiness, coma, paralysis, seizures, ataxia, organic psychoses)
- Vomiting
- Coma (following the acute phase of illness)

- Sensory alterations

Diagnostic findings
- Blood studies identify the virus, confirming the diagnosis.
- CSF analysis identifies the virus.
- Lumbar puncture discloses CSF pressure is elevated and, despite inflammation, the fluid is commonly clear. WBC count and protein levels in CSF are slightly elevated, but the glucose level remains normal.
- EEG reveals abnormalities such as generalized slowing of waveforms.
- CT scan may be ordered to rule out cerebral hematoma.

Nursing diagnoses
- Disturbed thought processes
- Hyperthermia
- Impaired physical mobility

Treatment
- ET intubation and mechanical ventilation
- I.V. fluids
- NG tube feedings or TPN

Drug therapy options
- Anticonvulsant: phenytoin (Dilantin), phenobarbital (Luminal)
- Antiviral: acyclovir (Zovirax) (effective only against herpes encephalitis; effective only if administered before the onset of coma)
- Analgesic and antipyretic: aspirin or acetaminophen (Tylenol) to relieve headache and reduce fever
- Diuretic: furosemide (Lasix) or mannitol (Osmitrol) to reduce cerebral swelling
- Corticosteroid: dexamethasone (Decadron) to reduce cerebral inflammation and edema
- Laxative: bisacodyl (Dulcolax)
- Sedative: lorazepam (Ativan) for restlessness
- Stool softener: docusate (Colace)

Patient care goals
- The client will have appropriate thought processes.
- The client will exhibit temperature within normal limits.
- The client will have improved physical mobility.

Nursing interventions
During the acute phase of the illness
- Assess neurologic function often. Observe the client's mental status and cognitive abilities. *Changes in the*

client's mental status and cognitive abilities indicate that tissue within the brain has become edematous.

● Maintain adequate fluid intake *to prevent dehydration,* but avoid fluid overload, *which may increase cerebral edema.* Measure and record intake and output accurately *to assess fluid status.*

● Maintain a patent I.V. line for administration of acyclovir by slow I.V. infusion only. The client must be well-hydrated and the infusion given over 1 hour *to avoid kidney damage.* Watch for adverse effects, such as nausea, diarrhea, pruritus, and rash, and adverse effects of other drugs *to prevent complications.* Check the infusion site often *to avoid infiltration and phlebitis.*

● Carefully position the client *to prevent joint stiffness and neck pain,* and turn him often *to prevent skin breakdown.*

● Assist with ROM exercises *to maintain joint mobility.*

● Maintain adequate nutrition *to meet increased metabolic needs and promote healing.* It may be necessary to give the client small, frequent meals or to supplement these meals with NG tube or parenteral feedings.

● Give a stool softener or mild laxative *to prevent constipation and to minimize the risk of increased ICP from straining during defecation.*

● Provide good mouth care *to prevent breakdown of the oral mucous membrane.*

● Maintain a quiet environment *to promote comfort and decrease stimulation, which can cause ICP to rise.* Darkening the room *may decrease photophobia and headache.*

● If the client naps during the day and is restless at night, plan daytime activities *to minimize napping and to promote sleep at night.*

● Provide emotional support and reassurance *because the client is apt to be frightened by the illness and frequent diagnostic tests.*

● Reassure the client and his family that behavioral changes caused by encephalitis usually disappear *to decrease anxiety.*

Evaluation

● The client has appropriate thought processes.
● The client has a normal temperature.
● The client has returned to baseline physical mobility.

Guillain-Barré syndrome

GUILLAIN-BARRÉ SYNDROME, also known as infectious polyneuritis, Landry's syndrome, and acute idiopathic polyneuritis, is an acute, rapidly progressive, and potentially fatal form of polyneuritis (inflammation of several peripheral nerves at once) that causes muscle weakness and mild distal sensory loss.

Recovery is spontaneous and complete in about 95% of clients, although mild motor or reflex deficits in the feet and legs may persist. The prognosis is best when symptoms clear between 15 and 20 days after onset.

Possible causes

● Cell-mediated immune response with an attack on peripheral nerves in response to a virus
● Demyelination of the peripheral nerves
● Respiratory infection

Data collection findings

● Muscle weakness (ascending from the legs to arms)
● Dysphagia (difficulty swallowing) or dysarthria (poor speech caused by impaired muscular control)
● Facial diplegia (affecting like parts on both sides of the face; possibly accompanied by ophthalmoplegia [ocular paralysis])
● Hypertonia (excessive muscle tone) and areflexia (absence of reflexes)
● Paresthesia
● Stiffness and pain in the form of a severe "charley horse"
● Weakness of the muscles supplied by cranial nerve XI, the spinal accessory nerve (these muscles affect shoulder movement and head rotation)

Diagnostic findings

● A history of preceding febrile illness (usually a respiratory tract infection) and typical clinical features suggest Guillain-Barré syndrome.
● CSF protein level begins to rise, peaking in 4 to 6 weeks. The CSF WBC count remains normal but, in severe disease, CSF pressure may rise above normal.
● Blood studies reveal a CBC that shows leukocytosis with the presence of immature forms early in the illness, but blood study results soon return to normal.
● EMG may show repeated firing of the same motor unit, instead of widespread sectional stimulation.
● Nerve conduction velocities are slowed soon after paralysis develops. Diagnosis must rule out similar diseases such as acute poliomyelitis.

Nursing diagnoses

● Ineffective breathing pattern
● Impaired physical mobility
● Anxiety

Treatment

- ET intubation or tracheotomy if the client has difficulty clearing secretions or mechanical ventilation, if necessary
- NG tube feedings or TPN
- I.V. fluid therapy
- Specialty bed or support surfaces
- Plasmapheresis

Drug therapy options

- Corticosteroid: prednisone (Deltasone)
- Antiarrhythmic: propranolol (Inderal), atropine
- Anticoagulant: heparin, warfarin (Coumadin)

Patient care goals

- The client will maintain adequate ventilation.
- The client will return to baseline motor ability.
- The client will use available support systems and develop adequate coping mechanisms.

Nursing interventions

- Watch for ascending sensory loss, which precedes motor loss. Also, monitor vital signs and LOC *to detect disease progression.*
- Assess and treat respiratory dysfunction *to prevent respiratory arrest.* If respiratory muscles are weak, assist with vital capacity recordings. Use of a respirometer with a mouthpiece or a facemask for bedside testing *ensures rapid measurement.*
- Be alert for signs of rising partial pressure of carbon dioxide ($Paco_2$) (confusion, tachypnea) *to detect early signs of hypoventilation and avoid treatment delay.*
- Auscultate for breath sounds to detect early changes in respiratory function, and encourage coughing and deep breathing *to mobilize secretions and prevent atelectasis.*
- Begin respiratory support at the first sign of dyspnea (in adults, a vital capacity less than 800 ml) or a decreasing partial pressure of arterial oxygen (Pao_2) *to prevent hypoxemia.*
- If respiratory failure becomes imminent, assist with establishment of an emergency airway with an ET tube *to prevent organ damage from anoxia.*
- Give meticulous skin care *to prevent skin breakdown and contractures.*
- Establish a strict turning schedule; inspect the skin (especially the sacrum, heels, and ankles) for breakdown, and reposition the client every 2 hours. *These measures prevent skin breakdown and pressure ulcer development.*
- After each position change, stimulate circulation by carefully massaging pressure points. Also, use foam, gel, or alternating-pressure pads at points of contact *to prevent skin breakdown.*
- Perform passive ROM exercises within the client's pain limits, perhaps using a Hubbard tank. Remember that the proximal muscle groups of the thighs, shoulders, and trunk will be the most tender and cause the most pain on passive movement and turning. *Passive ROM exercises maintain joint function.*
- When the client's condition stabilizes, change to gentle stretching and active assistance exercises *to strengthen muscles and maintain joint function.*
- Assess the client for signs of dysphagia (coughing, choking, "wet"-sounding voice, increased presence of rhonchi after feeding, drooling, delayed swallowing, regurgitation of food, and weakness in cranial nerve V, VII, IX, X, XI, or XII). *These measures help prevent aspiration.*
- Elevate the head of the bed, position the client upright and leaning forward when eating, feed semisolid food, and check the mouth for food pockets *to minimize aspiration.*
- Encourage the client to eat slowly and remain upright for 15 to 20 minutes after eating *to prevent aspiration.*
- If aspiration can't be minimized by diet and position modification, expect to provide NG feeding *to prevent aspiration and ensure that nutritional needs are met.*
- As the client regains strength and can tolerate a vertical position, be alert for postural hypotension. Monitor blood pressure and pulse rate during tilting periods and, if necessary, apply toe-to-groin elastic bandages or an abdominal binder *to prevent postural hypotension.*
- Inspect the client's legs regularly for signs of thrombophlebitis (localized pain, tenderness, erythema, edema, positive Homans' sign). *Thrombophlebitis is a common complication of Guillain-Barré syndrome.*
- Apply antiembolism stockings and give prophylactic anticoagulants as needed *to prevent thrombophlebitis.*
- If the client has facial paralysis, give eye and mouth care every 4 hours *to prevent corneal damage and breakdown of the oral mucosa.*
- Protect the corneas with isotonic eyedrops and conical eye shields *to prevent corneal injury.*
- Encourage adequate fluid intake (2,000 ml per day), unless contraindicated, *to prevent dehydration, constipation, and renal calculi formation.*
- Measure and record intake and output every 8 hours, and offer the bedpan every 3 to 4 hours *to monitor for urine retention.*
- Begin intermittent catheterization as needed *to relieve urine retention.* The client may need manual pressure on the bladder (Credé's maneuver) before he can urinate *be-*

NURSING PROCEDURE

Performing Credé's maneuver

Purpose

When lower motor neuron damage impairs the voiding reflex, the bladder may become flaccid or areflexic. Because the bladder fails to contract properly, urine collects inside it, causing distention. Credé's maneuver—application of manual pressure over the lower abdomen—promotes complete emptying of the bladder. After appropriate instruction, the client can perform the maneuver himself, unless he can't reach his lower abdomen or lacks sufficient strength and dexterity. Even when performed properly, however, Credé's maneuver isn't always successful and doesn't always eliminate the need for catheterization.

Credé's maneuver can't be used after abdominal surgery if the incision isn't completely healed. When a client uses Credé's maneuver, close monitoring of urine output is necessary to help detect possible infection from accumulation of residual urine.

Implementation

- Explain the procedure to the client.
- Wash your hands.
- If the client's condition permits, assist him onto the bedside commode. If not and the client's condition permits, place the client in Fowler's position and position the bedpan or urinal.
- Place your hands flat on the client's abdomen just below the umbilicus. Ask the female client to bend forward from the hips. Firmly stroke downward toward the bladder about six times to stimulate the voiding reflex.
- Place one hand on top of the other above the pubic arch. Press firmly inward and downward to compress the bladder and to expel residual urine.
- Some facilities require a physician's order for performing Credé's maneuver. This procedure shouldn't be performed on clients with normal bladder tone or bladder spasms.
- Record the date and time of the procedure, the amount of urine expelled, and the client's tolerance of the procedure.

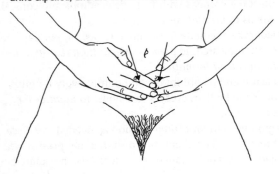

cause the abdominal muscles are weak. (See *Performing Credé's maneuver.*)

- Offer prune juice and a high-bulk diet *to prevent and relieve constipation.* If necessary, give daily or alternate-day suppositories (glycerin or bisacodyl) or Fleet enemas *to relieve constipation.*
- As needed, refer the client for physical therapy, occupational therapy, and speech therapy *to promote recovery.*

Evaluation

- The client has adequate ventilation as evidenced by a stable pulse oximetry and ABG levels.
- The client's joint mobility and ROM are at the same level as they were before the illness.
- The client demonstrates effective coping abilities for dealing with his illness.

Increased intracranial pressure

INTRACRANIAL PRESSURE (ICP) is the pressure that three different components — brain tissue (84%), CSF (12%), and cerebral blood volume (4%) — exert inside the rigid, unyielding skull. The Monro-Kellie doctrine states that, because of the limited space in the skull, an increase in any one component must cause a compensatory change in the volume of the others, by displacing or shifting CSF, increasing the absorption of CSF, or decreasing cerebral blood volume in order to maintain normal ICP of 5 to 15 mm Hg. Typically, these compensatory mechanisms keep the volume and pressure of these three components in a state of equilibrium, resulting in normal ICP.

When a pathologic condition causes these compensatory mechanisms to fail, ICP begins to increase. Increased ICP is characterized by pressure greater than 15 mm Hg and is potentially life threatening. Increasing pressure in the skull diminishes the functioning of various cranial areas and, if unrelieved, affects the vital centers. Aggressive treatment of increased ICP is thought to improve survival and function in clients who have a pathologic condition associated with increased ICP.

Possible causes
Increased brain volume
- Abscess
- Edema
- Neoplasm

Increased blood volume
- Decreased venous return
- Hemorrhage and hematoma formation

- Hypercapnia
- Hypoxemia
- Increased arterial blood flow
- Increased intrathoracic pressure
- Pooling of venous blood

Increased CSF flow
- Deficient CSF absorption
- Increased production of CSF
- Obstruction

Data collection findings
- Alterations in LOC
- Headache
- Motor, sensory, or reflex dysfunction
- Respiratory dysfunction
- Vomiting with or without nausea
- Oculomotor dysfunction
- Pupillary dysfunction
- Papilledema
- Posturing (decerebrate, decorticate)
- Brain herniation syndromes
- Cushing's phenomenon or response

Diagnostic findings
- CT scan, MRI, skull X-ray, or cerebral angiography reveals underlying pathology precipitating the signs and symptoms of increased ICP.
- Volume-pressure response test measures change in ICP induced by adding 1 ml of fluid or withdrawing 1 ml of CSF (normal response is 2 mm Hg or less increase in ICP; abnormal response is 2 mm Hg or more increase in ICP [indicates decreased compliance]).
- Pressure-volume index test is used to measure the amount of fluid necessary to cause a 10 mm Hg change in ICP (normal response is 25 ml; abnormal response is less than 10 ml and indicates decreased compliance).
- Positive emission tomography (PET) scan may reveal decreased cerebral metabolism and blood flow characteristics.
- Evoked potential studies are used to locate brain lesions and evaluate brain stem integrity.
- Transcranial Doppler ultrasonography may reveal decreased cerebral metabolism and blood flow characteristics.

Nursing diagnoses
- Decreased intracranial adaptive capacity
- Ineffective tissue perfusion (cerebral)
- Ineffective breathing pattern

Treatment
- Deliberate hyperventilation to maintain hypocapnia with $Paco_2$ of 25 to 30 mm Hg
- Restricted fluid intake
- 30- to 45-degree elevation of head of bed as well as avoidance of extreme neck flexion or turning, extreme hip flexion, Valsalva's maneuver, and isometric muscle contractions
- Maintenance of normothermia
- Hypothermia
- Control of noxious auditory, tactile, and visual environmental stimuli
- Avoidance of clustering of nursing care
- ICP monitoring (for example, with an epidural probe, a subarachnoid screw, or an intraventricular catheter)
- Craniotomy

Drug therapy options
- Analgesic: acetaminophen (Tylenol), codeine phosphate, or codeine sulfate
- Antipyretic: acetaminophen (Tylenol)
- Antishivering agent: chlorpromazine (Thorazine)
- Barbiturate: thiopental (Pentothal) or pentobarbital (Nembutal)
- Diuretic: ethacrynic acid (Edecrin), furosemide (Lasix), or mannitol (Osmitrol)
- Glucocorticoid: dexamethasone (Decadron)
- H_2-receptor antagonist: cimetidine (Tagamet), famotidine (Pepcid), or ranitidine (Zantac)
- Hyperosmolar agent: mannitol (Osmitrol) 20% or glycerol 10%
- Paralyzant: pancuronium (Pavulon)

Patient care goals
- The client will have an ICP of 5 to 15 mm Hg.
- The client won't have sustained increases in ICP during nursing interventions, monitoring activities, or nursing care activities.
- The client will regain a usual or an improved LOC, cognition, and motor-sensory function.
- The client will experience no preventable complications associated with increased ICP.

Nursing interventions
- Maintain a patent airway *to promote oxygenation of cerebral tissues.*
- Administer oxygen as ordered *to maintain a Pao_2 between 80 and 100 mm Hg, which promotes oxygenation of cerebral tissues.*

● Assist in monitoring ABG levels, *to help determine if Pao$_2$ is in the desired range and if Paco$_2$ is between 25 and 30 mm Hg, which is ideal for cerebral vasoconstriction and decreased blood flow and helps decrease ICP.*

● Assist with administration of medications (such as a hyperosmolar agent, diuretic, and glucocorticoid) *to reduce cerebral edema and increase serum osmolality, which causes water to move from extracellular brain tissue into the intravascular space. Excess body water is thus eliminated by pulling it from the brain and depositing it in the cardiovascular system.*

● Raise the head of the client's bed 30 to 45 degrees *to reduce edema of cerebral tissues by promoting cerebral venous drainage.*

● Assess neurologic status every 1 to 2 hours *to determine baseline and then to detect changes in neurologic status and signs and symptoms of increased ICP.*

● Avoid extreme flexion of the client's head and neck *to reduce edema of cerebral tissues and decrease ICP by promoting cerebral venous drainage.*

● Avoid extreme flexion of the client's hips *to prevent trapping of venous blood in the intra-abdominal space — which increases intra-abdominal and intrathoracic pressure — and reduce cerebral venous drainage.*

● Maintain a patent I.V. site for administration of medications (such as a paralyzant, an analgesic, and an antishivering drug) *to control posturing, restlessness, and shivering and to reduce the metabolic rate, consequently reducing the needs of the cerebral tissue.*

● Control noxious auditory, tactile, and visual stimuli in the client's environment *to prevent increases in ICP.*

Evaluation

● The client has an ICP of 5 to 15 mm Hg.

● The client doesn't have sustained increases in ICP during nursing interventions, monitoring activities, or nursing care activities.

● The client regains usual or improved LOC, cognition, and motor-sensory function.

● The client experiences no preventable complications associated with increased ICP.

Meningitis

In MENINGITIS, the brain and the spinal cord meninges become inflamed, usually as a result of bacterial infection. Such inflammation may involve all three meningeal membranes: the dura mater, arachnoid, and pia mater.

The prognosis is good and complications are rare, especially if the disease is recognized early and the infecting organism responds to antibiotics. The prognosis is poorer for infants and elderly people. Mortality is high in untreated meningitis.

Possible causes

● Bacterial infection (may occur secondary to bacteremia [especially from pneumonia, empyema, osteomyelitis, and endocarditis], sinusitis, otitis media, encephalitis, myelitis, or brain abscess)

● Head trauma (may follow a skull fracture, a penetrating head wound, lumbar puncture, or ventricular shunting procedure)

● Virus (in aseptic viral meningitis, which is usually mild and self-limiting)

● Fungal or protozoal infection (less common)

Data collection findings

● Malaise

● Chills

● Fever

● Headache

● Stiff neck and back

● Photophobia

● Positive Brudzinski's sign, in which the client flexes hips or knees when the nurse places her hands behind his neck and bends it forward (a sign of meningeal inflammation and irritation)

● Positive Kernig's sign (pain or resistance when the client's leg is flexed at the hip or knee while he's in a supine position)

● Vomiting

● Exaggerated deep tendon reflexes

● Visual alterations (diplopia — two images of a single object)

● Confusion

● Delirium

● Deep stupor

● Coma

● Increased ICP

● Irritability

● Opisthotonos (a spasm in which the back and extremities arch backward so that the body rests on the head and heels)

● Petechial, purpuric, or ecchymotic rash on the lower part of the body (meningococcal meningitis)

● Seizures

● Twitching

Diagnostic findings

● A lumbar puncture shows elevated CSF pressure, cloudy or milky white CSF, high protein level, positive Gram stain and culture that usually identifies the infecting organism (unless it's a virus) and depressed CSF glucose concentration.

● Chest X-rays may reveal pneumonitis or lung abscess, tubercular lesions, or granulomas secondary to fungal infection.

● Sinus and skull films may help identify the presence of cranial osteomyelitis, paranasal sinusitis, or skull fracture.

● WBC count reveals leukocytosis.

● CT scan can rule out cerebral hematoma, hemorrhage, or tumor.

Nursing diagnoses

● Decreased intracranial adaptive capacity
● Hyperthermia
● Risk for injury

Treatment

● Bed rest
● Hypothermia
● I.V. fluid administration
● Oxygen therapy, possibly with ET intubation and mechanical ventilation

Drug therapy options

● Antibiotic: penicillin G (Pfizerpen), ampicillin (Omnipen), or nafcillin (Unipen); tetracycline (Achromycin V), or chloramphenicol (Chloromycetin), if allergic to penicillin
● Cardiac glycoside: digoxin (Lanoxin)
● Diuretic: mannitol (Osmitrol)
● Anticonvulsant: phenytoin (Dilantin), phenobarbital (Luminal)
● Analgesic or antipyretic: acetaminophen (Tylenol), aspirin
● Anesthetic: lidocaine (Xylocaine)
● Laxative: bisacodyl (Dulcolax)
● Stool softener: docusate (Colace)

Patient care goals

● The client will maintain normal ICP.
● The client will exhibit a normal temperature.
● The client will remain free from injury.

Nursing interventions

● Assess neurologic function often to detect early signs of increased ICP, such as plucking at the bedcovers, vomiting, seizures, and a change in motor function and vital signs. *Detecting early signs of increased ICP prevents treatment delay.*

● Watch for deterioration in the client's condition, *which may signal an impending crisis.*

● Monitor fluid balance. Maintain adequate fluid intake *to avoid dehydration without causing fluid overload, which may lead to cerebral edema.*

● Measure intake and output accurately and maintain safety of devices measuring CVP *to determine fluid volume status.*

● Suction the client only if necessary. Limit suctioning to 10 to 15 seconds per pass of the catheter. Suctioning stimulates coughing and Valsalva's maneuver; *Valsalva's maneuvers increase intrathoracic pressure, decrease cerebral venous drainage, and increase cerebral blood volume, resulting in increased ICP.*

● Hyperoxygenate the lungs with 100% oxygen for 1 minute before and after suctioning. Hypercapnia results in cerebral vasodilation, increased blood volume, and increased ICP. *Preoxygenation helps avoid hypoxemia and tissue ischemia.*

● Maintain I.V. site patency for administration of lidocaine if prescribed (it may also be prescribed to be given via the ET tube before suctioning). *Lidocaine suppresses the cough reflex, thereby preventing increases in ICP.*

● Watch for adverse reactions to I.V. antibiotics and other drugs *to prevent complications such as anaphylaxis.*

● Check the I.V. site often, and change the site according to facility policy *to avoid infiltration and phlebitis.*

● Position the client carefully *to prevent joint stiffness and neck pain.*

● Turn the client often, according to a planned positioning schedule *to prevent skin breakdown.*

● Assist with ROM exercises *to prevent contractures.*

● It may be necessary to provide small, frequent meals or supplement meals with NG tube or parenteral feedings *to maintain adequate nutrition and elimination.*

● Give the client a mild laxative or stool softener *to prevent constipation and to minimize the risk of increased ICP resulting from straining during defecation.*

● Ensure the client's comfort *to prevent rises in ICP.*

● Provide mouth care regularly *to prevent breakdown of the oral mucosa and to promote client comfort.*

● Maintain a quiet environment. *Auditory stimuli can contribute to increased ICP.*

● Darken the room *to decrease photophobia.*

● Relieve headache with a nonnarcotic analgesic, such as aspirin or acetaminophen. *Narcotics interfere with accurate neurologic assessment.*

- Provide reassurance and support. The client may be frightened by his illness and frequent lumbar punctures. *These measures decrease anxiety; emotional upsets may increase ICP.*
- Reassure the family that the delirium and behavior changes caused by meningitis usually disappear *to allay anxiety.*
- Follow strict sterile technique when treating clients with head wounds or skull fractures *to prevent meningitis.*

Evaluation

- The client has normal ICP and adequate cerebral perfusion.
- The client has a normal temperature.
- The client is free from injury.

Multiple sclerosis

MULTIPLE SCLEROSIS (MS) is a progressive degenerative disease that affects the myelin sheath surrounding the axons in the CNS. It's a leading cause of neurologic disability between ages 20 and 40.

MS is characterized by periods of exacerbation and remission:
- During periods of exacerbation, well-circumscribed areas of patchy demyelination, or plaques, are scattered along the myelin sheath. Conduction of nerve impulses along affected axons is slowed or inhibited, producing neurologic deficits.
- During periods of remission, the myelin sheath affected during exacerbation undergoes myelinization. Conduction of nerve impulses along affected axons returns to normal, and the neurologic deficits that developed during exacerbation are reversed. In most instances, however, recovery from each period of exacerbation is incomplete, causing a stepwise decline in neurologic function.

Possible causes

- Autoimmune response
- Cell-mediated immune reaction
- Environmental or genetic factors
- Infection by a slow, latent virus
- Susceptibility gene

Data collection findings

- Cerebellar dysfunction (signs and symptoms include ataxia, dysarthria, incoordination, tremor, vertigo)
- Cognitive dysfunction (signs and symptoms include deceased concentration and short-term memory, depression, difficulty finding words and learning new information, euphoria, and short attention span)
- Cranial nerve dysfunction (signs and symptoms include blind spots, blurred central vision, diplopia, dysphagia, facial weakness, faded colors, numbness, and pain)
- Motor dysfunction (signs and symptoms include abnormal gait, paralysis, spasticity, and weakness)
- Sensory dysfunction (symptoms include decreased proprioception and temperature perception, Lhermitte's sign, and paresthesia)
- Bowel and bladder dysfunction (signs and symptoms include constipation; fecal incontinence and urgency; nocturia; urinary frequency, hesitancy, incontinence, and urgency; urine retention)
- Sexual dysfunction (signs and symptoms include decreased libido, orgasmic ability, and genital sensation [women]; ejaculatory, erectile, and orgasmic dysfunction and fatigue [men])

Diagnostic findings

- CSF analysis may reveal elevation of oligoclonal bands of immunoglobulin G, protein, Υ-globulin, myelin basic protein, and lymphocytes.
- CT scan or MRI may reveal plaques and demyelination in the CNS or an underlying pathology that precipitate the signs and symptoms of MS.
- Evoked potentials may reveal slowing or absence of nerve conduction along the visual, auditory, and somatosensory pathways.
- PET scan may reveal altered locations and patterns of cerebral glucose metabolism.
- EMG may reveal slowing of nerve conduction.

Nursing diagnoses

- Impaired physical mobility
- Disturbed body image
- Self-care deficit: Bathing or hygiene, dressing or grooming, or toileting
- Interrupted family processes

Treatment

- High-fiber diet adjusted for the client's ability to chew or swallow
- Active or passive ROM exercises
- Dietary consultation
- Physical therapy
- Speech therapy
- Plasmapheresis (for antibody removal)

Drug therapy options

- Cholinergic: bethanechol (Urecholine)
- Glucocorticoid: corticotropin, dexamethasone (Decadron), prednisone (Deltasone)
- Immunosuppressant: cyclophosphamide (Cytoxan), interferon beta-1b (Betaseron), methotrexate (Folex)
- Skeletal muscle relaxant: baclofen (Lioresal), dantrolene (Dantrium)

Patient care goals

- The client will retain a usual or an improved level of neurologic functioning.
- The client will develop maximal self-care abilities and physical mobility and an effective means of communication within the limits imposed by MS.
- The client will experience no preventable complications associated with MS.
- The client will develop strategies to effectively cope with health problems and body image disturbances associated with MS.

Nursing interventions

- Assess neurologic status and vital signs, at least once every 8 hours, *to determine baseline and detect changes.*
- Encourage the client to eat a high-fiber diet, adjusted for his ability to chew or swallow *to promote adequate nutritional status, meet metabolic needs, and promote bowel regularity.*
- Consult a speech therapist *to evaluate and treat communication or swallowing problems.*
- Assess gag reflex and ability to swallow *to prevent aspiration of food particles.*
- Monitor weight on a weekly basis *to determine nutritional status.*
- Encourage fluid intake of 2½ qt (2.4 L) every 24 hours, unless contraindicated, *to promote normovolemia and optimal urinary function.*
- Institute a bowel and bladder program *to promote urinary and fecal continence.*
- Encourage communication *to promote independence and self-esteem.*
- Administer prescribed medications on schedule *to maintain therapeutic drug levels and an optimal level of neurologic functioning.*
- Consult both a physical and an occupational therapist *to evaluate which adaptive assistive devices the client may need to independently and safely perform activities of daily living (ADLs).*
- Provide uninterrupted rest periods *to help conserve energy, reduce the client's oxygen demand, reduce fatigue, and*

restore the client to an optimal level of neurologic functioning.

- Perform active or passive ROM exercises *to maintain joint mobility and prevent contractures.*
- Encourage the client to express feelings about changes in his body image and neurologic functioning *to help him cope with body changes caused by MS.*

Evaluation

- The client retains a usual or an improved level of neurologic functioning.
- The client develops maximal self-care abilities and physical mobility and an effective means of communication within the limits imposed by MS.
- The client experiences no preventable complications associated with MS.
- The client develops strategies to effectively cope with health problems and body image disturbances associated with MS.

Myasthenia gravis

MYASTHENIA GRAVIS (MG) is a chronic, progressive neuromuscular disorder that affects normal conduction of nerve impulses across the neuromuscular junction. Under normal circumstances, the neurotransmitter ACh is released from storage vesicles in the axonal ending. ACh then diffuses across the synaptic cleft between the axonal ending and the muscle fiber, attaches to ACh receptor sites located primarily on the peaks of the junctional folds of the muscle fiber, and stimulates the muscle fiber to contract. The enzyme acetylcholinesterase then destroys the ACh, thus terminating nerve impulse conduction across the neuromuscular junction.

Clients with MG have a normal amount of ACh available at the neuromuscular junction, but the structure of the junction is altered. Between 60% and 90% of those clients have antibodies to ACh receptor sites, strongly indicating an autoimmune mechanism. These antibodies change the structure of the neuromuscular junction by accelerating the degeneration of ACh receptor sites. The outcome of this process is a reduction of the absolute number of functioning ACh receptor sites by 70% to 80%, development of a decreased number of shallow junctional folds, and a widened synaptic cleft. These structural changes result in the typical symptoms of MG: weakness and abnormal fatigability of skeletal muscles — especially those involved in ocular movements, facial expression, respiration, chewing, and swallowing — that's exacerbated by exercise and relieved by rest.

Possible causes
- Autoimmune disease (antibodies to ACh receptors found in 60% to 90% of clients with MG)

Data collection findings
- Muscle weakness and fatigue (typically muscles are strongest in the morning but weaken throughout the day, especially after exercise)
- Blurred vision
- Difficulty chewing
- Diminished vital capacity
- Diplopia
- Drooling
- Dysarthria
- Dysphagia
- Dyspnea
- Facial droop
- Flat facial affect
- Nasal regurgitation
- Nasal, monotone speech
- Ptosis
- Shallow, slowed respirations
- Soft or inaudible voice
- Strabismus

Diagnostic findings
- EMG may reveal a decrease in amplitude of muscle contraction with progressive stimulation.
- Chest X-ray or CT scan may reveal thymoma or hyperplasia of the thymus gland.
- I.V. drug challenge with neostigmine (Prostigmin) or edrophonium (Tensilon) may relieve symptoms in clients with MG.
- Blood chemistry test results may reveal ACh receptor antibody levels and elevated thyroid function tests.

Nursing diagnoses
- Impaired physical mobility
- Ineffective breathing pattern
- Risk for aspiration
- Ineffective coping
- Disturbed body image

Treatment
- Oxygen therapy
- Intermittent positive-pressure breathing (IPPB) and chest physiotherapy
- Mechanical ventilation and suctioning
- Active or passive ROM exercises

- Small, frequent high-calorie meals and high-calorie snacks and supplements adjusted for the client's ability to chew or swallow
- Dietary consultation
- Physical therapy
- Speech therapy
- Plasmapheresis (in clients with severe exacerbation) to remove circulating ACh receptor antibodies
- Thymectomy to remove thymoma or thymic hyperplasia, which is suspected of synthesizing ACh receptor antibodies

Drug therapy options
- Anticholinesterase inhibitor: neostigmine (Prostigmin), pyridostigmine (Mestinon)
- Glucocorticoid: corticotropin, dexamethasone (Decadron), prednisone (Deltasone)
- Immunosuppressant: azathioprine (Imuran), cyclophosphamide (Cytoxan)

Patient care goals
- The client will retain a usual or an improved level of functioning of affected muscles.
- The client will develop maximal self-care abilities and physical mobility and an effective means of communication within the limits imposed by MG.
- The client will experience no preventable complications associated with MG.
- The client will develop strategies to effectively cope with health problems and body image disturbances associated with MG.

Nursing interventions
- Maintain a patent airway and administer oxygen *to promote oxygenation of tissues.*
- Encourage the client to cough and deep breathe *to help mobilize secretions in the airway.*
- Provide IPPB and chest physiotherapy as prescribed *to mobilize secretions in the airway and expand the lungs.*
- Have emergency intubation equipment readily available. *Respiratory muscle weakness may be severe enough in a myasthenic crisis to require emergency intubation and mechanical ventilation.*
- Assess neurologic status at least once every 8 hours, or as indicated, *to determine baseline and to detect changes in neurologic status as well as early signs and symptoms of myasthenic or cholinergic crisis.*
- Assess respiratory status at least once every 8 hours, or as indicated, *to determine baseline and to detect changes*

in respiratory status as well as early signs and symptoms of respiratory distress resulting from respiratory muscle weakness during a myasthenic crisis.

● Assess the client's gag reflex and ability to swallow *to prevent aspiration and to determine the extent of the neurologic deficit.*

● Administer prescribed medications on schedule *to maintain continuous therapeutic drug levels and an optimal level of neurologic functioning.*

● Plan activities early in the day or during energy peaks that follow administration of medications *to ensure that the client is at an optimal level of neurologic functioning during these activities.*

● Encourage the client to eat small, frequent, high-calorie meals and high-calorie snacks and supplements, adjusted for his ability to chew or swallow, *to help conserve energy, promote adequate nutritional status, and meet metabolic demands.*

● Consult a speech therapist *to evaluate the client's ability to communicate and swallow and to determine an effective regimen for doing both.*

● Monitor weight weekly *to help determine the client's nutritional status.*

● Consult a physical therapist and an occupational therapist *to evaluate which adaptive assistive devices the client may need to independently and safely perform ADLs.*

● Assess the client for signs and symptoms of a myasthenic or cholinergic crisis. A myasthenic crisis can occur as a result of undermedication and a cholinergic crisis can occur as a result of overmedication.

● Encourage the client to express his feelings about changes in his body image *to reduce his tendency to suppress or repress those feelings and to help him cope.*

Evaluation

● The client retains a usual or an improved level of functioning of affected muscles.

● The client develops maximal self-care abilities and physical mobility and an effective means of communication within the limits imposed by MG.

● The client experiences no preventable complications associated with MG.

● The client develops strategies to effectively cope with health problems associated with MG.

FAST FACT

A client with MG can develop cholinergic crisis due to overmedication. Expect to see these muscarinic or nicotinic effects of cholinergic (anticholinesterase) drugs:

● abdominal cramping
● constricted pupils
● diaphoresis
● diarrhea
● fasciculations of eyes and mouth
● increased salivation.

Parkinson's disease

PARKINSON'S DISEASE is a CNS disorder that results in widespread, progressive degeneration of dopamine-producing cells of the substantia nigra in the brain and, consequently, a decrease in the level of the neurotransmitter dopamine.

When dopamine levels are normal, the excitatory cholinergic pathways and the inhibitory dopaminergic pathways are usually balanced, so the client can control or limit voluntary motor movement. However, when dopamine levels are decreased, the pathways are unbalanced, so the client can't control or limit voluntary motor movement, resulting in the signs and symptoms of Parkinson's disease: tremors, muscular rigidity, bradykinesia, akathisia, dyskinesia, weakness, and fatigue. These signs and symptoms typically occur when 70% of the dopamine-producing cells in the substantia nigra have degenerated.

Possible causes

● Drug therapy (for example, with methyldopa or reserpine)

● Metabolic conditions (for example, Huntington's chorea and Wilson's disease)

● Neurotoxins

● Postencephalitis

● Structural conditions (for example, basal ganglia infarction, hydrocephalus, repeated head trauma, tumors)

Data collection findings

● Akathisia
● Bradykinesia
● Cogwheel, plastic, or lead pipe rigidity
● Difficulty swallowing
● Drooling

- Dyskinesia
- Dysphagia
- Fatigue
- Flexed trunk and stooped posture
- Hypophonia
- Dysarthria
- Masklike facies with wide-open, fixed staring eyes
- Muscular rigidity
- Restricted chest wall movement
- Shuffling gait
- Small handwriting
- Tremors (pill-rolling, resting)
- Weakness

Diagnostic findings

- Diagnosis of Parkinson's disease is made on the basis of a comprehensive history and physical examination; there are no specific diagnostic tests for Parkinson's disease.
- The following tests may be ordered to reveal whether another underlying pathology is precipitating the signs and symptoms of Parkinson's disease:
  – skull X-rays
  – CT scan
  – MRI
  – EEG
  – EMG
  – urinalysis
  – CSF analysis
  – drug screen.

Nursing diagnoses

- Impaired physical mobility
- Risk for injury
- Disturbed body image
- Ineffective coping

Treatment

- Small, frequent high-calorie meals and high-calorie snacks and supplements adjusted for the client's ability to chew or swallow
- Active or passive ROM exercises
- Dietary consultation
- Occupational therapy
- Physical therapy
- Speech therapy
- Stereotactic neurosurgery (for example, thalamotomy or pallidotomy)

Drug therapy options

- Anticholinergic: trihexyphenidyl (Artane)
- Antihistamine: diphenhydramine (Benadryl)
- Antiviral agent: amantadine (Symmetrel)
- Dopaminergic agent: benztropine (Cogentin), carbidopa-levodopa (Sinemet), levodopa (Larodopa)
- Dopamine agonist: bromocriptine (Parlodel), pergolide (Permax)
- Monoamine oxidase inhibitor: selegiline (Deprenyl)
- Antispasmodic: procyclidine (Kemadrin)
- Antidepressant: amitriptyline (Elavil)

Patient care goals

- The client will retain a usual or an improved level of neurologic functioning.
- The client will develop maximal self-care abilities and physical mobility and an effective means of communication within the limits imposed by Parkinson's disease.
- The client will experience no preventable complications associated with Parkinson's disease.
- The client will develop strategies to effectively cope with health problems and body image disturbances associated with Parkinson's disease.

Nursing interventions

- Assess neurologic status at least once every 8 hours *to determine baseline and detect changes in neurologic status.*
- Encourage the client to eat small, frequent, high-calorie meals and high-calorie snacks and supplements, adjusted for his ability to chew or swallow, *to promote adequate nutritional status and to meet his metabolic needs.*
- Consult a speech therapist *to evaluate the client's ability to communicate and swallow and to determine an effective regimen for doing both.*
- Assess the client's gag reflex and ability to swallow *to prevent aspiration of food particles.*
- Monitor the client's weight weekly *to determine nutritional status.*
- Provide ample time for communicating *to decrease the client's frustration and to promote independence and self-esteem.*
- Administer prescribed medications on schedule *to maintain continuous therapeutic drug levels and an optimal level of neurologic functioning.*
- Consult a physical therapist and an occupational therapist *to evaluate which adaptive assistive devices the client may need to independently and safely perform ADLs.*
- Provide ample time for the client to perform activities of daily living and to move around *to decrease the client's*

frustration and promote safety, independence, and self-esteem.

● Manipulate the environment (for example, by removing clutter) *to promote client safety and prevent injury.*

● Encourage the client to express his feelings about changes in his body image *to reduce his tendency to suppress or repress those feelings and to help him cope.*

Evaluation

● The client retains a usual or an improved level of neurologic functioning.

● The client develops maximal self-care abilities and physical mobility and an effective means of communication within the limits imposed by Parkinson's disease.

● The client experiences no preventable complications associated with Parkinson's disease.

● The client develops strategies to effectively cope with health problems and body image disturbances associated with Parkinson's disease.

Seizure disorders (epilepsy)

A seizure is an uncontrolled discharge of neurons in the cerebral cortex. It interferes with normal CNS function, altering sensation, behavior, movement, perception, or consciousness. This alteration may be as brief as a blank stare, lasting a second, or long-lasting as a tonic-clonic seizure, lasting several minutes, accompanied by loss of consciousness, bowel and bladder incontinence, and respiratory cessation. Signs and symptoms depend on the region of the cerebral cortex in which the seizure originates and the path of spread.

Epilepsy is defined as recurrent seizures. It isn't a disease but rather a sign of a CNS disorder. Epilepsy can be classified as partial (seizure begins in a local area), generalized (associated with loss of consciousness; convulsive or nonconvulsive, bilateral without focal onset), or unclassified (because of inadequate data). (See *Classifying seizures,* page 322.)

Possible causes
Structural factors

● Cerebrovascular disorder (such as embolism, hemorrhage, or ischemia)

● Head trauma

● Infection (such as brain abscess, encephalitis, meningitis, or opportunistic lesions from acquired immune deficiency syndrome)

● Space-occupying lesions (such as arteriovenous malformation [AVM], neurofibromatosis, primary and metastatic brain tumors, or subdural hematoma)

Metabolic-nutritional factors

● Acidosis

● Amino acid or fat metabolism disorder

● Drug withdrawal (for example, alcohol, barbiturates, or diazepam [Valium])

● Electrolyte or water imbalance (for example, hypocalcemia, hypocapnia, hypoglycemia, hyponatremia)

● Hypoxia

● Pyridoxine deficiency

● Toxins and toxic factors (such as heavy metals, street drugs, systemic disorders [such as toxemia and uremia], and toxic levels of any drug)

Genetic factors

● Chromosomal abnormalities

Data collection findings

● Aura just before onset of the seizure (client reports unusual tastes, feelings, or odors)

● Eyes deviating to a particular side or blinking

● Irregular breathing with spasms

● Usually unresponsiveness during tonic-clonic muscular contractions (and possibly incontinence)

● Possible disorientation to time and place, drowsiness, and lack of coordination (immediately after a seizure)

Diagnostic findings

● EEG may reveal abnormal patterns of electrical activity.

● CT scan or MRI may reveal that an underlying pathology precipitated the seizures.

● ABG levels may reveal acidosis, hypocapnia, or hypoxia.

● CSF analysis may point to increased ICP or infection (for example, meningitis) as the underlying pathology that precipitated the seizures.

● Blood chemistry test results may reveal acidosis, elevated prescription drug levels, hypoglycemia, hyponatremia, toxic conditions (such as uremia), or toxic substances (such as cocaine or heavy metals).

Nursing diagnoses

● Risk for injury

● Ineffective airway clearance

● Risk for aspiration

● Disturbed body image

Classifying seizures

Seizures can take various forms depending on their origin and whether they're localized to one area of the brain (as occurs in partial seizures) or in both hemispheres (as happens in generalized seizures). This chart describes each type of seizure and lists common signs and symptoms.

TYPE	CLIENT DESCRIPTION	SIGNS AND SYMPTOMS
Partial		
Simple partial	Symptoms confined to one hemisphere	May have motor (change in posture), sensory (hallucinations), or autonomic (flushing, tachycardia) symptoms; no loss of consciousness
Complex partial	Begins in one focal area but spreads to both hemispheres (more common in adults)	Loss of consciousness; aura of visual disturbances; postictal symptoms
Generalized		
Absence (petit mal)	Sudden onset; lasts 5 to 10 seconds; can have 100 daily; precipitated by stress, hyperventilation, hypoglycemia, fatigue; differentiated from daydreaming	Loss of responsiveness but continued ability to maintain posture control and not fall; twitching eyelids; lip smacking; no postictal symptoms
Myoclonic	Movement disorder (not a seizure); seen as client awakens or falls asleep; may be precipitated by touch or visual stimuli; focal or generalized; symmetrical or asymmetrical	No loss of consciousness; sudden, brief, shocklike involuntary contraction of one muscle group
Clonic	Opposing muscles contract and relax alternately in rhythmic pattern; may occur in one limb more than others	Mucus production
Tonic	Muscles are maintained in continuous contracted state (rigid posture)	Variable loss of consciousness; pupils dilate; eyes roll up; glottis closes; possible incontinence; may foam at mouth
Tonic-clonic (grand mal, major motor)	Violent total body seizure	Aura; tonic first (20 to 40 seconds); clonic next; postictal symptoms
Atonic	Drop and fall attack; needs to wear protective helmet	Loss of posture tone
Akinetic	Sudden brief loss of muscle tone or posture	Temporary loss of consciousness
Miscellaneous		
Febrile	Seizure threshold lowered by elevated temperature; only one seizure per fever; common in 4% of population under age 5; occurs when temperature is rapidly rising	Lasts less than 5 minutes; generalized, transient, and nonprogressive; doesn't generally result in brain damage; EEG is normal after 2 weeks
Status epilepticus	Prolonged or frequent repetition of seizures without interruption; results in anoxia and cardiac and respiratory arrest	Consciousness not regained between seizures; lasts more than 30 minutes

Treatment

- Supportive oxygen therapy and suctioning, as needed (maintaining airway and preventing injury), until the seizure ends
- Cortical resection of epileptic focus
- Corpus callosotomy
- Anterior temporal lobe resection

Drug therapy options

- Barbiturate: phenobarbital (Luminol)
- Benzodiazepine: diazepam (Valium)
- Deoxybarbiturate: primidone (Mysoline)
- Hydantoin: phenytoin (Dilantin)
- Iminostilbene: carbamazepine (Tegretol)
- Miscellaneous drugs: felbamate (Felbatol), gabapentin (Neurontin), lamotrigine (Lamictal), valproic acid (Depakene), or vigabatrin (Sabril)
- Oxazolidinedione: trimethadione (Tridione)
- Succinimide: ethosuximide (Zarontin)

Patient care goals

- The client will regain usual or improved LOC, cognition, and motor-sensory function after and between seizures.
- The client will experience no preventable complications associated with seizures.
- The client will develop strategies to effectively cope with health problems and body image disturbances associated with seizures.

Nursing interventions

Before seizure

- If the client has a seizure disorder, institute seizure precautions *to prevent him from injuring himself during a seizure.*

During seizure

- Note the date, time of onset, and duration of the seizure as well as what the client was doing when the seizure started *to help diagnose the type of seizure and to develop a therapeutic treatment plan.*
- Provide privacy *to preserve the client's dignity and self-esteem during the seizure.*
- If the client is standing, lower him to a flat surface *so he doesn't injure himself.*
- Maintain a patent airway and administer oxygen *to promote oxygenation of the client's tissues.*
- Suction as needed *to clear secretions from the client's airway.*

- Turn the client's head to one side *to allow secretions to drain from his mouth.*
- Guide, if necessary, don't restrain, the movement of the client's limbs *to prevent injury to the client.*
- Note the seizure activity (including the body parts involved, sequence, character of movements, head and eye deviation, and behavior) *to help diagnose the type of seizure and develop a therapeutic treatment plan.*
- Administer prescribed medications on schedule *to maintain continuous therapeutic drug levels and an optimal level of neurologic functioning.*

After seizure

- Assess the client's vital signs and neurologic status *to detect changes from baseline.*
- Encourage the client to express feelings about changes in his body image *to help him cope with changes caused by the seizure disorder.*

Evaluation

- The client regains usual or improved LOC, cognition, and motor-sensory function after seizures.
- The client experiences no preventable complications associated with seizures.
- The client develops strategies to effectively cope with health problems and body image disturbances associated with seizures.

 SPOT CHECK

Would you expect all clients with epilepsy to have abnormal EEGs?

Answer: No. A normal EEG doesn't always exclude a diagnosis of epilepsy; conversely, an abnormal EEG doesn't always confirm the diagnosis. During a seizure, EEG abnormalities are present; between seizures, a client with epilepsy may show no abnormalities or abnormalities not characteristic of seizure disorders.

Spinal cord injury

SPINAL CORD INJURY usually results from a traumatic force to the vertebral column. This injury typically has lifelong consequences, not only for the client but also for family members and society.

Spinal cord injuries are classified by type, level, degree, mechanism, and force of injury:

- Types of injury are classified as concussion, contusion, laceration, transection, or hemorrhage.

- Levels of injury are classified as cervical, thoracic, or lumbar. An injury to the spinal cord at the cervical level may result in QUADRIPLEGIA. An injury to the spinal cord at the thoracic or lumbar level may result in PARAPLEGIA.
- Degrees of injury are classified as complete or incomplete:
– A complete injury initially results in flaccid paralysis and total loss of motor, sensory, reflex, and bowel and bladder function below the level of injury.
– An incomplete injury is a mixed pattern of motor, sensory, reflex, and bowel and bladder function below the level of injury because some spinal cord tracts remain intact.
- The major mechanisms of injury are acceleration, deceleration, deformation, axial loading or vertical compression, and penetration.
- The four forces of injury are flexion, extension, rotation, and compression.

After a spinal cord injury, necrosis and scar tissue form in the area of the traumatized spinal cord, resulting in typical signs and symptoms: varying, and commonly catastrophic, degrees of permanent neurologic deficits, depending on the specific nerve tracts damaged.

Possible causes
- Congenital anomalies
- Diving into shallow water
- Falling
- Gunshot wounds
- Infections
- Sports injuries
- Stab wounds
- Tumors
- Vehicular accidents

Data collection findings
- Complete or incomplete loss of the following functions below the level of the injury:
– Voluntary motor movement
– Pain, light touch, temperature, pressure, and proprioception
– Reflex activity
– Autonomic activity
– Localized pain or tenderness over the site of injury
– Bowel and bladder dysfunction
– Respiratory distress

Diagnostic findings
- CT scan or MRI may reveal changes in the spinal cord, vertebrae, and soft tissue surrounding the spine.

- Myelography may reveal blockage or disruption of the spinal canal.
- Spinal X-rays may reveal fracture, deformity, or displacement of vertebrae as well as soft-tissue masses such as hematomas.

Nursing diagnoses
- Impaired physical mobility
- Impaired gas exchange
- Powerlessness
- Disturbed body image

Treatment
- Immobilization, reduction, and alignment of injured area of spinal column (for example, Crutchfield, Vinke, or Gardner-Wells tongs with cervical traction, halo external fixation device, body jacket, Minerva jacket)
- Cervical traction
- Pin care
- Halo external fixation device care
- Bed rest on a firm surface (for example, on a kinetic, CircOlectric, or RotoRest bed or Stryker frame) until the client's condition stabilizes; then ambulation
- Oxygen therapy
- IPPB and chest physiotherapy
- Mechanical ventilation and suctioning
- Enteral nutrition through an enteral feeding tube (for example, gastrostomy, percutaneous gastrostomy [PEG], or percutaneous jejunostomy [PEJ]) or TPN, as prescribed
- High-protein, high-fiber diet
- Consultation with a dietitian
- Physical therapy
- Occupational therapy
- Antiembolism or sequential compression stockings
- Bowel and bladder program
- Surgery to stabilize the injured spine (for example, insertion of Harrington rods)

Drug therapy options
- Analgesic: acetaminophen (Tylenol), codeine
- Anticoagulant: heparin
- Anxiolytic: lorazepam (Ativan)
- Glucocorticoid: methylprednisolone (Solu-Medrol)
- H_2-receptor antagonist: cimetidine (Tagamet), famotidine (Pepcid), ranitidine (Zantac)
- Laxative: bisacodyl (Dulcolax)
- Muscle relaxant: dantrolene (Dantrium), baclofen (Lioresal)

Patient care goals

- The client will retain a usual or an improved level of neurologic functioning.
- The client will develop maximal self-care abilities and physical mobility within the limitations imposed by spinal cord injury.
- The client will experience no preventable complications associated with spinal cord injury.
- The client will develop strategies to effectively cope with health problems and body image disturbances associated with spinal cord injury.

Nursing interventions

- Immobilize, reduce, and align the injured area of the spinal column, using Crutchfield, Vinke, or Gardner-Wells tongs with cervical traction; a halo external fixation device; a body jacket; or a Minerva jacket *to prevent further trauma to the spinal column, spinal cord, and extension of the spinal cord injury.*
- If the client is in cervical traction, assess and clean the pin sites as prescribed *to detect signs and symptoms of infection* and make sure the weights are free-hanging — not lying on the floor or headboard.
- If the client is in a halo external fixation device, assess and clean the pin sites as prescribed; assess pins, bolts, and vest structure for looseness; keep a torque screwdriver readily available and in a secure place so that tension on bars can be adjusted; and keep an open-end wrench readily available and in a secure place so that bolts can be released and the vest temporarily removed in the case of cardiac arrest *to detect signs and symptoms of infection, to ensure that traction is being applied to the spinal column, and to allow access to the client's chest if CPR is required.*
- Provide bed rest on a firm surface (such as a kinetic, CircOlectric, or RotoRest bed or Stryker frame) *to keep the spinal column aligned while allowing you to move and turn the client.*
- Maintain a patent airway and administer oxygen *to promote oxygenation of tissues.*
- Assist the client with coughing and deep breathing *to mobilize secretions in the airway and expand the lungs.*
- Assess the client's neurologic status and vital signs every 1 to 2 hours initially and then every 4 hours when the client's condition becomes stable *to determine baseline and to detect changes in neurologic status and early signs and symptoms of spinal shock and to determine a possible need for changes in the treatment plan.*
- Encourage the client to eat a high-protein, high-fiber diet or, if necessary, administer enteral nutrition through an enteral feeding tube (for example, gastrostomy, PEG, or PEJ) or TPN *to promote adequate nutritional status, facilitate tissue healing, and meet metabolic demands.*
- Monitor the client's weight weekly *to determine nutritional status.*
- Provide urinary catheterization during the acute phase *to provide bladder decompression when spinal shock is likely.*
- Institute a bowel and bladder program *to promote urinary and fecal continence and to avoid stimuli that could trigger autonomic dysreflexia (AD).* (AD is an exaggerated sympathetic response to a noxious stimulus that occurs in clients with a spinal cord injury above T7. Signs and symptoms include extreme hypertension, pounding headache, flushing, diaphoresis, blurred vision, and bradycardia. Treatment consists of removing the noxious stimulus.)
- Assess the client for signs and symptoms of AD.
- Consult a physical therapist and an occupational therapist *to evaluate which adaptive assistive devices the client may need to independently and safely perform activities of daily living.*
- Perform active or passive ROM exercises *to help maintain joint mobility and prevent contractures.*
- Apply antiembolism or sequential compression stockings, as prescribed, *to promote venous return and prevent deep vein thrombosis of the lower extremities.*
- Assess the client for signs and symptoms of depression *to detect the need for possible intervention.*
- Encourage the client to express his feelings about changes in his body image *to reduce his tendency to suppress or repress those feelings and to help him cope.*
- Provide sexual counseling *to encourage the client to ask question and avoid misunderstandings.*

Evaluation

- The client retains a usual or an improved level of neurologic functioning.
- The client develops maximal self-care abilities and physical mobility within the limitations imposed by spinal cord injury.
- The client experiences no preventable complications associated with spinal cord injury.
- The client develops strategies to effectively cope with health problems and body image disturbances associated with the spinal cord injury.

Stroke

A STROKE, also known as a cerebrovascular accident or brain attack, is a sudden disruption in normal cerebral circulation from occlusion of an intracranial or extracranial blood vessel or hemorrhage in the brain from rupture of an intracranial blood vessel. No matter what the cause of a stroke, the extent of the cerebral ischemia, neuronal death, and subsequent neurologic impairment depends on numerous factors.

When a stroke results from occlusion of an intracranial or extracranial blood vessel, the location, size, and degree of occlusion and the adequacy of collateral circulation to the area of the brain supplied by the affected blood vessel have a significant impact on the client's recovery from the event. When a stroke results from hemorrhage in the brain from rupture of an intracranial blood vessel, the location, size, and mass of the hematoma and the adequacy of collateral circulation to the area of the brain affected by the hematoma have a significant impact on the client's recovery from the event. (See *Causes of stroke.*)

Possible causes
Embolism
- Air or fat emboli
- AF
- Cardiac arrhythmias
- Heart valve replacement
- Oral contraceptives

Thrombosis
- Atherosclerosis
- Diabetes mellitus
- Hyperlipidemia
- Hypertension
- Hypovolemia
- Obesity

Causes of stroke

This illustration shows the causes of stroke (cerebral hemorrhage, cerebral embolus, and cerebral thrombosis) and their locations in the central nervous system

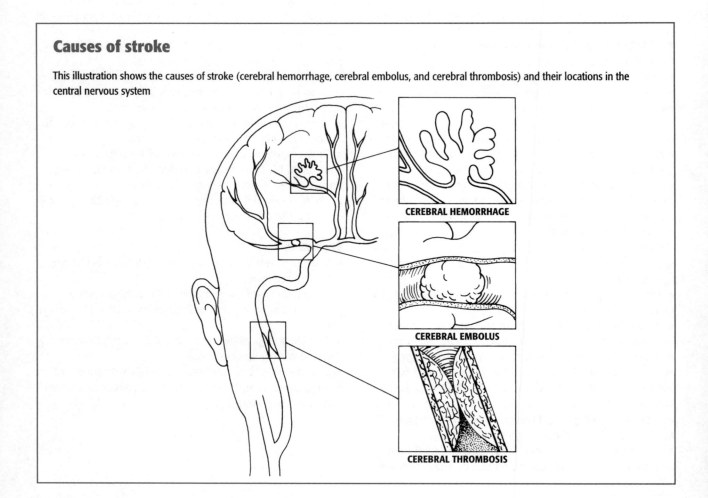

CEREBRAL HEMORRHAGE

CEREBRAL EMBOLUS

CEREBRAL THROMBOSIS

- Polycythemia
- Sedentary lifestyle
- Sickle cell anemia
- Smoking
- Stress
- TIA

Hemorrhage
- Aneurysm rupture
- Anticoagulants
- Aplastic anemia
- AVM rupture
- Hemophilia
- Hypertension
- Liver disease
- Metastatic brain tumor rupture
- Substance abuse (for example, cocaine)
- Vasopressors

Data collection findings
- Neurologic deficits (progressive or abrupt in onset)
- Altered LOC (wakefulness to coma)
- Headache
- Fever
- Nuchal rigidity
- Seizures (see *Stroke sites*)

Diagnostic findings
- CSF analysis, which isn't routinely done, may reveal bloody CSF with hemorrhagic stroke.
- Lumbar puncture, which isn't routinely done, may reveal increased CSF pressure.
- CT scan or MRI may reveal the site of infarction, hematoma, and shift of brain structures.
- Cerebral angiogram is used to identify collateral blood circulation and may reveal the site of rupture or occlusion.
- PET scan may reveal information on cerebral metabolism and blood flow characteristics.
- EEG may reveal abnormal electrical activity, such as focal slowing, which helps to locate the lesion or to assess the client's amount of brain wave activity.
- ECG may reveal AF as the source of emboli.
- Echocardiography may reveal thrombus on valvular heart structures and mural thrombi on the myocardial walls as the possible sources of emboli.
- Oculoplethysmography may reveal decreased intraocular systolic pressure and, thus, carotid blood flow.
- Transcranial Doppler ultrasonography may reveal decreased cerebral metabolism and characteristics of blood flow.

Stroke sites

Clinical features of stroke vary with the artery affected (and, consequently, the portion of the brain the artery supplies), the severity of damage, and the extent of collateral circulation that develops to help the brain compensate for decreased blood supply.

Typical arteries affected and their associated signs and symptoms are described here.

Middle cerebral artery
Injury to the middle cerebral artery causes aphasia, dysphasia, visual field cuts, and hemiparesis on the affected side (more severe in the face and arm than in the leg).

Carotid artery
If the carotid artery is affected, the client may develop weakness, paralysis, numbness, sensory changes, and visual disturbances on the affected side; altered level of consciousness, bruits, headaches, aphasia, and ptosis.

Vertebrobasilar artery
A stroke affecting the vertebrobasilar artery may lead to weakness on the affected side, numbness around the lips and mouth, visual field cuts, diplopia, poor coordination, dysphagia, slurred speech, dizziness, amnesia, and ataxia.

Anterior cerebral artery
If the anterior cerebral artery becomes affected, the client may develop confusion, weakness, and numbness (especially in the leg) on affected side, incontinence, loss of coordination, impaired motor and sensory functions, and personality changes.

Posterior cerebral arteries
If the posterior cerebral arteries are affected, the client may develop visual fields cuts, sensory impairment, dyslexia, coma, and cortical blindness. Usually, paralysis is absent.

- Blood chemistry study results may reveal decreased Hb level, HCT, and RBC count; increased PT, PTT, liver function test results, and cholesterol, triglycerides, and glucose levels; and positive sickle cell trait.

Nursing diagnoses
- Disturbed body image
- Disturbed sensory perception (visual, auditory, kinesthetic, gustatory, tactile, or olfactory, depending on the

area of the brain affected and extent of cerebral tissue affected)
- Disturbed thought processes
- Ineffective tissue perfusion (cerebral)
- Interrupted family processes

Treatment
- Oxygen therapy
- IPPB and chest physiotherapy
- Mechanical ventilation
- I.V. fluids
- Bed rest during the acute stage (until the client's condition stabilizes)
- Head of bed elevated 30 to 45 degrees, or as prescribed
- Active and passive ROM exercises
- Enteral nutrition through an enteral feeding tube (for example, gastrostomy, PEG or PEJ) or TPN
- Low-sodium diet, low-cholesterol, and low-fat diet adjusted for the client's ability to chew and swallow
- Dietary consultation
- Physical therapy
- Speech therapy
- Antiembolism or sequential compression stockings, as prescribed
- Bowel and bladder program
- Carotid endarterectomy, embolization of AVM, clipping of aneurysm, evacuation of hematoma

Drug therapy options
- Antipyretic: acetaminophen (Tylenol)
- Analgesic: acetaminophen (Tylenol), codeine phosphate, codeine sulfate
- Anticoagulant: heparin, ticlopidine (Ticlid), warfarin (Coumadin)
- Antiplatelet aggregation drug: acetylsalicylic acid (ASA), dipyridamole (Persantine)
- Anticonvulsant: phenytoin (Dilantin)
- Antihypertensive: nifedipine (Procardia)
- Diuretic: furosemide (Lasix)
- Glucocorticoid: dexamethasone (Decadron)
- H_2-receptor antagonist: cimetidine (Tagamet), famotidine (Pepcid), ranitidine (Zantac)
- Thrombolytic enzyme: tissue plasminogen activator for embolic or thrombotic stroke

Patient care goals
- The client will regain a usual or an improved LOC, cognition, and motor-sensory function.
- The client will develop maximal self-care abilities and physical mobility and an effective means of communication within the limitations imposed by the stroke.
- The client will experience no preventable complications associated with a stroke.
- The client will develop strategies to effectively cope with health problems and body image disturbances associated with a stroke.

Nursing interventions
- Maintain a patent airway and administer oxygen, as prescribed, *to help promote oxygenation of cerebral tissues.*
- Encourage the client to cough and deep breathe *to help mobilize secretions in the airway and expand the lungs.*
- Monitor pulse oximetry and ABG levels, as prescribed, *to evaluate the effectiveness of gas exchange and ventilatory effort.*
- Make sure the client maintains bed rest during the acute phase *to conserve his energy, reducing the oxygen demands of cerebral tissues and the body, and to restore the client to an optimal level of neurologic functioning.*
- Assess neurologic status every 1 to 2 hours initially and then every 4 hours when the client's condition becomes stable. Determine the baseline and then detect changes in neurologic status.
- Maintain nothing-by-mouth status and possible NG decompression during the acute phase *to help prevent gastric distention, nausea, and vomiting.*
- Encourage the client to eat a low-sodium, low cholesterol and, if needed, low-fat diet. The diet should be adjusted for his ability to chew and swallow and determined in collaboration with the registered dietitian *to promote nutritional status, facilitate tissue healing, and meet metabolic demands.*
- If necessary, administer enteral nutrition through an enteral feeding tube (for example, gastrostomy, PEG, or PEJ) or maintain safety of central venous access for TPN, as prescribed, *until oral intake is sufficient to meet metabolic demands.*
- Consult a speech therapist *to evaluate the client's ability to communicate and swallow.*
- Assess gag reflex and ability to swallow *to prevent aspiration of food particles.*
- Institute a bowel and bladder program *to help promote urinary and fecal continence.*
- Administer I.V. fluids as prescribed *to help promote normovolemia and electrolyte balance.*
- Monitor intake and output *to help detect the need for early intervention for fluid volume overload or deficit.*
- Assist in administration of prescribed medications *to help the client maintain continuous therapeutic drug levels and an optimal level of neurologic functioning.*

CLINICAL SITUATION

Caring for a client after a stroke

A 68-year-old African-American male had a stroke due to a right cerebral thrombosis 1 week ago that resulted in left hemiplegia. He's a history instructor at the local community college. His hobby is wood carving, and he spends hours each week working in his garden. The client is also an active member of his church. For the past 2 years, he has been taking medication for hypertension, but his wife reports that he often forgets to take it and that his blood pressure was high at his last physical examination. She tells the nursing staff that she has never had to worry about her husband's health before and that she wants to learn everything she can to care for him at home. However, she says that her husband was always the one to make the decisions and pay the bills. She adds that the children, grandchildren, neighbors, and family pastor want to see her husband back at home as soon as possible.

What are three appropriate nursing diagnoses for this situation?
● Ineffective tissue perfusion (cerebral) (related to disruption of blood flow)
● Interrupted family processes (related to the change in the client's function and needs secondary to stroke)
● Disturbed body image (related to residual deficits caused by stroke)

Questions for further thought
● Would you expect the client to have difficulty with his speech? Why?
● What considerations must be included when planning for the client's discharge to the home and community?
● What would you reply if, after you've completed passive range-of-motion exercises on the client's left arm, he states, "I just ignore that part of my body; it doesn't work anyway."

● Consult a physical therapist and an occupational therapist *to evaluate which adaptive assistive devices the client may need to independently and safely perform ADLs.*
● Perform active or passive ROM exercises *to help the client maintain joint mobility and prevent contractures.*
● Apply antiembolism or sequential compression stockings, as prescribed, *to promote venous return and prevent deep vein thrombosis of lower extremities.*
● Institute seizure precautions *to prevent the client from injuring himself during a seizure.*

● Encourage the client to express his feelings about changes in his body image *to reduce his tendency to suppress or repress those feelings and to help him cope.*

Evaluation
● The client regains a usual or an improved LOC, cognition, and motor-sensory function.
● The client develops maximal self-care abilities and physical mobility and an effective means of communication within the limitations imposed by the stroke.
● The client experiences no preventable complications associated with the stroke.
● The client develops strategies to effectively cope with health problems and body image disturbances associated with the stroke. (See *Caring for a client after a stroke*.)

Trigeminal neuralgia

TRIGEMINAL NEURALGIA is a painful disorder of one or more branches of the fifth cranial (trigeminal) nerve that produces paroxysmal attacks of excruciating facial pain. Attacks are precipitated by stimulation of a trigger zone, a hypersensitive area of the face.

This disorder occurs mostly in people over age 40, in women more commonly than men, and on the right side of the face more commonly than the left. Trigeminal neuralgia can subside spontaneously, with remissions lasting from several months to years. The disorder is also called *tic douloureux.*

Possible causes
Although the cause remains undetermined, trigeminal neuralgia may:
● reflect an afferent reflex phenomenon located centrally in the brain stem or more peripherally in the sensory root of the trigeminal nerve
● be related to compression of the nerve root by posterior fossa tumors, middle fossa tumors, or vascular lesions (subclinical aneurysm), although such lesions usually produce simultaneous loss of sensation
● occasionally be a manifestation of MS or herpes zoster.

Data collection findings
● Searing pain in the facial area

Triggers
● Light touch to a sensitive area of the face (trigger zone)
● Exposure to hot or cold temperatures
● Eating, smiling, or talking
● Drinking hot or cold beverages

Diagnostic findings
● Observation during the examination shows the client favoring (splinting) the affected area. To ward off a painful attack, the client typically holds his face immobile when talking. He may also leave the affected side of his face unwashed and unshaven.
● Skull X-rays, tomography, and CT scan rule out sinus or tooth infections, and tumors.

Nursing diagnoses
● Acute pain
● Powerlessness
● Anxiety

Treatment
● Percutaneous radio frequency procedure, which causes partial root destruction and relieves pain
● Microsurgery for vascular decompression
● Percutaneous electrocoagulation of nerve rootlets, under local anesthesia

Drug therapy options
● Anticonvulsant: carbamazepine (Tegretol) or phenytoin (Dilantin) to temporarily relieve or prevent pain

Patient care goals
● The client will experience increased comfort and relief from pain.
● The client will identify triggers that intensify the disorder and develop methods to control them.
● The client will use available support systems to cope with the effects of the disorder.

Nursing interventions
● Observe and record the characteristics of each attack, including the client's protective mechanisms *to gain information for developing the treatment plan.*
● Provide adequate nutrition in small, frequent meals at room temperature *to ensure nutritional needs are met. Temperature extremes may cause an attack.*
● If the client is receiving carbamazepine, watch for cutaneous and hematologic reactions (erythematous and pruritic rashes, urticaria, photosensitivity, exfoliative dermatitis, leukopenia, agranulocytosis, eosinophilia, aplastic anemia, thrombocytopenia) and, possibly, urine retention and transient drowsiness. *Identifying adverse reactions early helps to limit complications.*
● For the first 3 months of carbamazepine therapy, CBC and liver function should be monitored weekly, then monthly thereafter. Warn the client to immediately report

fever, sore throat, mouth ulcers, easy bruising, or petechial or purpuric hemorrhage. *Hematologic toxicity is rare but serious.*
● If the client is receiving phenytoin, watch for adverse effects, including ataxia, skin eruptions, gingival hyperplasia, and nystagmus. *Early detection of adverse reactions limits complications with early intervention.*
● After resection of the first division of the trigeminal nerve, tell the client to avoid rubbing his eyes and using aerosol spray. Advise him to wear glasses or goggles outdoors and to blink often *to prevent injury.*
● After surgery to sever the second or third division, tell the client to avoid hot foods and drinks, which could burn his mouth, and to chew carefully *to avoid biting his mouth.*
● Advise the client to place food in the unaffected side of his mouth when chewing, to brush his teeth often, and to see a dentist twice per year to detect cavities. *Cavities in the area of the severed nerve won't cause pain.*
● After surgical decompression of the root or partial nerve dissection, check neurologic and vital signs often *to detect early signs of postoperative complications.*
● Reinforce natural avoidance of stimulation (air, heat, cold) of trigger zones (lips, cheeks, gums) *to prevent further episodes.*

Evaluation
● The client reports adequate pain control.
● The client demonstrates appropriate measures to control exacerbation of his disorder.
● The client displays appropriate coping mechanisms.

RESPIRATORY SYSTEM

The respiratory system is made up of the lungs and the structures that conduct air to and from the lungs and are involved in related functions. The major function of the respiratory system is gas exchange.

Respiratory structure and function
During gas exchange, air is taken into the body by inhalation and travels through respiratory passages to the lungs. In the lungs, oxygen (O_2) diffuses into the blood and carbon dioxide (CO_2) is removed by exhalation.

Lungs and related structures

As a unit, the lungs are composed of three lobes on the right side and two lobes on the left side. The respiratory process involves the lungs and related structures, such as the nose and mouth, trachea, bronchi, and alveoli.

● The nose and mouth allow airflow into and out of the body. They also humidify inhaled air, which reduces irritation of the mucous membranes. Within the nose, the nares (nostrils) contain olfactory receptor sites, providing for the body's sense of smell.

● The paranasal sinuses are air-filled, cilia-lined cavities within the nose. Their function is to trap particles of foreign matter that might interfere with respiration.

● The pharynx serves as a passageway to the digestive and respiratory tracts. The pharynx maintains air pressure in the middle ear and also contains a mucosal lining. This lining humidifies and warms inhaled air and traps foreign particles.

● The larynx, also known as the *voice box,* connects the upper and lower airways. It contains vocal cords that produce sounds. The larynx also initiates the cough reflex, which is one of the respiratory system's defense mechanisms.

● The trachea contains C-shaped cartilaginous rings composed of smooth muscle. It connects the larynx to the bronchi.

● The trachea branches into the right and left bronchi, the large air passages that lead to the right and left lungs. The right main bronchus is slightly larger and more vertical than the left.

● As they pass into the lungs, the bronchi form smaller branches called *bronchioles,* which branch into terminal bronchioles and alveoli.

● Alveoli are clustered microscopic sacs enveloped by capillaries. The lungs contain millions of alveoli, in which gas exchange occurs. The alveoli contain a coating of surfactant, which reduces surface tension, keeps the alveoli from collapsing, and facilitates gas exchange.

● The lungs regulate air exchange by a concentration gradient in the alveoli. In the alveoli, gases move from an area of high concentration to an area of low concentration. Because the concentration of carbon dioxide is greater in the alveoli, it diffuses out into the lungs and is exhaled. Because the lungs contain a greater concentration of oxygen, oxygen diffuses out of the lungs and into the alveoli and then travels through the bloodstream to the rest of the body.

● Pleurae are membranes that cover the lungs and line the thoracic cavity. The visceral pleura covers the lungs; the parietal pleura covers the thoracic cavity. Pleural fluid lubricates the pleurae to reduce friction during respiration.

RESPIRATORY DISORDERS

Major respiratory disorders include acute respiratory failure, adult respiratory distress syndrome (ARDS), asphyxia, asthma, atelectasis, chronic bronchitis, COPD, emphysema, legionnaires' disease, lung cancer, lung resection, pleural effusion and empyema, pleurisy, *Pneumocystis carinii* pneumonia (PCP), pneumonia, pneumothorax and hemothorax, pulmonary embolism, and TB.

Acute respiratory failure

In ACUTE RESPIRATORY FAILURE, the respiratory system can neither adequately supply the body with the oxygen it needs nor adequately remove carbon dioxide. Respiratory failure occurs when Pao_2 is 50 mm Hg or less or $Paco_2$ is 50 mm Hg or greater with pH 7.25 or less.

Acute respiratory failure can be classified as ventilatory failure or oxygenation failure:

● Ventilatory failure is characterized by alveolar hypoventilation.

● Oxygenation failure is characterized by ventilation-perfusion mismatching (blood flow to areas of the lung with reduced ventilation or ventilation to lung tissue that's experiencing reduced blood flow) or physiologic shunting (blood moving from the right side of the heart to the left without being oxygenated).

Possible causes

● Abdominal or thoracic surgery
● Anesthesia
● ARDS
● Atelectasis
● Brain tumors
● COPD
● Drug overdose
● Encephalitis
● Flail chest
● Guillain-Barré syndrome
● Head trauma
● Hemothorax
● Meningitis
● MS
● Muscular dystrophy
● MG
● Pleural effusion

- Pneumonia
- Pneumothorax
- Poliomyelitis
- Polyneuritis
- Pulmonary edema
- Pulmonary embolism
- Stroke

Data collection findings

- Adventitious breath sounds, including crackles, pleural friction rub, rhonchi, and wheezing
- Difficulty breathing, shortness of breath, dyspnea, tachypnea, orthopnea
- Cough, sputum production, hemoptysis
- Decreased respiratory excursion
- Accessory muscle use
- Retractions
- Tachycardia
- Chest pain
- Change in mentation
- Anxiety
- Nasal flaring
- Fatigue
- Cyanosis
- Diaphoresis

Diagnostic findings

- ABG levels show hypoxemia, acidosis, alkalosis, and hypercapnia.
- Chest X-ray shows pulmonary infiltrates, interstitial edema, and atelectasis.
- Hematology reveals increased WBC count and ESR.
- Lung scan shows ventilation-perfusion ratio mismatches.
- Sputum study identifies the causative organism.

Nursing diagnoses

- Ineffective breathing pattern
- Ineffective airway clearance
- Anxiety

Treatment

- Chest physiotherapy, postural drainage (position the client in a prone or supine position, with the foot of the bed elevated higher than the head for postural drainage), and incentive spirometry
- Chest tube insertion if pneumothorax develops from high positive end-expiratory pressure (PEEP) administration

- High-calorie, high-protein diet and decreased or increased fluid intake, depending on the cause
- Oxygen therapy, intubation, and mechanical ventilation (possibly with PEEP)

Drug therapy options

- Analgesic: morphine
- Antibiotic (infecting organism determines drug used)
- Anticoagulant: heparin, warfarin (Coumadin)
- Anxiolytic: lorazepam (Ativan)
- Bronchodilator: aminophylline, terbutaline (Brethine), theophylline (Theo-Dur); via nebulizer: albuterol (Proventil), ipratropium (Atrovent), metaproterenol (Alupent)
- Diuretic: furosemide (Lasix)
- H_2-blocker: cimetidine (Tagamet), famotidine (Pepcid), ranitidine (Zantac), nizatidine (Axid)
- Neuromuscular blocker: atracurium (Tracrium), pancuronium (Pavulon), vecuronium (Norcuron)
- Steroid: hydrocortisone (Solu-Cortef), methylprednisolone (Solu-Medrol)

Patient care goals

- The client will maintain an open airway.
- The client will verbalize fears and concerns related to breathing difficulties.
- The client will have adequate oxygenation.

Nursing interventions

- Assess respiratory status *to detect early signs of compromise and hypoxemia.*
- Monitor and record intake and output *to detect fluid volume excess,* which may lead to pulmonary edema.
- Track laboratory test results. Report deteriorating ABG values, such as a decrease in Pao_2 levels and an increase in $Paco_2$ levels. *Low Hb levels and HCT reduce the blood's oxygen-carrying capacity. Electrolyte abnormalities may result from diuretic use.*
- Monitor pulse oximetry *to detect a drop in arterial oxygen saturation (Sao_2).*
- Monitor and record vital signs. *Tachycardia and tachypnea may indicate hypoxemia.*
- Monitor and record the color, consistency, and amount of sputum *to determine hydration status, effectiveness of therapy, and presence of infection.*
- Administer oxygen *to reduce hypoxemia and relieve respiratory distress.*
- Monitor mechanical ventilation *to prevent complications and optimize Pao_2.*

NURSING PROCEDURE

Performing oronasopharyngeal suction

Purpose

In oronasopharyngeal suction, a suction catheter is inserted through the mouth or nostril to remove secretions from the pharynx. Used to maintain a patent airway, this procedure helps clients who can't clear their airways effectively by coughing and expectoration, such as unconscious and severely debilitated clients. The procedure should be done as often as necessary, depending on the client's condition.

Because the catheter may inadvertently slip into the lower airway or esophagus, oronasopharyngeal suction is a sterile procedure that requires sterile equipment. However, clean technique may be used for a tonsil-tip suction device. In fact, an alert client can use a tonsil-tip suction device himself to remove secretions.

Nasopharyngeal suctioning should be used with caution in clients who have nasopharyngeal bleeding or spinal fluid leakage into the nasopharyngeal area, trauma clients, clients who are receiving anticoagulant therapy, and clients who have blood dyscrasias; these conditions increase the risk of bleeding.

Implementation

- Explain the procedure to the client even if he's unresponsive.
- Wash your hands.
- Position the client in semi-Fowler's or high Fowler's position.
- Turn on the suction from the wall or portable unit, and set the pressure according to your facility's policy (usually between 80 and 120 mm Hg).
- Occlude the end of the connecting tubing *to check suction pressure.*
- Using strict sterile technique, open the suction catheter kit or the packages containing the sterile catheter, disposable container, and gloves. Put on the gloves; consider your dominant hand sterile and your nondominant hand nonsterile. Using your nondominant hand, pour saline solution into the sterile container.
- With your nondominant hand, place a small amount of water-soluble lubricant on the sterile area.
- Pick up the catheter with your dominant (sterile) hand, and attach it to the connecting tubing. Use your nondominant hand to control the suction valve while your dominant hand manipulates the catheter.
- Instruct the client to cough and breathe slowly and deeply several times before beginning suction.

For nasal insertion

- Raise the tip of the client's nose with your nondominant hand *to straighten the passageway and facilitate catheter insertion.* Without applying suction, gently insert the suction catheter into the client's naris. Roll the catheter between your fingers *to help it advance through the turbinates.* Continue to advance the catheter approximately 5″ to 6″ (12.5 to 15 cm) until you reach the pool of secretions or the client begins to cough.

For oral insertion

- Without applying suction, gently insert the catheter into the client's mouth. Advance it 3″ to 4″ (7.5 to 10 cm) along the side of the client's mouth until you reach the pool of secretions or the client begins to cough. Suction both sides of the client's mouth and pharyngeal area.
- Using intermittent suction, withdraw the catheter from either the mouth or the nose with a continuous rotating motion *to minimize invagination of the mucosa into the catheter's tip and side ports.* Apply suction for only 10 to 15 seconds at a time *to minimize tissue trauma.*
- Between passes, wrap the catheter around your dominant hand *to prevent contamination.*
- If secretions are thick, clear the lumen of the catheter by dipping it in normal saline solution and applying suction.
- Repeat the procedure until gurgling or bubbling sounds stop and respirations are quiet.
- After completing suctioning, pull your sterile glove off over the coiled catheter. Discard both gloves and the container of water.
- Flush the connecting tubing with normal saline solution.
- Document the procedure, being sure to include the client's tolerance and the color, consistency, and amount of secretions suctioned.

- Provide suctioning; assist with turning, coughing, and deep breathing; and perform chest physiotherapy and postural drainage *to facilitate removal of secretions.* (See *Performing oronasopharyngeal suction.*)

- Make sure the client maintains bed rest *to reduce the amount of oxygen required.*
- Keep the client in semi-Fowler's or high Fowler's position *to promote chest expansion and ventilation.*

- Maintain diet restrictions. *Fluid restrictions and a low-sodium diet may be necessary to avoid fluid overload.*
- Assist with administration of medications as prescribed *to treat infection, dilate airways, and reduce inflammation.*
- Monitor the chest tube system *to assess for lung reexpansion.*

Evaluation

- The client demonstrates decreased anxiety with improved ventilation.
- The client breathes without difficulty.
- The client has adequate oxygenation.

SPOT CHECK

A client experiencing acute respiratory failure is most likely to demonstrate:

A. hypocapnia, hypoventilation, and hyperoxemia.

B. hypocapnia, hyperventilation, and hyperoxemia.

C. hypercapnia, hyperventilation, and hypoxemia.

D. hypercapnia, hypoventilation, and hypoxemia.

Answer: D. Acute respiratory failure is marked by hypercapnia (elevated arterial carbon dioxide), hypoventilation, and hypoxemia (subnormal oxygen).

Adult respiratory distress syndrome

In ADULT RESPIRATORY DISTRESS SYNDROME (ARDS), fluid builds up in the lungs and causes them to stiffen. This impairs breathing, thereby reducing the amount of oxygen in the capillaries that supply the lungs. In severe cases, the syndrome can cause an unmanageable and ultimately fatal lack of oxygen. However, people who recover may have little or no permanent lung damage.

Possible causes

- Aspiration
- Decreased surfactant production
- Fat emboli
- Fluid overload
- Neurologic injuries
- Oxygen toxicity
- Respiratory tract infection
- Sepsis
- Shock
- Trauma

Data collection findings

- Crackles, decreased breath sounds, rhonchi
- Dyspnea or tachypnea
- Cyanosis
- Cough
- Anxiety
- Restlessness

Diagnostic findings

- ABG levels show respiratory acidosis, metabolic acidosis, and hypoxemia that doesn't respond to increased fraction of inspired oxygen (FIO_2).
- Blood culture reveals the infectious organism.
- Chest X-ray shows bilateral infiltrates (in early stages) and lung fields with a ground-glass appearance and, with irreversible hypoxemia, massive consolidation of both lung fields (in later stages).
- Sputum study reveals the infectious organism.

Nursing diagnoses

- Impaired gas exchange
- Ineffective breathing pattern
- Ineffective tissue perfusion (cardiopulmonary)

Treatment

- Bed rest with prone positioning, if possible, and passive ROM exercises
- Chest physiotherapy, postural drainage, and suction
- Restricted fluid intake or, if intubated, nothing by mouth
- Extracorporeal membrane oxygenation if available
- Intubation and mechanical ventilation using PEEP or pressure-controlled inverse ratio ventilation
- Oxygen therapy
- Transfusion therapy: platelets, packed RBCs

Drug therapy options

- Analgesic: morphine
- Antacid: aluminum hydroxide gel (AlternaGEL)
- Antibiotic (infecting organism determines which drug is used)
- Anticoagulant: heparin (Liquaemin Sodium)
- Diuretic: ethacrynic acid (Edecrin), furosemide (Lasix)
- Exogenous surfactant: beractant (Survanta)
- Mucosal barrier fortifier: sucralfate (Carafate)
- Neuromuscular blocker: pancuronium (Pavulon), vecuronium (Norcuron)
- Steroid: hydrocortisone (Solu-Cortef), methylprednisolone (Solu-Medrol)

Patient care goals

- The client will have improved oxygenation.
- The client won't have difficulty breathing.

Nursing interventions

- Assess respiratory, cardiovascular, and neurologic status *to detect evidence of hypoxemia, such as tachycardia, tachypnea, and irritability.*
- Monitor pulse oximetry continuously *to determine the effectiveness of therapy.*
- Monitor blood chemistry test results. *A decrease in Hb levels and HCT affects the oxygen-carrying capacity of the blood. An increase in WBC count suggests an infection such as pneumonia.* Monitor platelet count, fibrinogen level, PT, and PTT *to detect disseminated intravascular coagulation, a complication of ARDS.*
- Monitor and record intake and output *to determine fluid status and hemodynamic variables.*
- Monitor mechanical ventilation (high PEEP increases the risk for pneumothorax) *to increase Pao_2 without raising Fio_2, thereby reducing risk of oxygen toxicity,* and provide suction as necessary *to aid removal of secretions.*
- Make sure the client maintains bed rest with prone positioning, if possible, *to promote oxygenation.*
- Maintain fluid restrictions *to reduce fluid volume overload.*
- Provide turning, chest physiotherapy, and postural drainage *to promote drainage and keep airways clear.*
- Keep the client in high Fowler's position *to promote chest expansion.*
- Maintain the patency of the central line for administration of TPN or give enteral feedings, as appropriate, *to prevent respiratory muscle impairment and maintain nutritional status.*
- Administer medications as prescribed *to optimize respiratory and hemodynamic status.*
- Organize nursing care *to allow rest periods to conserve energy and to avoid overexertion and fatigue.*
- Weigh the client daily *to detect fluid retention.*
- Encourage the client to express his feelings about fear of suffocation *to reduce anxiety and, therefore, oxygen demands.*

Evaluation

- The client has adequate oxygenation.
- The client breathes without difficulty.

Asphyxia

In ASPHYXIA, interference with respiration leads to insufficient oxygen and accumulating carbon dioxide in the blood and tissues. Asphyxia leads to cardiopulmonary arrest and is fatal without prompt treatment.

Possible causes

- Extrapulmonary obstruction, such as tracheal compression from a tumor, strangulation, trauma, or suffocation
- Hypoventilation as a result of narcotic abuse, medullary disease, hemorrhage, pneumothorax, respiratory muscle paralysis, or cardiopulmonary arrest
- Inhalation of toxic agents, such as carbon monoxide poisoning, smoke inhalation, and excessive oxygen inhalation
- Intrapulmonary obstruction, such as airway obstruction, severe asthma, foreign body aspiration, pulmonary edema, pneumonia, and near-drowning

Data collection findings

- Agitation
- Central and peripheral cyanosis (cherry-red mucous membranes in late-stage carbon monoxide poisoning)
- Dyspnea
- Altered respiratory rate (apnea, bradypnea, occasional tachypnea)
- Decreased breath sounds
- Anxiety
- Confusion leading to coma
- Fast, slow, or absent pulse
- Seizures

Diagnostic findings

- ABG measurement indicates decreased Pao_2 (less than 60 mm Hg) and increased $Paco_2$ (greater than 50 mm Hg).
- Chest X-rays may show a foreign body, pulmonary edema, or atelectasis.
- Pulmonary function tests may indicate respiratory muscle weakness.
- Pulse oximetry reveals decreased Hb saturation of oxygen.
- Toxicology tests may show drugs, chemicals, or abnormal Hb.

Nursing diagnoses

- Impaired gas exchange
- Impaired spontaneous ventilation
- Risk for suffocation

Treatment
- Bronchoscopy (for extraction of a foreign body)
- Gastric lavage (for poisoning)
- Oxygen therapy, which may include ET intubation and mechanical ventilation

Drug therapy options
- Narcotic antagonist: naloxone (Narcan) for narcotic overdose

Patient care goals
- The client will maintain adequate ventilation and oxygenation.
- The client will remain free from injury caused by suffocation.

Nursing interventions
- Assess cardiac and respiratory status *to detect early signs of compromise.*
- Position the client upright, if the client's condition permits, *to promote lung expansion and improve oxygenation.*
- Reassure the client during treatment *to ease anxiety associated with respiratory distress.*
- Give prescribed medications *to promote ventilation and oxygenation.*
- Suction carefully as needed and encourage deep breathing *to mobilize secretions and maintain airway patency.*
- Closely monitor vital signs and laboratory test results *to guide treatment.*

Evaluation
- The client has adequate gas exchange as evidenced by stable pulse oximetry and ABG.
- The client has a safe environment and is free from injury related to suffocation.

Asthma

ASTHMA is a form of chronic obstructive airway disease in which the bronchial linings overreact to various stimuli, causing episodic spasms and inflammation that severely restrict the airways. Symptoms range from mild wheezing and labored breathing to life-threatening respiratory failure.

Asthma can be extrinsic, intrinsic, or both. Extrinsic (atopic) asthma is caused by sensitivity to specific external allergens. Intrinsic (nonatopic) asthma is caused by a reaction to internal, nonallergic factors.

Possible causes
Extrinsic asthma
- Allergens (pollen, dander, dust, sulfite food additives)

Intrinsic asthma
- Endocrine changes
- Noxious fumes
- Respiratory infection
- Stress
- Temperature and humidity

Data collection findings
- Chest tightness
- Dyspnea
- Wheezing, primarily on expiration but also sometimes on inspiration
- Absent or diminished breath sounds during severe obstruction
- Tachypnea
- Tachycardia
- Productive cough with thick mucus
- Prolonged expiration
- Use of accessory muscles
- Absence of symptoms between attacks (usually)

Diagnostic findings
- ABG analysis in acute severe asthma shows decreased Pao_2 and decreased, normal, or increased $Paco_2$.
- Blood tests: Serum immunoglobulin E (IgE) may increase from an allergic reaction; CBC may reveal increased eosinophil count.
- Chest X-ray shows hyperinflated lungs with air trapping during an attack.
- Pulmonary function tests during attacks show decreased forced expiratory volumes that improve with therapy and increased residual volume and total lung capacity.
- Skin tests may identify allergens.

Nursing diagnoses
- Ineffective airway clearance
- Impaired gas exchange
- Ineffective therapeutic regimen management

Treatment
- Desensitization to allergens
- Intubation and mechanical ventilation if respiratory status worsens
- Oxygen therapy at 2 L/minute
- Fluid intake up to 3,000 ml/day as tolerated

Drug therapy options

- Antacid: aluminum hydroxide gel (AlternaGEL)
- Antibiotic: according to sensitivity of infective organism
- Antileukotriene: zileuton (Zyflo), zafirlukast (Accolate)
- Beta-adrenergic drug: epinephrine hydrochloride (Adrenalin chloride), salmeterol (Serevent)
- Bronchodilator: terbutaline (Brethine), aminophylline (Aminophyllin), theophylline (Theo-Dur); via nebulizer: albuterol (Proventil), ipratropium (Atrovent), metaproterenol (Alupent)
- Respiratory inhalant: cromolyn (Intal)
- Steroid: hydrocortisone (Solu-Cortef), methylprednisolone (Solu-Medrol)
- Steroid (via nebulizer): beclomethasone (Vanceril), triamcinolone (Azmacort)

Patient care goals

- The client will maintain a patent airway.
- The client will maintain adequate ventilation.
- The client and family members will indicate verbally or through demonstration that they learned what was taught.

Nursing interventions

- Administer low-flow humidified oxygen *to reduce inflammation of the airways, ease breathing, and increase Sao_2.*
- Administer medications as prescribed *to reduce inflammation and obstruction of airways.* Auscultate lungs for improved breath sounds. Observe for complications of drug therapy.
- Encourage the client to express feelings about fear of suffocation *to reduce anxiety.* As breathlessness and hypoxemia are relieved, anxiety should be reduced.
- Allow activity as tolerated, with rest periods *to reduce the work of breathing and to reduce oxygen demands.*
- Assess respiratory status *to determine the effectiveness of therapy,* such as clear breath sounds and improved airflow, pulmonary function tests, Sao_2, and ease of breathing. Louder wheezing may be heard as airways respond to therapy and open up. As the condition improves and airflow increases, wheezing should diminish and breath sounds improve.
- Assist with turning, coughing, deep breathing, and breathing retraining *to mobilize and clear secretions. Pursed-lip and diaphragmatic breathing promote more effective ventilation.*
- Keep the client in high Fowler's position *to improve ventilation.*

- Maintain the client's diet and administer small, frequent feedings *to reduce pressure on the diaphragm and to increase caloric intake.*
- Encourage fluids *to treat dehydration* and liquefy secretions *to facilitate their removal.*
- Monitor and record the color, amount, and consistency of sputum. *Changes in sputum characteristics may signal respiratory infection.*
- Monitor and record vital signs *to assess overall condition.* Tachycardia may indicate worsening asthma or drug toxicity. Hypertension may indicate hypoxemia. Fever may signal infection.
- Monitor laboratory studies *to identify potential problems.* An increase in WBC count may signal infection. Eosinophilia may indicate an allergic response. Drug levels may reveal toxicity.
- Provide chest physiotherapy, postural drainage, incentive spirometry, and suction *to aid in the removal of secretions.*

Evaluation

- The client has adequate gas exchange as evidenced by stable pulse oximetry and ABG levels.
- The client and family exhibit appropriate knowledge of the therapeutic regimen.

Atelectasis

ATELECTASIS is marked by incomplete expansion of lobules (clusters of alveoli) or lung segments, which may result in partial or complete lung collapse. The collapsed areas are unavailable for gas exchange; blood that lacks oxygen passes through unchanged, thereby producing hypoxia.

Atelectasis may be chronic or acute. It occurs to some degree in many clients who undergo upper abdominal or thoracic surgery. The prognosis depends on prompt removal of the airway obstruction, relief of hypoxia, and re-expansion of the collapsed lung.

FAST FACT

Atelectasis can cause hypoxemia and acute respiratory failure. Additionally, static secretions from atelectasis may lead to pneumonia.

Possible causes

- Bronchial occlusion by mucus plugs, as in clients with COPD, bronchiectasis, or cystic fibrosis or those who smoke heavily

- CNS depression
- External compression, such as from upper abdominal surgical incisions, rib fractures, pleuritic chest pain, tight dressings around the chest, or obesity
- Occlusion by foreign bodies, bronchogenic carcinoma, and inflammatory lung disease
- Prolonged immobility

Data collection findings
- Diminished or bronchial breath sounds
- Dyspnea

In severe cases
- Severe dyspnea
- Cyanosis
- Diaphoresis
- Anxiety
- Substernal or intercostal retraction
- Tachycardia
- Hyperinflation of unaffected areas of the lung
- Peripheral circulatory collapse

Diagnostic findings
- Chest X-ray shows characteristic horizontal lines in the lower lung zones and, with segmental or lobar collapse, characteristic dense shadows commonly associated with hyperinflation of neighboring lung zones (in widespread atelectasis).

Nursing diagnoses
- Impaired gas exchange
- Ineffective breathing pattern
- Risk for infection

Treatment
- Bronchoscopy
- Chest physiotherapy
- Surgery or radiation therapy to remove an obstructing neoplasm

Drug therapy options
- Analgesic: morphine
- Bronchodilator: albuterol (Proventil)
- Mucolytic inhalation therapy: acetylcysteine (Mucomyst)

Patient care goals
- The client will maintain a patent airway.
- The client will maintain adequate ventilation.
- The client will remain free from infection.

Nursing interventions
- Encourage postoperative and other high-risk clients to cough and deep-breathe every 1 to 2 hours *to prevent atelectasis.*
- Hold a pillow tightly over the incision; teach the client this technique as well to minimize pain during coughing exercises in postoperative clients. Gently reposition these clients often and help them walk as soon as possible *to prevent atelectasis.*
- Administer adequate analgesics to control pain. *Pain may prevent the client from taking deep breaths, which leads to atelectasis.*
- During mechanical ventilation, maintain tidal volume at 10 to 15 ml/kg of the client's body weight *to ensure adequate lung expansion.* The sigh mechanism on the ventilator may be used if appropriate to intermittently increase tidal volume at the rate of 10 to 15 sighs per hour.
- Use an incentive spirometer *to encourage deep inspiration through positive reinforcement.* Teach the client how to use the spirometer and encourage him to use it every 1 to 2 hours.
- Humidify inspired air and encourage adequate fluid intake *to mobilize secretions.* Use postural drainage and chest percussion *to promote loosening and clearance of secretions.*
- If the client is intubated or uncooperative, provide suctioning as needed *to maintain a clear airway.* Use sedatives with discretion *because they depress respirations and cough reflex and suppress sighing.*
- Assess breath sounds and ventilatory status frequently and be alert for changes *to prevent respiratory compromise.*
- Encourage the client to stop smoking, lose weight, or both, as needed. Refer him to appropriate support groups for help *to modify risk factors.*
- Provide reassurance and emotional support *because the client may be frightened by his limited breathing capacity.*

Evaluation
- The client has adequate ventilation and oxygenation.
- The client doesn't exhibit any signs of infection.

Chronic bronchitis
CHRONIC BRONCHITIS, a form of COPD, results from irritants and infections that increase mucus production, impair airway clearance, and cause irreversible narrowing of the small airways. This causes a severe ventilation-perfusion imbalance, leading to hypoxemia and carbon dioxide retention.

Possible causes
- Airborne irritants and pollutants
- Chronic respiratory infections
- Smoking

Data collection findings
- Dyspnea
- Increased sputum production
- Productive cough
- Prolonged expiration
- Rhonchi, wheezes
- Use of accessory muscles
- Weight gain, edema, jugular vein distention
- Finger clubbing, later in the disease

Diagnostic findings
- ABGs show decreased Pao_2 and normal or increased $Paco_2$.
- Chest X-ray shows hyperinflation and increased bronchovascular markings.
- ECG shows atrial arrhythmias, peaked P waves in leads II, III, and aV_F and, occasionally, right ventricular hypertrophy.
- Pulmonary function tests may reveal increased residual volume, decreased vital capacity and forced expiratory volumes, and normal static compliance and diffusion capacity.
- Sputum culture may reveal many microorganisms and neutrophils.

Nursing diagnoses
- Ineffective airway clearance
- Ineffective breathing pattern
- Activity intolerance

Treatment
- Chest physiotherapy, postural drainage, and incentive spirometry
- Dietary changes, including establishing a diet high in protein, vitamin C, calories, and nitrogen
- Fluid intake up to 3,000 ml/day, if not contraindicated
- Intubation and mechanical ventilation if respiratory status deteriorates
- Oxygen therapy at 2 to 3 L/minute
- Ultrasonic or mechanical nebulizer treatments

Drug therapy options
- Antacid: aluminum hydroxide gel (AlternaGEL)
- Antibiotic (according to sensitivity of infective organism)
- Bronchodilator: terbutaline (Brethine), aminophylline (Aminophyllin), theophylline (Theo-Dur); via nebulizer: albuterol (Proventil), ipratropium (Atrovent), metaproterenol (Alupent)
- Diuretic: furosemide (Lasix) for edema
- Expectorant: guaifenesin (Robitussin)
- Influenza and Pneumovax vaccines
- Steroid: hydrocortisone (Solu-Cortef), methylprednisolone (Solu-Medrol)
- Steroid (via nebulizer): beclomethasone (Vanceril), triamcinolone (Azmacort)

Patient care goals
- The client will maintain adequate ventilation.
- The client will identify measures to prevent or reduce fatigue.

Nursing interventions
- Administer low-flow oxygen. *Because clients with chronic bronchitis have chronic hypercapnia, they have a hypoxic respiratory drive. Higher flow rates may eliminate this hypoxic respiratory drive. Low flow rates may not eliminate this drive.*
- Administer medications as prescribed *to relieve symptoms and prevent complications.*
- Allow activity as tolerated *to avoid fatigue and reduce oxygen demands.*
- Assess respiratory status, ABG levels, and pulse oximetry *to detect respiratory compromise, severe hypoxemia, and hypercapnia.*
- Assist with turning, coughing, and deep breathing *to mobilize secretions and facilitate removal.*
- Assist with diaphragmatic and pursed-lip breathing *to strengthen respiratory muscles.*
- Keep the client in high Fowler's position *to improve ventilation.*
- Maintain the client's diet and administer small, frequent feedings *to avoid fatigue when eating and to reduce pressure on the diaphragm from a full stomach.*
- Monitor and record the color, amount, and consistency of sputum. *Changes in sputum characteristics may signal respiratory infection.*
- Monitor and record cardiovascular status and vital signs *to assess for complications.* Edema, jugular vein distention, tachycardia, and an elevated CVP suggest right-sided heart failure. An irregular pulse may indicate an arrhythmia caused by altered ABGs. Tachycardia and tachypnea may indicate hypoxemia.
- Monitor laboratory studies *to identify potential problems.* Follow drug levels for evidence of toxicity. Elec-

trolyte imbalances may occur with use of diuretics. Reduced Hb level and HCT affect the oxygen-carrying capacity of the blood.

● Monitor intake and output and daily weights *to detect fluid overload associated with right-sided heart failure. Dehydration impairs the removal of secretions.*

● Provide chest physiotherapy, postural drainage, incentive spirometry, and suction *to aid in removal of secretions.*

● Weigh the client daily *to detect edema caused by right-sided heart failure.*

Evaluation

● The client has adequate ventilation as exhibited by stable ABG levels.

● The client reports less incidence of fatigue.

Chronic obstructive pulmonary disease

CHRONIC OBSTRUCTIVE PULMONARY DISEASE (COPD), also known as *chronic airflow limitation,* is a group of conditions that obstruct pulmonary air outflow, resulting in air being trapped in the alveoli.

Chronic obstructive bronchitis, a productive cough persisting for 3 months of the year for at least 2 consecutive years, causes inflamed airways that lead to increased mucus production and bronchospasms. Mucus plugs trap air, resulting in alveolar hyperinflation. Clients with severe chronic bronchitis usually have severe hypoxemia and polycythemia, with HCT values from 50% to 55%.

Emphysema, characterized by enlargement of the alveoli distal to the terminal bronchioles, leads to alveolar wall destruction, obstructed expiratory airflow, and irreversible loss of lung elasticity. Emphysema causes less hypoxemia than chronic bronchitis does, and HCT values commonly are normal.

Asthma, marked by a widespread airway narrowing in response to various stimuli, is considered COPD only if airway obstruction becomes irreversible.

Possible causes

● Airborne irritants and pollutants
● Allergens
● Alpha$_1$-antitrypsin deficiency
● Chronic respiratory tract infection
● Smoking

Data collection findings

● Anatomic changes, such as barrel chest and clubbing, in late disease

● Cor pulmonale (right-sided heart failure)
● Cough (evaluate character, frequency, and time of day)
● Decreased breath sounds, hyperresonant breath sounds on percussion, and wheezing
● Dyspnea
● Jugular vein distention
● Peripheral edema
● Posturing (leaning forward)
● Prolonged expiration
● Pursed-lip breathing
● Risk factors
● Sputum (amount, color, and consistency)
● Accessory muscle use

Diagnostic findings

● Pulmonary function tests, especially spirometry, reveal diminished lung function.
● Chest X-ray provides baseline norms; in late disease, the client's diaphragm appears flat.
● ABG levels show hypercapnia and hypoxemia. Bicarbonate levels may increase to compensate for chronic hypercapnia and the resultant respiratory acidosis.
● CBC shows elevated Hb level and HCT.
● Pulse oximetry may show a decrease in Sao$_2$, which indicates impending hypoxia.
● ECG shows signs of right ventricular hypertrophy in late disease.

Nursing diagnoses

● Ineffective airway clearance
● Impaired gas exchange
● Fatigue
● Chronic low self-esteem

Treatment

● Chest physiotherapy, postural drainage, and incentive spirometry
● Fluid intake up to 3,000 ml/day if not contraindicated by heart failure
● Oxygen therapy at 2 to 3 L/minute and transtracheal therapy (for home)
● Diet high in protein, vitamin C, calories, and nitrogen (clients with advanced disease may require a diet that's low in carbohydrates and high in fat)

Drug therapy options

● Alpha$_1$-antitrypsin
● Antacid: aluminum hydroxide gel (AlternaGEL)
● Antibiotic (infecting organism determines which drug is used)

- Bronchodilator: aminophylline (Aminophyllin), terbutaline (Brethine), theophylline (Theo-Dur); by nebulizer: albuterol (Proventil), ipratropium (Atrovent), metaproterenol (Alupent)
- Diuretic: furosemide (Lasix)
- Expectorant: guaifenesin (Robitussin)
- Steroid: hydrocortisone (Solu-Cortef), methylprednisolone (Solu-Medrol); by nebulizer: beclomethasone (Vanceril), triamcinolone (Azmacort)
- Influenza and Pneumovax vaccines

Patient care goals

- The client will maintain adequate gas exchange.
- The client will remain free from infection.
- The client will establish an effective breathing pattern.
- The client will have an adequately clear airway.
- The client will understand why he should avoid respiratory irritants.

Nursing interventions

- Assess respiratory status and ABG and pulse oximetry studies *to evaluate oxygenation.* Administer low-flow oxygen if indicated, usually 1 to 2 L per minute in 24% to 28% concentrations.

  FAST FACT

Some clients with emphysema respond only to low oxygen tension. Giving these clients too much oxygen reduces the drive to breathe and contributes to respiratory failure.

- Monitor cardiovascular status *to detect arrhythmias related to hypoxia or adverse reaction to medications.*
- Encourage the client to drink plenty of fluids, and weigh him daily *to monitor for fluid overload and right-sided heart failure.*
- Monitor and record color, amount, and consistency of sputum; *change may indicate infection.*
- Monitor electrolyte levels, blood counts, and drug levels *for indications of a possible toxic reaction.*
- Administer medications as prescribed *to relieve symptoms and prevent complications.*
- Encourage activity as tolerated *to help the client avoid fatigue.*
- Provide chest physiotherapy—including, postural drainage and percussion, incentive spirometry, and suction—as needed, *to aid in secretion removal.*

Evaluation

- The client stops smoking and obtains a job with little or no exposure to respiratory irritants.
- The client remains free from respiratory tract infection.
- The client regularly practices breathing exercises, and his breathing efficiency increases.

Emphysema

EMPHYSEMA is a form of COPD in which recurrent pulmonary inflammation damages and eventually destroys the alveolar walls, creating large air spaces. This breakdown leaves the alveoli unable to recoil normally after expanding and, upon expiration, results in bronchiolar collapse. This traps air in the lungs, leading to overdistention and reduced gas exchange.

Possible causes

- Deficiency of $alpha_1$-antitrypsin
- Smoking

Data collection findings

- Dyspnea
- Pursed-lip breathing
- Decreased breath sounds
- Prolonged expiration
- Accessory muscle use
- Anorexia and weight loss
- Barrel chest
- Finger clubbing, late in the disease

Diagnostic findings

- ABG analysis shows reduced Pao_2, with normal $Paco_2$ until late in the disease.
- Chest X-ray in advanced disease reveals a flattened diaphragm, reduced vascular markings in the lung periphery, enlarged anteroposterior chest diameter, and a vertical heart.
- CBC shows increased Hb level late in disease when the client has severe persistent hypoxia.
- ECG shows tall, symmetrical P waves in leads II, III, and aV_F, vertical QRS axis, and signs of right ventricular hypertrophy late in disease.
- Pulmonary function tests show increased residual volume, total lung capacity, and compliance as well as decreased vital capacity, diffusing capacity, and expiratory volumes.

Nursing diagnoses

- Impaired gas exchange
- Fatigue
- Imbalanced nutrition: Less than body requirements

Treatment

- Chest physiotherapy, postural drainage, and incentive spirometry
- Dietary changes, including establishing a diet high in protein, vitamin C, calories, and nitrogen
- Fluid intake up to 3,000 ml/day, if not contraindicated by heart failure
- Intubation and mechanical ventilation if respiratory status deteriorates
- Oxygen therapy at 2 to 3 L/minute and transtracheal therapy (for home)
- Ultrasonic or mechanical nebulizer treatments
- Lung volume reduction surgery

Drug therapy options

- Alpha$_1$-antitrypsin therapy
- Antacid: aluminum hydroxide gel (AlternaGEL)
- Antibiotic (according to sensitivity of infective organism)
- Bronchodilator: terbutaline (Brethine), aminophylline (Aminophyllin), theophylline (Theo-Dur); via nebulizer: albuterol (Proventil), ipratropium (Atrovent), metaproterenol (Alupent)
- Diuretic (to reduce edema): furosemide (Lasix)
- Expectorant: guaifenesin (Robitussin)
- Influenza and Pneumovax vaccines
- Steroid: hydrocortisone (Solu-Cortef), methylprednisolone (Solu-Medrol)
- Steroid (via nebulizer): beclomethasone (Vanceril), triamcinolone (Azmacort)

Patient care goals

- The client will maintain a patent airway and adequate ventilation.
- The client will identify measures to prevent or reduce fatigue.
- The client will consume adequate daily calories as required.

Nursing interventions

- Administer low-flow oxygen *because emphysema clients have chronic hypercapnia, so they have a hypoxic respiratory drive. Higher flow rates may eliminate this hypoxic respiratory drive. Low flow rates may not eliminate this drive.*
- Administer medications as prescribed *to relieve symptoms and prevent complications.*
- Allow activity as tolerated *to avoid fatigue and reduce oxygen demands.*
- Assess respiratory status, ABG levels, and pulse oximetry *to detect respiratory compromise, severe hypoxemia, and hypercapnia.*
- Monitor and record cardiovascular status and vital signs *to assess for complications.* An irregular pulse may indicate an arrhythmia caused by altered ABG levels. Tachycardia and tachypnea may indicate hypoxemia. Late in the disease, pulmonary hypertension may lead to right ventricular hypertrophy and right-sided heart failure. Jugular vein distention, edema, hypotension, tachycardia, S$_3$ heart sound, a loud pulmonic component of S$_2$, heart murmurs, and hepatojugular reflux may be present.
- Assist with turning, coughing, and deep breathing *to mobilize secretions and facilitate removal.*
- Assist with diaphragmatic and pursed-lip breathing *to strengthen respiratory muscles.*
- Keep the client in high Fowler's position *to improve ventilation.*
- Maintain the client's diet and administer small, frequent feedings *to avoid fatigue when eating.* Small meals relieve pressure on the diaphragm and allow fuller lung movement.
- Monitor and record the color, amount, and consistency of sputum. *Changes in sputum may signal respiratory infection.*
- Monitor laboratory studies *to identify potential problems.* Follow drug levels for evidence of toxicity. Electrolyte imbalances may occur with diuretic use. Reduced Hb level and HCT affect the oxygen-carrying capacity of the blood.
- Monitor intake and output and daily weights *to detect fluid overload associated with right-sided heart failure.* Dehydration may impair the removal of secretions.

- Encourage fluids, unless contraindicated, *to liquefy secretions.*
- Provide chest physiotherapy, postural drainage, incentive spirometry, and suction *to aid in the removal of secretions.*
- Weigh the client daily *to detect edema caused by right-sided heart failure.*

Evaluation

- The client has adequate gas exchange as exhibited by stable ABG levels.
- The client reports increased energy and tolerance of ADLs.
- The client maintains stable weight.

Legionnaires' disease

LEGIONNAIRES' DISEASE is an acute bronchopneumonia, an inflammation of the lungs that begins in the terminal bronchioles. It's produced by a fastidious, gram-negative bacillus (rod-shaped bacterium).

Legionnaires' disease derives its name from the peculiar, highly publicized disease that struck 182 people (29 of whom died) at an American Legion convention in Philadelphia in July 1976.

This disease may occur epidemically or sporadically, usually in late summer or early fall. Its severity ranges from a mild illness, with or without pneumonitis, to multilobar pneumonia, with a mortality as high as 15%. A milder, self-limiting form (Pontiac fever) subsides within a few days but leaves the client fatigued for several weeks; this form mimics legionnaires' disease but produces few or no respiratory symptoms, no pneumonia, and no fatalities.

Possible cause

- *Legionella pneumophila*

Data collection findings

- Cough that's initially nonproductive but that can eventually produce grayish, nonpurulent, blood-streaked sputum
- Fever
- Recurrent chills
- Malaise
- Generalized weakness
- Bradycardia
- Headache
- Diffuse myalgias
- Anorexia
- Diarrhea
- Mental sluggishness
- Amnesia

Diagnostic findings

- Blood tests show leukocytosis, increased ESR, increased liver enzyme levels (alanine aminotransferase, aspartate aminotransferase, alkaline phosphatase), and hyponatremia.
- Chest X-ray shows patchy, localized infiltration, which progresses to multilobar consolidation (usually involving the lower lobes), pleural effusion and, in fulminant disease, opacification of the entire lung.
- Direct immunofluorescence of *L. pneumophila* and indirect fluorescent serum antibody testing compare findings from initial blood studies with findings from those done at least 3 weeks later. A convalescent serum sample showing a fourfold or greater rise in antibody titer for *L. pneumophila* confirms the diagnosis.
- Sputum test eliminates other organisms.

Nursing diagnoses

- Impaired gas exchange
- Ineffective tissue perfusion (cardiopulmonary)
- Hyperthermia

Treatment

- Oxygen therapy, which may require intubation and mechanical ventilation

Drug therapy options

- Antibiotic: erythromycin (Erythrocin), rifampin (Rifadin), tetracycline (Achromycin V)
- Antipyretic: acetaminophen (Tylenol), aspirin
- Inotropic agent: dopamine (Intropin)

Patient care goals

- The client will have adequate gas exchange.
- The client will cough effectively.
- The client will remain normothermic.

Nursing interventions

- Closely monitor the client's respiratory status. Evaluate chest wall expansion, depth and pattern of respirations, cough, and chest pain *to detect respiratory decompensation.*
- Continually monitor the client's vital signs, pulse oximetry or ABG values, LOC, and dryness and color of the lips and mucous membranes. Watch for signs of shock

(decreased blood pressure, thready pulse, diaphoresis, clammy skin) *to avoid crisis.*

● Keep the client comfortable; avoid chills and exposure to drafts, *which increase metabolic demands.* Provide mouth care frequently. If necessary, apply soothing cream to the nostrils *to promote comfort and prevent skin breakdown.*

● Replace fluid and electrolytes as needed *to maintain homeostasis.* The client with renal failure may require dialysis.

● Provide mechanical ventilation and other respiratory therapy as needed *to promote oxygenation.*

● Give antibiotics as necessary to eradicate infection, and observe carefully for adverse effects *to prevent complications.*

Evaluation

● The client has adequate gas exchange as evidenced by stable pulse oximetry and ABG levels.

● The client maintains a normal temperature.

Lung cancer

In LUNG CANCER, unregulated cell growth and uncontrolled cell division result in the development of a neoplasm. Cancer may also reach the lungs due to metastasis from other organs, mainly the liver, brain, bone, kidneys, and adrenal glands.

Four histologic types of lung cancer are:

● squamous cell (epidermoid) — a slow-growing cancer that originates from bronchial epithelium; metastasizes late to the surrounding area but may cause bronchial obstruction

● adenocarcinoma — a moderately growing cancer located in peripheral areas of the lung; metastasizes through the bloodstream to other organs

● large-cell anaplastic — a very fast-growing cancer associated with early and extensive metastasis; more common in peripheral lung tissue

● small-cell (oat cell cancer) — a very fast-growing cancer that metastasizes very early through lymph vessels and the bloodstream to other organs.

Possible causes

● Cigarette smoking

● Exposure to environmental pollutants

● Exposure to occupational pollutants

Data collection findings

● Cough

● Hemoptysis

● Weight loss and anorexia

● Chest pain

● Chills, fever

● Dyspnea

● Wheezing

● Weakness and fatigue

Diagnostic findings

● Bronchoscopy reveals a positive biopsy.

● Chest X-ray shows lesion or mass.

● Lung scan shows a mass.

● Open lung biopsy reveals a positive biopsy.

● Sputum study reveals positive cytology for cancer cells.

Nursing diagnoses

● Impaired gas exchange

● Activity intolerance

● Acute pain

Treatment

● Dietary changes, including establishing a high-protein, high-calorie diet and providing small, frequent meals

● Incentive spirometry

● Laser photocoagulation

● Oxygen therapy, intubation and, if the condition deteriorates, mechanical ventilation

● Radiation therapy

● Resection of the affected lobe (lobectomy) or lung (pneumonectomy)

Drug therapy options

● Analgesic: morphine, fentanyl (Sublimaze)

● Antiemetic: prochlorperazine (Compazine), ondansetron (Zofran)

● Antineoplastic: cyclophosphamide (Cytoxan), doxorubicin (Adriamycin), cisplatin (Platinol), vincristine (Oncovin)

● Diuretic: furosemide (Lasix), ethacrynic acid (Edecrin)

Patient care goals

● The client will maintain adequate ventilation.

● The client will carry out ADLs without weakness or fatigue.

● The client will express feelings of comfort and decreased pain.

Caring for the client with lung cancer

A 55-year-old male client is diagnosed with lung cancer and is to receive radiation and chemotherapy. He expresses extreme anxiety over his diagnosis and treatment.

How can you reduce some of this client's anxiety?

Urge the client to express his concerns. Answer all questions honestly. Include family members or significant others in the discussion. Explain all procedures that the client will experience. Reassure the client that adverse effects will be treated and that the client's comfort is of utmost importance. Suggest that the client and family contact the American Cancer Society for information on local support groups.

Questions for future thought

- What measures could be taken to decrease anxiety concerning future surgery for lung cancer?
- How would decreasing anxiety improve the client's recovery?

Nursing interventions

- Assess respiratory status *to detect respiratory complications. Cyanosis may suggest respiratory failure; an increase in sputum production may suggest an infection.*
- Assess the client's pain and administer analgesics as prescribed. *Assessment allows for care plan modification as needed.*
- Monitor and record vital signs *to assess for complications.* Tachycardia and tachypnea may indicate hypoxemia. An elevated temperature suggests an infection.
- Monitor and record intake and output *to assess fluid status.*
- Track laboratory values *to identify potential problems.* Monitor for bleeding, infection, and electrolyte imbalance due to effects of chemotherapy. A low WBC count increases the risk of infection. Low platelets increase the risk of bleeding. Electrolyte abnormalities, especially hypercalcemia, may also occur.
- Monitor pulse oximetry values and report a drop in oxygen saturation *to avoid hypoxemia.*
- Administer oxygen *to maintain tissue oxygenation.*

- Encourage fluids and administer I.V. fluids *to provide hydration and liquefy secretions to facilitate removal. Drinking moistens mucous membranes.*
- Provide suctioning, and assist with turning, coughing, and deep breathing *to facilitate removal of secretions.*
- Keep the client in semi-Fowler's position *to maximize ventilation.*
- Prepare the client for TPN administration or enteral feeding, as indicated, *which optimizes his nutrition and bolsters the immune system.*
- Administer medications as prescribed to treat the cancer and provide pain relief.
- Encourage the client to express feelings about changes in his body image and fear of dying *to reduce anxiety.*
- Provide mouth care *to improve comfort and reduce the risk of stomatitis* (for the client undergoing chemotherapy). Provide skin care *to minimize the adverse effects of radiation therapy.*
- Provide rest periods *to enhance tissue oxygenation.*

Evaluation

- The client has adequate gas exchange as evidenced by stable pulse oximetry and ABG results.
- The client reports ability to perform ADLs without fatigue.
- The client reports adequate pain control.

(See *Caring for the client with lung cancer.*)

Lung resection

Lung resection may involve removal of an entire lung, a lobe, or a segment. In segmental resection, one or more segments are removed and as much functioning lung tissue as possible is retained. Lung resections are done to treat bronchiectasis, lung abscess, and lung cancer.

Possible causes

- Bronchiectasis (recurrent inadequately treated infections)
- Cigarette smoke
- Lung abscess (aspiration, pneumonia)
- Lung cancer
- Mucoviscidosis (for example, cystic fibrosis)
- Obstruction (by foreign body, tumor, or stenosis) in association with recurrent infection
- Occupational and environmental pollutants

Data collection findings
- Cough
- Hemoptysis
- Dyspnea
- Wheezing
- Fever and chills
- Weakness and fatigue
- Weight loss and anorexia
- Chest pain

Diagnostic findings
- Chest X-ray shows a lesion or mass, evidence of abscess, or bronchiectasis.
- Bronchoscopy with biopsy is positive.
- Sputum cytology is positive for cancer cells.
- Pulmonary function tests determine the ability of the remaining lung tissue to meet the client's respiratory needs.

Nursing diagnoses
- Impaired gas exchange
- Ineffective airway clearance
- Acute pain
- Anxiety

Treatment
- High-protein, high-calorie diet and small, frequent meals
- Incentive spirometry
- Oxygen therapy, intubation and, if the client's condition deteriorates, mechanical ventilation
- Chest tubes

Drug therapy options
- Analgesic: morphine, fentanyl (Sublimaze)
- Antiemetic: ondansetron (Zofran), prochlorperazine (Compazine)
- Antineoplastic: cisplatin (Platinol), cyclophosphamide (Cytoxan), doxorubicin (Adriamycin), vincristine (Oncovin)
- Diuretic: ethacrynic acid (Edecrin), furosemide (Lasix)

Patient care goals
- The client's lung will reexpand without difficulty.
- The client will maintain an effective breathing pattern.
- The client won't hemorrhage after surgery.
- The client will maintain full ROM of the shoulder on the affected side.

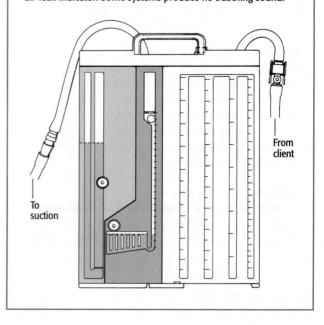

Disposable drainage systems

Commercially prepared disposable drainage systems combine drainage collection, water seal, and suction control in one unit (as shown here). These systems ensure client safety with positive- and negative-pressure relief valves and have a prominent air-leak indicator. Some systems produce no bubbling sound.

To suction

From client

- The client will be discharged with pain controlled and with knowledge of ways to prevent infection and further lung compromise.

Nursing interventions
Preoperative
- Assess respiratory status *to detect respiratory compromise.*
- Make sure the client receives nothing by mouth 8 hours before bronchoscopy and until gag reflex returns afterward *to prevent aspiration.*
- Teach the client about chest tubes, incentive spirometry, coughing and deep breathing, and pain medication *to reduce anxiety and improve compliance with the treatment regimen.*

Postoperative
- Monitor respiratory status, pulse oximetry, and vital signs *to detect signs of infection, hypoxia, and respiratory or cardiac failure.*

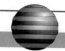

CLINICAL SITUATION

Caring for the client with hemoptysis

A female client, age 60, was admitted to the hospital with a cough and hemoptysis. A lesion was detected by X-ray. After a bronchoscopy, the client undergoes segmental resection of a coin-size lesion in the lower lobe of her right lung.

After lung resection, the client has a chest tube attached to a three-chamber chest drainage system. During the night, she becomes disoriented, gets out of bed, and steps on the drainage device, causing it to crack open and lose its seal.

Which nursing diagnoses apply to the client?
- Acute pain (related to the surgery)
- Anxiety (related to the diagnosis and surgery)
- Impaired gas exchange (related to potential postoperative complications)
- Ineffective airway clearance (related to anesthesia and postoperative discomfort)

What should the nurse do if the chest drainage system cracks open?
When a chest drainage system cracks open, the closed system between the pleural space and the device is broken. This allows air to move through the tubing into the pleural space. The nurse should immediately place the distal end of the tube in sterile water, closing the system again. The tube shouldn't be clamped because it increases pressure against the pleural space. It's inappropriate to attach the drain directly to wall suction. The nurse should call the physician *after* correcting the problem.

Questions for further thought
- Why is encouraging deep breathing an appropriate nursing intervention for a client with a chest tube?
- What are appropriate outcomes for this client at the time of discharge?

- Monitor intake and output *to assess fluid status.*
- Track laboratory values *to assess for signs of infection and electrolyte imbalance.*
- Administer oxygen as needed *to maintain tissue oxygenation.*

- Administer I.V. fluids and encourage the client to drink fluids, as tolerated, *to maintain hydration and liquefy secretions.*
- Provide suctioning as needed, and assist with turning, coughing, and deep breathing *to facilitate removal of secretions.*
- Place the client in semi-Fowler's position *to maximize ventilation.*

Care of chest tube
- Check for water level fluctuation in the water-seal chamber, *which indicates patency.*
- Check for bubbling in the water seal. *If surgery exposed raw lung tissue, bubbling may be normal with coughing and expiration. Continuous bubbling may indicate a leak in the system.*
- If water is used in the suction chamber, check for continuous bubbling, *which indicates that the system is working properly.* If a waterless suction system is used, make sure that the suction dial is set correctly.
- Maintain the drainage system below chest level *to preserve the water seal and prevent reflux.*
- Reinforce connections with tape *to avoid kinks* and keep the tubing straight.
- If the client has drainage, measure and mark the level each time vital signs are taken. Immediately report any amount greater than the established range, which varies depending on the type of surgery. (See *Disposable drainage systems.*)

Evaluation
- The client's pain is controlled.
- The client's lung reexpands without complication, and the chest tube is removed.
- The client has full ROM on the affected side.
- The client's respiratory status is at the optimum level based on remaining lung function.
- The client verbalizes measures to prevent infection and further lung compromise.

(See *Caring for the client with hemoptysis.*)

Pleural effusion and empyema

PLEURAL EFFUSION is an excess of fluid in the pleural space (the thin space between the lung tissue and the membranous sac that protects it). Normally, the pleural space contains a small amount of extracellular fluid that lubricates the pleural surfaces. Increased production or inadequate removal of this fluid results in pleural effusion.

EMPYEMA is the accumulation of pus and necrotic tissue in the pleural space. Blood and chyle may also collect in this space, resulting in HEMOTHORAX and CHYLOTHORAX, respectively.

Possible causes

- Bacterial or fungal pneumonitis or empyema
- TB
- Chest trauma
- Hepatic disease with ascites
- Collagen disease (lupus erythematosus and rheumatoid arthritis)
- Heart failure
- Infection in the pleural space
- Malignancy
- Myxedema
- Pancreatitis
- Hypoalbuminemia
- Peritoneal dialysis
- Pulmonary embolism with or without infarction
- Subphrenic abscess

Data collection findings

- Pleuritic chest pain
- Dyspnea
- Decreased breath sounds
- Fever
- Malaise

Diagnostic findings

- Chest X-ray shows radiopaque fluid in dependent regions.
- Thoracentesis shows LD levels less than 200 IU and protein levels less than 3 g/dl (in transudative effusions); ratio of protein in pleural fluid to serum greater than or equal to 0.5, LD in pleural fluid greater than or equal to 200 IU, and ratio of LD in pleural fluid to LD in serum greater than 0.6 (in exudative effusions); and acute inflammatory WBCs and microorganisms (in empyema).
- Tuberculin skin test rules out TB as the cause.

Nursing diagnoses

- Impaired gas exchange
- Hyperthermia
- Risk for infection

Treatment

- Thoracentesis to remove fluid
- Thoracotomy if thoracentesis is ineffective

Drug therapy options

- Antibiotic for empyema (according to sensitivity of causative organism)

Patient care goals

- The client will maintain adequate ventilation.
- The client will remain free from signs and symptoms of infection.
- The client will remain normothermic.

Nursing interventions

- Explain thoracentesis to the client before the procedure *to allay his anxiety.* Tell the client to expect a stinging sensation from the local anesthetic and a feeling of pressure when the needle is inserted.
- Instruct the client to tell you immediately if he feels uncomfortable or has trouble breathing during the procedure. *Difficulty breathing may indicate pneumothorax, which requires immediate chest tube insertion.*
- Reassure the client during thoracentesis *to allay anxiety.*
- Remind the client to breathe normally and to avoid sudden movements, such as coughing and sighing, *to prevent improper needle placement.*
- Monitor vital signs and watch for syncope *to prevent injury.*
- Watch for respiratory distress or pneumothorax (sudden onset of dyspnea, cyanosis) after thoracentesis *to detect complications of thoracentesis.*
- Administer oxygen *to improve oxygenation.*
- Administer antibiotics *to treat empyema.*
- Encourage the client to perform deep-breathing exercises *to promote lung expansion.* Also encourage use of an incentive spirometer *to promote deep breathing.*
- Assist with providing meticulous chest tube care, and use sterile technique for changing dressings around the tube insertion site in empyema *to prevent infection at the insertion site.*
- Ensure chest tube patency by watching for bubbles in the underwater seal chamber *to prevent respiratory distress resulting from chest tube obstruction.*
- Record the amount, color, and consistency of tube drainage *to monitor the effectiveness of treatment.*
- Assist with arranging visiting nurse referrals for clients who will be discharged with the tube in place *to ensure that the healing process is evaluated.*

Evaluation

- The client has adequate gas exchange as evidenced by a stable pulse oximetry and ABG levels.
- The client has no complications caused by infection.
- The client has a normal temperature.

Pleurisy

Also known as *pleuritis*, PLEURISY is inflammation of the visceral and parietal pleurae, the serous membranes that line the inside of the thoracic cage and envelop the lungs.

Possible causes

- Cancer
- Chest trauma
- Dressler's syndrome
- Pneumonia
- Pulmonary infarction
- Rheumatoid arthritis
- Systemic lupus erythematosus
- TB
- Uremia
- Viruses

Data collection findings

- Sharp, stabbing pain that increases with respiration
- Pleural friction rub (a coarse, creaky sound heard during late inspiration and early expiration)
- Dyspnea

Diagnostic findings

Although diagnosis generally rests on the client's history and the nurse's respiratory assessment, diagnostic tests help rule out other causes and pinpoint the underlying disorder.

- ECG rules out CAD as the source of the client's pain.
- Chest X-rays identify pneumonia.

Nursing diagnoses

- Ineffective breathing pattern
- Acute pain
- Activity intolerance

Treatment

- Bed rest
- Thoracentesis (for pleurisy with pleural effusion)

Drug therapy options

- Analgesic: oxycodone and acetaminophen (Percocet)
- Anti-inflammatory: indomethacin (Indocin)

Patient care goals

- The client will maintain adequate gas exchange.
- The client will express feelings of comfort and pain relief.
- The client will demonstrate skill in conserving energy while carrying out ADLs to tolerance level.

Nursing interventions

- Stress the importance of bed rest and plan your care *to allow the client as much uninterrupted rest as possible.*
- Administer antitussives and pain medication as necessary *to relieve cough and pain.*
- If the pain requires a narcotic analgesic, warn the client about to be discharged to avoid overuse *because such medication depresses coughing and respiration.*
- Encourage the client to cough and apply firm pressure at the pain site during coughing exercises *to minimize pain.*

Evaluation

- The client has adequate gas exchange as evidenced by stable pulse oximetry and ABG levels.
- The client reports adequate pain control.
- The client reports increased activity level.

Pneumocystis carinii pneumonia

The microorganism *Pneumocystis carinii* is part of the normal flora in most healthy people. However, in the immunocompromised client, *P. carinii* becomes an aggressive pathogen. PNEUMOCYSTIS CARINII PNEUMONIA (PCP) is an opportunistic infection strongly associated with HUMAN IMMUNODEFICIENCY VIRUS (HIV) infection.

PCP occurs in up to 90% of HIV-infected clients in the United States at some point during their lifetime. It's the leading cause of death in these clients. Disseminated infection doesn't occur.

PCP is also associated with other immunocompromised conditions, including organ transplantation, LEUKEMIA, and lymphoma.

Possible causes

- *P. carinii*

Data collection findings

- Generalized fatigue
- Low-grade, intermittent fever
- Nonproductive cough
- Shortness of breath
- Dyspnea
- Tachypnea
- Anorexia
- Weight loss

Diagnostic findings

- ABG studies detect hypoxia and an increased alveolar-arterial gradient.

- Chest X-ray may show slowly progressing, fluffy infiltrates and occasionally nodular lesions or a spontaneous pneumothorax, but these findings must be differentiated from findings in other types of pneumonia or ARDS.
- Fiberoptic bronchoscopy confirms PCP.
- Gallium scan may show increased uptake over the lungs even when the chest X-ray appears relatively normal.
- Histologic studies confirm *P. carinii*. In clients with HIV infection, initial examination of a first morning sputum specimen (induced by inhaling an ultrasonically dispersed saline mist) may be sufficient; however, this technique is usually ineffective in clients without HIV infection.

Nursing diagnoses
- Impaired gas exchange
- Imbalanced nutrition: Less than body requirements
- Risk for infection

Treatment
- Diet therapy to maintain adequate nutrition
- Oxygen therapy, which may include ET intubation and mechanical ventilation

Drug therapy options
- Antibiotic: co-trimoxazole (Bactrim), pentamidine (NebuPent)

Patient care goals
- The client will maintain adequate oxygenation.
- The client will have adequate daily calorie intake.
- The client will remain free from infection.

Nursing interventions
- Frequently assess the client's respiratory status, and monitor ABG levels every 4 hours *to detect early signs of hypoxemia.*
- Administer oxygen therapy as necessary. Encourage the client to ambulate and to perform deep-breathing exercises and incentive spirometry *to facilitate effective gas exchange.*
- Administer antipyretics as required *to relieve fever.*
- Monitor intake and output and daily weight *to evaluate fluid balance.* Replace fluids as necessary *to correct fluid volume deficit.*
- Prepare the client for administration of antimicrobial drugs as required. *Pentamidine is never given I.M. because it can cause pain and sterile abscesses.* Administration of the I.V. drug form should be done slowly over 60 minutes *to reduce the risk of hypotension.*

- Monitor the client for adverse reactions to antimicrobial drugs. If he's receiving co-trimoxazole, watch for nausea, vomiting, rash, bone marrow suppression, thrush, fever, hepatotoxicity, and anaphylaxis. If he's receiving pentamidine, watch for cardiac arrhythmias, hypotension, dizziness, azotemia, hypocalcemia, and hepatic disturbances. *These measures detect problems early to avoid crisis.*
- Provide diversional activities and coordinate health care team activities *to allow adequate rest periods between procedures.*
- Supply nutritional supplements as needed. Encourage the client to eat a high-calorie, protein-rich diet. Offer small, frequent meals if the client can't tolerate large amounts of food. *These measures ensure that the client's nutritional intake meets his metabolic needs.*
- Provide a relaxing environment, eliminate excessive environmental stimuli, and allow ample time for meals *to reduce anxiety.*
- Give emotional support and help the client identify and use meaningful support systems *to promote emotional well-being.*

Evaluation
- The client has adequate gas exchange as evidenced by stable pulse oximetry and ABG levels.
- The client maintains an appropriate weight.
- The client is free from infection.

Pneumonia

PNEUMONIA refers to a bacterial, viral, parasitic, or fungal infection that causes inflammation of the alveolar spaces. In pneumonia, microorganisms enter alveolar spaces through droplet inhalation, resulting in inflammation and an increase in alveolar fluid. Ventilation decreases as secretions thicken.

Possible causes
- Aspiration
- Chemical irritants
- Organisms, such as *Escherichia coli*, *Haemophilus influenzae*, *Staphylococcus aureus*, *Pneumocystis carinii*, *Streptococcus pneumoniae*, and *Pseudomonas*

Data collection findings
- Shortness of breath
- Dyspnea
- Tachypnea
- Accessory muscle use

CLINICAL SITUATION

Caring for the client with pneumonia

A 60-year-old female client presents with complaints of malaise, productive cough, fever with chills, and pleuritic chest pain. Her white blood cell count indicates leukocytosis in bacterial pneumonia and a normal or low count in viral or mycoplasmal pneumonia.

Which diagnostic measures should be taken to confirm a diagnosis of pneumonia?
A. Chest X-ray, urinalysis (UA), bronchoscopy
B. Chest X-ray, sputum and blood culture, complete blood count (CBC)
C. Throat culture, CBC, arterial blood gas
D. Throat culture, UA, chest X-ray
Answer: B. Chest X-ray discloses infiltrates, confirming the diagnosis. Sputum specimen for Gram stain and culture and sensitivity shows acute inflammatory cells, and can direct antibiotic therapy. Blood cultures reflect bacteremia and help to determine the causative organism.

Which nursing diagnoses would be appropriate when caring for the client with pneumonia?
● Imbalanced nutrition: Less than body requirements
● Impaired gas exchange
● Ineffective airway clearance
● Acute pain
● Risk for deficient fluid volume
● Risk for infection

Questions for further thought
● What measures would decrease the incidence of pneumonia in the elderly, pediatric, or immunosuppressed client?
● What teaching should be done to maximize oxygenation in the client with pneumonia?

● Sputum production that's rusty, green, or bloody with pneumococcal pneumonia and yellow-green with bronchopneumonia
● Fever and chills
● Crackles, rhonchi, pleural friction rub on auscultation
● Cough
● Malaise
● Pleuritic pain
● Restlessness
● Confusion

Diagnostic findings
● ABG levels show hypoxemia and respiratory alkalosis.
● Chest X-ray shows pulmonary infiltrates.
● Hematology study shows increased WBCs and ESR.
● Sputum study identifies organism.

Nursing diagnoses
● Impaired gas exchange
● Ineffective airway clearance
● Imbalanced nutrition: Less than body requirements

Treatment
● Chest physiotherapy, postural drainage, and incentive spirometry

● Dietary changes, including establishing a high-calorie, high-protein diet and forcing fluids
● Intubation and mechanical ventilation if condition deteriorates
● Nutritional support, including enteral nutrition if the client requires intubation

Drug therapy options
● Antibiotic (according to organism sensitivity)
● Antipyretic: aspirin, acetaminophen (Tylenol)
● Bronchodilator: metaproterenol (Alupent), isoetharine (Bronkosol), albuterol (Proventil)

Patient care goals
● The client will maintain adequate ventilation and oxygenation.
● The client will consume a specific number of calories daily.

Nursing interventions
● Monitor and record intake and output. *Insensible water loss secondary to fever may cause dehydration.* (See *Caring for the client with pneumonia.*)

- Monitor laboratory studies. An elevated WBC count suggests infection. *Blood and sputum cultures may identify the causative agent.*
- Monitor pulse oximetry *to detect respiratory compromise.*
- Assess respiratory status *to detect early signs of compromise.*
- Monitor and record vital signs. An elevated temperature increases oxygen demands. *Hypotension and tachycardia may suggest hypovolemic shock.*
- Monitor and record the color, consistency, and amount of sputum. Sputum amount and consistency may indicate hydration status and the effectiveness of therapy. Foul-smelling sputum suggests respiratory infection.
- Administer oxygen *to help relieve respiratory distress.*
- Maintain the client's diet *to offset hypermetabolic state due to infection.*
- Force fluids to 3,000 ml per day and administer I.V. fluids *to help liquefy secretions to aid in their removal.*
- Provide suction and assist with turning, coughing, and deep breathing *to promote mobilization and removal of secretions.*
- Administer chest physiotherapy *to facilitate removal of secretions.*
- Administer medications as prescribed *to treat infection and improve ventilation.*
- Encourage the client to express feelings about fear of suffocation *to reduce anxiety.*
- Provide tissues and a bag for hygienic sputum disposal *to prevent the spread of infection.*
- Provide oral hygiene *to promote comfort and improve nutrition.*

Evaluation

- The client has adequate oxygenation as evidenced by stable pulse oximetry and ABG levels.
- The client maintains appropriate weight.

Pneumothorax and hemothorax

In PNEUMOTHORAX, loss of negative intrapleural pressure results in the collapse of the lung. Pneumothorax may be described as spontaneous, open, or tension:

- Spontaneous pneumothorax results from the rupture of a bleb.
- Open pneumothorax occurs when an opening through the chest wall allows air to flow between the pleural space and the outside of the body.
- Tension pneumothorax results from a buildup of air in the pleural space that can't escape.

In all cases, the surface area for gas exchange is reduced, resulting in hypoxia and hypercapnia.

In HEMOTHORAX, blood accumulates in the pleural space when a rib lacerates lung tissue or an intercostal artery. This compresses the lung and limits respiratory capacity. Hemothorax can also result from rupture of large or small pulmonary vessels.

Possible causes

- Blunt chest trauma
- Central venous catheter insertion
- Penetrating chest injuries
- Rupture of a bleb
- Thoracentesis
- Thoracic surgeries

Data collection findings

- Dyspnea
- Tachypnea
- Subcutaneous emphysema
- Cough
- Diminished or absent breath sounds unilaterally
- Sharp pain that increases with exertion
- Dullness on chest percussion (in the case of hemothorax and tension pneumothorax)
- Tracheal shift and decreased chest expansion unilaterally
- Anxiety
- Diaphoresis
- Pallor
- Hypotension (in the case of hemothorax)
- Tachycardia

Diagnostic findings

- ABG levels show respiratory acidosis and hypoxemia.
- Chest X-ray reveals pneumothorax or hemothorax.
- Ventilation-perfusion scintigraphy is decreased.
- Lung scan shows ventilation-perfusion ratio mismatches.

Nursing diagnoses

- Impaired gas exchange
- Ineffective breathing pattern
- Acute pain

Treatment

- Active ROM exercises to affected arm
- Blood transfusions for hemothorax as indicated
- Chest tube to water-seal drainage
- Incentive spirometry

- Occlusive dressing (for open pneumothorax)
- Oxygen therapy

Drug therapy options
- Analgesic: morphine

Patient care goals
- The client will maintain adequate ventilation.
- The client will achieve a normal breathing pattern.
- The client will express feelings of comfort and a decrease in pain.

Nursing interventions
- Monitor and record vital signs. *Hypotension, tachycardia, and tachypnea suggest tension pneumothorax.*
- Check the chest drainage system for air leaks *that can impair lung expansion.*
- Assess respiratory status *to identify possible complications.* Dyspnea, tachypnea, diminished breath sounds, subcutaneous emphysema, and accessory muscles use suggest accumulation of air in the pleural space.
- Monitor chest tube drainage to ensure proper placement. *An increase in the amount of bloody drainage suggests new bleeding or an increase in bleeding.* Check tubing for kinks if there's a sudden reduction in drainage.
- Assess cardiovascular status *to identify possible complications.* Tachycardia, hypotension, and jugular vein distention suggest tension pneumothorax.
- Assess the client's pain and administer medications as prescribed *to control pain.*
- Administer oxygen *to relieve respiratory distress caused by hypoxemia.*
- Assist with turning, coughing, deep breathing, and incentive spirometry *to enhance mobilization of secretions and prevent atelectasis.*
- Maintain chest tube to water-seal *to prevent air from entering the chest tube when the client inhales.*
- Keep the client in high Fowler's position *to enhance chest expansion.*

Evaluation
- The client has adequate gas exchange as evidenced by stable pulse oximetry and ABG levels.
- The client has a normal breathing pattern.
- The client reports adequate pain control.

Pulmonary embolism

A PULMONARY EMBOLISM results from an undissolved substance (such as fat, air, or thrombus) obstructing blood flow in the pulmonary vessels. The embolus travels from the venous circulation to the right side of the heart and pulmonary artery, obstructing blood flow and resulting in pulmonary hypertension and possible infarction.

Possible causes
- Abdominal, pelvic, or thoracic surgery
- Central venous catheter insertion
- Venous stasis
- Heart failure
- Flat long-bone fractures
- Prolonged bed rest
- Hypercoagulability
- Obesity
- Polycythemia vera
- Oral contraceptives
- Malignant tumors
- Pregnancy
- Sickle cell anemia
- Thrombophlebitis

Data collection findings
- Sudden onset of dyspnea, tachypnea, or crackles
- Chest pain
- Tachycardia
- Arrhythmias
- Hypotension
- Anxiety
- Cough
- Hemoptysis
- Fever

Diagnostic findings
- ABG levels show respiratory alkalosis and hypoxemia.
- Blood chemistry tests reveal increased LD level.
- Chest X-ray shows dilated pulmonary arteries, pneumoconstriction, and diaphragm elevation on the affected side.
- ECG shows tachycardia, nonspecific ST-segment changes, and right axis deviation.
- Pulmonary angiography shows the location of the embolism and a pulmonary artery filling defect.
- Lung scan shows ventilation-perfusion mismatch.

Nursing diagnoses
- Impaired gas exchange
- Ineffective tissue perfusion (cardiopulmonary)
- Anxiety

Treatment
● Bed rest with active and passive ROM and isometric exercises
● Vena cava filter insertion
● Oxygen therapy, intubation, and mechanical ventilation, if necessary

Drug therapy options
● Analgesic: morphine
● Anticoagulant: heparin (Liquaemin), followed by warfarin (Coumadin)
● Diuretic: furosemide (Lasix) if pulmonary edema develops
● Fibrinolytic: streptokinase (Streptase), urokinase (Abbokinase)

Patient care goals
● The client will have adequate gas exchange.
● The client will have improved tissue perfusion.
● The client will use support systems to assist with coping.

Nursing interventions
● Assess respiratory status *to detect respiratory distress.*
● Assess cardiovascular status for complications. An irregular pulse may signal arrhythmia caused by hypoxemia. If pulmonary embolism is caused by thrombophlebitis, temperature may be elevated.
● Monitor laboratory studies for possible problems. PTT should be maintained at 1½ to 2 times control in client receiving heparin. PT should be maintained at 1½ to 2 times control or INR at 2 to 3 for the client receiving warfarin. Monitor ABGs for evidence of pulmonary compromise.
● Maintain safety of equipment for monitoring CVP. *CVP may rise if right-sided heart failure develops.*
● Monitor and record intake and output *to detect fluid volume overload and renal perfusion.*
● Assess for positive Homans' sign *to detect thromboembolism as a cause of pulmonary embolus.*
● Administer oxygen *to enhance arterial oxygenation.*
● Assist with turning, coughing, and deep breathing *to mobilize secretions and clear airways.*
● Keep the client in high Fowler's position *to enhance ventilation.*
● Provide suctioning and monitor and record color, consistency, and amount of sputum *to assess for complications.* A productive cough and blood-tinged sputum may be present with pulmonary embolism.
● Administer I.V. fluids as ordered *to maintain hydration.*

● Administer medications as prescribed *to enhance tissue oxygenation.*

Evaluation
● The client has adequate gas exchange and cardiac perfusion as evidenced by stable vital signs.
● The client demonstrates calm behavior and appropriate coping skills.

Tuberculosis
TUBERCULOSIS (TB) is an airborne, infectious, communicable disease that can occur acutely or chronically. It occurs most commonly in lower socioeconomic groups and immigrants and is associated with overwork, poor nutrition, and overcrowding combined with poor ventilation. Individuals with immunosuppression (for example, cancer or HIV) are at increased risk.

Inhaled mycobacteria, carried by droplet nuclei, usually settle in alveolar lung tissue, where they begin an inflammatory process. Cell-mediated immunity to the mycobacteria develops within 3 to 6 weeks and arrests the disease. If the infection reactivates, the inflammatory process can lead to necrosis in the center of the inflamed area, causing caseation (a process that changes dead tissue into a cheeselike substance). The caseum may localize, undergo fibrosis, or excavate and form cavities, the walls of which are studded with multiplying mycobacteria. If this occurs, infected caseous debris may spread by the tracheobronchial tree to other areas throughout the lungs.

Possible causes
● *Mycobacterium tuberculosis*

Data collection findings
● Cough, hemoptysis, or mucoid sputum
● Dyspnea
● Low-grade fever
● Night sweats
● Crackles
● Fatigue
● Malaise
● Weight loss and anorexia
● Pleuritic chest pain

Diagnostic findings
● Chest X-ray shows active or calcified lesions.
● Hematology shows increased WBC count and ESR.
● Smear is positive for acid bacilli.
● Culture is positive for *M. tuberculosis.*

Medications for clients with tuberculosis

Streptomycin

- Streptomycin is an aminoglycoside antibiotic used in combination with other antituberculotic drugs. It's administered only by deep I.M. injection.
- Central nervous system depression syndrome has been reported in infants on high doses.
- Avoid direct contact with the drug because sensitization may occur.
- Monitor the client for ototoxicity and nephrotoxicity.

Isoniazid (INH)

- Isoniazid is used to treat clients with active tuberculosis and to prevent the disorder in high-risk clients.
- The oral form is best administered on an empty stomach.
- A client taking the drug should avoid tyramine- and histamine-containing foods.
- If the solution crystallizes, warm it to room temperature to dissolve the crystals.
- Monitor the client for visual changes.
- This drug causes vitamin B_6 deficiency. Monitor the client for paresthesia of the hands and feet, and administer pyridoxine.
- Monitor blood pressure for orthostatic hypotension.
- Monitor liver enzyme levels.
- Monitor weight.

Ethambutol (Myambutol)

- Ethambutol is an antituberculotic drug given with at least one other drug.
- Protect this drug from light, moisture, and heat.
- Monitor vision.
- Monitor hepatic and renal function.
- Monitor blood counts and serum uric acid levels.

Rifampin (Rifadin, Rimactane, Rofact)

- Rifampin is an antituberculotic drug given in combination with other antituberculotic drugs.
- Administer oral medication on an empty stomach.
- Monitor hepatic function.
- Monitor prothrombin time if the client is also taking an anticoagulant.
- Urine, feces, sputum, and sweat may be stained red-orange.
- Rifampin can decrease the effectiveness of oral contraceptives.

Pyrazinamide (Pyrazinamide, Tebrazid)

- Pyrazinamide may affect glycemic control in diabetics.
- Monitor hepatic function and uric acid levels.
- Encourage the client to drink plenty of fluids.

- Mantoux skin test result is positive. Induration is localized. The amount of induration considered positive ranges from 5 to 15 mm, depending on the risk category. Old infections may no longer be positive. A two-step method may be used to boost response.

Nursing diagnoses

- Ineffective airway clearance
- Ineffective health maintenance
- Imbalanced nutrition: Less than body requirements
- Deficient knowledge (client)

Treatment

- Standard airborne precautions (As long as the client is contagious, everyone entering the client's room must wear a respirator with high-efficiency particulate air filter or positive pressure air supplied.)
- Diet high in carbohydrates, protein, vitamins B_6 and C, and calories
- Chest physiotherapy, postural drainage, and incentive spirometry

Drug therapy options

- Directly observed combination therapy with isoniazid (Laniazid), rifampin (Rifadin), pyrazinamide (Pyrazinamide), and ethambutol (Myambutol). Streptomycin may be substituted for ethambutol but must be given by injection. (See *Medications for clients with tuberculosis.*)

Patient care goals

- The client will take medication as directed.
- The client will explain why medications are important.
- The client will explain ways to prevent organisms from spreading.
- The client's nutritional needs will be met.
- The client and contacts will remain free from active pulmonary disease.

Nursing interventions

- Provide negative pressure room *to prevent spread of infection.* (See *Guidelines for respiratory isolation,* page 356.)

> ## Guidelines for respiratory isolation
>
> ● Provide a private, negative-pressure room for the client, and keep the door closed.
> ● Wash your hands before entering and leaving the client's room.
> ● Use special handling procedures for sputum and secretions.
> ● Have the client wear a mask when being transported outside the room.
> ● Instruct everyone entering the client's room to wear a respirator with a high efficiency particulate filter while the client is contagious.

● Monitor respiratory status, vital signs, and laboratory test results *to detect signs of respiratory compromise and adverse reactions to drug therapy.*
● If ordered, perform chest physiotherapy *to help mobilize secretions.*
● Encourage frequent oral hygiene *to promote comfort and appetite.*
● Encourage the client to eat foods rich in protein, calcium, and vitamins C, D, and B complex *to improve nutritional status.*
● Encourage the client to drink plenty of fluids *to liquefy sputum.*
● Administer medications as prescribed *to avoid development of drug-resistant organisms.*
● Teach the client the importance of following a prescribed regimen *to promote compliance.*
● Advise the client to cover his mouth when coughing, sneezing, or raising sputum *to reduce droplet transmission.*

Evaluation
● The client understands and follows the medication regimen.
● The client maintains a normal weight.
● The client describes and demonstrates ways to prevent spread of TB.

MUSCULOSKELETAL SYSTEM

The musculoskeletal system has two main functions: to provide support and to produce movement. In addition, the musculoskeletal system protects internal tissues and organs, produces RBCs in the bone marrow, and stores mineral salts such as calcium.

Musculoskeletal structure and function

The musculoskeletal system is made up of the skeleton, skeletal muscles, and associated structures, such as tendons and ligaments.

Bones, muscles, and other structures
● The skeleton consists of 206 bones that work with the muscles to support and protect internal organs. The bones store calcium, magnesium, and phosphorus. Bone marrow produces RBCs.
● Skeletal muscles are attached to the bones by tendons and provide body movement and posture by tightening and shortening. They begin contracting when stimulated by a motor neuron, and derive energy for muscle contraction from hydrolysis of adenosine triphosphate to adenosine diphosphate and phosphate. The skeletal muscles relax with the breakdown of ACh by cholinesterase. Even then, they retain some contraction to maintain muscle tone.
● Ligaments and tendons are tough bands of collagen fibers. Ligaments connect bones to bones and encircle joints to add strength and stability. Tendons connect muscles to bones.
● Joints are formed by the articulation of two bone surfaces. Joints provide stabilization and permit locomotion. The degree of joint movement is called range of motion (ROM).
● The synovium is a membrane that lines a joint's inner surfaces. In conjunction with cartilage, the synovium reduces friction in joints through its production of synovial fluid.
● Cartilage is a specialized tissue that serves as a smooth surface for articulating bones. It absorbs shock to joints and serves as padding to reduce friction. Cartilage atrophies with limited ROM or in the absence of weight-bearing bursae (small sacs of synovial fluid).

MUSCULOSKELETAL DISORDERS

Disorders of the musculoskeletal system may be acute or chronic. Disorders include arm and leg fractures, carpal tunnel syndrome, compartment syndrome, gout, herniated disk, hip fracture, osteoarthritis, osteomyelitis, and osteoporosis.

Arm and leg fractures

Fractures of the arms and legs usually result from trauma and commonly cause substantial muscle, nerve, and other soft-tissue damage. The prognosis varies with the extent of disability or deformity, the amount of tissue and vascular damage, the adequacy of reduction and immobilization, and the client's age, health, and nutritional status.

Children's bones usually heal rapidly and without deformity. Bones of adults in poor health and with impaired circulation may never heal properly. Severe open fractures, especially of the femoral shaft, may cause substantial blood loss and life-threatening hypovolemic shock.

Possible causes
- Bone tumors
- Major trauma
- Osteoporosis

Data collection findings
- Discoloration
- Loss of function
- Pain
- Swelling
- Deformity
- Crepitus

Diagnostic findings
- Anteroposterior and lateral radiographs of the suspected fracture as well as radiographs of the joints above and below it confirm the diagnosis.

Nursing diagnoses
- Impaired physical mobility
- Acute pain
- Deficient fluid volume
- Anxiety

Treatment
Emergency care
- Splinting the limb above and below the suspected fracture
- Cold pack application and elevation of the extremity to reduce edema and pain
- Direct pressure to control bleeding in severe fractures that cause blood loss
- If blood loss occurs, fluid replacement as soon as possible to prevent hypovolemic shock

After confirming diagnosis
- Closed reduction (restoring displaced bone segments to their normal position)
- Open reduction during surgery to reduce and immobilize the fracture using rods, plates, and screws when closed reduction is impossible, usually followed by application of a plaster cast
- Immobilization with a splint, cast, or traction
- Skin or skeletal traction (if splint or cast fails to maintain the reduction)

Open fractures
- Surgery to repair soft-tissue damage
- Thorough debridement of the wound

Drug therapy options
- Analgesic: codeine, morphine, oxycodone and acetaminophen (Percocet)
- Prophylactic antibiotic: cefazolin (Ancef)
- Tetanus prophylaxis: tetanus toxoid

Patient care goals
- The client's fractured bone fragments will realign and unite.
- The client's fracture will heal without complications.
- The client will regain mobility over time.
- The client's fluid and electrolyte balance will be restored.
- The client will demonstrate decreased anxiety.

Nursing interventions
- Observe the client for signs of shock, such as rapid pulse, decreased blood pressure, pallor, and cool, clammy skin. Severe open fracture of a large bone such as the femur *can cause increased blood loss, leading to hypovolemic shock.*
- Assess the affected limb *for signs of compartment syndrome.* (See *Recognizing compartment syndrome,* page 358.)
- Administer I.V. fluids as needed *to replace fluid loss.*
- Offer reassurance. *With any fracture, the client is likely to be frightened and in pain.*
- Ease pain with analgesics as needed.
- Reassure the client and help him set realistic goals for recovery *to prevent frustration with the recovery process.*
- If the fracture requires long-term immobilization with traction, reposition the client often *to increase comfort and prevent pressure ulcers.* Assist with active ROM exercises *to prevent muscle atrophy.* Encourage deep breathing and coughing *to avoid hypostatic pneumonia.*

Recognizing compartment syndrome

Compartment syndrome occurs when the pressure within a muscle and its surrounding structures increases. If the pressure becomes greater than diastolic blood pressure, circulation can be impaired or interrupted completely. Tissue damage occurs after 30 minutes; after 4 hours, irreversible damage may occur.

Compartment syndrome, indicated by an inability to perform active movements and by increasing pain with passive movements, results from compromised arterial and venous circulation caused by hemorrhage into the muscle mass. The resultant edema increases venous pressure. Arterial circulation decreases, leading to anoxia and cell death in 6 to 8 hours if the venous pressure isn't decreased. Treatment (fasciotomy) involves cutting the fascia over affected muscles to permit muscle expansion. About 7 to 10 days later, when the swelling subsides, the muscle fascia can be closed secondarily or covered with a skin graft if the fascial opening is large.

● Make sure the immobilized client receives adequate fluid intake *to prevent urinary stasis and constipation.* Watch for signs of renal calculi, such as flank pain, nausea, and vomiting, *to ensure early recognition and treatment.*
● Provide good cast care *to avoid skin breakdown.* (See *Performing cast care.*)
● Encourage the client to start moving around as soon as possible *to prevent complications of immobility.* Help him walk. (Remember that the client who has been bedridden for some time may be dizzy at first.)
● Demonstrate how to use crutches properly *to prevent injury.*
● After cast removal, refer the client for physical therapy *to restore limb mobility.*

Evaluation

● The client experiences no complications from the injury or treatment.
● The client learns safe mobility techniques such as crutch walking.
● The client is discharged home for recuperation and bone healing.
● The client verbalizes acceptance of the injury and required treatment.
● The client's fluid and electrolyte balance is restored.

NURSING PROCEDURE

Performing cast care

Purpose

A cast is a hard mold that encases a body part, usually an extremity, to provide immobilization of bones and surrounding tissue. It can be used to treat injuries (including fractures), correct orthopedic conditions (such as deformities), or promote healing after general or plastic surgery, amputation, or nerve and vascular repair.

Swelling of an injured body part may occur, causing decreased circulation if the body part is confined in a cast. Skin care should be performed to detect any communication with rough cast edges that may disrupt skin integrity. Careful assessment of the cast appearance can also detect problems, such as bleeding, that may occur beneath the cast surface. Early detection of problems can decrease complications.

Implementation

● Support a plaster cast with pillows while it's drying (up to 72 hours, depending on cast size) *to maintain proper shape.* Keep the cast dry at all times.
● Mark on the cast the time and date of any drainage sites. Observe for increases in these sites, *which may indicate bleeding or infection beneath the cast.*
● Demonstrate to the client proper body mechanics for movement with larger casts.
● Perform regular neurovascular checks.
● Tell the client to report extreme pain or pressure beneath the cast. Note any drainage or fever, *which may indicate infection under the cast.*
● Check the skin along the edges of the cast and protect it as necessary.
● Allow family or friends to sign the cast — however, discourage covering large areas of the cast with markings because *this may obscure drainage sites.*

Carpal tunnel syndrome

CARPAL TUNNEL SYNDROME results from compression of the median nerve at the wrist, within the carpal tunnel. This nerve — along with blood vessels and flexor tendons — passes through to the fingers and thumb. Compression neuropathy causes sensory and motor changes in the median distribution of the hand. Carpal tunnel is the most common of the nerve entrapment syndromes.

Carpal tunnel syndrome usually occurs in women ages 30 to 60 and poses a serious occupational health problem. Assembly-line workers and packers, typists, and people who repeatedly use poorly designed tools are most likely to develop this disorder. Any strenuous use of the hands — sustained grasping, twisting, or flexing — aggravates this condition.

Possible causes
- Flexor tenosynovitis (commonly associated with rheumatic disease)
- Nerve compression
- Physical trauma
- Rheumatoid arthritis

Data collection findings
- Numbness, burning, or tingling
- Pain
- Weakness
- Atrophic nails
- Shiny, dry skin

Diagnostic findings
- Physical examination reveals decreased sensation to light touch or pinpricks in the affected fingers. Thenar muscle atrophy occurs in about half of carpal tunnel syndrome cases. The client exhibits positive Tinel's sign (tingling over the median nerve on light percussion). She also responds positively to Phalen's maneuver, in which holding the forearms vertically and allowing both hands to drop into complete flexion at the wrists for 1 minute reproduces symptoms of carpal tunnel syndrome.
- A blood pressure cuff inflated above systolic pressure on the forearm for 1 to 2 minutes provokes pain and paresthesia along the distribution of the median nerve.
- EMG detects a median nerve motor conduction delay of more than 5 msec.

Nursing diagnoses
- Chronic pain
- Impaired physical mobility
- Disturbed sensory perception (kinesthetic, tactile)

Treatment
- Resting the hands by splinting the wrist in neutral extension for 1 to 2 weeks (if a definite link has been established between the client's occupation and the development of carpal tunnel syndrome, she may have to seek other work)
- Correction of underlying disorder

- Surgical decompression of the nerve by resecting the entire transverse carpal tunnel ligament or by using endoscopic surgical techniques (neurolysis, or releasing of nerve fibers, may also be necessary)

Drug therapy options
- NSAID: indomethacin (Indocin), ibuprofen (Motrin), naproxen (Naprosyn)
- Corticosteroid injection: betamethasone (Celestone), hydrocortisone (Hydrocortone)

Patient care goals
- The client will express feelings of comfort and pain relief.
- The client will maintain joint mobility and ROM.
- The client will maintain tactile and kinesthetic sensation.

Nursing interventions
- Administer NSAIDs as needed *to reduce inflammation and pain.*
- Encourage the client to use her hands as much as possible *to maintain ROM.*
- If the client's dominant hand has been impaired, you may have to help with eating and bathing. *Mobility may be limited with carpal tunnel syndrome.*
- Regularly assess the client's degree of physical immobility *to evaluate the effectiveness of the current treatment plan.*
- After surgery, monitor vital signs and regularly check the color, sensation, and motion of the affected hand *to detect signs of compromised circulation.*
- Advise the client who is about to be discharged to occasionally exercise her hands. If her arm is in a sling, tell her to remove the sling several times per day and perform elbow and shoulder exercises *to maintain ROM.*

Evaluation
- The client reports adequate pain control.
- The client demonstrates functional joint mobility and ROM.
- The client reports decreased numbness and tingling and improved sensation.

Compartment syndrome
COMPARTMENT SYNDROME occurs when the pressure within a muscle and its surrounding structures increases. If the pressure becomes greater than diastolic blood pressure, circulation can be impaired or interrupted completely. Tis-

sue damage occurs after 30 minutes; after 4 hours, irreversible damage may occur.

If compartment syndrome is suspected, pressure within muscles is assessed by sticking a needle into the muscle. The needle is attached to an I.V. bag with tubing and a stopcock. Elevated pressure, as indicated by a blood pressure machine, indicates compartment syndrome.

Possible causes
- Application of a dressing or cast that's too tight
- Burns
- Closed fracture injury
- Crushing injuries
- Muscle swelling after exercise

Data collection findings
- Severe or increased pain in the affected area with stretching or muscle elevation that's unrelieved by narcotics
- Tense, swollen muscle
- Decreased movement, strength, and sensation
- Increased pain with muscle stretching
- Loss of distal pulse
- Numbness and tingling distal to the involved muscle
- Paralysis

Diagnostic findings
- Intracompartment pressure is elevated, as indicated by a blood pressure machine.

Nursing diagnoses
- Acute pain
- Impaired physical mobility
- Risk for peripheral neurovascular dysfunction

Treatment
- Fasciotomy
- Positioning affected extremity lower than the heart
- Removal of dressings or constrictive coverings of the area

Drug therapy options
- Narcotic analgesic: morphine

Patient care goals
- The client will express feelings of comfort and pain relief.
- The client will maintain muscle strength and ROM.
- The client will maintain peripheral circulation.

Nursing interventions
- Monitor vital signs *to detect early changes and prevent complications.*
- Monitor the affected extremity and perform neurovascular checks *to detect signs of impaired circulation.*
- Maintain the extremity in a position lower than the heart *to ensure adequate circulation and to reduce pressure.*
- Assess the client for pain and anxiety *because stress may lead to vasoconstriction.*
- Administer medications as ordered *to maintain or improve the client's condition.*
- Perform dressing changes after the fasciotomy and reinforce dressings frequently *to facilitate monitoring of the extremity.* (A large amount of bloody drainage should be expected.)

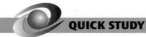 **QUICK STUDY**

Numbers to remember for compartment syndrome: 30 to 4
Tissue damage occurs after 30 minutes; permanent damage occurs after 4 hours.

Evaluation
- The client reports adequate pain control.
- The client has appropriate muscle strength and ROM.
- The client has adequate peripheral circulation.

Gout

GOUT is a metabolic disease marked by urate deposits in the joints, which cause painfully arthritic joints. It can strike any joint but favors those in the feet and legs. Primary gout usually occurs in men older than age 30 and in postmenopausal women. Secondary gout occurs in older people.

Gout follows an intermittent course and commonly leaves clients free from symptoms for years between attacks. Gout can lead to chronic disability or incapacitation and, rarely, severe hypertension and progressive renal disease. The prognosis is good with treatment.

Possible causes
- Genetic predisposition
- Increased uric acid

Data collection findings
- Inflamed, painful joints
- Hypertension
- Back pain

NURSING PROCEDURE

Applying heat therapy

Purpose

Heat applied directly to the client's body raises tissue temperature and enhances the inflammatory process by causing vasodilation and increasing local circulation. This promotes leukocytosis, suppuration, drainage, and healing. Heat also increases tissue metabolism, reduces pain caused by muscle spasm, and decreases congestion in deep visceral organs.

Direct heat may be dry or moist. Dry heat can be delivered at a higher temperature and for a longer time. Devices for applying dry heat include the hot-water bottle, electric heating pad, K pad, and chemical hot pack.

Moist heat softens crusts and exudates, penetrates deeper than dry heat, is less drying to the skin, produces less perspiration, and usually is more comfortable for the client. Devices for applying moist heat include warm compresses for small body areas and warm packs for large areas.

Direct heat treatment can't be used on a client at risk for hemorrhage. It's also contraindicated if the client has a sprained limb in the acute stage (because vasodilation would increase pain and swelling) or if he has a condition associated with acute inflammation such as appendicitis. Direct heat should be applied cautiously to pediatric and elderly clients and to clients with impaired renal, cardiac, or respiratory function; arteriosclerosis or atherosclerosis; or impaired sensation. It should be applied with extreme caution to heat-sensitive areas, such as scar tissue and stomas.

Implementation

- Check the physician's order and assess the client's condition.
- Position the client comfortably in the bed.
- Explain the procedure to the client and tell him not to lean or lie directly on the heating device *because this reduces air space and increases the risk of burns.* Warn him against adjusting the temperature of the heating device or adding hot water to a hot-water bottle. Advise him to report pain immediately and to remove the device if necessary.
- Take the client's temperature, pulse, and respiration *to serve as a baseline.* If heat treatment is being applied to raise the client's body temperature, monitor temperature, pulse, and respirations throughout the application.
- Expose only the treatment area *because vasodilation will make the client feel chilly.*
- Be sure to time heat therapies and apply for the ordered amount of time.
- *Because tissue damage may result from direct heat application,* monitor the temperature of the heating device carefully. Assess frequently the condition of the client's skin under the heat application device.

Applying a hot-water bottle, an electric heating pad, a K pad, or a chemical hot pack

- Before applying the heating device, press it against your inner forearm *to test its temperature and heat distribution.* If it heats unevenly, obtain a new device.
- Apply the device to the treatment area and, if necessary, secure it with tape or roller gauze.
- Check the client for tolerance and skin reaction.

Applying a warm compress or pack

- Place a linen-saver pad under the site.
- Remove the warm compress or pack from the bowl or basin. (Use sterile forceps throughout the procedure if needed.)
- Wring excess solution from the compress or pack. *Excess moisture increases the risk of burns.*
- Apply the compress gently to the affected site. After a few seconds, check for tolerance and skin reaction.
- Apply a waterproof covering (sterile if necessary) to the compress. Secure it with tape or roller gauze *to prevent it from slipping.*
- Place a hot-water bottle, K pad, or chemical hot pack over the compress and waterproof covering *to maintain the correct temperature.*
- Record the time and date of heat application including type, temperature or heat setting, duration, and site of application; the client's temperature, pulse, respirations, and skin condition before, during, and after treatment; signs of complications; and the client's tolerance of the treatment.

Diagnostic findings

- Arthrocentesis reveals the presence of monosodium urate monohydrate crystals or needlelike intracellular crystals of sodium urate in synovial fluid taken from an inflamed joint or a tophus.
- Blood studies show serum uric acid level above normal. The urine uric acid level is usually higher in secondary gout than in primary gout.
- X-ray examination results are normal initially. X-rays show damage of the articular cartilage and subchondral

NURSING PROCEDURE

Applying cold therapy

The application of cold constricts blood vessels; inhibits local circulation, suppuration, and tissue metabolism; relieves vascular congestion; slows bacterial activity in infections; reduces body temperature; and may act as a temporary anesthetic during brief, painful procedures. Because treatment with cold also relieves inflammation, reduces edema, and slows bleeding, it may provide effective initial treatment after eye injuries, strains, sprains, bruises, muscle spasms, and burns. Cold doesn't reduce existing edema, however, because it inhibits reabsorption of excess fluid.

Cold may be applied in dry or moist forms, but ice shouldn't be placed directly on a client's skin because it may further damage tissue. Moist application is more penetrating than dry because moisture facilitates conduction. Devices for applying cold include an ice bag or collar, K pad (which can produce cold or heat), and chemical cold packs and ice packs. Devices for applying moist cold include cold compresses for small body areas and cold packs for large areas.

Apply cold treatments cautiously on clients with impaired circulation, on children, and on elderly or arthritic clients because of the risk of ischemic tissue damage.

Apply cold immediately after an injury to minimize edema. Although colder temperatures can be tolerated for a longer time when the treatment site is small, don't continue any application for longer than 1 hour to avoid reflex vasodilation. The application of temperatures below 59° F (15° C) also causes local reflex vasodilation.

Implementation
- Check the physician's order and assess the client's condition.
- Explain the procedure to the client, provide privacy, and make sure the room is warm and free from drafts. Wash your hands thoroughly.
- Record the client's temperature, pulse, and respirations *to serve as a baseline.*

- Expose only the treatment site *to avoid chilling the client.*
- Be sure to time all cold therapies and apply for the ordered amount of time.
- *Because tissue damage may result from direct heat application,* monitor the temperature of the cold device carefully. Frequently assess the condition of the client's skin under the cold application device.

Applying an ice bag or collar, a K pad, or a chemical cold pack
- Place the covered cold device on the treatment site.
- Refill or replace the cold device as necessary *to maintain the correct temperature.* Change the protective cover if it becomes wet.

Applying a cold compress or pack
- Place a linen-saver pad under the site.
- Remove the compress or pack from the water, and wring it out *to prevent dripping.* Apply it to the treatment site.
- Cover the compress or pack with a waterproof covering *to provide insulation and to keep the surrounding area dry.* Secure the covering with tape or roller gauze *to prevent it from slipping.*
- Check the application site frequently for signs of tissue intolerance and note complaints of burning or numbness. If these symptoms develop, discontinue treatment and notify the physician.
- Change the compress or pack as needed *to maintain the correct temperature.* Remove it after the prescribed treatment period (usually 20 minutes).
- Record the time, date, and duration of cold application; type of device used (ice bag or collar, K pad, or chemical cold pack); site of application; temperature or temperature setting; client's temperature, pulse, and respirations before and after application; skin appearance before, during, and after application; signs of complications; and the client's tolerance of treatment.

---

bone in chronic gout and outward displacement of the overhanging margin from the bone contour.

Nursing diagnoses
- Chronic pain
- Impaired physical mobility
- Risk for injury

Treatment
- Bed rest
- Immobilization and protection of the inflamed joints
- Local application of heat and cold
- Diet changes (with the goal of weight loss)

Drug therapy options
- Analgesic: acetaminophen (Tylenol)
- Antigout drug: colchicine, allopurinol (Zyloprim)
- Uricosuric drug: probenecid (Benemid), sulfinpyrazone (Anturane)
- Alkalinizing drug: sodium bicarbonate
- Corticosteroid: betamethasone (Celestone), hydrocortisone (Hydrocortone)

Patient care goals
- The client will express feelings of comfort and pain relief.
- The client will maintain joint mobility and ROM.
- The client will remain free from injury.

Nursing interventions
- Encourage bed rest but use a bed cradle *to keep bedcovers off extremely sensitive, inflamed joints.*
- Give pain medication as needed, especially during acute attacks, *to promote comfort.*
- Apply hot or cold packs to inflamed joints *to promote comfort.* (See *Applying heat therapy,* page 361, and *Applying cold therapy.*)
- Administer anti-inflammatory medication and other drugs *to decrease inflammation and increase excretion of uric acid.*
- Be alert for GI disturbances with colchicine administration *to prevent complications.*
- Urge the client to drink plenty of fluids (up to 2 qt [2 L] per day) *to prevent formation of renal calculi.*
- When forcing fluids, record intake and output accurately *to detect fluid volume excess.*
- Be sure to monitor serum uric acid levels regularly *to evaluate the effectiveness of the treatment plan.*
- Alkalinize urine with sodium bicarbonate or another agent, as needed, *to prevent renal calculi formation.*
- Make sure the client understands the importance of having serum uric acid levels checked periodically *to help ensure compliance.*
- Advise the client receiving allopurinol, probenecid, and other drugs to immediately report adverse effects, such as drowsiness, dizziness, nausea, vomiting, urinary frequency, and dermatitis, *to prevent complications.*
- Warn the client taking probenecid or sulfinpyrazone to avoid aspirin and other salicylates. *Their combined effect causes urate retention.*
- Inform the client that long-term colchicine therapy is essential during the first 3 to 6 months of treatment with

uricosuric drugs or allopurinol *to prevent further acute attacks.*

Evaluation
- The client reports adequate pain control.
- The client demonstrates adequate joint mobility and ROM.
- The client doesn't experience injury.

Herniated disk

In herniated disk (herniated nucleus pulposus), the intervertebral disk ruptures, causing a protrusion of the nucleus pulposus (the soft, central portion of a spinal disk) into the spinal canal. (See *What happens when a disk herniates?*) This causes compression of the spinal cord or nerve roots resulting in pain, numbness, and loss of motor function. Neurologic deficits experienced vary in relation to level of spinal cord involved with lumbosacral levels L4, L5, S1 and cervical levels C5, C6, C7 being the most common levels involved. Herniation typically occurs on only one side due to vertical support provided by the longitudi-

---

What happens when a disk herniates?

The spinal column is made up of vertebra that are separated by cartilage called *disks*. Within each disk is a soft, gelatinous center (nucleus pulposus) that acts as a cushion during vertebral movement. When there's severe trauma or strain or intervertebral joint degeneration, the outer ring of the disk or anulus fibrosus can weaken or tear, and the nucleus pulposus is forced through this opening. The extruded disk can impinge on the spinal nerve root or the spinal cord.

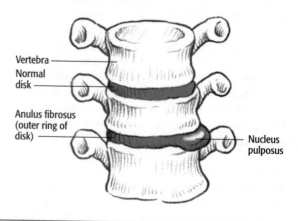

Surgeries for ruptured disk

Laminectomy or hemilaminectomy
A laminectomy or hemilaminectomy consists of removing the vertebral lamina (wing) to gain access to the disk area. The disk pieces are then removed from the annulus, the cartilage ring between the vertebrae. After a laminectomy, the client can get up (on the same day, if able) and move with minimal restriction. Recovery proceeds fairly steadily after the ruptured disk pieces are removed, relieving nerve pressure and pain. The client should be taught proper lifting techniques to prevent additional trauma and exercises to strengthen back and abdominal muscles after discharge.

Spinal fusion
A spinal fusion involves laminectomy to remove the ruptured disk pieces followed by placement of bone inserts (grafts), screws, or pins to fuse the vertebral segments solidly. After spinal fusion, the client may require bed rest for 1 to 3 days or more, depending on the fusion type. At times, a client may need a brace, which helps stabilize the fused parts for the lengthy healing time required (9 to 12 months for solid fusion). Postoperatively, the client must be positioned with the logrolling maneuver and will have limited ability to bend when the fusion heals.

Chemonucleolysis
Chemonucleolysis is the dissolution of ruptured disk pieces by injecting chymopapain, an enzyme from the papaya plant, into the affected disk. The enzyme dissolves the disk, which is replaced with scar tissue. Chymopapain can elicit severe anaphylactic responses and may result in death. Preoperative preparation includes obtaining a thorough allergy history and administering I.V. preoperative corticosteroids, antihistamines, and cimetidine (Tagamet) to block histamine release.

  Postoperatively, the client may have back muscle spasms of varying intensity and duration. Pain relief may be temporary, with pain returning 6 or more months later, possibly from scar tissue formation. The verdict is out on this controversial procedure's effectiveness and safety. Although initial enthusiasm for chemonucleolysis appears to be waning, the procedure is still being performed. For some clients, results have been good; other clients have resorted to laminectomy.

Microdiskectomy
Microdiskectomy is similar to laminectomy but requires an incision measuring 1″ to 3″ (2.5 to 7.5 cm); only the disk fragments are removed, and recovery is faster. Sometimes, multiple operations are required because of retained disk fragments.

---

nal ligament. Subsequently, pain and neurologic deficits are usually experienced on only one side of the body.

Possible causes
- Accidents or trauma
- Congenital or developmental bone deformity
- Degeneration of disk

Data collection findings
Cervical area
- Neck pain that radiates down the arm to the hand
- Neck stiffness
- Weakness of affected upper extremities with numbness and tingling of the hand
- Atrophy of biceps and triceps

Lumbosacral area
- Acute pain in the lower back radiating across the buttock and down the leg
- Pain on ambulation
- Weakness, numbness, and tingling of the foot and leg
- Straightening of normal lumbar curve with scoliosis away from the affected side

Diagnostic findings
- Deep tendon reflexes are depressed or absent in the affected extremity.
- EMG shows spinal nerve involvement.
- Lasègue's sign is positive.
- MRI depicts disk bulges and protrusions.
- Myelography and contrast-enhanced CT show compression of spinal cord.
- Radiography shows narrowing of disk space.

Nursing diagnoses
- Acute pain
- Impaired physical mobility

Treatment
- Bed rest with active and passive ROM and isometric exercises
- Diet that includes increased fiber and fluids
- Heating pad and moist, hot compresses
- Orthopedic devices, including back brace and cervical collar
- Transcutaneous electrical nerve stimulation
- Laminectomy, spinal fusion, chemonucleolysis, or microdiskectomy (see *Surgeries for ruptured disk*)

CLINICAL SITUATION

Caring for the client with a compression fracture

A 40-year-old male construction worker is hospitalized after falling from a scaffold. He complains of bilateral numbness of his fourth and fifth toes and pain that radiates down his buttocks and the back of his thighs. Radiographs indicate that the client has a compression fracture of the fourth lumbar vertebra (L4). He's admitted to the orthopedic unit for further evaluation and treatment.

Describe the appropriate conservative treatment for the client with a compression fracture.

Conservative treatment includes bed rest with active and passive range-of-motion and isometric exercises; heating pad and moist, hot compresses; orthopedic devices; and transcutaneous electrical nerve stimulation.

Name potential surgical interventions for the client with a compression fracture.

Surgical intervention may include laminectomy, spinal fusion, chemonucleolysis, or microdiskectomy.

Questions for further thought

● Why does the nurse need to continue to assess *all* body systems?

● What are some key assessments when checking the client's neurovascular status? What findings could indicate progression of symptoms?

● What should be included in client teaching if the client is placed in a body cast?

Drug therapy options

● Corticosteroid: cortisone (Cortone)
● Fecal softeners or fiber stimulant: docusate sodium (Colace), psyllium (Metamucil)
● Muscle relaxant: cyclobenzaprine (Flexeril), diazepam (Valium)
● Narcotic analgesic: codeine, meperidine, morphine, oxycodone (OxyContin)
● NSAID: diclofenac sodium (Voltaren), diflunisal (Dolobid), flurbiprofen (Ansaid), ibuprofen (Motrin), indomethacin (Indocin), naproxen (Naprosyn), piroxicam (Feldene), rofecoxib (Vioxx), sulindac (Clinoril)

Patient care goals

● The client will regain musculoskeletal and neurologic tissue function without complications.
● The client will understand the implications of a spinal injury and will participate in rehabilitation.

Nursing interventions

● Assess neurovascular status *to determine baseline and detect early changes.*
● Monitor and record vital signs, intake and output, and results of laboratory studies *to detect changes in the client's condition.*
● Maintain the client's diet and increase fluid intake *to maintain hydration.*
● Keep the client in semi-Fowler's position with moderate hip and knee flexion *to promote comfort.*

● Administer medications as prescribed *to maintain or improve the client's condition.*
● Encourage the client to express feelings about changes in his body image and about fears of disability *to help the client resolve feelings.*
● Provide skin and back care *to promote comfort and prevent skin breakdown.*
● Turn the client every 2 hours using the logrolling technique *to prevent injury.*
● Continue bed rest and body alignment *to maintain joint function and prevent neuromuscular deformity.*
● Maintain traction, braces, and cervical collar *to prevent further injury and promote healing.*
● Promote independence in ADLs *to maintain self-esteem.*

Evaluation

● The client is regaining full motor and sensory functions in the limb as healing continues.
● The client regains limited mobility initially, working up to full rehabilitation. (See *Caring for the client with a compression fracture.*)

Hip fracture

A fracture occurs when too much stress is placed on the bone in relation to its stress tolerance. As a result, the bone breaks and local tissue becomes injured causing muscle spasm, edema, hemorrhage, compressed nerves, and ecchymosis.

Sites of hip fractures include intracapsular (within the capsule of the femur), extracapsular (outside the capsule of the femur), intertrochanteric (within the trochanter), or subtrochanteric (below the trochanter).

Possible causes
- Aging
- Bone tumors
- Cushing's syndrome
- Immobility
- Malnutrition
- Multiple myeloma
- Osteomyelitis
- Osteoporosis
- Steroid therapy
- Trauma (especially falls)

Data collection findings
- Shorter appearance and outward rotation of affected leg resulting in limited or abnormal ROM
- Edema and discoloration of surrounding tissue
- Pain in the affected hip and leg that's exacerbated by movement
- History of a fall or other trauma to the bones

Diagnostic findings
- CT scan for complicated fractures pinpoints abnormalities.
- Hematologic studies show decreased Hb level and HCT.
- Radiography reveals a break in the continuity of the bone.

Nursing diagnoses
- Acute pain
- Deficient fluid volume
- Impaired physical mobility

Treatment
- Abductor splint or trochanter roll between legs to prevent loss of alignment
- Isometric exercises, such as quadriceps setting and flexing the calf muscles
- Physical therapy to teach the client non-weight-bearing transfers and to work with changes in weight-bearing status
- Skin traction, such as Buck's extension or Russell traction (see *Types of skin traction*)
- Surgical immobilization or joint replacement

Drug therapy options
- Narcotic analgesia: codeine, meperidine, morphine
- NSAID: ibuprofen (Motrin), naproxen (Naprosyn)

Patient care goals
- The client won't experience complications from injury or treatment.
- The client will increase physical mobility through use of a walker.
- The client will use appropriate supportive services, such as physical therapy and home health care.

Nursing interventions
- Assess neurovascular and respiratory status. Most important, check for compromised circulation, hemorrhage, and neurologic impairment in the affected extremity and pneumonia in the bedridden client *to detect changes and prevent complications.*
- Monitor and record vital signs, intake and output, and results of laboratory studies *to detect early changes in the client's condition.*
- Maintain the client's diet and increase fluid intake *to maintain hydration.*
- Keep the client in a flat position with the foot of the bed elevated 25 degrees when in traction *to prevent further injury.*
- Keep the legs abducted *to prevent dislocation of the hip joint.*
- Avoid hip flexion greater than 90 degrees *to prevent dislocation of the hip joint.*
- Administer medications as prescribed *to improve or maintain the client's condition.*
- Provide skin care, and logroll the client every 2 hours *to maintain skin integrity and prevent pressure ulcers.*
- Assist with coughing, deep breathing, and incentive spirometry *to maintain patent airway.*
- Keep the hip extended *to prevent further injury and maintain circulation.*
- Promote independence in ADLs *to promote self-esteem.*
- Provide active and passive ROM and isometric exercises for unaffected limbs *to maintain joint mobility.*
- Provide an over-the-bed trapeze *to promote independence in self-care.*
- Maintain traction at all times *to ensure proper body alignment and promote healing.*
- Keep side rails up *to prevent injury.*
- Provide appropriate sensory stimulation with frequent reorientation *to reduce anxiety.*

Types of skin traction

TRACTION TYPE	APPLICATION SITE	WEIGHT	CARE FACTORS
Buck's extension	Arm or leg (one or both)	5 to 7 lb per extremity	● Clean and dry the skin. Make sure the client has no open cuts or wounds. ● Make sure equipment (tape, bandages, traction straps, or boot) is new (when appropriate) and functioning properly. ● Remove the traction apparatus to care for and observe tissues. ● Keep the client recumbent *to obtain the most effective traction.* ● Teach the client how to use traction at home.
Russell traction	Leg only (one or both)	5 to 10 lb per leg	● Arrange pulleys and ropes, and determine the weight by applying the principle "for every force in one direction, there's an equal force in the opposite direction." ● Loosen the knee sling for care and observation. ● Keep the client recumbent. ● Remove the traction to care for the client (always check with the physician before removing it).
Bryant's traction	One or both legs (usually both)	Varies—enough weight to raise the buttocks off the bed	● Use for client's under 35 lb. ● Position both legs at 90-degree angles to the buttocks. ● Position the client's buttocks slightly off the bed *to ensure correct amount of pull.* ● Supervise the client closely *to maintain the recumbent position.* ● Remove the traction to provide care, according to the physician's orders or institutional policy (requires two people, with one gently maintaining manual traction). ● Teach the client and his family how to use this traction at home.
Pelvic belt	Around abdomen and pelvis, like a girdle	20 to 35 lb	● Use for conservative low-back pain and possible ruptured disk. ● Use traction intermittently and never at night. ● Keep the client recumbent, with knees and hips flexed at 45-degree angles. ● Teach the client how to use traction at home.
Pelvic sling	Under the pelvis like a hammock	20 to 35 lb	● Use for pelvic bone fractures. ● Advise the client to stay in the sling except when it's removed for care. ● Wean the client from the sling *to prevent dependency.* ● Keep the sling clean and dry *to prevent pressure areas.* ● Position the client's buttocks slightly off the bed *to ensure correct use of the sling.* ● One person can remove the client from the sling, but two are needed to reapply it *to center the client properly.*

(continued)

Types of skin traction *(continued)*

TRACTION TYPE	APPLICATION SITE	WEIGHT	CARE FACTORS
Head halter	Under the chin and around the skull base	5 to 15 lb (8 to 10 lb most common)	• Use for neck muscle disorders, degenerative cervical conditions, and (rarely) cervical vertebral fractures. • Explain that the pull comes mostly from the occipital area of the halter, not from the chin. • Tell the client that pressure exerted on the chin reverts to the temporomandibular joint, causing pain and soreness when chewing. • Remove the client from the traction for care before inserting skull tongs (if the client has a fractured cervical vertebra, only the physician removes the traction). • Show the client (especially one with arthritis) how to use traction at home. • Avoid pressure exerted over the facial nerve by a halter that's too small or incorrectly applied.
90°-90° (ninety-ninety)	Lower legs and thighs	5 to 15 lb	• Relieves lumbosacral muscle spasms by applying the principle of 90-degree angle of knees and hips. • Keep the client flat in bed while in this traction. • Use traction intermittently, and usually not at night.
Dunlop's	Humerus	8 to 15 lb	• Use for humeral fractures *to decrease muscle spasms and align bone fragments.* • Hold the client's forearm in Buck's extension vertically, with the elbow at a 90-degree angle to the arm *for most effective traction.* • Keep the client recumbent *for effective traction.*
Cotrel's	Head halter to the head and a pelvic belt to the pelvis	15 to 30 lb for pelvic belt; 8 to 15 lb for head halter	• Use to assist straightening scoliotic curvature (commonly used before brace application or surgical correction). • Maintain the client flat in bed so that the spine is pulled lengthwise in opposite directions by the head halter and pelvic belt. • Use intermittently, but not at night unless curvature and muscle spasms are severe.

• Encourage increased fiber, fluids, and activity as allowed as well as medication, as needed, *to prevent constipation.*
• Provide diversional activities *to promote self-esteem.*
• Apply antiembolism stockings or sequential compression device *to promote venous circulation.*

 QUICK STUDY

Remember, don't **CFR** a **THR.** That means don't:
Cross
Flex
Rotate
a
Total
Hip
Replacement.

Evaluation

● The client doesn't experience complications from the injury or treatment.
● The client can use a walker effectively to increase mobilization.
● The client uses supportive services appropriately.

Osteoarthritis

OSTEOARTHRITIS, also known as *degenerative joint disease*, is characterized by degeneration of cartilage in weight-bearing joints, such as the spine, knees, and hips. It occurs when cartilage softens with age, narrowing the joint space. This allows bones to rub together, causing pain and limiting joint movement.

Osteoarthritis can be primary or secondary. Primary osteoarthritis, a normal part of aging, results from metabolic, genetic, chemical, and mechanical factors. Secondary osteoarthritis usually follows an identifiable cause, such as obesity and congenital deformity, and leads to degenerative changes. A client suffering from rheumatoid arthritis who is receiving long-term corticosteroid therapy is also at risk for osteoarthritis. (See *Comparing rheumatoid arthritis and osteoarthritis.*)

Possible causes

● Aging
● Congenital abnormalities
● Joint trauma
● Obesity

Data collection findings

● Crepitation
● Enlarged, edematous joints
● Heberden's nodes
● Increased pain in damp, cold weather and late in day
● Joint stiffness
● Limited ROM
● Pain relieved by resting joints
● Smooth, taut, shiny skin

Diagnostic findings

● Arthroscopy reveals bone spurs and narrowing of joint space.
● Radiography shows joint deformity, narrowing of joint space, and bone spurs.

Nursing diagnoses

● Impaired physical mobility
● Activity intolerance
● Chronic pain

Treatment

● Joint-protective exercises, such as walking, swimming, and water aerobics
● Canes or walkers
● Cold therapy
● Low-calorie diet if the client is over optimal weight
● Heat therapy
● Isometric exercises
● Joint replacement

Comparing rheumatoid arthritis and osteoarthritis

RHEUMATOID ARTHRITIS	OSTEOARTHRITIS
● Systemic disease: affects multiple body systems	● Local disease of joints only
● Affects synovial membranes initially, then other joint structures	● Affects cartilage initially, then other joint structures
● Affects symmetrical joints bilaterally; affects proximal joints and smaller joints most commonly	● Asymmetrical joint involvement; distal joints and larger weight-bearing joints most likely to be involved
● Multiple subcutaneous nodules under skin surfaces, not in joints	● Bony enlargements of distal joints common (Heberden's nodes)
● Dislocations, subluxations (partial dislocations), and deformities common (swan neck and boutonnière deformities of joints)	● Dislocation and subluxation uncommon; deformity from bony outgrowths
● Signs of inflammation: heat, fever, swelling, malaise, elevated erythrocyte sedimentation rate	● No systemic signs of inflammation; joints may be swollen but rarely hot
● Three times more common in women than in men; affects those ages 30 to 55	● Not gender-specific; affects those age 45 and older

Drug therapy options

- Analgesic: aspirin
- NSAID: diclofenac (Voltaren), diflunisal (Dolobid), flurbiprofen (Ansaid), ibuprofen (Motrin), indomethacin (Indocin), naproxen (Naprosyn), piroxicam (Feldene), sulindac (Clinoril)

Patient care goals

- The client's joint mobility will improve.
- The client will maintain or improve mobility by participating in joint-protective exercises.
- The client will have less pain.

Nursing interventions

- Assess musculoskeletal status *to determine baseline and detect changes.*
- Assess pain. *Correlating the client's pain with the time of day and visits may be useful in modifying tasks.*
- Keep joints extended *to prevent contractures and maintain joint mobility.*
- Administer medications as prescribed *to relieve pain and encourage mobility.*
- Assess for increased bleeding or bruising tendency *to facilitate early intervention for adverse drug effects.*
- Urge the client to express feelings about changes in body image *to promote effective communication about changes.*
- Provide rest periods *to conserve energy.*
- Maintain calorie count *to promote nutrition and healing and keep weight within normal limits.*
- Provide moist compresses and paraffin baths (heat therapy) as prescribed *to promote comfort.*
- Teach proper body mechanics *to prevent injury.*
- Provide passive ROM exercises *to maintain joint mobility.*

Evaluation

- The client demonstrates improved mobility of joints.
- The client expresses decreased amount of pain.

 SPOT CHECK

When assessing a client with osteoarthritis of the knees, when are you most likely to detect crepitation?
Crepitus is a grating sensation associated with degenerative joint disease and it can be felt or heard. You're most likely to detect it during palpation of the affected joint.

Osteomyelitis

OSTEOMYELITIS is a pyogenic (pus-producing) bone infection. It may be chronic or acute and commonly results from a combination of local trauma — usually quite trivial but resulting in hematoma formation — and an acute infection originating elsewhere in the body. Although osteomyelitis commonly remains localized, it can spread through the bone to the marrow, cortex, and periosteum (the membrane that covers the bone).

Acute osteomyelitis is usually a blood-borne disease that most commonly affects rapidly growing children. Chronic osteomyelitis (rare) is characterized by multiple draining sinus tracts and metastatic lesions.

Osteomyelitis occurs more commonly in children than adults — and particularly in boys — usually as a complication of an acute, localized infection. The most common sites in children are the lower end of the femur and the upper ends of the tibia, humerus, and radius. In adults, the most common sites are the pelvis and vertebrae, generally the result of contamination associated with surgery or trauma.

Possible causes

- Exposure to disease-causing organisms

Data collection findings

- Pain
- Tenderness
- Swelling

Diagnostic findings

- Blood cultures identify the causative organism.
- ESR is elevated.
- WBC count shows leukocytosis.
- Bone scan shows infection site.

Nursing diagnoses

- Activity intolerance
- Acute and chronic pain
- Impaired physical mobility

Treatment

- Early surgical drainage to relieve pressure buildup and formation of sequestrum — dead bone that has separated from sound bone
- High-protein diet with extra vitamin C
- Immobilization of the affected bone by plaster cast, traction, or bed rest
- I.V. fluids

Drug therapy options

- Antibiotic: large doses of I.V. antibiotics, usually a penicillinase-resistant penicillin, such as nafcillin (Unipen) and oxacillin (Bactocill), or a cephalosporin such as cefazolin (Ancef) after blood cultures are taken
- Analgesic: ibuprofen (Motrin), oxycodone and acetaminophen (Percocet)

Patient care goals

- The client will perform ADLs within the confines of the disease.
- The client will express feelings of comfort and pain relief.
- The client will maintain joint mobility and ROM.

Nursing interventions

- Use strict sterile technique when changing dressings and irrigating wounds *to prevent infection.*
- If the client is in skeletal traction for compound fractures, cover insertion points of pin tracks with small, dry dressings, and tell him not to touch the skin around the pins and wires *to prevent infection.*
- Monitor I.V. fluids *to maintain adequate hydration as necessary.*
- Provide a diet high in protein and vitamin C *to promote healing.*
- Assess vital signs and wound appearance daily and monitor daily for new pain, *which may indicate secondary infection.*
- Support the affected limb with firm pillows. Keep the limb level with the body — don't let it sag — *to prevent injury.*
- Provide good skin care. Turn the client gently every 2 hours *to prevent skin breakdown,* and watch for signs of developing pressure ulcers *to ensure early intervention and treatment.*
- Provide good cast care. Support the cast with firm pillows and "petal" the edges with pieces of adhesive tape or moleskin to smooth rough edges *to prevent skin breakdown, which may lead to infection.*
- Check circulation and drainage. If a wet spot appears on the cast, circle it with a marking pen and note the time of appearance on the cast. Be aware of how much drainage is expected. Check the circled spot at least every 4 hours. Watch for enlargement. *These measures help detect early signs of hemorrhage.*
- Protect the client from mishaps, such as jerky movements and falls, which may threaten bone integrity *to prevent injury.*

- Be alert for sudden pain, crepitus, or deformity. Watch for sudden malposition of the limb *to detect fracture.*
- Provide emotional support and appropriate diversions *to reduce anxiety.*

Evaluation

- The client reports the ability to adequately perform ADLs.
- The client reports adequate pain control.
- The client demonstrates adequate joint mobility and ROM.

Osteoporosis

In OSTEOPOROSIS, a metabolic bone disorder, the rate of bone resorption accelerates while the rate of bone formation slows down, causing a progressive loss of bone mass. Bones affected by this disease lose calcium and phosphate salts and thus become porous, brittle, and abnormally vulnerable to fracture.

Osteoporosis may be primary or secondary to an underlying disease. Primary osteoporosis is typically called *senile* or *postmenopausal osteoporosis* because it most commonly develops in elderly, postmenopausal women. Secondary osteoporosis results from an underlying condition, such as hyperparathyroidism or long-term corticosteroid therapy.

FAST FACT

In osteoporosis, bone deteriorates faster than the body can restore it.

Possible causes

- Decreased hormonal function
- Lack of weight bearing secondary to paralysis
- Long-term corticosteroid therapy
- Negative calcium balance

Data collection findings

- Compression fractures of spine or Colles' fracture of wrist
- Height loss
- Kyphosis
- Pain

Diagnostic findings

- Bone biopsy specimen shows a thin and porous, but otherwise normal-looking, bone.

- Dual or single photon absorptiometry, which aids assessment of the extremities, hips, and spine, reveals decreased bone mass.
- Serum calcium, phosphorus, and alkaline phosphatase levels are within reference limits, but parathyroid hormone level may be increased.
- Radiographs show degeneration in the lower thoracic and lumbar vertebrae; the vertebral bodies appear flattened and may look more dense than normal.

Nursing diagnoses
- Risk for injury
- Impaired physical mobility
- Chronic pain

Treatment
- Physical therapy of gentle exercise and activity
- Supportive devices for weakened vertebrae
- Balanced diet high in vitamin D, calcium, and protein

Drug therapy options
- Analgesic: aspirin, indomethacin (Indocin)
- Antihypercalcemic drug: etidronate (Didronel)
- Hormonal agent: calcitonin (Calcimar), conjugated estrogen (Premarin)
- Vitamin D supplements

Patient care goals
- The client will remain free from injury.
- The client will decrease bone resorption through exercise, diet, and medication.

Nursing interventions
- Focus on the client's fragility, stressing careful positioning, ambulation, and prescribed exercises *to prevent injury.*
- Provide a balanced diet high in such nutrients as vitamin D, calcium, and protein *to support skeletal metabolism.*
- Administer analgesics and heat *to relieve pain.*
- Advise the client to sleep on a firm mattress *to promote comfort* and to avoid excessive bed rest *to slow disease progression.*
- Make sure the client knows how to wear a back brace *to prevent back injury.*
- Encourage appropriate exercises *to help slow disease progression.*

Evaluation
- The client has an established exercise program of at least 1 hour weekly.

- The client doesn't exhibit signs of further bone loss.
- The client remains free from injury.

INTEGUMENTARY SYSTEM

The integumentary system protects the body's inner organs. It also helps regulate body temperature through function of the sweat glands.

Integumentary structure and function

Skin, hair, nails, and certain glands make up the integumentary system:
- The skin provides the first line of defense against microorganisms and is composed of three layers:
  – epidermis (outer layer), which contains keratinocytes and melanocytes
  – dermis (middle layer), a collagen layer that supports the epidermis, contains nerves and blood vessels, and is the origin of hair, nails, sebaceous glands, eccrine sweat glands, and apocrine sweat glands
  – hypodermis (third layer), which is composed of loose connective tissue filled with fatty cells and provides heat, insulation, shock absorption, and a reserve of calories (also known as *subcutaneous tissue*)
- Hair also provides protection and coverage for most of the body, with the exception of the palms, lips, soles of the feet, nipples, penis, and labia.
- The nails, protecting the tips of the fingers and toes, are composed of dead cells filled with keratin.

The integumentary system contains three types of glands:
- sebaceous (oil) glands, which lubricate hair and the epidermis and are stimulated by sex hormones
- eccrine sweat glands, which regulate body temperature through water secretion
- apocrine sweat glands, which are located in the axilla, nipple, anal, and pubic areas and secrete odorless fluid (decomposition of this fluid by bacteria causes odor).

INTEGUMENTARY DISORDERS

Major integumentary disorders include atopic dermatitis, burns, herpes zoster, pressure ulcers, psoriasis, and skin cancer.

Atopic dermatitis

ATOPIC DERMATITIS is a chronic skin disorder characterized by superficial skin inflammation and intense itching. It may also be called *atopic eczema* or *infantile eczema*.

Atopic dermatitis may be associated with other atopic diseases, such as bronchial asthma and allergic rhinitis. It usually develops in infants and toddlers between ages 1 month and 1 year, commonly in those with strong family histories of atopic disease. These children commonly acquire other atopic disorders as they grow older.

Typically, this form of dermatitis flares and subsides repeatedly before finally resolving during adolescence. However, it can persist into adulthood.

Possible causes
- Chemical irritants
- Food allergies
- Genetic predisposition
- Immune dysfunction (possibly linked to elevated serum IgE levels or defective T-cell function)
- Infections (with *Staphylococcus aureus*)

Data collection findings
- Characteristic location of lesions in areas of flexion and extension, such as the neck, antecubital fossa (behind the elbow), popliteal folds (posterior surface of the knee), and behind the ears
- Erythematous lesions that eventually become scaly and lichenified
- Excessive dry skin
- Hyperpigmentation
- Skin eruptions

Diagnostic findings
- Serum IgE levels are commonly elevated in patients with atopic dermatitis; however, this finding isn't diagnostic.

Nursing diagnoses
- Impaired skin integrity
- Disturbed body image
- Anxiety

Treatment
- Washing lesions with water and a little soap
- Environmental control of offending allergens

Drug therapy options
- Antihistamine: hydroxyzine (Atarax)
- Corticosteroid ointment: hydrocortisone (Dermacort)

Patient care goals
- The client will exhibit improved or healed lesions or wounds.
- The client will express feelings about his changed body image.
- The client will use support systems to assist with coping mechanisms.

Nursing interventions
- Warn that antihistamines used to relieve daytime itching may cause drowsiness *to prevent injury.*
- If nocturnal itching interferes with sleep, suggest methods for inducing natural sleep, such as drinking a glass of warm milk, *to prevent overuse of sedatives.* If these methods don't work, antihistamines may be used *to relieve itching and cause drowsiness.*
- Help the client set up an individual schedule and plan for daily skin care *to help the client cope with the chronic condition and promote compliance.*
- Instruct the client to bathe in plain water. (He may have to limit bathing, depending on the severity of the lesions.) Tell him to bathe with a special nonfatty soap and tepid water (96° F [35.6° C]), to avoid using soap when lesions are acutely inflamed, and to limit baths or showers to 5 to 7 minutes. *These measures prevent worsening of the condition.*
- For scalp involvement, advise the client to shampoo frequently and to apply a corticosteroid solution to the scalp afterward *to improve skin integrity.*
- Advise the patient to keep his fingernails short *to limit excoriation and secondary infections caused by scratching.*
- Advise the patient to lubricate the skin after a shower or bath *to prevent excessive dryness.*
- Apply occlusive dressings (such as plastic film) over a corticosteroid cream intermittently as necessary *to help clear lichenified skin.*
- Be careful not to show anxiety or revulsion when touching the lesions during treatment. Help the client accept his altered body image, and encourage him to verbalize his feelings. *Coping with disfigurement is extremely difficult, especially for children and adolescents.*

Evaluation
- The client displays healing lesions.
- The client demonstrates a positive attitude regarding his self-image.
- The client demonstrates appropriate coping abilities.

Burns

A burn is a destruction of skin that causes loss of intracellular fluid and electrolytes. A burn is characterized as first, second, third, or fourth degree, depending on the extent (area) and degree (depth) of the burn (most burns include a combination of degrees):

- A first-degree (superficial partial-thickness) burn involves the epidermal layer.
- A second-degree (dermal partial-thickness) burn involves the epidermal and dermal layers.
- A third-degree (full-thickness) burn involves epidermal, dermal, subcutaneous layers, and nerve endings.

- A fourth-degree burn involves deeply charred subcutaneous tissue down to muscle and bone.

The Rule of Nines is a method used to estimate the percentage of a person's body that has been burned. In this method, a person's skin area is divided into several sections, each representing 9% (or multiples of 9%) of the total body area. By observing the size and location of a burn and assigning the appropriate body percentage, the nurse can roughly determine what percentage of a client's body has been burned. (See *Emergency burn care.*)

The Lund and Browder chart is a more accurate method of estimating body surface area that has been

---

Emergency burn care

Nursing behaviors

- Stop the burning process.
- *Chemical burn* – Remove clothes if splattered; flush burned areas with cool, clean water for 10 to 15 minutes. Wear double gloves.
- *Thermal burn* – Remove objects that retain heat (such as rings and medals). Remove the client's clothes, if dirty, and cover the client with clean cloths or dressings, moistening them for easy removal.
- *Electrical burn* – Monitor vital functions of the brain, heart, and lungs. The human body is electrolytic (it conducts electricity). Make sure the current is off.
- Prevent infection.
- Determine the extent and degree of tissue burned.

Nursing rationales

- Flushing the area dilutes the chemicals and washes them away. Wearing double gloves aids in avoiding contact with the chemical.
- Electricity that passes through the body (the body will have an entrance and exit site) affects all body systems.
- Because skin is the body's first line of defense against infecting organisms, its disruption by burning predisposes the client to infection, which is the major cause of death among burn victims. When caring for a burned client, always use sterile techniques and equipment. Cover the burn area to keep it soil-free, prevent heat loss, and protect exposed nerve endings, thereby decreasing pain.
- The Rule of Nines is a formula used to estimate body surface area burned. The body is visually divided into percentages: 9% to the head and each arm, 18% to each leg and to the posterior and anterior trunk, and 1% to the perineum. The percentages of burned areas are added to estimate the percent of total body surface area burned. When used for children, the age and size are considered, but this isn't done for adults, making it a valid guideline only in an emergency.

Depth of burns

- *Partial thickness* – superficial; epidermis only (for example, sunburn-marked reddening from dilated dermal blood vessels)
- *Deep* – between dermis and epidermis; plasma leakage from dilated vessels, and blisters of plasma fluid between the skin layers
- *Full thickness* – complete damage of epidermis, dermis, and skin appendages (sweat glands, sebaceous glands, and hair follicles); burned areas appear black, brownish, and leathery and fail to heal (reepithelialize) without grafting

RULE OF NINES

burned because it accounts for changes in body proportion that occur with age. The greater accuracy of this method helps the nurse better determine a client's exact fluid replacement requirements after a burn injury.

Possible causes
- Chemical: acids, alkalies, vesicants
- Electrical: lightning, electrical wires
- Mechanical: friction
- Radiation: X-rays, sun, nuclear
- Thermal: flame, frostbite, scald

Data collection findings
First-degree burn
- Erythema
- Edema
- Pain
- Blanching

Second-degree burn
- Pain
- Oozing, fluid-filled vesicles
- Erythema
- Shiny, wet subcutaneous layer after vesicles rupture

Third-degree burn
- Eschar
- Edema
- Little or no pain

Fourth-degree burn
- Deeply charred subcutaneous tissue, muscle, and bone

 QUICK STUDY

When assessing a burn victim, obtain an **AMPLE** history, including:

Allergies
Medications
Past medical history
Last meal
Events surrounding the injury.

Diagnostic findings
- A 24-hour urine collection specimen shows decreased creatinine clearance and negative nitrogen balance.
- ABG analysis shows metabolic acidosis.

- Blood chemistry test results show an increased potassium level and decreased sodium, albumin, complement fixation, immunoglobulin levels.
- Hematologic study results show increased Hb level and HCT and decreased fibrinogen, platelets, and WBC count.
- Urine chemistry results show hematuria and myoglobinuria.
- Visual examination is used to estimate the extent of burn (determined by Rule of Nines and Lund and Browder chart).

Nursing diagnoses
- Acute pain
- Risk for infection
- Deficient fluid volume
- Impaired gas exchange
- Disturbed body image

Treatment
- Biological dressings
- Diet high in protein, fat, calories, and carbohydrates with small, frequent feedings
- Early excisional therapy
- Escharotomy (surgical excision of burned tissue)
- I.V. therapy, including hydration and electrolyte replacement (I.V. administration is gauged according to the amount of fluid it takes to maintain a urine output of 30 to 50 ml/hour)
- Protective isolation to protect the client from infection
- Skin grafts
- Splints to maintain proper joint position and to prevent contractures
- Transfusion therapy of fresh frozen plasma, platelets, packed RBCs, and plasma
- Withholding of oral food and fluids until allowed

Drug therapy options
- Analgesic: morphine
- Antacid: aluminum hydroxide gel (AlternaGEL), magnesium and aluminum hydroxide (Maalox)
- Antianxiety: lorazepam (Ativan)
- Antibiotic: gentamicin (Garamycin)
- Anti-infective: mafenide (Sulfamylon), povidone-iodine (Betadine), silver sulfadiazine (Silvadene), silver nitrate
- Antitetanus: tetanus toxoid
- Colloid: albumin 5% (Albuminar-5)
- Diuretic: mannitol (Osmitrol)
- Histamine antagonist: cimetidine (Tagamet), famotidine (Pepcid), nizatidine (Axid), ranitidine (Zantac)
- Mucosal barrier fortifier: sucralfate (Carafate)

● Sedative: oxazepam (Serax)
● Vitamin: phytonadione (AquaMEPHYTON), cyanocobalamin (vitamin B_{12})

Patient care goals
● The client will heal without infection or complications.
● The client will maintain an adequate airway and adequate oxygenation.
● The client's fluid, electrolyte, and cellular balances will be restored.
● The client's self-concept will be restored without lasting deficits.

Nursing interventions
● Assess respiratory status. Upper airway injury is common with burns to the face, neck, and chest. *Edema may narrow the airways.*
● Assess fluid status. *Hypovolemia is indicated by a decreasing LOC, urine output less than 30 ml/hour, blood pressure less than 90/60 mm Hg, heart rate greater than 100 beats/minute, dry mucous membranes, and delayed capillary refill.*
● If the client underwent skin grafting, keep pressure off the donor side *to maintain blood flow to the site and to promote wound healing.*
● Monitor for signs of infection *to determine if the treatment plan must be altered.*
● Assess the effectiveness of pain medication *to promote comfort.*
● Monitor and record vital signs, fluid intake and output, laboratory studies, hemodynamic variables, stool for occult blood, specific gravity, calorie count, daily weight, neurovascular checks, and pulse *to detect complications.*
● Assess bowel sounds *to determine motility of the GI tract.*
● Monitor I.V. fluids *to maintain hydration and replace fluid loss.*
● Administer oxygen *to meet cellular demands.*
● Provide suctioning; assist with turning, coughing, and deep breathing; and perform chest physiotherapy and postural drainage *to maintain the client's airway.*
● Maintain the position, patency, and low suction of the NG tube *to prevent vomiting.*
● Prepare the client for TPN or enteral feedings *to meet the client's increased metabolic demands.*
● Administer medications as prescribed *to maintain or improve the client's condition.*
● Encourage the client to express feelings about disfigurement, immobility from scarring, and a fear of dying *to encourage coping.*

● Provide treatments, such as ROM exercises, Hubbard tank (for immersing the client), bed cradle, splints, and Jobst clothing, *to maintain ROM and prevent complications.*
● Elevate the affected extremities *to promote venous drainage and decrease edema.*
● Maintain a warm environment during the acute period *because the client can't regulate body temperature.*
● Maintain protective precautions *to prevent the transmission of infection to the client.*
● Provide skin and mouth care *to promote comfort.*

Evaluation
● The client regains skin integrity and is free from infection.
● The client returns to social roles and accepts his altered body image.
● The client maintains fluid and nutritional status.
● The client maintains optimal oxygenation.

Herpes zoster
HERPES ZOSTER, also known as shingles, is an acute viral infection of nerve structures caused by varicella zoster. Affected areas include the spinal and cranial sensory ganglia and posterior gray matter of the spinal cord. Herpes zoster produces localized vesicular skin lesions confined to a dermatome and severe neurologic pain in peripheral areas innervated by nerves arising in the inflamed root ganglia.

Possible causes
● Cytotoxic drug-induced immunosuppression
● Debilitating disease
● Exposure to varicella zoster
● Hodgkin's disease

Data collection findings
● Unilaterally clustered skin vesicles along peripheral sensory nerves on the trunk, thorax, or face
● Erythema
● Pruritus
● Malaise
● Neuralgia
● Severe deep pain
● Fever
● Anorexia
● Edematous skin
● Headache
● Paresthesia

Diagnostic findings
- Skin study identifies the organism.
- Visual examination shows vesicles along the peripheral sensory nerves.

Nursing diagnoses
- Impaired skin integrity
- Acute pain
- Risk for infection

Treatment
- No specific treatment (primary goal is to relieve itching and pain)

Drug therapy options
- Analgesic: acetaminophen (Tylenol) with codeine
- Antianxiety agent: lorazepam (Ativan), hydroxyzine (Vistaril)
- Antipruritic: diphenhydramine (Benadryl)
- Antiviral agent: acyclovir (Zovirax), famciclovir (Famvir), valacyclovir (Valtrex)
- Nerve blocker: lidocaine (Xylocaine)

Patient care goals
- The client will exhibit improved or healed lesions or wounds.
- The client will express feelings of comfort and pain relief.
- The client will remain free from signs and symptoms of infection.

Nursing interventions
- Assess neurologic status *to determine baseline and detect changes.*
- Assess pain and note the effectiveness of analgesics *to promote comfort and evaluate the need for a change in the current treatment plan.*
- Monitor and record vital signs, laboratory results, and cranial nerve function *to assess baseline and detect changes.*
- Administer medications as directed *to maintain or improve the client's condition.*
- Encourage the client to express feelings about changes in his physical appearance and the recurrent nature of the illness *to help him adapt to his illness.*
- Prevent scratching and rubbing of affected areas *to prevent infection.*

Evaluation
- The client displays healing lesions.
- The client reports adequate pain control.
- The client doesn't display signs or symptoms of infection.

Pressure ulcers
Pressure ulcers are localized areas of cellular necrosis that occur most commonly in skin and subcutaneous tissue over bony prominences. These ulcers may be superficial, caused by local skin irritation with subsequent surface maceration, or deep, originating in underlying tissue. Deep lesions commonly go undetected until they penetrate the skin but, by then, subcutaneous damage has occurred.

Possible causes
- Pressure, particularly over bony prominences

Data collection findings
Stage 1
- Nonblanchable erythema of intact skin
- Skin discoloration
- Warmth and hardness

Stage 2
- Abrasion
- Blister
- Partial-thickness skin loss involving the epidermis and dermis
- Shallow crater

Stage 3
- Deep crater with or without undermining of adjacent tissue
- Full-thickness skin loss involving damage or necrosis of subcutaneous tissue that may extend down to, but not through, underlying fasciae

Stage 4
- Damage to muscle, bone, tendon, or joint
- Full-thickness skin loss with extensive destruction
- Tissue necrosis

Diagnostic findings
- Visual inspection reveals pressure ulcer.
- Wound culture and sensitivity tests identify the infecting organism.

What are the characteristics of a stage 3 pressure ulcer?
● Deep crater with or without undermining of adjacent tissue
● Full-thickness skin loss involving damage or necrosis of subcutaneous tissue that may extend down to, but not through, underlying fasciae

Nursing diagnoses
● Impaired skin integrity
● Imbalanced nutrition: Less than body requirements
● Impaired physical mobility

Treatment
● High-protein, high-calorie diet in small frequent feedings; parenteral or enteral feedings if the client is unable or unwilling to take adequate nutrients orally
● Topical wound care according to the facility's protocol
● Wound debridement; tissue flap

Patient care goals
● The client will have improved nutritional status.
● The client will have evidence of pressure ulcer healing.
● The client will increase his physical mobility.

Nursing interventions
● Assess skin integrity and watch for signs of infection *to detect complications.*
● Check the bedridden client for possible changes in skin color, turgor, temperature, and sensation *to prevent further skin breakdown.*
● Reposition the client every 2 hours *to prevent pressure ulcers.*
● Use a special mattress, bed cradle, or other device *to avoid skin breakdown.*
● Provide meticulous skin care and check bony prominences *to reduce the chance of pressure ulcer development.*
● Provide wound care *to promote healing.*
● Maintain the client's diet and encourage oral fluid intake *to promote wound healing.*
● Provide ROM exercises *to promote joint mobility.*

Evaluation
● The client has intact skin integrity.
● The client has improved physical mobility.
● The client has adequate nutritional intake.

Psoriasis
PSORIASIS is a chronic, recurrent disease marked by epidermal proliferation. Lesions appear as erythematous papules and plaques covered with silver scales; they vary widely in severity and distribution.

Although this disorder most commonly affects young adults, it may strike at any age, including infancy. Psoriasis is characterized by recurring partial remissions and exacerbations.

Possible causes
● Genetic predisposition

Data collection findings
● Itching
● Lesions (red and usually forming well-defined patches)
● Pustules
● Characteristic location of lesions: scalp, chest, elbows, knees, back, buttocks
● Pain
● Patches, consisting of silver scales that flake off or thicken and cover the lesions
● Arthritic symptoms

Diagnostic findings
● Skin biopsy is positive for the disorder.
● Blood studies reveal elevated serum uric acid level in severe cases, due to accelerated nucleic acid degradation, but indications of gout are absent.

Nursing diagnoses
● Impaired skin integrity
● Risk for infection
● Disturbed body image

Treatment
● Tar, wet dressings, or oatmeal baths
● Ultraviolet (UV) light to retard cell production (may be used in conjunction with psoralen plus ultraviolet A [PUVA] therapy)

Drug therapy options
● Corticosteroid ointment: hydrocortisone (Dermacort)
● Corticosteroid: intralesional steroid injections
● Antipsoriatic agent: calcipotriene (Dovonex), anthralin (Drithocreme)
● Antihypocalcemic agent: calcitriol (Rocaltrol)
● Antineoplastic agent: methotrexate (Folex)

Patient care goals

- The client will exhibit improved or healed lesions or wounds.
- The client will remain free from signs and symptoms of infection.
- The client will express feelings about his changed body image.

Nursing interventions

- Make sure the client understands his prescribed therapy; provide written instructions *to promote compliance and avoid confusion.*
- Watch for adverse reactions, especially allergic reactions to anthralin, atrophy and acne from steroids, and burning, itching, nausea, and squamous cell epitheliomas from PUVA *to prevent complications.*
- Initially evaluate the client on methotrexate weekly (and later monthly) for RBC, WBC, and platelet counts *because cytotoxins may cause hepatic or bone marrow toxicity.* Liver biopsy may be done to assess the effects of methotrexate.
- Caution the client receiving PUVA therapy to stay out of the sun on the day of treatment and to protect his eyes with sunglasses that screen UVA for 24 hours after treatment. Tell him to wear goggles during exposure to this light. *These measures protect the client from injury caused by excessive UVA exposure.*
- Be aware that psoriasis can cause psychological problems. Assure the client that psoriasis isn't contagious and, although exacerbations and remissions occur, they're controllable with treatment. However, make sure he understands there's no cure. *Appropriate teaching helps the client develop healthy coping strategies.*
- Help the client learn to cope with stressful situations *because stressful situations tend to exacerbate psoriasis.*

Evaluation

- The client displays healing lesions.
- The client doesn't display signs or symptoms of infection.
- The client demonstrates a positive attitude regarding his self-image.

Skin cancer

Skin cancer is a malignant primary tumor of the skin. There are three types:

- Basal cell epithelioma is a tumor commonly caused by prolonged exposure to the sun.
- Melanoma is a neoplasm that arises from melanocytes. Melanoma spreads through the lymph and vascular systems and metastasizes to the lymph nodes, skin, liver, lungs, and CNS.
- Squamous cell carcinoma is a slow-growing cancer that causes airway obstruction, cough, and sputum production.

Possible causes

- Chemical irritants
- Friction or chronic irritation
- Heredity
- Immunosuppressive drugs
- Infrared heat or light
- Precancerous lesions, such as leukoplakia, nevi, and senile keratoses
- Radiation
- UV rays

Data collection findings

- Change in color, size, or shape of preexisting lesion
- Irregular, circular bordered lesion with hues of tan, black, or blue (melanoma)
- Local soreness
- Oozing, bleeding, crusting lesion
- Pruritus
- Small, red, nodular lesion that begins as an erythematous macule or plaque with indistinct margins (squamous cell carcinoma)
- Waxy nodule with telangiectasis (basal cell epithelioma)

Diagnostic findings

- Skin biopsy specimen shows cancer cells.

 FAST FACT

Remember, a change in color, size, or shape of a skin lesion may indicate a cancerous growth.

Nursing diagnoses

- Risk for infection
- Anxiety
- Disturbed body image

Caring for the client with a cancerous lesion

A 62-year-old female client recently had a cancerous lesion diagnosed by results of a circular skin punch procedure.

For which of the following should the nurse observe immediately after the procedure?

A. Infection
B. Dehiscence
C. Hemorrhage
D. Swelling

Answer: C. The nurse's main concern after a circular skin punch procedure is to monitor for bleeding. Dehiscence is more likely in larger wounds such as surgical wounds of the abdomen or thorax. Infection is a later possible effect of a skin punch, and swelling is a normal reaction associated with any event that traumatizes the skin.

What teaching should the nurse include regarding skin care?

The client should be taught to:
● avoid contact with chemical irritants
● use sunblock and layered clothing when outdoors
● self-monitor for lesions and moles that don't heal or that change characteristics
● have moles that are subject to chronic irritation removed.

Questions for further thought
● What are appropriate outcomes for this client after the procedure?
● What types of statements indicate that the client understands necessary precautions?

Treatment
● Chemosurgery with zinc chloride
● Cryosurgery with liquid nitrogen
● Curettage and electrodesiccation
● Radiation therapy

Drug therapy options
● Alkylating agent: carmustine (BiCNU), dacarbazine (DTIC-Dome)
● Antiemetic: prochlorperazine (Compazine), ondansetron (Zofran)
● Antimetabolite: fluorouracil (Adrucil)
● Antineoplastic: hydroxyurea (Hydrea), vincristine (Oncovin)
● Immunotherapy for melanoma: bacillus Calmette-Guérin (BCG) vaccine

Patient care goals
● The client will accept body image changes related to lesion removal.
● The client will remain free from infection.
● The client will have decreased anxiety regarding the treatment and outcome of lesion removal. (See *Caring for the client with a cancerous lesion.*)

Nursing interventions
● Monitor a skin punch biopsy site for *bleeding.*

● Assess lesions. *Regular assessment prevents recurrence.*
● Monitor and record vital signs *to determine baseline and detect changes.*
● Prepare the client for administration of medications as prescribed *to maintain and improve his condition.*
● Encourage the client to express feelings about changes in his body image and a fear of dying *to help him cope.*
● Provide postchemotherapy and postradiation nursing care *to promote healing.*

Evaluation
● The client has decreased anxiety and expresses acceptance of the outcome of cancer treatment.
● The client doesn't demonstrate signs of infection.

ENDOCRINE SYSTEM

The endocrine system is a complex network of hormone-secreting structures that regulate metabolism and other body processes.

Endocrine structure and function
The endocrine system consists of glands, which are made up of specialized cell clusters, and hormones, which are

released by the glands and act as chemical transmitters throughout the body.

Glands and hormones

The primary structures of the endocrine system include the hypothalamus, pituitary gland, thyroid gland, parathyroid glands, adrenal glands, and pancreas.

Hypothalamus

The hypothalamus controls temperature, respiration, and blood pressure. Its functions affect the emotional states. The hypothalamus also produces hypothalamic-stimulating hormones, which affect the inhibition and release of pituitary hormones.

Pituitary gland

The pituitary gland is composed of anterior and posterior lobes. Each lobe produces various hormones that affect the body.

Anterior lobe

The anterior lobe of the pituitary gland secretes:
- follicle-stimulating hormone, which stimulates graafian follicle growth and estrogen secretion in women
- luteinizing hormone, which induces ovulation and development of the corpus luteum in women and stimulates testosterone secretion in men
- corticotropin, also called *adrenocorticotropic hormone*, which stimulates the secretion of hormones from the adrenal cortex
- thyroid-stimulating hormone (TSH), which regulates the thyroid gland's secretory activity
- growth hormone, which is an insulin antagonist that stimulates the growth of cells, bones, muscle, and soft tissue.

Posterior lobe

The posterior lobe of the pituitary gland secretes:
- vasopressin (antidiuretic hormone [ADH]), which helps the body retain water
- oxytocin, which stimulates uterine contractions during labor and milk secretion in lactating women.

Thyroid gland

The thyroid gland accelerates growth and cellular reactions, including basal metabolic rate. TSH controls hormones released by the thyroid gland. The thyroid gland produces thyrocalcitonin, triiodothyronine (T_3), and thyroxine (T_4), which are necessary for growth and development.

Parathyroid gland

The parathyroid gland secretes parathyroid hormone (parathormone), which regulates calcium and phosphorus levels and promotes the resorption of calcium from bones.

Adrenal glands

The adrenal glands include the adrenal cortex and the adrenal medulla.

Adrenal cortex

The adrenal cortex secretes three major hormones:
- glucocorticoids (cortisol, cortisone, and corticosterone), which mediate the stress response, promote sodium and water retention and potassium secretion, and suppress corticotropin secretion
- mineralocorticoids (aldosterone and deoxycorticosterone), which promote sodium and water retention and potassium secretion
- sex hormones (androgens, estrogens, and progesterone), which develop and maintain secondary sex characteristics and libido.

Adrenal medulla

The adrenal medulla secretes two hormones:
- norepinephrine, which regulates generalized vasoconstriction
- epinephrine, which regulates instantaneous stress reaction and increases metabolism, blood glucose levels, and cardiac output.

Pancreas

The pancreas is an accessory gland of digestion. It has exocrine and endocrine functions:
- In its exocrine function, it secretes digestive enzymes (amylase, lipase, and trypsin). Amylase breaks down starches into smaller carbohydrate molecules. Lipase breaks down fats into fatty acids and glycerol. Trypsin breaks down proteins. Note that exocrine glands discharge secretions through a duct; the pancreas secretes enzymes into the duodenum through the pancreatic duct.
- In its endocrine function, the pancreas secretes hormones (insulin, glucagon, and somatostatin) from the islets of Langerhans. Insulin regulates fat, protein, and carbohydrate metabolism and decreases blood glucose levels by promoting glucose transport into cells. Glucagon increases blood glucose levels by promoting hepatic glyconeogenesis. Somatostatin inhibits the release of insulin, glucagon, and somatotropin. Note that endocrine glands discharge secretions into the blood or lymph.

ENDOCRINE DISORDERS

Major endocrine disorders include Addison's disease, Cushing's syndrome, diabetes insipidus, diabetes mellitus, hyperthyroidism, hypothyroidism, pancreatic cancer, thyroid cancer, and thyroiditis.

Addison's disease

ADDISON'S DISEASE, also known as *adrenal hypofunction,* occurs when the adrenal gland fails to secrete sufficient mineralocorticoids, glucocorticoids, and androgens.

ADDISONIAN CRISIS (adrenal crisis) is a critical deficiency of mineralocorticoids and glucocorticoids. It generally occurs in clients who have chronic adrenal insufficiency and follows acute stress, sepsis, trauma, surgery, or omission of steroid therapy. It's a medical emergency that necessitates immediate, vigorous treatment.

Possible causes
- Autoimmune disease
- Histoplasmosis
- Idiopathic atrophy of adrenal glands
- Metastatic lesions from lung cancer
- Pituitary hypofunction
- Surgical removal of adrenal glands
- Trauma
- TB

Data collection findings
- Hypoglycemia
- Weakness and lethargy
- Bronzed skin pigmentation of nipples, scars, and buccal mucosa
- Depression and personality changes
- Anorexia, diarrhea, and nausea
- Orthostatic hypotension
- Weight loss
- Dehydration and thirst
- Decreased pubic and axillary hair

Diagnostic findings
- Blood chemistry reveals decreased HCT; decreased Hb, cortisol, glucose, sodium, chloride, and aldosterone levels; and increased BUN and potassium levels.
- Basal metabolic rate is decreased.
- ECG demonstrates prolonged PR and QT intervals.
- Fasting blood glucose reveals hypoglycemia.
- Urine chemistry shows decreased 17-ketosteroids and 17-hydroxycorticosteroids.

Nursing diagnoses
- Imbalanced nutrition: Less than body requirements
- Risk for infection
- Decreased cardiac output

Treatment
- High-carbohydrate, high-protein, high-sodium, low-potassium diet in small, frequent feedings before steroid therapy; high-potassium and low-sodium diet while on steroid therapy
- In adrenal crisis, I.V. hydrocortisone administered promptly along with 3 to 5 L of normal saline solution

Drug therapy options
- Antacid: magnesium and aluminum hydroxide (Maalox)
- Glucocorticoid: cortisone (Cortone), hydrocortisone (Solu-Cortef)
- Mineralocorticoid: fludrocortisone (Florinef)
- Vasopressor: phenylephrine (Neo-Synephrine)

SPOT CHECK

Clients receiving long-term therapy with corticosteroids must not abruptly stop taking the drug but must have the dosage gradually reduced. What's the rationale for this?
Answer: An abrupt withdrawal of corticosteroids may trigger addisonian crisis. Gradual withdrawal of the medication will prevent this situation because the body will produce some corticosteroids.

Patient care goals
- The client will have normal serum cortisol and blood glucose levels.
- The client will understand how to take medications.
- The client will remain hemodynamically stable.
- The client will be free from injury.

Nursing interventions
- Maintain a patent I.V. site for administration of I.V. hydrocortisone and saline solution promptly if the client is in adrenal crisis *to reverse shock and hyponatremia.*
- Assess fluid balance (and tell the client to increase fluid intake in hot weather) *to prevent addisonian crisis, which may be precipitated by salt or fluid loss in hot weather and during exercise.*
- Monitor and record vital signs, intake and output, urine specific gravity, and laboratory studies *to assess for deficient fluid volume.*
- Maintain the client's diet *to promote nutritional balance.*

- Monitor I.V. fluids *to maintain hydration and prevent addisonian crisis.*
- Weigh the client daily *to determine nutritional status and detect fluid loss.*
- Administer medications as prescribed *to maintain or improve the client's condition.*
- Don't allow the client to sit up or stand quickly *to avoid orthostatic hypotension.*
- Assist with ADLs and maintain a quiet environment *to conserve energy and decrease metabolic demands.*

Evaluation
- The client has normal serum cortisol and glucose levels.
- The client takes medications correctly and verbalizes understanding of the potential adverse effects.
- The client doesn't demonstrate signs and symptoms of infection.

Cushing's syndrome

CUSHING'S SYNDROME, also known as *hypercortisolism,* is the hyperactivity of the adrenal cortex. It results in excessive secretion of glucocorticoids, particularly cortisol, and may also result in an increase in mineralocorticoids and sex hormones.

Possible causes
- Adenoma or carcinoma of the adrenal cortex or pituitary gland
- Excessive or prolonged administration of glucocorticoids or corticotropin
- Exogenous secretion of corticotropin by malignant neoplasms in the lungs or gallbladder
- Hyperplasia of the adrenal glands
- Hypothalamic stimulation of the pituitary gland

Data collection findings
- Weight gain, especially truncal obesity, buffalo hump, and moonface
- Hypertension
- Muscle wasting
- Fragile skin
- Amenorrhea
- Mood swings
- Acne
- Decreased libido
- Ecchymosis
- Edema
- Gynecomastia
- Hirsutism
- Pain in joints
- Poor wound healing
- Enlarged clitoris
- Purple striae on abdomen
- Recurrent infections
- Weakness and fatigue

QUICK STUDY

Remember the signs of Cushing's syndrome are *cushioning* of the face, neck, and trunk from fat.

Diagnostic findings
- Blood chemistry studies show increased cortisol, aldosterone, sodium, corticotropin, and glucose levels and decreased potassium level.
- CT scan shows pituitary or adrenal tumors.
- Dexamethasone suppression test shows no decrease in 17-hydroxycorticosteroids.
- Glucose tolerance test shows hyperglycemia.
- Hematology shows increased WBC and RBC counts and decreased eosinophil count.
- MRI shows pituitary or adrenal tumors.
- Ultrasonography shows pituitary or adrenal tumors.
- Urine chemistry shows increased 17-hydroxycorticosteroids and 17-ketosteroids, decreased urine specific gravity, and glycosuria.
- Radiography shows pituitary or adrenal tumor and osteoporosis.

Nursing diagnoses
- Disturbed body image
- Excess fluid volume
- Risk for injury

Treatment
- Hypophysectomy or bilateral adrenalectomy
- Low-sodium, low-carbohydrate, low-calorie, high-protein, and high-potassium diet
- Radiation therapy

Drug therapy options
- Adrenal suppressant: aminoglutethimide (Cytadren), metyrapone (Metopirone)
- Insulin or oral antidiabetic agents: acetohexamide (Dymelor), chlorpropamide (Diabinese), glipizide (Glucotrol), glyburide (DiaBeta, Micronase), tolazamide (Tolinase), tolbutamide (Orinase)
- Diuretic: ethacrynic acid (Edecrin), furosemide (Lasix)

- Potassium supplement: potassium chloride (K-Lor), potassium gluconate (Kaon)

Patient care goals
- The client will have adequate metabolic function and normal fluid and electrolyte balance.
- The client will be free from injury and complications.
- The client will gain a positive self-image.

Nursing interventions
- Perform postoperative care *to prevent complications*.
- Assess fluid balance and edema *to detect fluid deficit or overload*.
- Monitor and record vital signs, intake and output, urine specific gravity, fingersticks, urine glucose and ketones, and laboratory studies. *Altered parameters may indicate altered fluid or electrolyte status*.
- Apply antiembolism stockings *to promote venous return and prevent thromboembolism formation*.
- Maintain the client's diet *to maintain nutritional status*.
- Maintain standard precautions *to protect the client from infection*.
- Provide meticulous skin care and reposition the client every 2 hours *to prevent skin breakdown*.
- Limit water intake *to prevent excess fluid volume*.
- Weigh the client daily *to detect fluid retention*.
- Administer medications as prescribed *to maintain or improve the client's condition*.
- Encourage the client to express feelings about changes in his body image and sexual function *to help him cope effectively*.
- Provide rest periods *to prevent fatigue*.
- Provide postradiation nursing care *to prevent complications*.

Evaluation
- The client's electrolyte levels have returned to normal.
- The client's blood glucose level remains within reference limits.
- The client is coping with an altered body image.
- The client remains free from infection and trauma.

Diabetes insipidus

DIABETES INSIPIDUS stems from a deficiency of ADH (vasopressin) secreted by the posterior lobe of the pituitary gland. Decreased ADH reduces the ability of distal and collecting renal tubules in the kidneys to concentrate urine, resulting in excessive urination, excessive thirst, and excessive fluid intake.

Possible causes
- Brain surgery
- Idiopathy
- Head injury
- Meningitis
- Trauma to the posterior lobe of the pituitary gland
- Tumor of the posterior lobe of the pituitary gland

Data collection findings
- Polyuria (greater than 5 L/day)
- Polydipsia (excessive thirst, consumption of 4 to 40 L/day)
- Dehydration
- Fatigue
- Headache
- Muscle weakness and pain
- Tachycardia
- Weight loss

Diagnostic findings
- Blood chemistry shows decreased ADH by radioimmunoassay and increased potassium, sodium, and osmolality levels.
- Urine chemistry shows urine specific gravity less than 1.004, osmolality 50 to 200 mOsm/kg, decreased urine pH, and decreased sodium and potassium levels.

Nursing diagnoses
- Deficient fluid volume
- Impaired oral mucous membrane
- Deficient knowledge (diabetes insipidus)

Treatment
- I.V. therapy: hydration (when first diagnosed, intake and output must be matched milliliter to milliliter to prevent dehydration) and electrolyte replacement
- Regular diet with restriction of foods that exert a diuretic effect

Drug therapy options
- ADH replacement: vasopressin (Pitressin), lypressin (Diapid)
- ADH stimulant: carbamazepine (Tegretol)

Patient care goals
- The client's fluid volume will remain within normal limits.
- The client's oral mucous membranes will remain intact.
- The client will have knowledge of his illness.

Nursing interventions

- Assess fluid balance *to avoid dehydration.*
- Monitor and record vital signs, intake and output (urine output should be measured every hour when first diagnosed), urine specific gravity (check every 1 to 2 hours when first diagnosed), and laboratory studies *to assess for fluid volume deficit.*
- Maintain the client's diet *to maintain nutritional balance.*
- Force fluids *to keep intake equal to output and to prevent dehydration.*
- Administer I.V. fluids *to replace fluid and electrolyte loss.*
- Maintain the patency of the indwelling urinary catheter *to allow an accurate measure of urine output.*
- Administer medications as prescribed to enable the client *to concentrate urine and prevent dehydration.*
- Weigh the client daily *to detect fluid loss.*

Evaluation

- The client has adequate intake and output values.
- The client has intact oral mucous membranes.
- The client relates appropriate knowledge of his illness.

SPOT CHECK

Which nursing diagnosis is most likely for a client with an acute episode of diabetes insipidus?
A. Imbalanced nutrition: Less than body requirements
B. Deficient fluid volume
C. Impaired gas exchange
D. Ineffective tissue perfusion (cerebral)
Answer: B. Diabetes insipidus causes a pronounced loss of intravascular volume. The most prominent risk to the client is deficient fluid volume. Nutrition, gas exchange, and tissue perfusion are risks as a result of the deficient fluid volume caused by diabetes insipidus.

Diabetes mellitus

DIABETES MELLITUS is a chronic disorder resulting from a disturbance in the production, action, and rate of insulin utilization. There are several types of diabetes mellitus:
- Type 1 (insulin-dependent diabetes mellitus) usually develops in childhood.
- Type 2 (non-insulin-dependent diabetes mellitus) usually develops after age 30.
- Gestational diabetes mellitus occurs with pregnancy.

- Secondary diabetes mellitus is induced by trauma, surgery, pancreatic disease, or medications and can be treated as type 1 or type 2.

Factors that increase blood glucose include glucocorticoids, epinephrine, glucagon, somatotropin, emotional stress, pregnancy with multiple births, surgery or trauma, and obesity (overeating). Factors that decrease blood glucose include insulin, exercise, and decreased food intake. (See *Major complications of diabetes mellitus,* page 386.)

Possible causes

- Autoimmune disease
- Blockage of insulin supply
- Cushing's syndrome
- Exposure to chemicals
- Failure of the body to produce insulin
- Genetics
- Hyperpituitarism
- Hyperthyroidism
- Infection
- Medications
- Pregnancy
- Receptor defect in normally insulin-responsive cells
- Stress
- Surgery
- Trauma

Data collection findings

- Polyuria
- Weakness
- Polydipsia
- Polyphagia
- Weight loss
- Dehydration
- Acetone breath
- Anorexia
- Atrophic muscles
- Blurred vision
- Fatigue
- Kussmaul's respirations
- Flushed, warm, smooth, shiny skin
- Multiple infections and boils
- Pain
- Mottled extremities
- Paresthesia
- Peripheral and visceral neuropathies
- Poor wound healing
- Retinopathy
- Sexual dysfunction

Major complications of diabetes mellitus

Arteriosclerosis

Assess for ulcers on the legs, lack of sensation in the legs and feet, angina pectoris, pyelonephritis and reduced renal function, and retinopathy (observe for visual impairment). Note that the client should undergo an annual vision examination by an ophthalmologist. The diabetic client is susceptible to peripheral vascular disease, neuropathy, and early coronary artery disease. Glomerulosclerosis is a common complication. Retinopathy is the major cause of acquired blindness in diabetic adults. With severely impaired vision, the client may require modifications in self-care management.

Metabolic acidosis

Diabetic ketoacidosis, more common in type 1 diabetes, has a slow onset. It results from acute insulin deficiency, causing acidosis from metabolism of fats (ketone bodies). Assess for dehydration caused by polyuria and hypovolemia as well as acid-base imbalance and electrolyte changes caused by acidosis and ketone excretion. Determine the client's blood glucose level and assess the client's history for recent infection, severe stress, and noncompliance with insulin therapy. Depending on the severity of the acidosis, the client may need I.V. insulin, plasma expanders *to prevent shock,* and electrolyte replacement. Monitor the client's blood glucose level frequently *to assess progress.* Teach the client how *to avoid recurrence* by adhering to the planned diet, exercise, and medication program.

Hyperosmolar hyperglycemic nonketotic syndrome

The client with type II diabetes is at risk for hyperosmolar hyperglycemic nonketotic syndrome, a life-threatening complication that occurs when an elevated blood glucose level leads to severe dehydration and electrolyte imbalance. Treatment resembles that for ketoacidosis; however, correcting dehydration is even more important.

Hypoglycemia (insulin reaction)

Assess the client for hunger, anxiety, blurred vision, sweating, and tremors. Unconsciousness can occur if the blood glucose level falls below 50 mg/dl. Provide a source of rapidly absorbed carbohydrate (for example, 4 oz of orange juice, regular soda pop, or five Life-Savers). If the client can't swallow, administer 25 ml of 50% glucose by I.V. bolus as ordered. (Glucagon, which converts glycogen stored in the liver to glucose, can also be administered to a client who can't swallow; for example, a family member can administer glucagon I.M. to an unconscious client. When the client regains consciousness, the family member should provide small, frequent meals.) Monitor the blood glucose level *to prevent relapse.* Teach the client *to avoid hypoglycemia* by regulating diet, exercise, and insulin or oral hypoglycemic drugs.

Diagnostic findings

- Blood chemistry shows increased glucose, potassium, chloride, ketone, cholesterol, and triglyceride levels; decreased carbon dioxide level; and pH less than 7.4.
- Fasting blood glucose level is increased (126 mg/dl or greater).
- Glycosylated Hb assay (Hb A_{1c}) is increased.
- Glucose tolerance test results show hyperglycemia.
- Two-hour postprandial blood glucose level shows hyperglycemia (greater than 200 mg/dl).
- Urine chemistry shows increased glucose and ketone levels.

Nursing diagnoses

- Risk for deficient fluid volume
- Risk for impaired skin integrity
- Risk for infection
- Deficient knowledge (diabetes mellitus)

Treatment

- Dietary restrictions
- Exercise
- Pancreas transplant
(See *Treating clients with diabetes.*)

Drug therapy options

- Insulin or oral antidiabetic agent: acetohexamide (Dymelor), chlorpropamide (Diabinese), glipizide (Glucotrol), glyburide (DiaBeta, Micronase), tolazamide (Tolinase), tolbutamide (Orinase)
- Vitamin and mineral supplement

Patient care goals

- The client will be able to cope with lifestyle changes caused by his diabetes mellitus and its associated therapy.
- The client won't experience complications resulting from not understanding or adhering to the appropriate therapy.

● The client's blood glucose level, Hb A$_{1c}$ level, and body weight will approach acceptable levels.

Nursing interventions

● Assess acid-base and fluid balance *to monitor for signs of hyperglycemia.*

● Monitor for signs of hypoglycemia (vagueness, slow cerebration, dizziness, weakness, pallor, tachycardia, diaphoresis, seizures, and coma), ketoacidosis (acetone breath, dehydration, weak or rapid pulse, Kussmaul's respirations), and hyperosmolar coma (polyuria, thirst, neurologic abnormalities, stupor) *to ensure early intervention and prevent complications.*

● Be prepared to treat hypoglycemia; immediately give carbohydrates in the form of fruit juice, hard candy, or honey. If the client is unconscious, prepare him for I.V. glucagon or dextrose administration *to prevent neurologic complications.*

● Maintain a patent I.V. line for administration of I.V. fluids, insulin and, usually, potassium replacement for ketoacidosis or hyperosmolar coma *to reduce the risk of potentially life-threatening complications.*

● Monitor and record vital signs, intake and output, fingersticks for blood glucose, and laboratory studies *to assess fluid and electrolyte balance.*

● Monitor wound healing *to assess for infection.*

● Maintain the client's diet *to prevent complications of diabetes,* such as hyperglycemia and hypoglycemia.

● Force fluids *to keep the client hydrated.*

● Administer medications as prescribed. *Diabetic control requires a dynamic balance between diet, antidiabetic agent, and exercise.*

● Encourage the client to express feelings about his diet, medication regimen, and body image changes *to facilitate coping mechanisms.*

● Encourage exercise as tolerated *to prevent long-term complications of diabetes.*

● Weigh the client weekly *to determine nutritional status.*

● Provide meticulous skin and foot care. Clients with diabetes are at increased risk for infection from impaired leukocyte activity. *These health care practices minimize the risk of infection and promote early detection of health problems.*

● Maintain a warm, quiet environment *to provide rest and reduce metabolic demands.*

● Foster independence *to promote self-esteem.*

● Determine the client's compliance with diet, exercise, and medication regimens *to help develop appropriate interventions.*

Treating clients with diabetes

Effective treatment for clients with diabetes optimizes blood glucose level and decreases complications. In type 1 diabetes (insulin-dependent), treatment includes insulin replacement, meal planning, and exercise. Current forms of insulin replacement include single-dose, mixed-dose, split-mixed-dose, and multiple-dose regimens. The multiple-dose regimen may use an insulin pump.

Insulin action

Insulin may be rapid-acting (Humalog), fast-acting (Regular), intermediate-acting (NPH and Lente), long-acting (ultralente), or a premixed combination of fast-acting and intermediate-acting. Insulin may be derived from beef, pork, or human sources. Purified human insulin is used commonly today.

Personalized meal plan

Treatment for clients with either type of diabetes also requires a meal plan to meet nutritional needs, to control blood glucose levels, and to help the client reach and maintain his ideal body weight. In type 1 diabetes, the calorie allotment may be high, depending on the client's growth stage and activity level. Weight reduction is a goal for the obese client with type 2 diabetes (non-insulin dependent).

Other treatments

Exercise is also useful in managing type 2 diabetes because it increases insulin sensitivity, improves glucose tolerance, and promotes weight loss. In addition, clients with type 2 diabetes may need oral antidiabetic drugs to stimulate endogenous insulin production and increase insulin sensitivity at the cellular level.

Long-term treatments

Treatment for clients with long-term complications may include dialysis or kidney transplantation for renal failure, photocoagulation for retinopathy, and vascular surgery for large vessel disease. Pancreas transplantation is also an option.

 SPOT CHECK

What are some signs of hypoglycemia?
Signs of hypoglycemia include vagueness, slow cerebration, dizziness, weakness, pallor, tachycardia, diaphoresis, seizures, and coma.

Evaluation
- The client verbalizes knowledge of his medication regimen, diet, and potential complications of the disease.
- The client remains free from infection.
- The client demonstrates adequate skin care.
- The client's blood studies are within acceptable limits and his weight is well controlled.

Hyperthyroidism

HYPERTHYROIDISM is the increased synthesis of thyroid hormone. It can result from overactivity (Graves' disease) or a change in the thyroid gland (toxic nodular goiter).

Possible causes
- Autoimmune disease
- Psychological or physiologic stress
- Infection
- Pituitary tumors
- Thyroid adenomas
- Genetic

Data collection findings
- Anxiety and mood swings
- AF
- Dyspnea
- Bruit or thrill over thyroid
- Diaphoresis
- Palpitations
- Diarrhea
- Fine hand tremors
- Flushed, smooth skin
- Hyperhidrosis
- Increased hunger
- Increased systolic blood pressure
- Heat intolerance
- Tachycardia
- Exophthalmos
- Tachypnea
- Weakness
- Weight loss

Diagnostic findings
- Blood chemistry shows increased T_3, T_4, and free T_4 levels and decreased TSH and cholesterol levels.
- Radioactive iodine uptake is increased.
- Thyroid scan shows nodules.

Nursing diagnoses
- Activity intolerance

Nursing care after thyroidectomy

Keep these crucial points in mind when caring for the client who has undergone thyroidectomy:
- Keep the client in Fowler's position *to promote venous return from the head and neck and to decrease oozing into the incision.*
- Watch for signs of respiratory distress (tracheal collapse, tracheal mucus accumulation, and laryngeal edema).
- Note that vocal cord paralysis can cause respiratory obstruction, with sudden stridor and restlessness.
- Keep a tracheotomy tray at the client's bedside for 24 hours after surgery and be prepared to assist with emergency tracheotomy, which may be necessary.
- Assess for signs of hemorrhage.
- Assess for hypocalcemia (tingling and numbness of the extremities, muscle twitching, cramps, laryngeal spasm, and positive Chvostek's and Trousseau's signs), which may occur when parathyroid glands are damaged.
- Keep calcium gluconate available for emergency I.V. administration.
- Be alert for signs of thyroid storm (tachycardia, hyperkinesis, fever, vomiting, and hypertension).

- Risk for imbalanced body temperature
- Risk for injury

Treatment
- High-protein, high-carbohydrate, high-calorie diet restricting such stimulants as coffee and caffeine
- Radiation therapy
- Thyroidectomy

Drug therapy options
- Adrenergic-blocking agent: guanethidine (Ismelin), propranolol (Inderal), reserpine (Serpalan)
- Antithyroid agent: methimazole (Tapazole), propylthiouracil (Propyl-Thyracil)
- Cardiac glycoside: digoxin (Lanoxin)
- Glucocorticoid: cortisone (Cortone), hydrocortisone (Solu-Cortef)
- Iodine preparation: potassium iodide (SSKI), radioactive iodine
- Sedative: oxazepam (Serax)
- Vitamin: ascorbic acid (vitamin C), thiamine (vitamin B_1)

Patient care goals
- The client will be free from toxic effects of thyroid hormone.
- The client will feel rested and comfortable.
- The client will understand the recommended treatment.
- The client will be hemodynamically stable.

Nursing interventions
- Assess cardiovascular status for signs of hyperthyroidism, such as tachycardia, increased blood pressure, palpitations, and atrial arrhythmias. Presence of these signs may require a change in the treatment regimen.
- Assess fluid balance for signs of fluid volume deficit.
- Monitor and record vital signs, intake and output, and laboratory studies *to detect early changes and guide treatment.*
- Maintain the client's diet *to promote adequate nutrition.*
- Avoid stimulants, such as drugs and foods that contain caffeine, *to reduce or eliminate arrhythmias.*
- Monitor I.V. fluids *to promote hydration.*
- Administer medications as prescribed *to maintain or improve the client's condition.*
- Weigh the client daily *to provide consistent readings.*
- Provide postoperative nursing care *to promote healing and prevent complications.* (See *Nursing care after thyroidectomy.*)
- Provide rest periods and a quiet, cool environment *to reduce metabolic demands and promote comfort.*
- Provide skin and eye care *to prevent complications.*
- Encourage the client to express feelings about changes in his body image *to reduce anxiety and facilitate coping mechanisms.*
- Provide postradiation nursing care *to prevent complications associated with treatment.*

Evaluation
- The client's weight and vital signs are within normal limits.
- The client verbalizes understanding and follows the recommended treatment.
- The client tolerates increased activity.

Hypothyroidism

Hypothyroidism, which affects women more commonly than men, occurs when the thyroid gland fails to produce sufficient thyroid hormone. This causes an overall decrease in metabolism.

Possible causes
- Hashimoto's thyroiditis
- Malfunction of pituitary gland
- Overuse of antithyroid drugs
- Thyroidectomy
- Use of radioactive iodine

Data collection findings
- Fatigue
- Coarse hair and alopecia
- Hypothermia
- Constipation
- Menstrual disorders
- Weight gain
- Anorexia (as the disorder progresses)
- Mental sluggishness
- Dry, flaky skin and thinning nails
- Cold intolerance
- Decreased diaphoresis
- Edema
- Hypersensitivity to narcotics, barbiturates, and anesthetics
- Thick tongue and swollen lips

Diagnostic findings
- Blood chemistry shows decreased T_3, T_4, and sodium levels and increased TSH and cholesterol levels.
- Radioactive iodine uptake is decreased.

Nursing diagnoses
- Activity intolerance
- Decreased cardiac output
- Ineffective coping

Treatment
- High-fiber, high-protein, low-calorie diet

Drug therapy options
- Stool softener: docusate sodium (Colace)
- Thyroid hormone replacement: levothyroxine (Synthroid), liothyronine (Cytomel)

Patient care goals
- The client will resume a normal activity level.
- The client will remain hemodynamically stable.
- The client will understand the recommended lifelong treatment.

CLINICAL SITUATION

Caring for the client with hypothyroidism

A 65-year-old male client recently retired after 50 years as a butcher. He has gradually become lethargic and usually sits all day. His physician has diagnosed his condition as hypothyroidism.

How would the client's condition be confirmed?

Laboratory tests could confirm hypothyroidism. The thyroid-stimulating hormone level would be increased and triiodothyronine and thyroxine levels would be decreased.

Why should the nurse instruct the client to monitor his pulse rate?

A rapid pulse rate may indicate signs of drug toxicity. Other adverse reactions include palpitations, nervousness, increased blood pressure, weight loss, heat intolerance, and insomnia.

How should sedatives be prescribed for this client?

A client with hypothyroidism should be given sedatives at one-half to one-third the normal dose *to prevent complications.*

Questions for further thought

● What are appropriate nursing diagnoses for this client?
● What effects does thyroid hormone replacement have on a client's metabolism? Why would that put a client who is susceptible to cardiac problems (such as angina) at risk?

Nursing interventions

● Avoid sedation. Administer one-half to one-third the normal dose of sedatives or narcotics *to prevent complications.* (See *Caring for the client with hypothyroidism.*) Clients taking warfarin (Coumadin) with levothyroxine may require lower doses of warfarin because levothyroxine enhances warfarin's effects.
● Assess fluid balance *to determine fluid volume deficit or excess.*
● Check for constipation and edema *to detect early changes.*
● Monitor and record vital signs, intake and output, and laboratory studies *to determine fluid status.*
● Maintain the client's diet *to facilitate nutritional balance.*
● Force fluids *to maintain hydration.*
● Administer medications as prescribed *to maintain or improve the client's condition.*
● Encourage the client to express feelings of depression *to promote coping mechanisms.*
● Encourage physical activity and mental stimulation *to enhance self-esteem.*
● Provide a warm environment *to promote comfort because the client with hypothyroidism may be sensitive to cold.*
● Turn the client every 2 hours and provide skin care *to prevent skin breakdown.*

● Provide frequent rest periods *because clients diagnosed with hypothyroidism are commonly fatigued.*

Evaluation

● The client has stable vital signs.
● The client resumes his previous activity level.
● The client verbalizes understanding of the chronic illness and required treatment.

Pancreatic cancer

Pancreatic cancer progresses rapidly and is deadly. Treatment is rarely successful because the disease has usually widely metastasized by the time it's diagnosed. Therapeutic care focuses on helping the client and family come to terms with the end of life.

Pancreatic tumors are almost always adenocarcinomas and most arise in the head of the pancreas. Tumors of the body and tail of the pancreas and of the islet cells are less common. The two main tissue types are cylinder cell and large, fatty, granular cell.

Possible causes

● Smoking
● Foods high in fat and protein
● Food additives
● Industrial chemicals, such as naphthalene, benzidine, and urea

Data collection findings

- Dull, intermittent epigastric pain (early in disease)
- Continuous pain that radiates to the right upper quadrant or dorsolumbar area (may be colicky, dull or vague, and unrelated to activity or posture)
- Anorexia
- Nausea
- Vomiting
- Diarrhea
- Jaundice
- Rapid, profound weight loss
- Palpable mass in the subumbilical or left hypochondrial region

Diagnostic findings

- Percutaneous fine-needle aspiration biopsy of the pancreas may detect tumor cells.
- Laparotomy with a biopsy allows definitive diagnosis.
- Ultrasound and CT scan can identify a mass but not its histology.
- Angiography can reveal a tumor's vascular supply.
- MRI shows tumor size and location in great detail.
- Blood studies reveal increased serum bilirubin, increased serum amylase and lipase, prolonged PT, elevated alkaline phosphatase (with biliary obstruction), and elevated aspartate aminotransferase and alanine aminotransferase (when liver cell necrosis is present).
- Fasting blood glucose may indicate hyperglycemia or hypoglycemia.
- Plasma insulin immunoassay shows measurable serum insulin in the presence of islet-cell tumors.
- Stool studies may show occult blood if ulceration in the GI tract or ampulla of Vater has occurred.
- Tumor markers for pancreatic cancer, including carcinoembryonic antigen, alpha fetoprotein, and serum immunoreactive elastase I, are elevated.

Nursing diagnoses

- Ineffective breathing pattern
- Acute pain
- Imbalanced nutrition: Less than body requirements

Treatment

- Blood transfusion
- I.V. fluid therapy
- Total pancreatectomy (surgical removal of the pancreas)
- Cholecystojejunostomy (surgical anastomosis of the gallbladder and the jejunum)
- Choledochoduodenostomy (surgical anastomosis of the common bile duct and the duodenum)
- Choledochojejunostomy (surgical anastomosis of the common bile duct and the jejunum)
- Whipple's operation or pancreatoduodenectomy (excision of the head of the pancreas along with the encircling loop of the duodenum)
- Gastrojejunostomy (surgical creation of an anastomosis between the stomach and the jejunum)
- Radiation therapy

Drug therapy options

- Antineoplastic combination: fluorouracil (Adrucil), streptozocin (Zanosar), ifosfamide (IFEX), and doxorubicin (Adriamycin)
- Antibiotic: cefmetazole (Zefazone) to prevent infection and relieve symptoms
- Anticholinergic: propantheline (Pro-Banthine) to decrease GI tract spasm and motility and reduce pain and secretions
- H_2-receptor antagonist: cimetidine (Tagamet), ranitidine (Zantac), famotidine (Pepcid), nizatidine (Axid)
- Diuretic: furosemide (Lasix) to mobilize extracellular fluid from ascites
- Insulin to provide an adequate exogenous insulin supply after pancreatic resection
- Narcotic analgesic: morphine, meperidine (Demerol), codeine (can lead to biliary tract spasm and increase common bile duct pressure; used when other methods fail)
- Pancreatic enzyme: pancrelipase (Pancrease)
- Vitamin K: phytonadione (AquaMEPHYTON)
- Stool softener: docusate (Colace)
- Laxative: bisacodyl (Dulcolax)

Patient care goals

- The client's breathing pattern will remain within 5 breaths of baseline.
- The client will express feelings of comfort and pain relief.
- The client will have improved nutritional status.

Nursing interventions
Before surgery

- Ensure that the client is medically stable, particularly regarding nutrition (this may take 4 to 5 days). If the client can't tolerate oral feedings, TPN and I.V. fat emulsions may be required *to correct deficiencies and maintain a positive nitrogen balance.*
- Educate the client about the necessity of blood transfusions *to combat anemia,* vitamin K *to overcome prothrombin deficiency,* antibiotics *to prevent postoperative infec-*

tion, and gastric lavage as necessary *to maintain gastric decompression.*

● Tell the client about expected postoperative procedures and expected adverse effects of radiation and chemotherapy *to allay anxiety.*

After surgery

● Watch for and report complications, such as fistula, pancreatitis, fluid and electrolyte imbalance, infection, hemorrhage, skin breakdown, nutritional deficiency, hepatic failure, renal insufficiency, and diabetes *to ensure early detection and treatment of complications.*

● If the client is receiving chemotherapy, treat adverse effects symptomatically *to promote client comfort and prevent complications.*

Throughout illness

● Monitor fluid balance, abdominal girth, metabolic state, and weight daily to determine fluid volume status. Replace nutrients I.V., orally, or by NG tube *to combat weight loss.* Impose dietary restrictions such as a low-sodium or fluid retention diet as required *to combat weight gain (due to ascites).* Maintain a 2,500 calorie diet for the client *to meet increased nutritional needs.*

● Serve small, frequent, nutritious meals by enlisting the dietitian's services *to help the client meet increased metabolic demands.*

● Administer an oral pancreatic enzyme at mealtimes if needed *to aid digestion.*

● Administer laxatives, stool softeners, and cathartics as required; modify diet; and increase client fluid intake *to prevent constipation.*

● Position the client properly at mealtime and help him walk when he can *to increase GI motility.*

● Administer pain medication, antibiotics, and antipyretics, as necessary.

● Watch for signs of hypoglycemia or hyperglycemia; administer glucose or an antidiabetic agent as necessary *to prevent complications of hypoglycemia or hyperglycemia.* Monitor blood glucose levels *to detect early signs of hypoglycemia or hyperglycemia.*

● Provide meticulous skin care *to avoid pruritus and necrosis.*

● Watch for signs of upper GI bleeding; test stools and vomitus for occult blood and keep a flow sheet of Hb and HCT values *to prevent hemorrhage.*

● Promote gastric vasoconstriction with prescribed medication *to control active bleeding.* Replace any fluid loss *to prevent hypovolemia.*

● Ease discomfort from pyloric obstruction with an NG tube *to provide gastric decompression.*

● Apply antiembolism stockings and assist in ROM exercises *to prevent thrombosis.* If thrombosis occurs, elevate the client's *legs to promote venous return* and give an anticoagulant or aspirin as required *to decrease blood viscosity and prevent further thrombosis.*

Evaluation

● The client has a stable breathing pattern.
● The client reports adequate pain control.
● The client has improved nutritional status as evidenced by laboratory values.

Thyroid cancer

Thyroid cancer is a malignant, primary tumor of the thyroid. It doesn't affect thyroid hormone secretion. (See *Anaplastic thyroid cancer.*)

Possible causes

● Chronic overstimulation of the pituitary gland
● Chronic overstimulation of the thymus gland
● Neck radiation

Data collection findings

● Enlarged thyroid gland
● Painless, firm, irregular, and enlarged thyroid nodule or mass
● Hoarseness
● Dysphagia
● Dyspnea
● Palpable cervical lymph nodes

Diagnostic findings

● Blood chemistry shows increased calcitonin, serotonin, and prostaglandin levels.
● Radioactive iodine uptake shows a "cold," or nonfunctioning, nodule.
● Thyroid biopsy shows cytology positive for cancer cells.
● Thyroid function test is normal.

Nursing diagnoses

● Anxiety
● Impaired swallowing
● Acute pain

Treatment

● High-protein, high-carbohydrate, high-calorie diet with supplemental feedings

Anaplastic thyroid cancer

The most disfiguring, destructive, and deadly form of thyroid cancer, anaplastic carcinoma has the poorest prognosis. Although this tumor rarely metastasizes to distant organs, its rapid growth and size produce severe anatomic distortion of nearby structures. Treatment usually consists of total thyroidectomy, which seldom is successful.

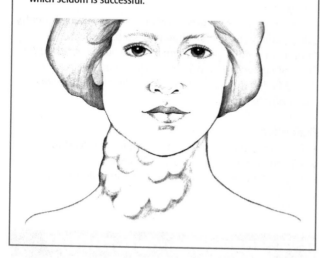

- Radiation therapy
- Thyroidectomy (total or subtotal); total thyroidectomy and radical neck excision

Drug therapy options
- Antiemetic: prochlorperazine (Compazine), ondansetron (Zofran)
- Chemotherapy: chlorambucil (Leukeran), doxorubicin (Adriamycin), vincristine (Oncovin)
- Thyroid hormone replacement: levothyroxine (Synthroid), liothyronine (Cytomel), thyroglobulin (Proloid)

Patient care goals
- The client will use available support systems to help with coping mechanisms.
- The client won't aspirate.
- The client will express feelings of comfort and pain relief.

Nursing interventions
- Assess respiratory status for signs of airway obstruction. A tracheotomy set should be kept at the bedside *because swelling may cause airway obstruction.*

- Assess the client's ability to swallow *to maintain a patent airway.*
- Provide postoperative thyroidectomy care *to promote healing and prevent postoperative complications.*
- Monitor and record vital signs, intake and output, and laboratory studies *to determine baseline and detect early changes that may occur with hemorrhage, airway obstruction, or hypocalcemia.*
- Administer medications as prescribed *to maintain or improve the client's condition.*
- Maintain the client's diet *to improve nutritional status.*
- Encourage the client to express his feelings *to facilitate coping mechanisms.*
- Provide postchemotherapy and postradiation nursing care *to prevent and treat complications associated with therapy.*

Evaluation
- The client demonstrates appropriate coping mechanisms in dealing with illness.
- The client doesn't display signs and symptoms of aspiration.
- The client reports adequate pain control.

Thyroiditis

THYROIDITIS is inflammation of the thyroid gland. It may occur in various forms: autoimmune thyroiditis or Hashimoto's (long-term inflammatory disease), subacute or granulomatous thyroiditis or de Quervain's (self-limiting inflammation), and silent thyroiditis (least common).

Possible causes
- Antibodies to thyroid antigens
- Bacterial invasion
- Mumps, influenza, coxsackievirus, or adenovirus infection

Data collection findings
- Thyroid enlargement
- Fever
- Pain
- Tenderness and reddened skin over the gland

Diagnostic findings
Autoimmune thyroiditis
- Blood studies show high titers of thyroglobulin and microsomal antibodies present in serum.

Subacute granulomatous
● Laboratory tests show elevated ESR, increased thyroid hormone levels, decreased thyroidal radioactive iodine uptake.

Chronic infective and noninfective
● Laboratory studies show varied findings, depending on underlying infection or other disease.

Nursing diagnoses
● Risk for infection
● Acute pain
● Disturbed body image

Treatment
● Partial thyroidectomy to relieve tracheal or esophageal compression in Riedel's thyroiditis

Drug therapy options
● Thyroid hormone replacement: levothyroxine (Synthroid) for accompanying hypothyroidism
● Analgesic and anti-inflammatory agent: indomethacin (Indocin) for mild subacute granulomatous thyroiditis
● Beta-adrenergic blocker: propranolol (Inderal) for transient thyrotoxicosis

Patient care goals
● The client won't have signs and symptoms of infection.
● The client will express feelings of comfort and pain relief.
● The client will express a positive image of himself.

Nursing interventions
Before thyroidectomy
● Obtain a client history *to identify underlying diseases that may cause thyroiditis, such as TB and a recent viral infection.*
● Check vital signs and examine the client's neck for unusual swelling, enlargement, or redness *to detect disease progression and signs of airway occlusion.*
● Provide a liquid diet if the client has difficulty swallowing, especially when due to fibrosis, *to aid swallowing and prevent aspiration.*
● If the neck is swollen, measure and record the circumference daily *to monitor progressive enlargement.*
● Check for signs of thyrotoxicosis (nervousness, tremor, weakness), which commonly occur in subacute thyroiditis. *Checking for early signs avoids treatment delay.*

After thyroidectomy
● Check vital signs every 15 to 30 minutes until the client's condition stabilizes. Stay alert for signs of tetany secondary to accidental parathyroid injury during surgery. Keep 10% calcium gluconate available for I.M. use if needed. *These measures help prevent serious postoperative complications.*
● Assess dressings frequently for excessive bleeding *to detect signs of hemorrhage.*
● Watch for signs of airway obstruction, such as difficulty talking and increased swallowing; keep tracheotomy equipment handy. *The airway may become obstructed because of postoperative edema; tracheotomy equipment should be handy to avoid treatment delay if airway becomes obstructed.*

Evaluation
● The client doesn't have further signs of infection.
● The client reports adequate pain control.
● The client demonstrates a positive attitude toward himself.

EYE, EAR, NOSE, AND THROAT

The senses of sight, hearing, smell, and taste allow us to communicate with others, connect with the world around us, and take pleasure in life.

Sensory structure and function
The structures discussed here include the sensory organs (the eyes, ears, and nose) and the throat.

Eye
About 70% of all sensory information reaches the brain through the eyes. Each eye is composed of external and internal structures. External structures include the eyelid, conjunctiva (a thin, transparent mucous membrane that lines the lid), lacrimal apparatus (which lubricates and protects the cornea and conjunctiva by producing and absorbing tears), extraocular muscles (which hold the eyes parallel to create binocular vision), and the eyeball itself.

The eye also contains numerous internal structures. Some of the most important include:
● iris — a thin, circular pigmented muscular structure in the eye that gives color to the eye and divides the space between the cornea and lens into anterior and posterior chambers

- cornea — a smooth, transparent tissue that works with the sclera to give the eye its shape
- pupil — the circular aperture in the iris that changes size as the iris adapts to light entering the eye
- lens — a biconvex, avascular, colorless, and transparent structure suspended behind the iris by the ciliary zonulae
- vitreous body — a clear, transparent, avascular, gelatinous fluid that fills the space in the posterior portion of the eye and maintains the transparency and form of the eye
- retina — a thin, semitransparent layer of nerve tissue that lines the eye wall
- retinal cones — visual cell segments responsible for visual acuity and color discrimination
- retinal rods — visual cell segments responsible for peripheral vision under decreased light conditions
- optic nerve — located at the posterior portion of the eye that transmits visual impulses from the retina to the brain.

Ear

The ears are composed of three sections: external, middle, and inner. The external ear includes the pinna (auricle) and external auditory canal. It's separated from the middle ear by the tympanic membrane.

The middle ear, known as the *tympanum*, is an air-filled cavity in the temporal bone. It contains three small bones (malleus, incus, and stapes).

The inner ear, known as the *labyrinth*, is the portion of the ear that consists of the cochlea, vestibule, and semicircular canals.

Nose

The nose is more than the sensory organ of smell. It also plays a key role in the respiratory system by filtering, warming, and humidifying inhaled air. The lower two-thirds of the external nose consists of flexible cartilage, and the upper one-third is rigid bone. Posteriorly, the internal nose merges with the pharynx. Anteriorly, it merges with the external nose.

The internal and external parts of the nose are divided vertically by the nasal septum, which is straight at birth and in early life but becomes slightly deviated or deformed in almost every adult. Only the posterior end, which separates the posterior nares, remains constantly in the midline. Kiesselbach's area, the most common site of nosebleeds, is located in the anterior portion of the septum.

Air entering the nose passes through the vestibule, which is lined with coarse hair that helps filter dust. Olfactory receptors lie above the vestibule in the roof of the nasal cavity and the upper one-third of the septum. Known as the olfactory region, this area is rich in capillaries and mucus-producing goblet cells that help warm, moisten, and clean inhaled air. Because of its rich blood supply, the nasal mucosa is redder than the oral mucosa.

Farther along the nasal passage are the superior, middle, and inferior turbinates. Separated by grooves called *meatus*, the curved bony turbinates and their mucosal covering ease breathing by warming, filtering, and humidifying inhaled air.

The sinuses serve as resonators for sound production and provide mucus. Four pairs of paranasal sinuses open into the internal nose, including the:
- maxillary sinuses, located on the cheeks below the eyes
- frontal sinuses, located above the eyebrows
- ethmoidal and sphenoidal sinuses, located behind the eyes and nose in the head.

Throat

The throat is composed of various structures:
- The nasopharynx is continuous with the nasal passage and is located behind and above the soft palate.
- The oropharynx extends from the soft palate to just above the hyoid bone.
- The laryngopharynx is located above the larynx and is the lower part of the pharynx.
- Located within the throat are the hard and soft palates, the uvula, and the tonsils.
- The mucous membrane lining the throat is usually smooth and bright pink to light red.

EYE, EAR, NOSE, AND THROAT DISORDERS

Major eye, ear, nose, and throat disorders include cataracts, conjunctivitis, corneal abrasion, deviated septum, glaucoma, laryngeal cancer, Ménière's disease, otosclerosis, and retinal detachment.

Cataract

A cataract occurs when the normally clear, transparent crystalline lens in the eye becomes opaque. With age, lens fibers become more densely packed, making the lens less transparent and giving the lens a yellowish hue. These changes result in vision loss.

A cataract usually develops first in only one eye but, in many cases, is followed by the development of a cataract in the other eye. Cataracts are removed surgically by intracapsular or extracapsular extraction followed by artificial intraocular lens implantation.

Possible causes

- Aging
- Anterior uveitis
- Blunt or penetrating trauma
- Congenital
- Diabetes mellitus
- Hypoparathyroidism
- Long-term steroid treatment
- Radiation exposure
- Ultraviolet light exposure

Data collection findings

- Disabling glare
- Distorted images
- Gradual dimmed or blurred vision
- Poor vision at night and in bright sunlight
- Red reflex lost as cataract matures
- Yellow, gray, or white pupil

Diagnostic findings

- Ophthalmoscopy or slit-lamp examination is used to confirm the diagnosis by revealing a dark area in the normally homogeneous red reflex.

Nursing diagnoses

- Disturbed sensory perception (visual)
- Impaired physical mobility
- Risk for injury

Treatment

- Intracapsular or extracapsular cataract extraction with intraocular lens implant

Patient care goals

- The client will have a safe postoperative course.
- The client will take steps to prevent infection and reduce intraocular pressure (IOP).

Nursing interventions

- Provide a safe environment for the client. Orient the client to his surroundings *to reduce the risk of injury.*
- Modify the environment to help the client meet self-care needs by placing items on the unaffected side *to discourage movement or positions that would apply pressure to the operative site or cause increased IOP.*
- Caution the client not to rub the eyes *to decrease the risk of infection and damage to the surgical site.*

- Enforce eye care *to prevent increased IOP,* including no bending, straining during defecation, coughing, sneezing, or squeezing eyes shut.
- Provide sensory stimulation (such as large print or tapes) *to help compensate for vision loss.*

Evaluation

- The client can perform required eye care.
- The client knows how to prevent infection and increased IOP.

Conjunctivitis

CONJUNCTIVITIS is characterized by inflammation of the conjunctiva, the delicate membrane that lines the eyelid and covers the exposed surface of the eyeball. It may result from infection, allergy, or chemical reactions.

Conjunctivitis is common. Bacterial and viral conjunctivitis are highly contagious but are also self-limiting after a couple of weeks' duration. Chronic conjunctivitis may result in degenerative changes to the eyelid.

Possible causes

- Bacterial — *Staphylococcus aureus, Streptococcus pneumoniae, Neisseria gonorrhoeae, N. meningitidis*
- Chlamydial — *Chlamydia trachomatis* (inclusion conjunctivitis)
- Viral — adenovirus types 3 and 7; Type 1 herpes simplex virus
- Allergic reactions to pollen, grass, topical medications, air pollutants, and smoke
- Fungal infections (rare)
- Occupational irritants (acids and alkalies)
- Parasitic diseases caused by *Phthirus pubis* or *Schistosoma haematobium*
- Rickettsial diseases (Rocky Mountain spotted fever)

Data collection findings

- Itching
- Burning
- Excessive tearing
- Mucopurulent discharge
- Hyperemia (engorgement) of the conjunctiva, sometimes accompanied by discharge and tearing

Diagnostic findings

- Culture and sensitivity tests identify the causative bacterial organism and indicate appropriate antibiotic therapy.

Nursing diagnoses

- Disturbed sensory perception (visual)
- Risk for infection
- Disturbed body image

Treatment

- Cold compresses to relieve itching for allergic conjunctivitis
- Warm compresses to treat bacterial or viral conjunctivitis

Drug therapy options

- Antiviral agent: vidarabine ointment (Vira-A) or oral acyclovir (Zovirax), if herpes simplex is the cause
- Corticosteroid: dexamethasone (Maxidex), fluorometholone (Fluor-Op Ophthalmic)
- Mast cell stabilizer: cromolyn (Opticrom) for allergic conjunctivitis
- Topical antibiotic according to sensitivity of infective organism, if cause is bacterial

Patient care goals

- The client will have improved visual ability.
- The client will prevent the spread of infection to other individuals.
- The client will have a positive body image.

Nursing interventions

- Teach proper hand-washing technique *because certain forms of conjunctivitis are highly contagious.*
- Stress the risk of spreading infection to family members by sharing washcloths, towels, and pillows. Warn against rubbing the infected eye, *which can spread the infection to the other eye and to other persons. These measures prevent the spread of infection.*
- Apply warm compresses and therapeutic ointment or drops. Don't irrigate the eye; *this will spread infection.*
- Have the client wash his hands before he uses the medication, and use clean washcloths or towels frequently *so he doesn't infect the other eye.*
- Teach the client to instill eyedrops and ointments correctly — without touching the bottle tip to his eye or lashes — *to prevent the spread of infection.*
- Stress the importance of safety glasses for the client who works near chemical irritants *to prevent further episodes of conjunctivitis.*
- Notify public health authorities if cultures show *N. gonorrhoeae. Public health authorities track sexually transmitted diseases.*

Evaluation

- The client has returned to baseline visual acuity.
- The client demonstrates safe practices to avoid transmission of infection.
- The client has a positive body image.

Corneal abrasion

A CORNEAL ABRASION is a scratch on the surface epithelium of the cornea, the dome-shaped transparent structure in front of the eye. This type of eye injury is commonly caused by a foreign body, such as a cinder or piece of dirt, or by improper use of a contact lens.

Possible causes

- Improper use of contact lens
- Trauma caused by a foreign body (such as a cinder or a piece of dust, dirt, or grit)

Data collection findings

- Burning
- Redness
- Increased tearing
- Sensation of "something in the eye"
- Pain disproportionate to the size of the injury
- Change in visual acuity (depending on the size and location of the injury)

Diagnostic findings

- Staining the cornea with fluorescein stain confirms the diagnosis — the injured area appears green when examined with a flashlight.
- Slit-lamp examination discloses the depth of the abrasion.

Nursing diagnoses

- Acute pain
- Risk for infection
- Disturbed sensory perception (visual)

Treatment

- Irrigation with saline solution
- Pressure patch (a tightly applied eye patch)
- Removal of a deeply embedded foreign body with a foreign body spud, using a topical anesthetic

Drug therapy options

- Antibiotic: sulfisoxazole (Gantrisin)
- Cycloplegic agent: tropicamide (Ocu-Tropic)

Patient care goals
● The client will express feelings of comfort and pain relief.
● The client will remain free from signs and symptoms of infection.
● The client will regain visual function.

Nursing interventions
● Assist with examination of the eye. Check visual acuity before beginning treatment *to assess visual loss from injury.*
● If the foreign body is visible, carefully irrigate the eye with normal saline solution *to wash away the foreign body without damaging the eye.*
● Tell the client with an eye patch to leave the patch in place for 6 to 8 hours *to protect the eye from further corneal irritation when the client blinks.*
● Warn the client with an eye patch that wearing a patch alters depth perception, so advise caution in everyday activities, such as climbing stairs or stepping off a curb, *to prevent injury.*
● Reassure the client that the corneal epithelium usually heals in 24 to 48 hours *to allay anxiety.*
● Stress the importance of instilling prescribed antibiotic eyedrops *because an untreated corneal infection can lead to ulceration and permanent loss of vision.*
● Emphasize the importance of safety glasses *to protect the eyes from flying fragments.*

Evaluation
● The client reports adequate pain control.
● The client doesn't display signs or symptoms of infection.
● The client has regained baseline visual acuity.

Deviated septum
Deviated septum is a shift of the nasal septum from the midline, which is common in adults. This shift may be severe enough to obstruct the passage of air through the nostrils; however, with surgery, the prognosis is good.

Possible causes
● Nasal trauma
● Shift of the septum from one side to the other during growth

Data collection findings
● Difficulty breathing through the nostrils
● Dry, cracked, or crusted nasal mucosa

● Ecchymosis from trauma
● Edema in the nasal mucosa
● Feeling of fullness in the face
● Recurring epistaxis, infection, sinusitis, and headache
● Shortness of breath

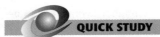 **QUICK STUDY**

Remember that a "deviated" septum may cause a "deviation" from normal breathing.

Diagnostic findings
● Radiography reveals nasal fracture and a deviated septum.
● Skull radiographs are used to rule out skull fracture.

Nursing diagnoses
● Ineffective airway clearance
● Acute pain
● Risk for infection
● Anxiety

Treatment
● Reconstruction of the nasal septum, rhinoplasty, or septoplasty to relieve nasal obstruction
● Vasoconstrictors, nasal packing, or cauterization to control hemorrhage

Drug therapy options
● Analgesic: acetaminophen (Tylenol), ibuprofen (Motrin)
● Decongestant: pseudoephedrine (Sudafed)

Patient care goals
● The client will exhibit adequate breathing patterns.
● The client will be able to breathe through the nose after packing is removed.
● The client will experience no complications.

Nursing interventions
● Encourage verbalization of concerns and answer questions *to allay anxiety.*
● *To relieve nasal congestion*, instill normal saline solution and provide a humidifier.
● If the client experiences epistaxis, elevate the head of the bed, compress the outer nose, and apply ice packs *to alleviate bleeding.*
● Postoperatively, place a small ice bag over the eyes and nose intermittently *to reduce facial edema and pain.*

- Provide good mouth care *because the client will be breathing through the mouth.*
- Warn the client not to blow the nose for 48 hours after the packing is removed *to decrease the risk of bleeding.*
- Limit physical activity for 2 to 3 days postoperatively *to reduce the risk of injury.*
- Allow verbalization of feelings regarding changes in appearance *to decrease anxiety.*

Evaluation

- The client maintains a patent airway.
- The client's surgery is successful and presents no complications.
- The client can correctly explain postoperative care.

Glaucoma

In GLAUCOMA, the client experiences visual field loss due to damage to the optic nerve resulting from increased IOP. If left untreated, glaucoma can lead to blindness.

There are two types of glaucoma: open-angle and angle-closure. In open-angle glaucoma, increased IOP is caused by overproduction of, or obstructed outflow of, AQUEOUS HUMOR. In angle-closure glaucoma, there's an obstructed outflow of aqueous humor due to anatomically narrow angles. (See *Normal flow of aqueous humor.*)

Possible causes

- Diabetes mellitus
- Family history of glaucoma
- Long-term steroid treatment
- Previous eye trauma or surgery
- Race (blacks have a higher incidence)
- Uveitis

Data collection findings

Chronic open-angle glaucoma

- Initially asymptomatic
- Atrophy and cupping of optic nerve head
- Increased IOP
- Narrowed field of vision
- Possible asymmetric involvement

Acute angle-closure glaucoma

- Acute ocular pain
- Blurred vision
- Dilated pupil
- Halo vision
- Increased IOP
- Nausea and vomiting

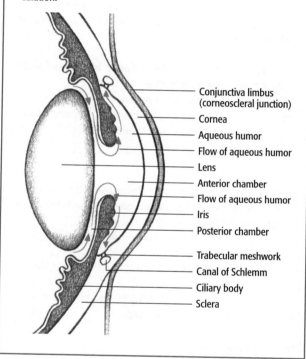

Normal flow of aqueous humor

Aqueous humor, a plasmalike fluid produced by the ciliary epithelium of the ciliary body, flows from the posterior chamber to the anterior chamber through the pupil. Here it flows peripherally and filters through the trabecular meshwork to the canal of Schlemm, through which the fluid ultimately enters venous circulation.

- Conjunctiva limbus (corneoscleral junction)
- Cornea
- Aqueous humor
- Flow of aqueous humor
- Lens
- Anterior chamber
- Flow of aqueous humor
- Iris
- Posterior chamber
- Trabecular meshwork
- Canal of Schlemm
- Ciliary body
- Sclera

Diagnostic findings

- Gonioscopy reveals if angle is open or closed.
- Ophthalmoscopy shows atrophy and cupping of the optic nerve head.
- Perimetry shows a decreased field of vision.
- Tonometry shows increased IOP.

Nursing diagnoses

- Acute pain
- Anxiety
- Disturbed sensory perception (visual)
- Risk for injury

Treatment

Chronic open-angle glaucoma

- Reduction of IOP by decreasing aqueous humor production with medication

---

CLINICAL SITUATION

Caring for the client with primary open-angle glaucoma

A 55-year-old female client sees halos around lights and has had mild pain in both eyes for several weeks. She works as a bookkeeper and lives alone. Primary open-angle glaucoma was previously diagnosed. She arrives at the ambulatory surgical unit on the morning she's scheduled for a laser trabeculoplasty. She'll be discharged the same day.

What postoperative measures should be stressed to the client before she goes home?
Be sure to stress the following information:
- Wear an eye shield or eyeglasses to protect the affected eye.
- Adjust the home environment to avoid injury.

- Report eye pain not relieved by analgesics that's accompanied by nausea or decreased vision.
- Adhere to instructions for the proper administration of eye medications.
- Keep follow-up appointments with the health care provider.

Questions for further thought
- Based on the client's medical condition, what assessment findings would the nurse anticipate?
- Why should the nurse caution the client to avoid bending, sneezing, straining, and coughing after the procedure?

- Argon laser trabeculoplasty (for those who don't respond to drug therapy) to create an opening for outflowing aqueous humor

Acute angle-closure glaucoma
- An ocular emergency that requires immediate treatment to decrease IOP
- Laser iridectomy or surgical iridectomy if pressure doesn't decrease with drug therapy

Drug therapy options
Chronic open-angle glaucoma
- Alpha-adrenergic agonist: brimonidine (Alphagan)
- Beta-adrenergic antagonist: timolol (Timoptic)

Acute angle-closure glaucoma
- Cholinergic: pilocarpine

Patient care goals
- The client's vision will improve and pain will decrease.
- The client will be able to perform postoperative self-care.
- The client will take steps to prevent infection and reduce IOP. (See *Caring for the client with primary open-angle glaucoma.*)

Nursing interventions
- Explain the disease process or surgical procedure *to reduce the client's anxiety.*

- Assess eye pain and administer medication as prescribed. *Medication reduces pain and may control disease progression.*
- Provide a safe environment. *Orienting the client to the surroundings reduces the risk of injury.*
- Modify the environment *to meet the client's self-care needs.*
- During an acute episode, limit activities that increase IOP *to reduce the risk of complications.*
- Advise the client to wear an eye shield or eyeglasses *to protect the affected eye.*
- Tell the client to report eye pain that isn't relieved by analgesics and is accompanied by nausea or decreased vision *to prevent complications.*
- Make sure the client understands the discharge instructions and proper administration of eye medications *to ensure self-care.*
- Encourage the client to express feelings about changes in his body image *to aid acceptance of vision loss.*

Evaluation
- The client accurately explains the medication regimen.
- The client plans to modify his lifestyle as necessary to cope effectively with glaucoma.
- The client's vision is improved.

Laryngeal cancer

Laryngeal cancer occurs in several forms: An intrinsic cancerous tumor that's on the true vocal cords tends not to spread because underlying connective tissues lack lymph nodes. An extrinsic tumor is on some other part of the larynx and tends to spread easily. Squamous cell carcinomas constitute about 95% of laryngeal tumors. Laryngeal cancer is nine times more common in men than in women, and most victims are between ages 50 and 65.

Possible causes

- Unknown

Risk factors

- Smoking
- Alcoholism
- Chronic inhalation of noxious fumes
- Familial disposition

Data collection findings

Findings depend on the tumor's location and size:
- stage I — local throat irritation or hoarseness
- stages II or III — hoarseness; possible sore throat and voice down to whisper
- stage IV — pain radiating to the ear, dysphagia, dyspnea, palpable neck mass or cervical lymph nodes

Diagnostic findings

- Laryngoscopy allows visualization of the tumor.
- Chest radiograph reveals metastasis.
- Laryngeal CT scan shows lymph node metastasis.
- Biopsy results reveal the type of cancer.
- Laryngography is used to define the tumor and its borders.

Nursing diagnoses

- Impaired verbal communication
- Acute pain
- Impaired gas exchange
- Imbalanced nutrition: Less than body requirements
- Anxiety

Treatment

Early lesions

- Laser surgery or radiation therapy

Advanced lesions

- Laser surgery
- Radiation therapy
- Chemotherapy

Drug therapy options

- Analgesic: morphine (MS Contin)

Patient care goals

- The client will have an unobstructed airway.
- The client's family and friends will provide emotional support.
- The client's nutrition will be adequate to meet his needs.
- The client will have adequate pain control.

Nursing interventions

- Provide supportive psychological care preoperatively and postoperatively *to help prevent complications.*
- Encourage the client to express his concerns and to choose an alternative method of communication *to decrease anxiety.*

After total laryngectomy

- Position the client on his side and elevate the head of the bed 30 to 45 degrees *to relieve pressure on the operative site.*
- Provide adequate humidification *to prevent crusting on the stoma and skin breakdown.*
- Monitor vital signs, especially temperature, *to assess for complications; an elevated temperature may indicate infection.*
- Give analgesics *to relieve discomfort.*

Evaluation

- The client maintains a patent airway.
- The client's skin lesions and stoma have healed without signs of infection.
- The client communicates effectively.
- The client's pain is minimal.
- The client maintains adequate nutrition.
- The client has an increased sense of well-being.

Ménière's disease

MÉNIÈRE'S DISEASE is a dysfunction in the labyrinth (the part of the ear that produces balance) that produces severe vertigo, sensorineural hearing loss, and tinnitus. It usually affects adults, men slightly more commonly than women, between ages 30 and 60. After multiple attacks over several years, this disorder leads to residual tinnitus and hearing loss. This disorder may also be called *endolymphatic hydrops.*

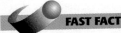
FAST FACT

In Ménière's disease, an increase in the amount of fluid in the labyrinth increases pressure in the inner ear and leads to a disruption of the client's sense of balance.

Possible causes
- Autonomic nervous system dysfunction that produces a temporary constriction of blood vessels supplying the inner ear
- Overproduction or decreased absorption of endolymph, which causes endolymphatic hydrops or endolymphatic hypertension, with consequent degeneration of the vestibular and cochlear hair cells

Data collection findings
- Severe vertigo
- Tinnitus
- Feeling of fullness or blockage in the ear
- Severe nausea
- Vomiting
- Sweating
- Giddiness
- Nystagmus
- Sensorineural hearing loss

Diagnostic findings
- Electronystagmography, electrocochleography, a CT scan, MRI, and X-rays of the internal meatus may be necessary for differential diagnosis.
- Audiometric studies indicate a sensorineural hearing loss and loss of discrimination and recruitment.

Nursing diagnoses
- Disturbed sensory perception (auditory)
- Powerlessness
- Risk for injury

Treatment
- Restrict sodium intake to less than 2 g per day.
- Surgery to destroy the affected labyrinth (if medical treatment fails, destruction of the labyrinth permanently relieves symptoms but at the expense of irreversible hearing loss)

Drug therapy options
- Anticholinergic: atropine (may stop an attack in 20 to 30 minutes)
- Cardiac stimulant: epinephrine (Adrenalin)
- Diuretic to prevents excess fluid in the labyrinth (long-term management)
- Antihistamine: possibly diphenhydramine (Benadryl) in a severe attack
- Antihistamine: meclizine (Antivert), dimenhydrinate (Dramamine) for milder attacks (may also be administered as part of prophylactic therapy)
- Sedative: phenobarbital (Luminal), diazepam (Valium) as part of prophylactic therapy

Patient care goals
- The client will regain hearing or develop alternate means of communication.
- The client will use available support systems to develop coping abilities to deal with the disorder.
- The client will remain free from injury.

Nursing interventions
In a facility
- Advise the client against reading and exposure to glaring lights *to reduce dizziness.*
- Keep the side rails of the client's bed up *to prevent falls.* Tell him not to get out of bed or walk without assistance *to prevent injury.*
- Instruct the client to avoid sudden position changes and tasks that vertigo makes hazardous *because an attack can begin quite rapidly.*

Before surgery
- If the client is vomiting, record fluid intake and output and characteristics of vomitus *to prevent dehydration.* Administer antiemetics as necessary, and give small amounts of fluid frequently *to prevent vomiting.*

After surgery
- Record intake and output carefully *to monitor fluid status and direct the treatment plan.*
- Tell the client to expect dizziness and nausea for 1 to 2 days after surgery *to relieve anxiety.*
- Give prophylactic antibiotics and antiemetics as required *to decrease the chance of infection and combat nausea.*

Evaluation
- The client has appropriate communication abilities.
- The client demonstrates appropriate coping behaviors.
- The client hasn't experienced injury.

Otosclerosis

Otosclerosis is characterized by overgrowth of the ear's spongy bone around the oval window and stapes footplate. This overgrowth curtails movement of the stapes in the oval window, preventing sound from being transmitted to the cochlea and resulting in conductive hearing loss.

Possible causes
- Familial tendency

Data collection findings
- Progressive hearing loss
- Tinnitus

Diagnostic findings
- Audiometric testing confirms hearing loss.

Nursing diagnoses
- Disturbed sensory perception (auditory)
- Impaired verbal communication
- Risk for infection
- Anxiety

Treatment
- Hearing aid (air conduction aid with molded ear insert receiver)
- Stapedectomy and insertion of a prosthesis to restore partial or total hearing

Drug therapy options
- Antibiotics postoperatively to prevent infection

Patient care goals
- The client will communicate effectively with others.
- The client will experience no complications.
- The client will be physically and emotionally prepared for surgery.

Nursing interventions
- Don't shout, particularly if the client uses a hearing aid *because hearing aids increase sensitivity to loud noises.*
- Monitor vital signs and monitor the dressing postoperatively for signs of bleeding *to detect complications.*
- Develop alternative means of communication *to decrease anxiety and communicate effectively with the client.*
- If the client has speech limitations or can't understand you, use gestures, allow time for responses, repeat words if necessary, remain calm, and avoid distractions *to communicate effectively with the client.*

- Tell the client that hearing may not be immediately restored postoperatively due to edema and packing *to decrease anxiety.*

Evaluation
- The client's surgery was successful and without complications.
- The client can explain postoperative care correctly.
- The client accurately describes measures to prevent infection.

SPOT CHECK

Why doesn't hearing improve immediately after a stapedectomy? Immediately after stapedectomy, the client experiences some postoperative edema. Also, packing must remain in place for a short time after surgery.

Retinal detachment

RETINAL DETACHMENT is the separation of the retina from the choroid (the middle vascular coat of the eye between the retina and the sclera). It occurs when the retina develops a hole or tear and the vitreous seeps between the retina and choroid. If left untreated, retinal detachment can lead to vision loss.

Possible causes
- Aging
- Diabetic neovascularization
- Familial tendency
- Hemorrhage
- Inflammatory process
- Myopia
- Trauma
- Tumor

Data collection findings
- Blurred vision worsening as the detachment increases
- Painless change in vision (floaters caused by blood cells in the vitreous humor and flashes of light as the vitreous humor pulls on the retina)
- Photopsia (recurrent flashes of light)
- With progression of detachment, painless vision loss that may be described as a veil, curtain, or cobweb that eliminates part of the visual field

Diagnostic findings
- Indirect ophthalmoscopy shows retinal tear or detachment.
- Slit-lamp examination reveals retinal tear or detachment.
- Ultrasound shows retinal tear or detachment in the presence of a cataract.

Nursing diagnoses
- Disturbed sensory perception (visual)
- Risk for injury
- Anxiety

Treatment
- Complete bed rest and restriction of eye movement to prevent further detachment
- Cryopexy, if there's a hole in the peripheral retina
- Laser therapy, if there's a hole in the posterior portion of the retina
- Scleral buckling to reattach the retina

Patient care goals
- The client will remain free from injury.
- The client will understand the treatment options.
- The client will be free from permanent visual impairment.

Nursing interventions
- Assess visual status and functional vision in the unaffected eye *to determine self-care needs.*
- Prepare the client for surgery by explaining possible surgical interventions and techniques *to alleviate some of the client's anxiety.*
- Postoperatively instruct the client to lie on his back or on his unoperated side *to reduce IOP on the affected side.*
- Discourage straining during defecation, bending down, and hard coughing, sneezing, or vomiting *to avoid activities that increase IOP.*
- Provide assistance with ADLs *to minimize frustration and strain.*
- Assist with ambulation, as needed, *to help the client remain independent.*
- Approach the client from the unaffected side *to avoid startling him.*
- Orient the client to his environment *to reduce the risk of injury.*

Evaluation
- The client remains free from injury.
- The client understands all discharge instructions.
- The client's vision is restored.

HEMATOLOGIC AND IMMUNE SYSTEMS

The hematologic and immune systems are closely related. The immune system consists of specialized cells and structures that defend the body against invasion by harmful organisms or chemical toxins. The hematologic system also functions as an important part of the body's defenses. Blood transports the components of the immune system throughout the body. In addition, blood delivers oxygen and nutrients to all tissues and removes wastes. Immune system cells and blood cells originate in the bone marrow. Blood components play a vital role in transporting electrolytes and regulating acid-base balance.

Hematologic and immune structure and function
The key structures of the immune system are:
- lymph nodes
- thymus
- spleen
- tonsils.
  The key structures of the hematologic system are:
- blood
- bone marrow.

Lymphatic vessels and nodes
Lymphatic vessels include capillaries that are permeable to large molecules. Lymphatic vessels prevent edema by moving fluid and proteins from interstitial spaces to venous circulation. Lymph nodes are patches of lymphatic tissue regionally dispersed throughout the body in clusters. They filter lymph fluid as it flows through the lymphatic vessels. These clusters include:
- cervical nodes — drain the head and neck
- axillary nodes — drain the upper extremities and chest
- inguinal nodes — drain the lower extremities and genitals.

  Lymph is a clear fluid resembling plasma. Lymph is composed of water, the end product of cell metabolism; protein; and electrolytes.

Thymus
The thymus gland is located in the neck. This structure forms thymosin, which is involved in the development of lymphocytes and T CELLS.

Spleen

The spleen, the largest lymphoid organ, is a collection of lymph tissue. The spleen destroys bacteria entering by the splenic artery. It filters blood rather than lymph and also serves as a blood reservoir. Lymphocytes and monocytes are located in the spleen. The spleen traps formed particles, which are destroyed in the spleen by leukocytes.

Tonsils

Tonsils are a large collection of lymph nodes in the oropharynx that filter pathogens entering the mouth or nose. There are three sets of tonsils: palatine, pharyngeal, and lingual.

Blood

Blood is composed of several components, including erythrocytes, thrombocytes, leukocytes, and plasma.

Erythrocytes

ERYTHROCYTES (also called red blood cells or RBCs) are formed in the bone marrow and contain Hb. Oxygen binds with Hb to form oxyhemoglobin, which is transported throughout the body.

Thrombocytes

THROMBOCYTES (also called platelets) are formed in the bone marrow and function in the coagulation of blood. They are produced from fragments of megakaryocytes.

Leukocytes

LEUKOCYTES (also called white blood cells or WBCs) are formed in the bone marrow and lymphatic tissue and include nuclei. They are white because they lack Hb. WBCs provide protection from infection by phagocytosis (engulfing, digesting, and destroying microorganisms).

Plasma

PLASMA is the liquid portion of the blood and is composed of water, proteins (albumin and globulin), glucose, and electrolytes.

Blood type

A person's BLOOD TYPE is determined by a system of antigens located on the surface of RBCs. The four blood types are:
- A antigen
- B antigen
- AB (both A and B) antigens
- O (no antigens).

Because group O negative lacks certain antigens, it can be transfused in limited amounts in an emergency to indi-

viduals of other blood types. People with that blood type are called *universal donors.* A person with AB negative lacks certain antigens and can receive blood from people of other blood types. This person is sometimes called a *universal recipient.*

The antigen Rh factor is found on the RBCs of approximately 85% of people. A person with the Rh factor is said to have Rh-positive blood. A person without the factor is Rh-negative. A person may receive blood only from a person with the same Rh factor.

Bone marrow

Bone marrow is involved in blood cell production. Hematopoiesis is carried out by red marrow and produces erythrocytes, leukocytes, and thrombocytes. Red bone marrow is a source of stem cells that differentiate into the three previously mentioned cells.
- Some stem cells evolve into lymphocytes; lymphocytes may become B CELLS or T cells.
- Other stem cells evolve into monocytes or megakaryocytes (thrombocytes [platelets]).

Immune system

In cell-mediated immunity, T cells respond directly to antigens (foreign substances such as bacteria or toxins that induce antibody formation). This response involves destruction of target cells — such as virus-infected cells and cancer cells — through secretion of lymphokines (lymph proteins). Examples of cell-mediated immunity are rejection of transplanted organs and delayed immune responses that fight disease.

T cells

T cells can be killers, helpers, or suppressors:
- Killer cells bind to the surface of the invading cell, disrupt the membrane, and destroy it by altering its internal environment.
- Helper cells stimulate T and B cells to mature, enhancing the immune response.
- Suppressor cells reduce the humoral response when the antigen is destroyed.

B cells

B cells act differently from T cells to recognize and destroy antigens. B cells are responsible for humoral or immunoglobulin-mediated immunity. B cells originate in the bone marrow and mature into plasma cells that produce antibodies (immunoglobulin molecules that interact with a specific antigen).

Immunoglobulins

There are five major classes of IMMUNOGLOBULIN:

● Immunoglobulin G (IgG) is found in the circulation and tissue spaces. It activates complement proteins.

● IgM is the first immunoglobulin produced during an immune response. It's too large to easily cross membrane barriers and is usually present only in the vascular system. It activates complement proteins.

● IgA is found mainly in body secretions, such as saliva, sweat, tears, mucus, bile, and colostrum. It defends against pathogens on body surfaces, especially those that enter the respiratory and GI tracts.

● IgD is found on the cell membrane of the surface of B cells. Its exact function is unknown; it may be active in antigen recognition.

● IgE is the antibody involved in immediate hypersensitivity reactions, or allergic reactions that develop within minutes of exposure to an antigen. IgE stimulates the release of mast cell granules, which contain histamine and heparin.

HEMATOLOGIC AND IMMUNE DISORDERS

Major immune disorders include ACQUIRED IMMUNODEFICIENCY SYNDROME (AIDS), anemia (aplastic, iron deficiency, pernicious, and sickle cell), ankylosing spondylitis, DISSEMINATED INTRAVASCULAR COAGULATION (DIC), hemophilia, Kaposi's sarcoma, leukemia, lymphoma, multiple myeloma, polycythemia vera, rheumatoid arthritis, scleroderma, SYSTEMIC LUPUS ERYTHEMATOSUS (SLE), and vasculitis.

Acquired immunodeficiency syndrome

AIDS is a defect in T cell–mediated immunity caused by HIV. AIDS places a client at significant risk for the development of potentially fatal opportunistic infections. A diagnosis of AIDS is based on laboratory evidence of HIV infection coexisting with one or more indicator diseases, such as herpes simplex virus, cytomegalovirus, mycobacteria, candidal infection, *Pneumocystis carinii* pneumonia, Kaposi's sarcoma, wasting syndrome, or dementia.

Possible causes

● Exposure to blood containing HIV (transfusions, contaminated needles, handling of blood, in utero)

● Exposure to semen and vaginal secretions containing HIV (sexual intercourse, handling of semen and vaginal secretions)

Data collection findings

● Anorexia, weight loss, recurrent diarrhea
● Disorientation, confusion, dementia
● Fatigue and weakness
● Fever
● Lymphadenopathy
● Malnutrition
● Night sweats
● Opportunistic infections
● Pallor

Diagnostic findings

● Blood chemistry shows increased transaminase, alkaline phosphatase, and gamma globulin levels and a decreased albumin level.
● CD4$^+$ T-cell level is less than 200 cells/mm^3
● Enzyme-linked immunosorbent assay (ELISA) shows positive HIV antibody titer.
● Hematologic studies show decreased WBCs, RBCs, and platelets.
● Western blot test result is positive.

Nursing diagnoses

● Ineffective protection
● Hopelessness
● Social isolation

Treatment

● Activity, including active and passive ROM exercises, as tolerated
● High-calorie, high-protein diet and small, frequent feedings
● Nutritional support, including TPN and enteral feedings, if necessary
● Plasmapheresis
● Respiratory treatments, including chest physiotherapy, postural drainage, and incentive spirometry
● Specialized air therapy bed
● Standard precautions
● Transfusion therapy, including fresh frozen plasma, platelets, and packed RBCs

Drug therapy options

● Antibiotic: co-trimoxazole (Bactrim)
● Antiemetic: prochlorperazine (Compazine)

● Antifungal: amphotericin B (Fungizone), fluconazole (Diflucan)

● Antiviral: acyclovir (Zovirax), aerosolized pentamidine (NebuPent), dapsone, didanosine (Videx), ganciclovir (Cytovene), pentamidine (Pentam 300), zidovudine (Retrovir, AZT)

● Interferon a-2a, recombinant (Roferon-A)

Medications used in combination to fight HIV

● Nonnucleoside reverse transcriptase inhibitor: delavirdine (Rescriptor), nevirapine (Viramune)

● Nucleoside reverse transcriptase inhibitor: lamivudine (Epivir), zalcitabine (Dideoxycytidine, ddC), zidovudine (Retrovir, AZT)

● Protease inhibitor: indinavir (Crixivan), nelfinavir (Viracept), ritonavir (Norvir), saquinavir (Invirase)

Patient care goals

● The client will remain free from infection and complications as long as possible.

● The client will identify a support system, be able to verbalize feelings, and learn lifestyle adjustments needed to cope with AIDS.

● The client will experience decreased feelings of isolation.

Nursing interventions

● Assess respiratory and neurologic systems *to detect AIDS-related dementia.* Other factors, such as anemia, fever, hypoxemia, and fluid balance, can affect neurologic status.

● Monitor and record vital signs *to detect evidence of compromise.*

● Monitor for opportunistic infections because *early treatment may limit complications.*

● Administer oxygen *to enhance oxygenation.*

● Provide incentive spirometry and assist with turning, coughing, and deep breathing *to mobilize and remove secretions.*

● Encourage fluids or administer I.V. fluids *to prevent dehydration.*

● Maintain the client's diet *to fight opportunistic infection and maintain weight.*

● Instruct client about TPN and enteral feedings if necessary *to bolster nutritional reserves and immune system.* (See *Nutrition and AIDS.*)

● Administer medications, as prescribed, *to reduce the risk of complications and halt reproduction of HIV.*

● Maintain client activity, as tolerated, *to encourage independence.*

Nutrition and AIDS

Certain clinical manifestations alter the nutritional status of your client with acquired immunodeficiency syndrome. Here are some that you should watch for:

● weight loss
– progressive and unexplained loss (wasting syndrome)
– massive loss (20 to 40 lb [9 to 18 kg]) with severe diarrhea
– reduced appetite secondary to malaise, depression, or drug therapy
– early satiety related to massive hepatomegaly or splenomegaly
● diarrhea (can be severe)
● other GI symptoms
– dysphagia
– steatorrhea
– lactose intolerance
– nausea and vomiting
– abdominal pain
– taste alterations
– malabsorption
– alterations in metabolism of nutrients.

Nutrition support
Include the following foods when planning meals to improve the nutritional status of your client.

For outpatient clients to supplement calories and protein
● Whole milk and cream
● Liberal use of butter, margarine, and mayonnaise
● Sauces and gravies
● Toppings (nuts, whipped cream, sour cream, frostings)
● Nonfat dry milk added to home-baked goods, hot cereals, soups, and desserts

For inpatient clients who have good appetite, minimal malabsorption, moderate diarrhea, and semisolid stool
● High calories
● High protein
● Low fat (about 3% of total calorie intake)
● Lactose-free dairy foods
● Oral food supplement

For inpatient clients with severe diarrhea
● Short-term use of the BRAT diet: Bananas, Rice, Apples, and Tea and Toast
● Oral food supplement

CLINICAL SITUATION

Caring for the client with HIV infection

A 30-year-old male client has a history of I.V. drug abuse. He arrives at the medical clinic complaining of shortness of breath, hacking cough, and loss of appetite. He has lost 20 lb (9.1 kg) during the past several months. Diagnostic testing reveals that he has Pneumocystis carinii *pneumonia and human immunodeficiency virus (HIV) infection. His CD4+ lymphocyte count has decreased from 220 cells/mm³ to 160/mm³.*

Can you identify at least four appropriate nursing diagnoses?

There are a number of appropriate nursing diagnoses for this client, including:

- Impaired gas exchange related to respiratory infection
- Imbalanced nutrition: Less than body requirements related to anorexia, weight loss, and possible GI manifestations
- Risk for infection related to impaired immunocompetence
- Diarrhea related to GI infection
- Activity intolerance related to weakness and air hunger
- Disturbed body image related to weight loss
- Impaired home maintenance management related to debilitation
- Social isolation related to possible rejection by peers
- Fear related to the disease's life-threatening consequences
- Disturbed sensory perception (visual) related to neurologic complications.

What steps could be taken to relieve respiratory distress?

Respiratory distress warrants immediate relief. Appropriate interventions include:

- administering oxygen to relieve hypoxemia present with extensive *Pneumocystis* infection
- instituting chest physiotherapy to mobilize secretions from the chest and help maintain a patent airway
- teaching the client diaphragmatic and pursed-lip breathing (breathing exercises enhance respirations)
- instructing the client to avoid smoking (smoking [and other forms of smoke] should be avoided to prevent further lung damage)
- administering antibiotics, such as co-trimoxazole and pentamidine (an antiprotozoal agent), as ordered, and monitoring the client for adverse effects (preventive treatment is recommended for a client whose CD4+ lymphocyte count drops below 200/mm³).

Questions for further thought

- Why is it so important to monitor for signs of immunosuppression?
- What should be included in instructions regarding sexual practices?

- Provide rest periods *to reduce oxygen demands and prevent fatigue.*
- Provide mouth care *to prevent infection, provide comfort, and enhance the taste of meals.*
- Maintain standard precautions *to avoid exposure to blood, body fluids, and secretions.*
- Provide pain medication as prescribed *to relieve pain and decrease anxiety.*
- Encourage the client to express feelings about changes in his body image, a fear of dying, and social isolation *to help him cope with chronic illness and reduce his anxiety.*
- Make referrals to community agencies for support *to enhance the client's quality of life and independence.*
- Monitor intake and output, daily weight, and urine specific gravity *for early recognition and treatment of dehydration.*
- Assess respiratory status *to detect complications, such as pneumonia and malignancies.*

- Monitor laboratory values *for early detection of complications.* Thrombocytopenia requires precautions *to prevent bleeding.* Leukopenia requires precautions *to prevent infection.*
- Review key teaching topics with the client *to ensure adequate knowledge about the condition and treatment,* including:
  – refraining from donating blood
  – avoiding use of alcohol and recreational drugs
  – using condoms during sexual intercourse
  – avoiding anal sex
  – getting laboratory testing performed every 3 months or as ordered
  – adhering to medication regimen
  – speaking with health care professional about vaccine status
  – cleaning drug paraphernalia with bleach (if using I.V. drugs).

Evaluation

- The client remains afebrile and exhibits no sign of infection, including wound, respiratory, skin, and oral infections.
- The client expresses feelings, learns coping skills, and can identify personal and community support systems.
- The client participates in care and unit activities as much as possible and maintains prior social relationships. (See *Caring for the client with HIV infection*.)

Anemia, aplastic

Aplastic anemia, also known as *pancytopenia*, results from suppression, destruction, or aplasia of the bone marrow. This damage to the bone marrow causes an inability to produce adequate amounts of erythrocytes, leukocytes, and platelets.

Possible causes

- Chemotherapy
- Drug-induced from chloramphenicol (Chloromycetin), phenylbutazone (Butazolidin), or phenytoin (Dilantin)
- Exposure to chemicals
- Idiopathy
- Radiation
- Viral hepatitis

Data collection findings

- Weakness and fatigue
- Purpura, petechiae, ecchymosis, and pallor
- Dyspnea or tachypnea
- Epistaxis
- Anorexia
- Gingivitis
- Headache
- Melena
- Multiple infections
- Fever
- Palpitations and tachycardia

Diagnostic findings

- Bone marrow biopsy specimen shows fatty marrow with reduction of stem cells.
- Fecal occult blood test result is positive.
- Hematologic studies show decreased granulocytes, thrombocytes, and RBCs.
- Peripheral blood smear shows pancytopenia.
- Urine chemistry reveals hematuria.

Nursing diagnoses

- Risk for infection
- Risk for deficient fluid volume
- Activity intolerance

Treatment

- Dietary changes, including establishing a high-protein, high-calorie, high-vitamin diet
- Tepid sponge baths and cooling blankets
- Transfusion of platelets and packed RBCs
- Genetic counseling

Drug therapy options

- Analgesic: ibuprofen (Motrin), acetaminophen (Tylenol)
- Androgen: fluoxymesterone (Halotestin), oxymetholone (Anadrol-50)
- Antibiotic, according to the sensitivity of the infecting organism
- Immunosuppressant: antithymocyte globulin (Atgam)
- Hematopoietic growth factor: epoetin alfa (Epogen)
- Human granulocyte colony-stimulating factor: filgastim (Neupogen)

Patient care goals

- The client will be free from complications caused by decreased activity.
- The client will maintain an adequate fluid balance.
- The client will remain free from infection.

Nursing interventions

- Assess respiratory status *to detect hypoxemia caused by low Hb levels.*
- Assess the client's vital signs *for signs of hemorrhage, infection, and activity intolerance.*
- Assess cardiovascular status *to detect arrhythmias or myocardial ischemia.*
- Monitor and record intake and output and urine specific gravity *to determine fluid balance.*
- Monitor laboratory values *to determine the effectiveness of therapy.*
- Assess stool, urine, and emesis *for occult blood loss caused by reduced platelet levels.* (See *Testing for occult blood*, page 410.)
- Monitor for infection, bleeding, and bruising caused by reduced levels of WBCs and platelets.
- Encourage fluids and administer I.V. fluids *to replace fluids lost by fever and bleeding.*
- Administer oxygen to improve tissue oxygenation *because low Hb levels reduce the oxygen-carrying capacity of blood.*

NURSING PROCEDURE

Testing for occult blood

Purpose

Invisible because of its minute quantity, fecal occult blood can be detected by microscopic analysis or chemical test for hemoglobin, such as the guaiac or orthotolidine tests. Small amounts of blood (2 to 2.5 ml/day) normally appear in the feces; these tests are designed to detect greater-than-normal quantities. This test can be used to detect GI bleeding and to aid early diagnosis of colorectal cancer.

Implementation

- Explain the purpose of the test to the client. Instruct him to avoid contaminating the stool specimen with toilet tissue or urine.
- Obtain a small specimen from two different areas of each stool *to allow for any variation in the distribution of blood.*
- Use a commercially prepared Hemoccult card and developer. Apply two drops of the chemical developer to the paper covering the sample. Note the color after 1 minute.
- Note the results. Results are normal if less than 2 ml of blood is present, and the test results in a green reaction; abnormal (positive for fecal occult blood), blue reaction that occurs within 30 to 60 seconds. If the blue color appears within this period, consider it strongly positive. However, a faint blue reaction is weakly positive and not necessarily abnormal. Test the next stool specimen.
- Document the appearance of the stool as well as the test results.

- Assist with turning, coughing, and deep breathing *to mobilize and remove secretions.*
- Maintain a patent I.V. site for administration of transfusion therapy, as prescribed, *to replace low blood components.*
- Administer medications, as prescribed, *to treat the disorder and prevent complications.*
- Maintain the client's diet *to promote RBC production and fight infection.*
- Encourage verbalization of concerns and fears *to allay the client's anxiety.*
- Alternate rest periods with activity *to conserve energy and reduce weakness caused by anemia.*

- Provide cooling blankets and tepid sponge baths for fever *to promote comfort and reduce metabolic demands.*
- Maintain protective precautions *to prevent infection and hemorrhage.*
- Provide mouth care before and after meals *to enhance the taste of meals.*
- Provide skin care *to prevent skin breakdown due to bed rest, dehydration, and fever.*
- Protect the client from falls, avoid giving him intramuscular (I.M.) injections, and avoid using hard toothbrushes and straight razors on the client *to reduce the risk of hemorrhage.*
- Review key teaching topics with the client *to ensure adequate knowledge about his condition and treatment,* including:
  – recognizing the early signs and symptoms of bleeding and infection
  – avoiding contact sports
  – wearing a medical identification bracelet
  – refraining from using over-the-counter medications
  – monitoring stool for occult blood
  – using an electric razor to avoid bleeding
  – refraining from taking aspirin.

Evaluation

- The client is afebrile and free from signs of infection, including respiratory infections and skin breakdown.
- The client has a balanced intake and output and normal vital signs.
- The client displays no complications from inactivity, such as skin breakdown or respiratory infections.

SPOT CHECK

What are three possible causes of aplastic anemia?
Three possible causes of aplastic anemia are chemotherapy, radiation, and viral hepatitis. (For other possible causes, see the list on page 409.)

Anemia, iron deficiency

IRON DEFICIENCY ANEMIA is a chronic, slowly progressing disease involving circulating RBCs. Iron deficiency results when an individual absorbs inadequate amounts of iron or loses excessive amounts (such as through chronic bleeding). This decreased iron affects the formation of Hb and RBCs which, in turn, decreases the oxygen-carrying capacity of the blood.

Possible causes
- Acute and chronic bleeding
- Alcohol abuse
- Drugs
- Gastrectomy
- Inadequate intake of iron-rich foods
- Malabsorption syndrome
- Menstruation
- Pregnancy
- Vitamin B_6 deficiency

Data collection findings
- Pallor
- Weakness and fatigue
- Sensitivity to cold
- Dizziness
- Dyspnea
- Palpitations
- Cheilosis (scalp and fissures of the lips)
- Koilonychia (spoon-shaped nails)
- Pale, dry mucous membranes
- Papillae atrophy of the tongue
- Stomatitis

Diagnostic findings
- Hematology shows decreased Hb level, HCT, iron, ferritin, reticulocytes, red cell indices, transferrin, and saturation; absent hemosiderin; and increased iron-binding capacity.
- Peripheral blood smear reveals microcytic and hypochromic RBCs.

Nursing diagnoses
- Activity intolerance
- Imbalanced nutrition: Less than body requirements
- Impaired gas exchange

Treatment
- Diet high in iron, roughage, and protein with increased fluids, avoiding teas and coffee, which reduce iron absorption
- Transfusion therapy with packed RBCs, if necessary
- Vitamins: pyridoxine (vitamin B_6), ascorbic acid (vitamin C)

Drug therapy options
- Antianemic: ferrous sulfate (Feosol), iron dextran (Dex-Ferrum)

Patient care goals
- The client will express feelings of increased energy.
- The client will maintain weight without further loss.
- The client will maintain adequate ventilation.

Nursing interventions
- Monitor intake and output *to detect fluid imbalances.*
- Monitor laboratory studies *to determine the effectiveness of therapy.*
- Assess cardiovascular and respiratory status *to detect decreased activity intolerance and dyspnea on exertion.*
- Monitor and record vital signs *to determine activity intolerance.*
- Monitor stool, urine, and emesis for occult blood *to identify the cause of anemia.*
- Administer oxygen, as necessary, *to treat hypoxemia caused by reduced Hb levels.*
- Provide a diet high in iron *to replace iron stores in the body.*
- Administer medications, as prescribed, *to replace iron stores in the body.* Administer iron injection deep into muscle using Z-track technique *to avoid subcutaneous irritation and discoloration from leaking drug.*
- Encourage fluids *to avoid dehydration.*
- Provide rest periods *to avoid fatigue and reduce oxygen demands.*
- Provide mouth, skin, and foot care *because the tongue and lips may be dry or inflamed and nails may be brittle.*
- Protect the client from falls caused by weakness and fatigue. *Falls may result in bleeding and bruising.*
- Keep the client warm *to enhance comfort.*

Evaluation
- The client reports increased energy and decreased periods of fatigue.
- The client has maintained a stable weight.
- The client has adequate ventilation as evidenced by normal respirations.

Anemia, pernicious
PERNICIOUS ANEMIA is a chronic, progressive, macrocytic anemia caused by a deficiency of intrinsic factor, a substance normally secreted by the stomach. Without intrinsic factor, dietary vitamin B_{12} can't be absorbed by the ileum, inhibiting normal deoxyribonucleic acid (DNA) synthesis and resulting in defective maturation of RBCs.

Possible causes

- Autoimmune disease
- Bacterial or parasitic infections
- Deficiency of intrinsic factor
- Gastric mucosal atrophy
- Genetics
- Lack of administration of vitamin B_{12} after small-bowel resection or total gastrectomy
- Malabsorption
- Prolonged iron deficiency

Data collection findings

- Weakness and fatigue
- Glossitis
- Sore mouth
- PARESTHESIA of the hands and feet
- Constipation or diarrhea
- Depression
- Delirium
- Dyspnea
- Mild jaundice of the sclera
- Pallor
- Paralysis
- Gait disturbances
- Tachycardia and palpitations
- Weight loss, anorexia, and dyspepsia

Diagnostic findings

- Blood chemistry test results reveal increased bilirubin and LD levels.
- Bone marrow aspiration specimen shows increased megaloblasts, few maturing erythrocytes, and defective leukocyte maturation.
- Gastric analysis shows hypochlorhydria.
- Hematology shows decreased Hb level and HCT.
- Peripheral blood smear reveals oval, macrocytic, hyperchromic erythrocytes.
- Romberg test result is positive.
- Schilling test result is positive.
- Upper GI series shows atrophy of the gastric mucosa.

Nursing diagnoses

- Imbalanced nutrition: Less than body requirements
- Impaired gas exchange
- Risk for injury

Treatment

- Establishing a diet high in iron and protein and restricting highly seasoned, coarse, or extremely hot foods
- Transfusion therapy with packed RBCs

- Vitamins: pyridoxine (vitamin B_6), ascorbic acid (vitamin C), cyanocobalamin (vitamin B_{12}), folic acid (vitamin B_9)

Drug therapy options

- Antianemic: ferrous sulfate (Feosol), iron dextran (DexFerrum)

Patient care goals

- The client will maintain an adequate diet.
- The client will demonstrate signs of adequate gas exchange.
- The client will identify precautions to prevent injury.

Nursing interventions

- Assess cardiovascular status to detect signs of compromise *because the heart works harder to compensate for the reduced oxygen-carrying capacity of the blood.*
- Monitor and record vital signs *to allow for early detection of compromise.*
- Monitor and record amount, consistency, and color of stools *to allow for early detection and treatment of diarrhea and constipation.*
- Maintain the client's diet *to ensure adequate intake of vitamins, iron, and protein.*
- Administer medications as prescribed. *Vitamin B_{12} injections are given monthly and are lifelong.*

QUICK STUDY

Remember that pernicious anemia results from a lack of vitamin B_{12} absorption, so it's easy to recall that vitamins are an important part of treating clients with this disorder.

- Maintain activity, as tolerated, *to avoid fatigue.*
- Provide mouth care before and after meals *for comfort and to reduce the risk of oral mucous membrane breakdown.*
- Use soft toothbrushes *to avoid injuring mucous membranes.*
- Maintain a warm environment *for client comfort.*
- Provide foot and skin care *because sensation in the feet may be reduced.*
- Prevent the client from falling *due to reduced coordination, paresthesia of the feet, and reduced thought processes.*
- Assess neurologic status *because poor memory and confusion increase the risk of injury.*
- Monitor laboratory studies *to determine the effectiveness of therapy.*

● Review key teaching topics with the *client to ensure adequate knowledge about his condition and treatment*, including:
– recognizing the signs and symptoms of skin breakdown
– altering ADLs to compensate for paresthesia
– complying with lifelong, monthly injections of vitamin B$_{12}$
– avoiding the use of heating pads and electric blankets.

Evaluation

● The client verbalizes the importance of maintaining a diet high in iron and protein and the necessity of taking vitamins and supplements as prescribed.
● The client has normal vital signs and exhibits no signs of respiratory distress.
● The client verbalizes the appropriate injury-preventing precautions, such as mouth care, protecting the extremities, and avoidance of falls.

Anemia, sickle cell

SICKLE CELL ANEMIA is a CONGENITAL hematologic disease that causes impaired circulation, chronic ill health, and premature death. Although it's most common in tropical Africa and in people of African descent, it also occurs in people from Puerto Rico, Turkey, India, the Middle East, and the Mediterranean.

In clients with sickle cell anemia, a change in the gene that encodes the beta chain of Hb results in a defect. This abnormal Hb is called HbS. When HYPOXIA occurs, the HbS in the RBCs becomes insoluble. The cells become rigid and rough, forming an elongated sickle shape and impairing circulation. Infection, stress, dehydration, and conditions that provoke hypoxia — strenuous exercise, high altitude, unpressurized aircraft, cold, and vasoconstrictive drugs — may all provoke periodic crisis. Crises can occur in different forms, including painful crisis, aplastic crisis, and acute sequestration crisis.

Possible causes

● Genetic inheritance (the disease results from homozygous inheritance of an autosomal recessive gene that produces a defective Hb molecule [HbS]); heterozygous inheritance results in sickle cell trait — people with this trait are carriers who can pass the gene to their offspring)

Data collection findings

● Aching bones
● Chronic fatigue
● Family history of the disease
● Frequent infections

● Tachycardia
● Unexplained dyspnea or dyspnea on exertion
● Jaundice
● Pallor
● Joint swelling
● Leg ulcers (especially on the ankles)
● Severe localized and generalized pain
● Unexplained PRIAPISM

Sickle cell crisis (general symptoms)
● Hematuria
● Irritability
● Lethargy
● Pale lips, tongue, palms, and nail beds
● Severe pain

Painful crisis (vaso-occlusive crisis, which appears periodically after age 5)
● Dark urine
● Low-grade fever
● Severe abdominal, thoracic, muscle, or bone pain
● Tissue anoxia and necrosis, caused by blood vessel obstruction by tangled sickle cells
● Worsening of jaundice

Aplastic crisis (generally associated with viral infection)
● Dyspnea
● Lethargy
● Sleepiness
● Markedly decreased bone marrow activity
● Pallor
● Possible coma
● RBC HEMOLYSIS

Acute sequestration crisis (rare; occurs in infants ages 8 months to 2 years)
● Hypovolemic shock caused by entrapment of RBCs in the spleen and liver
● Lethargy
● Liver congestion and enlargement
● Pallor
● Worsened chronic jaundice

Diagnostic findings
● Blood tests show low RBC counts, elevated WBC and platelet counts, decreased ESR, increased serum iron levels, decreased RBC survival, and reticulocytosis.
● Hb electrophoresis shows HbS.
● Hb levels may be low or normal.
● Stained blood smear shows sickled cells.

Nursing diagnoses

- Impaired gas exchange
- Acute pain
- Ineffective tissue perfusion (peripheral, renal)

Treatment

- Application of warm compresses for pain relief
- Blood transfusion therapy if Hb levels drop
- Iron and folic acid supplements to prevent anemia
- I.V. fluid therapy to prevent dehydration and vessel occlusion

Drug therapy options

- Analgesic: meperidine (Demerol) or morphine (MS Contin) to relieve pain from vaso-occlusive crises

Patient care goals

- The client will maintain adequate ventilation.
- The client will express feelings of comfort and pain relief.
- The client will have improved circulation.

Nursing interventions

- Provide emotional support *to allay the client's anxiety.*
- Refer the client for genetic counseling *to decrease his anxiety and help him understand the chances of passing the disease to his offspring.*
- Refer the client and his family to community support groups *to help them cope with the illness.*

During a crisis

- Apply warm compresses to painful areas and cover the client with a blanket. *Cold compresses and temperature can aggravate his condition.*
- Administer an analgesic-antipyretic, such as aspirin or acetaminophen, *for pain relief. (Additional pain relief may be necessary during an acute crisis.)*
- Maintain bed rest *to reduce the heart's workload and to reduce pain.*
- Maintain a patent I.V. site for administration of blood components (packed RBCs), as ordered, for aplastic crisis caused by bone marrow suppression.
- Administer oxygen *to enhance oxygenation and to reduce sickling.*
- Encourage fluid intake *to prevent dehydration, which can precipitate a crisis.*
- Administer prescribed I.V. fluids *to ensure fluid balance and renal perfusion.*
- Give antibiotics as ordered *to treat infection and avoid precipitating a crisis.*

Evaluation

- The client has adequate ventilation as evidenced by normal respiratory rate and effort.
- The client reports adequate pain control.
- The client doesn't display signs of diminished circulatory perfusion.

Ankylosing spondylitis

ANKYLOSING SPONDYLITIS is a chronic, usually progressive inflammatory disease that primarily affects the spine and adjacent soft tissue. Generally, the disease begins in the sacroiliac joints (between the sacrum and the ileum) and gradually progresses to the lumbar, thoracic, and cervical regions of the spine. Deterioration of bone and cartilage can lead to fibrous tissue formation and eventual fusion of the spine or peripheral joints.

Ankylosing spondylitis affects five times as many males as females. Progressive disease is well recognized in men, but the diagnosis is commonly overlooked in women, who tend to have more peripheral joint involvement.

Possible causes

- Familial tendency (strongly suggested)
- Possible link to underlying infection
- Presence of histocompatibility antigen (HLA-B27) and circulating immune complexes (suggests immunologic activity)
- Secondary ankylosing spondylitis possibly associated with reactive arthritis (Reiter's syndrome), psoriatic arthritis, or inflammatory bowel disease

Data collection findings

- Intermittent lower back pain (the first indication) usually most severe in the morning or after a period of inactivity
- Mild fatigue, fever, anorexia, or weight loss; unilateral acute anterior uveitis; aortic insufficiency and cardiomegaly; upper lobe pulmonary fibrosis (mimics tuberculosis)
- Stiffness and limited motion of the lumbar spine
- Symptoms that progress unpredictably (disease can go into remission, exacerbation, or arrest at any stage)
- Pain and limited expansion of the chest due to involvement of the costovertebral joints
- Pain or tenderness at tendon insertion sites (enthesitis), especially at the Achilles or patellar tendon
- Tenderness over the site of inflammation
- Peripheral arthritis involving the shoulders, hips, and knees

• Severe neurologic complications, such as cauda equina syndrome or paralysis, secondary to fracture of a rigid cervical spine or C1-C2 subluxation
• Kyphosis in advanced stages, caused by chronic stooping to relieve symptoms; hip deformity; and associated limited ROM

Diagnostic findings
• Confirmation requires characteristic X-ray findings, including blurring of the bony margins of joints in the early stage, bilateral sacroiliac involvement, patchy sclerosis with superficial bony erosions, eventual squaring of vertebral bodies, and "bamboo spine" with complete ANKYLOSIS.
• ESR and alkaline phosphatase and CK levels may be slightly elevated. A negative RF helps rule out rheumatoid arthritis, which produces similar symptoms.
• Typical symptoms, a family history, and the presence of HLA-B27 strongly suggest ankylosing spondylitis.

Nursing diagnoses
• Chronic pain
• Impaired physical mobility
• Activity intolerance

Treatment
• Good posture, stretching and deep-breathing exercises and, in some clients, braces and lightweight supports to delay further deformity (because ankylosing spondylitis progression can't be stopped)
• Long-term daily exercise program (essential to delay loss of function)
• Spinal wedge osteotomy to separate and reposition the vertebrae in case of severe spinal involvement (performed only on selected clients because of the risk of spinal cord damage and long convalescence)
• Surgical hip replacement in case of severe hip involvement

Drug therapy options
• Anti-inflammatory agent: aspirin, indomethacin (Indocin), sulfasalazine (Azulfidine), sulindac (Clinoril) to control pain and inflammation

Patient care goals
• The client will express feelings of comfort and pain relief.
• The client will maintain joint mobility and ROM.
• The client will perform ADLs within the confines of the disease.

Nursing interventions
• Offer support and reassurance. *Ankylosing spondylitis can be an extremely painful and crippling disease; the caregiver's main responsibility is to promote the client's comfort while preserving as much mobility as possible.* Keep in mind that the client's limited ROM makes simple tasks difficult.
• Administer medications as needed *to decrease inflammation and pain.*
• Apply local heat and provide massage *to relieve pain.* Assess mobility and degree of discomfort frequently *to monitor disease progression.*
• Teach and assist with daily exercises as *needed to maintain strength and function.* Stress the importance of maintaining good posture *to prevent kyphosis.*
• If treatment includes surgery, provide good postoperative care *to prevent postoperative complications, such as wound infection, thrombophlebitis, and pneumonia.*
• Comprehensive treatment should also reflect counsel from a social worker, visiting nurse, and dietitian *because ankylosing spondylitis is a chronic, progressively crippling condition.*

Evaluation
• The client reports adequate pain control.
• The client demonstrates adequate mobility.
• The client describes the ability to perform ADLs.

Disseminated intravascular coagulation

DIC, also called *consumption coagulopathy* and *defibrination syndrome,* occurs as a complication of diseases and conditions that accelerate clotting. This accelerated clotting process causes small blood vessel occlusion, organ necrosis, depletion of circulating clotting factors and platelets, and activation of the fibrinolytic system, which in turn can lead to severe hemorrhage.

Clotting in the microcirculation usually affects the kidneys and extremities but may occur in the brain, lungs, pituitary and adrenal glands, and GI mucosa. Other conditions, such as vitamin K deficiency, hepatic disease, and anticoagulant therapy, may cause a similar hemorrhage.

DIC is generally an acute condition but may be chronic in clients with cancer. The prognosis depends on early detection and treatment, the severity of the hemorrhage, and treatment of the underlying disease or condition.

Possible causes

- Disorders that produce necrosis: extensive burns and trauma, brain tissue destruction, transplant rejection, hepatic necrosis
- Infection (the most common cause): gram-negative or gram-positive septicemia; viral, fungal, or rickettsial infection; protozoal infection (falciparum malaria)
- Neoplastic disease: acute leukemia, metastatic carcinoma
- Obstetric complications, such as abruptio placentae, amniotic fluid embolism, and retained dead fetus

Data collection findings

- Abnormal bleeding without an accompanying history of a serious hemorrhagic disorder (petechiae, hematomas, ecchymosis, cutaneous oozing)
  - Oliguria
  - Shock
  - Dyspnea
  - Nausea
  - Vomiting
  - Severe muscle, back, and abdominal pain
  - Seizures
  - Coma

Diagnostic findings

- Blood tests show PT greater than 15 seconds; PTT greater than 80 seconds; fibrinogen levels less than 150 mg/dl; platelets less than 100,000/µl; fibrin degradation products greater than 100 µg/ml (in many cases); and a positive D-dimer test specific for DIC.

Nursing diagnoses

- Ineffective tissue perfusion (peripheral)
- Fatigue
- Risk for deficient fluid volume

Treatment

- Prompt recognition and treatment of the underlying disorder
- Bed rest
- Transfusion therapy, including fresh frozen plasma, platelets, packed RBCs

Drug therapy options

- Anticoagulant: heparin I.V. (controversial)

Patient care goals

- The client will maintain an adequate fluid balance.

- The client will exhibit signs of adequate tissue perfusion and no signs of hemorrhage.
- The client will exhibit a decreased level of fatigue.

Nursing interventions

- Don't scrub bleeding areas *to prevent clots from dislodging and causing fresh bleeding.* Use pressure, cold compresses, and topical hemostatic agents *to control bleeding.*
- Enforce complete bed rest during bleeding episodes. If the client is agitated, pad the side rails *to protect him from injury.*
- Check all I.V. and venipuncture sites frequently for bleeding. Apply pressure to the injection sites for at least 10 minutes. Alert other personnel to the client's tendency to hemorrhage. *These measures prevent hemorrhage.*
- Monitor intake and output hourly in acute DIC, especially if blood products are being administered, *to monitor the effectiveness of fluid volume replacement.*
- Watch for transfusion reactions and signs of fluid overload. Weigh dressings and linen and record drainage *to measure the amount of blood lost.* Weigh the client daily, particularly in renal involvement, *to monitor for fluid volume excess.*
- Watch for bleeding from the GI and genitourinary tracts *to detect early signs of hemorrhage.*
- Measure the client's abdominal girth at least once every 4 hours, and monitor closely for signs of shock *to detect intra-abdominal bleeding.*
- Monitor the results of serial blood studies (particularly HCT, Hb level, and coagulation times) *to guide the treatment plan.*
- Inform family members of the client's progress. Prepare them for his appearance (I.V. lines, NG tubes, bruises, dried blood). Provide emotional support to the client and his family. As needed, enlist the aid of a social worker, chaplain, and other members of the health care team in providing such support. *Providing support in a crisis situation reduces family members' anxiety.*
- Review key teaching topics with the client and family members *to ensure adequate knowledge about the condition and treatment,* including:
  – understanding the disorder and treatment options
  – preventing bleeding.

Evaluation

- The client has a balanced intake and output and normal vital signs.
- The client displays normal or maintained peripheral pulses, adequate color, and capillary refill.

● The client verbalizes decreased fatigue, energy-saving measures, and the need for rest.

Hemophilia

HEMOPHILIA is a hereditary bleeding disorder that affects only males and produces mild to severe abnormal bleeding. After a platelet plug develops at a bleeding site, the lack of clotting factor prevents the formation of a stable fibrin clot. Although hemorrhaging doesn't usually happen immediately, delayed bleeding is common. The severity of hemophilia and the client's prognosis vary with the degree of deficiency and the site of bleeding.

There are two types of hemophilia:
● hemophilia A, or classic hemophilia, (deficiency or nonfunction of factor VIII)
● hemophilia B, or Christmas disease, (deficiency or nonfunction of factor IX).

Possible causes
● Genetic inheritance (both types of hemophilia are inherited as X-linked recessive traits)

 FAST FACT

Hemophilia is an inherited X-linked recessive trait. A female carrier has a 50% chance of transmitting the trait to her daughter, making her a carrier, and a 50% chance of transmitting it to her son.

Data collection findings
Severe hemophilia
● Excessive bleeding after circumcision (in many cases, this is the first sign of the disease)
● Large subcutaneous and deep intramuscular hematomas
● Spontaneous or severe bleeding after minor trauma

Moderate hemophilia
● Occasional spontaneous bleeding
● Subcutaneous and intramuscular hematomas

Mild hemophilia
● No spontaneous bleeding
● Prolonged bleeding after major trauma or surgery (blood may ooze slowly or intermittently for up to 8 days after surgery)

All degrees of severity
● Hematemesis (bloody vomit)
● Hematomas on the extremities or torso
● Hematuria (bloody urine)
● History of prolonged bleeding after surgery, dental extractions, or trauma
● Joint tenderness
● Limited ROM
● Pain and swelling in a weight-bearing joint (such as the hip, knee, or ankle)
● Signs of decreased tissue perfusion, such as chest pain, confusion, cool and clammy skin, decreased urine output, hypotension, pallor, restlessness, anxiety, and tachycardia
● Signs of internal bleeding, such as abdominal, chest, or flank pain
● Tarry stools

Diagnostic findings
Hemophilia A
● Activated PTT is prolonged.
● Factor VIII assay reveals 0% to 25% of normal factor VIII.
● Platelet count and function, bleeding time, and PT are normal.

Hemophilia B
● Baseline coagulation result is similar to that of hemophilia A, with normal factor VIII.
● Factor IX assay shows deficiency.

Nursing diagnoses
● Risk for imbalanced fluid volume
● Ineffective tissue perfusion (cardiopulmonary)
● Impaired physical mobility
● Anxiety

Treatment
Hemophilia A
● Administration of cryoprecipitate antihemophilic factor (AHF) and lyophilized (dehydrated) AHF to encourage normal hemostasis (arrest of bleeding)
● Immediate notification of physician following injury, especially to the head, neck, or abdomen

Hemophilia B
● Administration of recombinant factor VIII and purified factor IX to promote hemostasis
● Immediate notification of physician following injury, especially injury to the head, neck, or abdomen

Drug therapy options

● Analgesics to control joint pain

Patient care goals

● The client will remain free from injury.
● The client will attain pain relief.
● The client will maintain joint mobility.

Nursing interventions

● Provide emotional support *because hemophilia is a chronic disorder.*
● Refer new clients to a hemophilia treatment center *for education, evaluation, and development of a treatment plan.*
● Refer clients and carriers for genetic counseling *to determine the risk of passing the disease to their offspring.*

During bleeding episodes

● Apply pressure to cuts and during epistaxis *to stop bleeding. Pressure is commonly the only treatment needed for surface cuts.*
● Apply cold compresses or ice bags and elevate the injured part *to control bleeding.*
● Maintain a patent I.V. site for administration of sufficient clotting factor or plasma, as ordered, *to promote hemostasis.* The body uses AHF in 48 to 72 hours, so repeat infusions may be necessary.
● Administer analgesics *to control pain.* Avoid I.M. injections *because they may cause hematomas at the injection site.* Aspirin and aspirin-containing medications are contraindicated *because they decrease platelet adherence and may increase bleeding.*

Bleeding into joint

● Immediately elevate the joint *to control bleeding.*
● Begin ROM exercises, if ordered, at least 48 hours after the bleeding has been controlled *to restore joint mobility.*
● Don't allow the client to bear weight on the affected joint until bleeding stops and swelling subsides *to prevent deformities due to hemarthrosis.*

After bleeding episodes and surgery

● Watch for signs of further bleeding *to detect and control bleeding as soon as possible.*
● Closely monitor PTT. *Prolonged times increase the risk of bleeding.*
● Review key teaching topics with the client and family members *to ensure adequate knowledge about the condition and treatment,* including:
– recognizing signs of severe internal bleeding

– knowing when to notify primary care provider; for example, after even a minor injury
– wearing a medical identification bracelet
– protecting a child from injury
– understanding the importance of medical follow-up
– understanding the risk of infection, such as hepatitis, from blood component administration
– caring for injuries
– administering blood factor components at home, as appropriate.

Evaluation

● The client remains injury-free and the client and family members verbalize steps to take to prevent injury.
● The client verbalizes that pain is relieved or controlled.
● The client demonstrates maintained mobility of the joint.

SPOT CHECK

If a client with hemophilia has an increased PTT, are bleeding tendencies decreased or increased?
Increased PTT indicates increased bleeding tendencies.

Kaposi's sarcoma

At one time, this cancer of the lymphatic cell wall was rare, occurring mostly in elderly Italian and Jewish men. The incidence of KAPOSI'S SARCOMA has risen dramatically along with the incidence of AIDS. Currently, it's the most common AIDS-related cancer.

Kaposi's sarcoma causes structural and functional damage. When associated with AIDS, it progresses aggressively, involving the lymph nodes, the viscera and, possibly, GI structures.

Possible causes

● Unknown, possibly related to immunosuppression

Data collection findings

● One or more obvious lesions in various shapes, sizes, and colors (ranging from red-brown to dark purple) appearing most commonly on the skin, buccal mucosa, hard and soft palates, lips, gums, tongue, tonsils, conjunctivae, and sclera
● Pain (if the sarcoma advances beyond the early stages or if a lesion breaks down or impinges on nerves or organs)

- Dyspnea (in cases of pulmonary involvement), wheezing, hypoventilation, and respiratory distress from bronchial blockage
- Edema from lymphatic obstruction

Diagnostic findings
- CT scan detects and evaluates possible metastasis.
- Tissue biopsy identifies the lesion's type and stage.

Nursing diagnoses
- Risk for infection
- Imbalanced nutrition: Less than body requirements
- Disturbed body image

Treatment
- High-calorie, high-protein diet
- Radiation therapy
- I.V. fluid therapy

Drug therapy options
- Chemotherapy: doxorubicin (Adriamycin), etoposide (VePesid), vinblastine (Velban), vincristine (Oncovin)
- Biological response modifier: interferon alfa-2b (ineffective in advanced disease)
- Antiemetic: trimethobenzamide (Tigan)

Patient care goals
- The client will remain free from signs and symptoms of infection.
- The client will maintain weight within an acceptable range.
- The client will express positive feelings about himself.

Nursing interventions
- Provide a referral for psychological counseling *to assist the client who is coping poorly.* Family members may also need help in coping with the client's disease and with associated demands that the disorder places on them.
- As appropriate, allow the client to participate in self-care decisions whenever possible, and encourage him to participate in self-care measures as much as he can. *Involving the client in the treatment plan helps him gain some sense of control over his situation.*
- Inspect the client's skin every shift. Look for new lesions and skin breakdown. If the client has painful lesions, help him into a more comfortable position *to alleviate pain and promote client comfort.*
- Administer pain medications. Suggest distractions, and help the client with relaxation techniques *to divert the client from his pain and promote comfort.*

- Urge the client to share his feelings, and provide encouragement *to help him adjust to changes in his appearance.*
- Monitor the client's weight daily *to evaluate if nutritional needs are being met.*
- Supply the client with high-calorie, high-protein meals. If he can't tolerate regular meals, provide frequent smaller meals. Consult with the dietitian, and plan meals around the client's treatment. Adverse reactions to medications and the disease itself may make it difficult for the client's nutritional intake *to meet his metabolic needs.*
- If the client can't take food by mouth, administer I.V. fluids *to maintain hydration.* Also, provide antiemetics *to combat nausea and encourage nutritional intake.*
- Be alert for adverse reactions to radiation therapy or chemotherapy — such as anorexia, nausea, vomiting, and diarrhea — and take steps to prevent or alleviate them. *Adverse reactions are common and can further compromise the client's condition.*
- Reinforce the explanation of treatments. Make sure the client understands which adverse reactions to expect and how to manage them *to ensure prompt intervention and treatment.* For example, during radiation therapy, instruct the client to keep irradiated skin dry *to avoid possible breakdown and subsequent infection.*
- Explain all prescribed medications, including possible adverse effects and drug interactions, *to promote compliance with the medication regimen.*
- Explain infection-prevention techniques and, if necessary, demonstrate basic hygiene measures *to prevent infection.* Advise the client not to share his toothbrush, razor, or other items that may be contaminated with blood. *These measures are especially important if the client also has AIDS because they prevent the spread of infection to others.*
- Encourage the client to set priorities, accept the help of others, and delegate nonessential tasks. Help the client plan daily periods of alternating activity and rest *to help him cope with fatigue.*
- Explain the proper use of assistive devices, when appropriate, *to ease ambulation and promote independence.*
- As appropriate, refer the client to support groups offered by the social services department *to promote emotional well-being.*
- If the client's prognosis is poor (less than 6 months to live), suggest immediate hospice care. *Hospice care provides much needed support to caregivers and helps the client through the dying process.*

Evaluation

- The client hasn't displayed signs or symptoms of infection.
- The client has maintained an acceptable weight.
- The client expresses a positive self-image.

Leukemia

LEUKEMIA is characterized by an uncontrolled proliferation of WBC precursors that fail to mature. Leukemia occurs when normal hemopoietic cells are replaced by leukemic cells in bone marrow. Immature forms of WBCs circulate in the blood, infiltrating the liver, spleen, and lymph nodes. Types of leukemia include:

- acute lymphocytic
- acute myelogenous
- chronic lymphocytic
- chronic myelocytic.

Possible causes

- Altered immune system
- Exposure to chemicals
- Genetics
- Radiation
- Virus

Data collection findings

- Enlarged lymph nodes, spleen, and liver
- Frequent infections
- Weakness and fatigue
- Epistaxis
- Fever
- Generalized pain
- Gingivitis and stomatitis
- Hematemesis
- Hypotension
- Jaundice
- Joint, abdominal, and bone pain
- Melena
- Night sweats
- Petechiae and ecchymoses
- Prolonged menses
- Tachycardia

Diagnostic findings

- Bone marrow biopsy reveals a large number of immature leukocytes.
- Hematology shows decreased HCT, Hb, RBCs, and platelets and increased ESR, immature WBCs, and pro-

CLINICAL SITUATION

Caring for the client with leukemia

A 25-year-old male client is seeing his health care provider because of his recent history of extreme fatigue and swollen glands in his neck. He has also had some spontaneous nose bleeds. The health care provider orders a complete blood count that reveals immature white blood cells. Then the health care provider orders a bone marrow biopsy.

What finding would most strongly support a diagnosis of acute leukemia?

A. Large number of immature lymphocytes
B. Large number of immature thrombocytes
C. Large number of immature reticulocytes
D. Large number of immature leukocytes

Answer: D. Leukemia is manifested by an abnormal overproduction of immature leukocytes in the bone marrow.

Questions for future thought

- What would you tell the client regarding bleeding tendencies?
- What symptoms would you warn the client about regarding infection?

longed bleeding time. (See *Caring for the client with leukemia.*)

Nursing diagnoses

- Imbalanced nutrition: Less than body requirements
- Chronic pain
- Risk for infection

Treatment

- High-protein, high-vitamin and high-mineral diet, involving soft, bland foods in small, frequent feedings
- Stem cell transplant
- Transfusion of platelets, packed RBCs, and whole blood

Drug therapy options

- Alkylating agent: busulfan (Myleran), chlorambucil (Leukeran)
- Antibiotic: doxorubicin (Adriamycin), plicamycin (Mithracin)

- Antimetabolite: fluorouracil (Adrucil), methotrexate (Folex)
- Antineoplastic: vinblastine (Velban), vincristine (Oncovin)
- Hematopoietic growth factor: epoetin alfa (Epogen)

Patient care goals

- The client will maintain weight within an acceptable range.
- The client will express feelings of comfort and pain relief.
- The client will remain free from signs and symptoms of infection.

Nursing interventions

- Monitor and record vital signs *to promptly detect deterioration in the client's condition.*
- Monitor intake, output, and daily weight *because body weight may decrease as a result of fluid loss.*
- Monitor laboratory studies *to help establish blood replacement needs, assess fluid status, and detect possible infection.*
- Monitor for bleeding. *Regular assessment may help anticipate or alleviate problems.*
- Place the client with epistaxis in an upright position leaning slightly forward *to reduce vascular pressure and prevent aspiration.*
- Monitor for infection. Damage to bone marrow may suppress WBC formation. Promptly report fever over 101° F (38.3° C) and decreased WBC counts *so that antibiotic therapy may be initiated.*
- Monitor oxygen therapy. *Oxygen therapy increases alveolar oxygen concentration and enhances arterial blood oxygenation.*
- Force fluids *to maintain adequate hydration.*
- Monitor the administration of I.V. fluids *to ensure replacement of lost fluid.*
- Encourage turning every 2 hours *to prevent venous stasis and skin breakdown.*
- Encourage coughing and deep breathing *to help remove secretions and prevent pulmonary complications.*
- Keep the client in semi-Fowler's position when in bed *to promote chest expansion and ventilation of basilar lung fields.*
- Maintain the client's diet *to provide necessary nutrition.*
- Prepare the client for TPN administration, if needed, *to provide the client with electrolytes, amino acids, and other nutrients tailored to his needs.*

- Maintain a patent I.V. site for administration of transfusion therapy as prescribed and monitor for adverse reactions. *Transfusion reactions may occur during blood administration and may further compromise the client's condition.*
- Administer medications as prescribed *to combat disease and promote wellness.*
- Provide gentle mouth and skin care *to prevent oral mucous membrane or skin breakdown.*
- Encourage the client to express his feelings about changes in his body image and fear of dying *to reduce anxiety.*
- Avoid giving the client I.M. injections and enemas and taking rectal temperature *to prevent bleeding.*

Evaluation

- The client has maintained an adequate weight.
- The client reports adequate pain control.
- The client hasn't displayed signs or symptoms of infection.

Lymphoma

LYMPHOMA can be classified as either HODGKIN'S DISEASE or MALIGNANT LYMPHOMA (also called non-Hodgkin's lymphoma).

In Hodgkin's disease, Reed-Sternberg cells proliferate in a single lymph node and travel contiguously through the lymphatic system to other lymphatic nodes and organs. (See *Progression of Hodgkin's disease.*)

In malignant lymphoma, tumors occur throughout lymph nodes and lymphatic organs in unpredictable patterns. Malignant lymphoma may be categorized as:
- lymphocytic
- histiocytic
- mixed cell types.

Progression of Hodgkin's disease

Hodgkin's disease occurs in four stages:
- Stage 1 – Disease occurs in a single lymph node region or single extralymphatic organ.
- Stage 2 – Disease occurs in two or more lymph nodes on the same side of the diaphragm or in an extralymphatic organ.
- Stage 3 – Disease spreads to both sides of the diaphragm and perhaps to an extralymphatic organ, the spleen, or both.
- Stage 4 – Disease disseminates.

Possible causes

- Environmental (Hodgkin's disease)
- Genetic (Hodgkin's disease)
- Immunologic
- Viral

Data collection findings

Hodgkin's disease

- Bone pain
- Dysphagia
- Dyspnea
- Edema and cyanosis of face and neck
- Enlarged, nontender, firm, and movable lymph nodes in lower cervical regions
- Predictable pattern of spread

Malignant lymphoma

- Less predictable pattern of spread
- Prominent, painless, generalized lymphadenopathy

Both lymphomas

- Anorexia and weight loss
- Cough
- Hepatomegaly
- Malaise and lethargy
- Night sweats
- Recurrent infection
- Recurrent, intermittent fever
- Severe pruritus
- Splenomegaly

Diagnostic findings

Hodgkin's disease

- Blood chemistry shows increased alkaline phosphatase.
- Chest radiograph reveals lymphadenopathy.
- Hematology shows decreased Hb level, HCT, and platelets and increased ESR, immature leukocytes, and gamma globulin.
- Lymph node biopsy specimen is positive for Reed-Sternberg cells.
- Lymphangiogram shows positive lymph node involvement.
- LD is increased.

Malignant lymphoma

- Bone marrow aspiration and biopsy specimens reveal small, diffuse lymphocytic or large, follicular-type cells.
- Chest radiograph reveals lymphadenopathy.

Nursing diagnoses

- Impaired tissue integrity
- Ineffective protection
- Risk for infection

Treatment

- Diet high in protein, calories, vitamins, minerals, iron, and calcium that consists of bland, soft foods
- Radiation therapy
- Transfusion of packed RBCs

Drug therapy options

Hodgkin's disease

- Chemotherapy: bleomycin (Blenoxane), dacarbazine (DTIC-Dome), doxorubicin (Adriamycin), mechloreth-amine (Mustargen), procarbazine (Matulane), vinblastine (Velban), vincristine (Oncovin)

Malignant lymphoma

- Chemotherapy: cyclophosphamide (Cytoxan), doxoru-bicin (Adriamycin), vincristine (Oncovin)

Patient care goals

- The client will be free from complications.
- The client will exhibit no signs of skin breakdown.
- The client will be free from infection.

Nursing interventions

- Monitor and record vital signs *to allow for early detection of complications.*
- Monitor intake and output and urine specific gravity. *Low urine output and high specific gravity indicate hypovolemia.*
- Monitor laboratory studies. *Electrolyte level, Hb levels, and HCT help indicate fluid status; WBC measurement may indicate bone marrow suppression.*
- Monitor for bleeding, infection, jaundice, and electrolyte imbalance *to detect complications associated with lymphoma.*
- Keep the client in semi-Fowler's position when in bed *to promote chest expansion and ventilation of basilar lung fields.*
- Administer oxygen. *Supplemental oxygen helps reduce hypoxemia.*
- Encourage turning every 2 hours *to prevent skin breakdown,* and encourage coughing and deep breathing *to help remove secretions and prevent pulmonary complications.*
- Provide mouth and skin care *to prevent the breakdown of the oral mucous membranes and skin.*

- Help the client maintain his diet *to ensure nutritional requirements are met.*
- Encourage fluids *to prevent dehydration and complications associated with chemotherapeutic drugs.*
- Monitor the administration of I.V. fluids as prescribed *to ensure replacement of lost fluid.*
- Administer medications as prescribed, and monitor for adverse effects *to prevent further complications.*
- Maintain a patent I.V. site for administration of transfusion therapy as prescribed, and monitor for adverse reactions. *Transfusion reactions during blood administration may further compromise the client's condition.*
- Provide rest periods *to enhance immune function and decrease weakness caused by anemia.*
- Encourage the client to express his feelings about changes in his body image and a fear of dying (indolent type of lymphoma isn't curable) *to allay the client's anxiety.*
- Review key teaching topics with the client *to ensure adequate knowledge about his condition and treatment,* including:
  – recognizing early signs and symptoms of motor and sensory deficits
  – increasing fluid intake
  – using only an electric razor
  – refraining from using over-the-counter medications (unless cleared by the physician)
  – contacting the American Cancer Society.

Evaluation

- The client displays no signs of complications, such as bleeding, dehydration, infection, jaundice, or hypoxemia.
- The client remains afebrile and exhibits no sign of infection, including wound, respiratory, skin, and oral infections.

Multiple myeloma

Multiple myeloma involves the abnormal proliferation of plasma cells. These plasma cells are immature and malignant and invade the bone marrow, lymph nodes, liver, spleen, and kidneys, triggering osteoblastic activity and leading to bone destruction throughout the body.

Possible causes

- Environmental
- Genetic
- Unknown

Data collection findings

- Anemia
- Thrombocytopenia
- Hemorrhage
- Constant, severe bone pain
- Headaches
- Hepatomegaly
- Multiple infections
- Pathologic fractures
- Skeletal deformities of the sternum and ribs
- Loss of height
- Back pain
- Renal calculi
- Splenomegaly
- Vascular insufficiency

 FAST FACT

A client with multiple myeloma may have bone demineralization and may lose large amounts of calcium into the urine and blood, resulting in renal calculi, nephrocalcinosis and, eventually, renal failure due to hypocalcemia.

Diagnostic findings

- Bence Jones protein is present in the urine.
- Blood chemistry tests show increased calcium, uric acid, BUN, and creatinine levels.
- Bone marrow biopsy specimen shows an increased number of immature plasma cells.
- Bone scan reveals increased uptake.
- Hematology shows decreased HCT, WBCs, and platelets and increased ESR.
- Immunoelectrophoresis shows monoclonal spike.
- Urine chemistry shows increased calcium and uric acid.
- Radiographs show diffuse, round, punched-out bone lesions; osteoporosis; osteolytic lesions of the skull; and widespread demineralization.

Nursing diagnoses

- Acute pain
- Chronic pain
- Impaired physical mobility
- Risk for infection

Treatment

- Allogenic bone marrow transplantation
- Diet that's high in protein, carbohydrates, vitamins, and minerals in small, frequent feedings

- Orthopedic devices, such as braces, splints, and casts
- Peritoneal dialysis and hemodialysis
- Radiation therapy
- Transfusion therapy, including packed RBCs

Drug therapy options

- Alkylating agent: melphalan (Alkeran), cyclophosphamide (Cytoxan)
- Analgesic: morphine (MS Contin)
- Androgen: fluoxymesterone (Halotestin)
- Antacid: magnesium hydroxide and aluminum hydroxide (Maalox), aluminum hydroxide (AlternaGEL)
- Antibiotic: doxorubicin (Adriamycin), plicamycin (Mithracin)
- Antiemetic: prochlorperazine (Compazine)
- Antigout agent: allopurinol (Zyloprim)
- Antineoplastic drug: vinblastine (Velban), vincristine (Oncovin)
- Diuretic: furosemide (Lasix)
- Glucocorticoid: prednisone (Deltasone)

Patient care goals

- The client will attain pain relief.
- The client will demonstrate maintained or improved mobility.
- The client will be free from signs of infection.

Nursing interventions

- Assess renal status *to detect renal calculi and renal failure secondary to hypercalcemia.*
- Monitor and record vital *signs to allow for early detection of complications.*
- Monitor intake and output, urine specific gravity, and daily weight *to identify fluid volume excess or deficit.*
- Monitor laboratory studies. *RBCs, WBCs, Hb, HCT, and platelets may be affected by chemotherapy.*
- Assess cardiovascular and respiratory status *to detect signs of compromise.*
- Assess bone pain *to determine the client's response to analgesics.*
- Monitor for infection and bruising *to detect complications.*
- Encourage the client to maintain a balanced diet *to ensure nutritional requirements are met.*
- Encourage fluids *to prevent dehydration and dilute calcium.*
- Monitor the administration of I.V. fluids *to ensure replacement of lost fluid and dilution of calcium and to prevent renal protein precipitation.*

- Assist with turning, coughing, and deep breathing *to mobilize and remove secretions.*
- Maintain patency of the I.V. site for administration of transfusion therapy as prescribed *to replace blood components.*
- Administer medications, as prescribed, and monitor for adverse effects *to prevent complications.*
- Maintain seizure precautions *to prevent injury.*
- Provide skin and mouth care *to prevent the breakdown of the oral mucous membranes and skin.*
- Alternate rest periods with activity *to prevent fatigue.*
- Prevent the client from falling *because he's vulnerable to fractures.*
- Move the client gently, keeping his body in alignment, *to prevent injury.*
- Apply and maintain braces, splints, and casts *to prevent injury and reduce pain.*
- Review key teaching topics with the client *to ensure adequate knowledge about his condition and treatment,* including:
  – exercising regularly, with particular attention to muscle-strengthening exercises
  – recognizing signs and symptoms of renal calculi, fractures, and seizures
  – avoiding lifting, constipation, and over-the-counter medications
  – monitoring stool for occult blood
  – using braces, splints, and casts
  – contacting the American Cancer Society.

Evaluation

- The client verbalizes that adequate pain relief is received with treatment.
- The client remains free from complications caused by immobility, demonstrates maintained or improved mobility, and verbalizes the appropriate use of splints or braces, and activities to maintain and improve muscle strength.
- The client is afebrile and free from such signs of infection (including respiratory infections) as skin breakdown.
- The client discusses appropriate precautions to take to prevent injury.

Polycythemia vera

POLYCYTHEMIA VERA is a chronic myeloproliferative disorder characterized by increased RBC mass, leukocytosis, thrombocytosis, and increased Hb concentration, with normal or increased plasma volume. It usually occurs in clients ages 40 to 60 and is most common among males of Jewish ancestry; it rarely affects children or blacks and doesn't appear to be familial. It may also be known as primary polycythemia, erythremia, polycythemia rubra vera, splenomegalic polycythemia, or Vaquez Osler disease.

The prognosis depends on the client's age at diagnosis, the treatment used, and complications. Mortality is high if polycythemia isn't treated or is associated with leukemia or myeloid metaplasia.

Possible causes
- Unknown (possibly due to a multipotential stem cell defect)

Data collection findings
- Congestion of the conjunctivae, retinas, and retinal veins
- Dizziness (vertigo)
- Dyspnea
- Feeling of fullness in the head
- Headache
- Hemorrhage
- Hypertension
- Pruritus
- Ruddy cyanosis of the nose
- Thrombosis of smaller vessels
- Tinnitus
- Vision disturbances (blurring, diplopia, engorged veins of fundus and retina)
- Weight loss

Diagnostic findings
- Blood test results show increased RBC mass and normal arterial oxygen saturation in association with splenomegaly or two of the following signs:
  - thrombocytosis
  - leukocytosis
  - elevated leukocyte alkaline phosphatase level
  - elevated serum vitamin B_{12} or unbound B_{12} binding capacity.
- WBC count is increased to 10,000 to 20,000 U/L.
- Platelets are increased to 1,000,000 U/L.
- HCT is increased to greater than 60% above normal.

Nursing diagnoses
- Ineffective tissue perfusion (cardiovascular)
- Deficient knowledge (client)

Treatment
- Phlebotomy (typically, 350 to 500 ml of blood is removed at variable intervals [depending on the client] until the client's HCT is reduced to the low-normal range)

Drug therapy options
- Chemotherapy: busulfan (Myleran), chlorambucil (Leukeran), melphalan (Alkeran)
- Myelosuppressive drug: hydroxyurea (Hydrea), radioactive phosphorus (^{32}P)
- Antigout agent: allopurinol (Zyloprim)

Patient care goals
- The client will have no signs of inadequate cardiovascular tissue perfusion.
- The client will verbalize knowledge about the disease, treatment course, and complications.

Nursing interventions
- Check blood pressure, pulse rate, and respiratory rate prior to and during phlebotomy *to monitor the client's tolerance of the procedure.*
- During phlebotomy, make sure the client is lying down comfortably *to prevent vertigo and syncope.*
- Stay alert for tachycardia, clamminess, or complaints of vertigo. If these effects occur, the procedure should be stopped. *These signs and symptoms indicate hypovolemia.*
- Immediately after phlebotomy, check the client's blood pressure and pulse rate. Have him sit up for about 5 minutes before allowing him to walk *to prevent vasovagal attack or orthostatic hypotension.* Also, give 24 oz (720 ml) of juice or water *to replace fluid volume lost during the procedure.*
- Tell the client to watch for and report signs or symptoms of iron deficiency (pallor, weight loss, weakness, glossitis). *After repeated phlebotomies, the iron deficiency will develop, which stabilizes RBC production and reduces the need for phlebotomy.*
- Keep the client active and ambulatory to prevent thrombosis. If bed rest is absolutely necessary, prescribe a daily program of both active and passive ROM exercises *to prevent thrombosis and maintain joint mobility.*
- Watch for complications, such as hypervolemia, thrombocytosis, and signs of an impending stroke (decreased sensation, numbness, transitory paralysis, fleeting blindness, headache, and epistaxis) *to ensure early treatment intervention.*
- Regularly examine the client closely for bleeding. Tell the client which bleeding sites are most common (such as the nose, gingivae, and skin) so he can check for bleeding. Advise the client to report abnormal bleeding promptly. *These measures decrease the risk of hemorrhage.*
- Give additional fluids, administer allopurinol, and alkalinize the urine *to compensate for increased uric acid production and prevent uric acid calculi.*

● If the client has symptomatic splenomegaly, suggest or provide small, frequent meals followed by a rest period *to prevent nausea and vomiting.*

● Report acute abdominal pain immediately *to avoid treatment delay.* Acute pain may signal splenic infarction, renal calculi, or abdominal organ thrombosis.

 SPOT CHECK

What can acute abdominal pain signify in a client with polycythemia vera?
Acute pain may signal splenic infarction, renal calculi, or abdominal organ thrombosis.

During myelosuppressive treatment

● Monitor CBC and platelet counts before and during therapy. Warn an outpatient who develops leukopenia that resistance to infection is low; advise the client to avoid crowds and watch for symptoms of infection. *These measures protect the client from life-threatening infection.*

● If leukopenia develops in a hospitalized client who needs reverse isolation, follow facility guidelines. If thrombocytopenia develops, tell the client to watch for signs of bleeding (blood in urine, nosebleeds, black stools) *to prevent hemorrhage.*

● Tell the client about possible adverse effects (nausea, vomiting, and the risk of infection) of alkylating agents *to allay his anxiety and ensure early treatment.*

● Watch for adverse reactions. If nausea and vomiting occur, begin antiemetic therapy and adjust the client's diet *to promote comfort.*

● Take a blood sample for CBC and platelet count before treatment with ³²P is begun. Use of ³²P requires radiation precautions *to prevent contamination.*

● Tell the client he will need to lie down during I.V. administration *to facilitate the procedure and prevent extravasation* and for 15 to 20 minutes afterward *to monitor the client's tolerance of the procedure.*

● Review key teaching topics with the client *to ensure adequate knowledge about condition and treatment,* including:
– understanding the disease process and treatment options
– understanding the importance of remaining as active as possible
– avoiding infection
– keeping the environment free from hazards that could cause falls
– using a safety razor to prevent bleeding

– preventing adverse reactions to treatment such as using antiemetics to prevent nausea and vomiting
– using community resources
– understanding warnings against fingerstick blood tests because of compromised circulation.

Evaluation

● The client displays a heart rate and blood pressure within normal range; warm, dry skin; and decreased dyspnea.

● The client demonstrates knowledge about the disease, treatment, and signs and symptoms that should be reported.

Rheumatoid arthritis

Believed to be an autoimmune disorder, RHEUMATOID ARTHRITIS is a systemic inflammatory disease that affects the synovial lining of the joints. Antibodies first attack the synovium of the joint, causing it to become inflamed and swollen. Eventually, the articular cartilage and surrounding tendons and ligaments are affected.

Inflammation of the synovial membranes is followed by formation of pannus (granulation tissue) and destruction of cartilage, bone, and ligaments. Pannus is replaced by fibrotic tissue and calcification, which causes subluxation of the joint. The joint becomes ankylosed — or fused — leaving a very painful joint and limited ROM.

Possible causes

● Autoimmune disease
● Genetic transmission

Data collection findings

● Symmetrical joint swelling (mirror image of affected joints)
● Painful, swollen joints; crepitus; and morning stiffness
● Fatigue
● Malaise
● Anorexia and weight loss
● Dry eyes and mucous membranes
● Enlarged lymph nodes
● Fever
● Leukopenia and anemia
● Limited ROM
● Paresthesia of the hands and the feet
● Pericarditis
● Raynaud's phenomenon
● Splenomegaly
● Subcutaneous nodules

Diagnostic findings
- Antinuclear antibody (ANA) test is positive.
- Hematology shows increased ESR, WBC, platelets, and anemia.
- RF test is positive.
- Serum protein electrophoresis shows elevated serum globulins.
- Synovial fluid analysis shows increased WBCs, increased volume and turbidity, and decreased viscosity and complement (C_3 and C_4 levels).
- X-rays reveal bone demineralization and soft-tissue swelling in early stages; in later stages, X-rays reveal a loss of cartilage, a narrowing of joint spaces, cartilage and bone destruction, and erosion, subluxations, and deformity.

Nursing diagnoses
- Chronic pain
- Activity intolerance
- Disturbed body image

Treatment
- Cold therapy during acute episodes
- Heat therapy to relax muscles and relieve pain for chronic disease
- Physical therapy (to forestall loss of joint function), passive ROM exercises, and observance of rest periods
- Weight control because obesity adds stress to joints
- Well-balanced diet

Drug therapy options
- Analgesic: aspirin
- Antacid: magnesium hydroxide and aluminum hydroxide (Maalox), aluminum hydroxide (Amphojel)
- Antimetabolite: methotrexate (Rheumatrex)
- Antirheumatic: hydroxychloroquine (Plaquenil)
- Glucocorticoid: prednisone (Deltasone) and hydrocortisone (Hydrocortone)
- Gold therapy: gold sodium thiomalate (Myochrysine)
- NSAID: indomethacin (Indocin), ibuprofen (Advil, Motrin), sulindac (Clinoril), piroxicam (Feldene), flurbiprofen (Ansaid), diclofenac (Voltaren), naproxen (Naprosyn), diflunisal (Dolobid)

Patient care goals
- The client will express feelings of comfort and pain relief.
- The client will attain the highest level of mobility possible within the confines of his disease.
- The client will express a positive image of himself.

Nursing interventions
- Monitor vital signs *to allow for early detection of complications.*
- Monitor neuromuscular status *to determine the client's capabilities.*
- Check joints for swelling, pain, and redness *to determine the extent of the disease and the effectiveness of treatment.*
- Monitor laboratory studies *to detect remissions and exacerbations.*
- Administer medications as prescribed *to enhance the treatment regimen.*
- Provide passive ROM exercises *to prevent joint contractures and muscle atrophy.*
- Splint inflamed joints *to maintain joints in a functional position and prevent musculoskeletal deformities.*
- Provide warm or cold therapy as prescribed *to help alleviate pain.*
- Provide skin care *to prevent skin breakdown.*
- Minimize environmental stress and plan rest periods *to help the client cope with the disease.*
- Encourage the client to express his feelings about changes in his body image *to help him express doubts and resolve concerns.*

Evaluation
- The client reports adequate pain control.
- The client demonstrates maximum mobility.
- The client displays a positive attitude regarding his self-image.

Scleroderma

SCLERODERMA is a diffuse connective tissue disease characterized by inflammatory and then degenerative and fibrotic changes in skin, blood vessels, synovial membranes, skeletal muscles, and internal organs (especially the esophagus, intestinal tract, thyroid, heart, lungs, and kidneys). The disease, also known as *progressive systemic sclerosis,* affects more women than men, especially between ages 30 and 50.

Possible causes
- Unknown

Data collection findings
- Signs and symptoms of Raynaud's phenomenon, such as blanching, cyanosis, and erythema of the fingers and toes in response to stress or exposure to cold
- Pain

- Stiffness
- Swelling of fingers and joints
- Taut, shiny skin over the entire hand and forearm
- Tight and inelastic facial skin, causing a masklike appearance and "pinching" of the mouth
- Slowly healing ulcerations on the tips of the fingers or toes that may lead to gangrene
- Cardiac and pulmonary fibrosis (in advanced disease)
- Renal involvement accompanied by malignant hypertension (the main cause of death)

Diagnostic findings
- Blood studies show slightly elevated ESR, positive RF in 25% to 35% of clients, and positive antinuclear antibody test.
- Chest X-rays show bilateral basilar pulmonary fibrosis.
- ECG reveals possible nonspecific abnormalities related to myocardial fibrosis.
- GI X-rays show distal esophageal hypomotility and stricture, duodenal loop dilation, small-bowel malabsorption pattern, and large diverticula.
- Hand X-rays show terminal phalangeal tuft resorption, subcutaneous calcification, and joint space narrowing and erosion.
- Pulmonary function studies show decreased diffusion and vital capacity.
- Skin biopsy may show changes consistent with the progress of the disease, such as marked thickening of the dermis and occlusive vessel changes.
- Urinalysis reveals proteinuria, microscopic hematuria, and casts (with renal involvement).

Nursing diagnoses
- Chronic pain
- Impaired physical mobility
- Impaired skin integrity

Treatment
- Palliative measures, such as physical therapy, to maintain function and promote muscle strength (currently, no cure exists for scleroderma)

Drug therapy
- Immunosuppressants: cyclosporine (Sandimmune), chlorambucil (Leukeran)

Patient care goals
- The client will express feelings of comfort and pain relief.

- The client will maintain maximum functional ability within the confines of disease.
- The client will maintain intact skin surfaces.

Nursing interventions
- Assess motion restrictions, pain, vital signs, intake and output, respiratory function, and daily weight *to monitor disease progression and guide the treatment plan.*
- Teach the client to monitor blood pressure at home and report increases above baseline. *Malignant hypertension is the main cause of death in clients diagnosed with scleroderma.*
- Warn against fingerstick blood tests because of compromised circulation.
- Help the client and family adjust to the client's new body image and to the limitations and dependence that these changes cause. *Clients and their families need time to adjust to the overwhelming effects of illness.*
- Help the client and family accept the fact that this condition is incurable. Encourage them to express their feelings, and help them cope with their fears and frustrations by offering information about the disease, its treatment, and relevant diagnostic tests. *Providing information helps to alleviate anxiety and provides the client with knowledge necessary for informed decision making.*
- Whenever possible, let the client participate in treatment by measuring her intake and output, planning her diet, assisting in dialysis, giving herself heat therapy, and doing prescribed exercises *to help her gain a sense of control over her condition.*
- Involve the client's family in treatment *to help the family overcome feelings of helplessness.*

Evaluation
- The client reports adequate pain control.
- The client demonstrates functional mobility.
- The client has intact skin integrity.

Systemic lupus erythematosus
SLE is an autoimmune disorder that involves most organ systems. It's chronic in nature and characterized by periods of exacerbation and remission.

In SLE, there's a depression of T-cell activity and an increase in the production of antibodies, specifically antibodies to DNA and ribonucleic acid and antierythrocyte, antinuclear, and antiplatelet antibodies. The immune response results in an inflammatory process involving the veins and arteries (vasculitis), which causes pain, swelling, and tissue damage in any area of the body.

Possible causes
- Autoimmune disease
- Drugs (procainamide [Pronestyl], hydralazine [Apresoline], and phenytoin [Dilantin]
- Genetic
- Viral
- Unknown

Data collection findings
- Fatigue
- Butterfly rash on face (rash may vary in severity from malar erythema to discoid lesions)
- Low-grade fever
- Migratory pain, stiffness, and joint swelling
- Photosensitivity
- Anorexia and weight loss
- Anemia
- Leukopenia
- Thrombocytopenia
- Erythema on palms
- Oral and nasopharyngeal ulcerations
- Alopecia
- Raynaud's phenomenon
- Lymphadenopathy
- Splenomegaly
- Hepatomegaly
- Renal involvement: glomerulonephritis and renal dysfunction and failure
- CNS involvement: impaired cognitive function, psychosis, depression, seizures, peripheral neuropathies, strokes, and organic brain syndrome
- Cardiac involvement: pleurisy, pericarditis, myocarditis, noninfectious endocarditis, and hypertension

Diagnostic findings
- ANA test is positive.
- Blood chemistry shows decreased complement fixation.
- Hematology shows decreased Hb, HCT, WBC, and platelets and an increased ESR.
- Lupus erythematosus cell preparation is positive.
- RF is positive.
- Urine chemistry shows proteinuria and hematuria.

Nursing diagnoses
- Ineffective breathing pattern
- Risk for infection
- Impaired mobility

Treatment
- Diet high in iron, protein, and vitamins (especially vitamin C)
- Hemodialysis or kidney transplant if renal failure occurs
- Limited exertion and maintenance of adequate rest
- Plasmapheresis

Drug therapy options
- Analgesic: aspirin
- Antianemic: ferrous sulfate (Feosol), ferrous gluconate (Fergon)
- Antirheumatic: hydroxychloroquine (Plaquenil)
- Cytotoxic drug: methotrexate (Folex) (these drugs may delay or prevent deteriorating renal status)
- Glucocorticoid: prednisone (Deltasone)
- Immunosuppressant: azathioprine (Imuran), cyclophosphamide (Cytoxan)
- NSAID: indomethacin (Indocin), ibuprofen (Motrin), sulindac (Clinoril), piroxicam (Feldene), flurbiprofen (Ansaid), diclofenac (Voltaren), naproxen (Naprosyn), diflunisal (Dolobid)

Patient care goals
- The client will maintain adequate ventilation.
- The client will remain fee from signs and symptoms of infection.
- The client will maintain joint mobility and ROM.

Nursing interventions
- Assess musculoskeletal status *to determine the client's baseline functional abilities.*
- Monitor renal status. Decreased urine output without lowered fluid intake may indicate decreased renal perfusion, a possible indication of decreased cardiac output.
- Monitor vital signs *to promptly determine if the client's condition is deteriorating and to evaluate the effectiveness of treatment.* Fever can signal an exacerbation.
- Provide prophylactic skin, mouth, and perineal care *to prevent skin and oral mucous membrane breakdown.*
- Administer medications as prescribed *to enhance the treatment regimen.*
- Maintain seizure precautions *to prevent client injury.*
- Monitor dietary intake *to help ensure adequate nutritional intake.*
- Minimize environmental stress and provide rest periods *to avoid fatigue and help the client to cope with illness.*
- Promote independence in ADLs *to help the client develop self-esteem.*
- Administer antiemetics *to alleviate nausea and vomiting.*

- Administer antidiarrheals as prescribed *to alleviate diarrhea.*
- Encourage the client to express feelings about changes in his body image and the chronic nature of the disease *to help him ventilate doubts and resolve concerns.*

SPOT CHECK

The nurse is preparing a client with SLE for discharge. Which information should she include in the teaching plan?
A. Exposure to sunlight will help control skin rashes.
B. There are no activity limitations between flare-ups.
C. Body temperature should be monitored.
D. Corticosteroids may be stopped when symptoms are relieved.
Answer: C. The client should monitor his temperature, because fever can signal an exacerbation and should be reported to the physician. Sunlight and other sources of UV light may precipitate severe skin reactions and exacerbate the disease. Fatigue can cause an SLE flare-up, and clients should be encouraged to pace activities and plan for rest periods. Corticosteroids must be gradually tapered because they can suppress the function of the adrenal gland. Abruptly stopping corticosteroids can cause adrenal insufficiency, a potentially life-threatening situation.

Evaluation
- The client has adequate ventilation as evidenced by normal respiratory effort.
- The client hasn't displayed signs or symptoms of infection.
- The client demonstrates functional mobility.

Vasculitis

VASCULITIS is a broad spectrum of disorders characterized by inflammation and necrosis of blood vessels. Its clinical effects depend on the vessels involved and reflect tissue ischemia caused by blood flow obstruction. Prognosis is also variable. For example, hypersensitivity vasculitis is usually a benign disorder limited to the skin, but the more extensive polyarteritis nodosa can be rapidly fatal.

Vasculitis can occur at any age, except for mucocutaneous lymph node syndrome, which occurs only during childhood. Vasculitis may be a primary disorder or secondary to other disorders, such as rheumatoid arthritis or SLE. The types of vasculitis are Wegener's granulomatosis, giant cell arteritis, and Takayasu's arteritis.

Possible causes
- Excessive levels of antigen
- High-dose antibiotic therapy
- Commonly associated with serious infectious disease, such as hepatitis B or bacterial endocarditis

Data collection findings
Wegener's granulomatosis
- Cough
- Fever
- Malaise
- Mild to severe hematuria
- Pulmonary congestion
- Anorexia
- Weight loss

Giant cell arteritis
- Fever
- Headache (associated with polymyalgia rheumatica syndrome)
- Jaw claudication
- Myalgia
- Visual changes

Takayasu's arteritis
- Malaise
- Arthralgias
- Pain or paresthesia distal to the affected area
- Bruits
- Syncope
- Stroke (with disease progression)
- Diplopia and transient blindness, if carotid artery is involved
- Heart failure (with disease progression)
- Loss of distal pulses
- Anorexia
- Nausea
- Night sweats
- Pallor
- Weight loss

Diagnostic findings
Wegener's granulomatosis
- Tissue biopsy shows necrotizing vasculitis with granulomatous inflammation.
- Blood studies show leukocytosis, elevated ESR, IgA, and IgG; low titer RF; circulating immune complexes (antineutrophil cytoplasmic antibody in more than 90% of clients)
- Renal biopsy shows focal segmental glomerulonephritis.

Giant cell arteritis
- Blood studies show decreased Hb level and elevated ESR.

- Tissue biopsy shows panarteritis with infiltration of mononuclear cells, giant cells within the vessel wall (seen in 50% of cases), fragmentation of the internal elastic lamina, and proliferation of intima.

Takayasu's arteritis
- Blood studies show decreased Hb level, leukocytosis, positive lupus erythematosus cell preparation, and elevated ESR.
- Arteriography shows calcification and obstruction of affected vessels.
- Tissue biopsy shows inflammation of adventitia and intima of vessels and thickening of vessel walls.

Nursing diagnoses
- Ineffective tissue perfusion (systemic)
- Acute pain
- Disturbed sensory perception (tactile)

Treatment
- Removal of identified environmental antigen
- Elimination of antigenic food, if identifiable

Drug therapy options
- Corticosteroid: prednisone (Deltasone)
- Antineoplastic: cyclophosphamide (Cytoxan)

Patient care goals
- The client will have improved tissue perfusion.
- The client will express feelings of comfort and pain relief.
- The client will have an improved sense of touch.

Nursing interventions
- Assess for dry nasal mucosa in clients with Wegener's granulomatosis. Instill nose drops *to lubricate the mucosa and help diminish crusting.* Alternatively, irrigate the nasal passages with warm normal saline solution *to combat drying.*
- Regulate environmental temperature *to prevent additional vasoconstriction caused by cold.*
- Monitor vital signs. Use a Doppler ultrasonic flowmeter, if available, *to auscultate blood pressure in clients with Takayasu's arteritis, in whom peripheral pulses are frequently difficult to palpate.*
- Monitor intake and output. Check daily for edema. Keep the client well-hydrated (3 L daily) *to reduce the risk of hemorrhagic cystitis associated with cyclophosphamide therapy.*
- Provide emotional *support to help the client and his family cope with an altered body image — the result of the* disorder or its therapy. *(For example, Wegener's granulomatosis may be associated with saddle nose, steroids may cause weight gain, and cyclophosphamide may cause alopecia.)*
- Monitor the client's WBC count during cyclophosphamide therapy *to prevent severe leukopenia.*

Evaluation
- The client displays improved systemic circulation and tissue perfusion.
- The client reports adequate pain control.
- The client has improved tactile perception.

GASTROINTESTINAL SYSTEM

The GI system is the body's food processing complex. This chapter provides a brief review of the structures of the GI system and some of the major disorders that affect it.

GI structure and function
The GI system includes the GI tract and its related structures, such as the tongue, as well as the liver and other accessory organs.

GI tract
The GI tract is basically a hollow, muscular tube through which food passes as it's digested. Accessory organs, such as the liver and pancreas, contribute substances that are vital to digestion.

Mouth and esophagus
The digestive process begins in the mouth, where a mechanical (tongue and teeth) and chemical (saliva) combination begins to break down food.

The esophagus transfers food from the oropharynx (behind the palate) to the stomach. The esophagus contains two structures, the epiglottis and the cardiac sphincter, that direct food into the stomach. The epiglottis closes to prevent food from entering the trachea; the cardiac sphincter closes to prevent reflux of gastric contents.

Stomach
The stomach is a hollow muscular pouch that secretes pepsin, mucus, and hydrochloric acid for digestion. In the stomach, food mixes with gastric juices to become chyme, which the stomach stores before parceling it into the small intestine. The stomach also secretes the intrinsic factor necessary for absorption of vitamin B_{12}.

Small intestine

The small intestine consists of the duodenum, jejunum, and ileum. Nearly all digestion takes place in the small intestine, which contains digestive agents, such as bile and pancreatic secretions. The small intestine is also lined with villi, which contain capillaries and lymphatics that transport nutrients from the small intestine to other parts of the body.

Large intestine

The large intestine consists of the ascending colon, transverse colon, descending colon, sigmoid colon, and rectum. It absorbs fluids and electrolytes, synthesizes vitamin K, and stores fecal material.

Liver and accessory organs

The liver is one of the largest organs of the body. Its many functions include:
- producing and conveying bile
- metabolizing carbohydrates, fats, and proteins
- synthesizing coagulation factors VII, IX, and X and prothrombin
- storing copper, iron, and vitamins A, D, E, K, and B_{12}
- detoxifying chemicals
- excreting bilirubin
- producing and storing glycogen
- promoting erythropoiesis when bone marrow production is insufficient.

Gallbladder

The gallbladder is a hollow, pear-shaped organ that stores bile and then delivers it through the cystic duct to the common bile duct.

Pancreas

The pancreas secretes three digestive enzymes: amylase, lipase, and trypsin. It also secretes the hormones insulin, glucagon, and somatostatin from the islets of Langerhans into the blood. In addition, the pancreas secretes large amounts of sodium bicarbonate, which neutralizes the acid in chyme.

GI DISORDERS

The major GI disorders include appendicitis, cholecystitis, cirrhosis, colorectal cancer, Crohn's disease, diverticular disease, esophageal cancer, gastric cancer, gastritis, gastroenteritis, gastroesophageal reflux disease (GERD), hepatitis, hiatal hernia, intestinal obstruction, irritable bowel syndrome, pancreatitis, peptic ulcer, peritonitis, and ulcerative colitis.

Appendicitis

APPENDICITIS is an inflammation of the appendix. Although the appendix has no known function, it regularly fills with and empties itself of food. Appendicitis occurs when the appendix becomes inflamed from ulceration of the mucosa or from obstruction of the lumen.

Possible causes
- Barium ingestion
- Fecal mass
- Stricture
- Viral infection

Data collection findings
- Anorexia
- Client lies in knee-bent position
- Constipation
- Generalized abdominal pain that becomes localized in the right lower abdomen (McBurney's point)
- Malaise
- Nausea and vomiting
- Sudden cessation of pain (indicates rupture)

Diagnostic findings
- Hematology shows a moderately elevated WBC count.

Nursing diagnoses
- Acute pain
- Imbalanced nutrition: Less than body requirements
- Risk for infection

Treatment
- Appendectomy
- I.V. fluids to prevent dehydration
- Nothing by mouth

Drug therapy options
- Analgesic: meperidine (Demerol), morphine (MS Contin) (administered only when diagnosis is confirmed)
- Antibiotic therapy

Patient care goals
- The client will experience pain relief.
- Fluid volume balance will be maintained.
- The client will remain free from infection.
- Skin integrity will remain intact.

Nursing interventions

- Assess GI status and pain. *Sudden cessation of pain preoperatively may indicate appendix rupture.*
- Monitor and record vital signs and intake and output *to determine fluid volume.*
- Administer I.V. fluids *to prevent dehydration.*
- Place the client in semi-Fowler's position *to reduce pain.*
- Maintain nothing-by-mouth status until bowel sounds return postoperatively; then advance the diet as tolerated *to promote healing and meet metabolic needs.*
- Assist the client with incentive spirometry, turning, coughing, and deep breathing *to mobilize secretions and promote lung expansion.*
- Monitor dressings for drainage and incision for infection postoperatively *to detect early signs of infection and prevent complications.*
- Review key teaching topics with the client and family members *to ensure adequate knowledge about condition and treatment,* including:
  – completing follow-up medical care
  – caring for incision
  – following activity restrictions
  – recognizing the signs and symptoms of infection.

Evaluation

- Adequate fluid and caloric intake is maintained.
- Skin integrity is intact without signs of infection.
- The client verbalizes knowledge of incision care and the importance of follow-up with physician.

Cholecystitis

CHOLECYSTITIS is an acute or chronic inflammation of the gallbladder most commonly associated with CHOLELITHIASIS. It occurs when an obstruction, such as calculi or edema, prevents the gallbladder from contracting when fatty foods enter the duodenum.

Based on the results of diagnostic studies, a client may undergo surgical removal of the stones in the bile duct and removal of the inflamed gallbladder by traditional cholecystectomy. (Some clients don't undergo surgical removal of gallstones.) (See *Alternative treatments for gallstones.*)

Clients who require gallbladder removal increasingly are undergoing laparoscopic cholecystectomy. In this ambulatory surgery, the surgeon makes four small incisions into the abdomen. Pain is minimal; the client is discharged the same day or on the 1st postoperative day and can resume activities after a few days. In contrast, with traditional cholecystectomy, the client typically is discharged in about 5 days. Postoperatively, the client may have a T tube in place. (For an illustration, see *T-tube placement,* page 434.)

Possible causes

- Cholelithiasis
- Estrogen therapy
- Infection of the gallbladder with *Escherichia coli*
- Obesity

Alternative treatments for gallstones

Extracorporeal shock wave lithotripsy

Extracorporeal shock wave lithotripsy is designed for a client with a small number of stones and mild to moderate symptoms. The client sits in a tank of water or holds a water-filled cushion against the appropriate place on the abdomen. Shock waves are sent through the water until the stones disintegrate (1 to 2 hours). The client is on a cardiac monitor throughout the procedure because shock waves must be coordinated with cardiac rhythm to prevent arrhythmias. After the procedure, observe the client for hematuria, hematoma, nausea, and biliary colic.

Endoscopic sphincterotomy

Endoscopic sphincterotomy uses an endoscope to remove stones from the common bile duct. After the procedure, monitor the client for bleeding, pain, and fever. Promote bed rest for 6 to 8 hours, and give the client nothing by mouth until the gag reflex returns.

Cholesterol dissolvent

Monoctanoin (Moctanin) is administered through a nasal biliary catheter to dissolve stones left in the bile duct after cholecystectomy. Dissolution may take 1 to 3 weeks. Observe the client for anorexia, nausea, vomiting, and abdominal pain.

Oral bile acids

Chenodiol (Chenix) and ursodiol (Actigall) are administered to dissolve small stones. Adverse effects include diarrhea (especially with chenodiol), elevation of hepatic enzymes, gastritis, and gastric ulcers. Dissolution takes between 6 months and 2 years, and the success rate is only about 30%.

T-tube placement

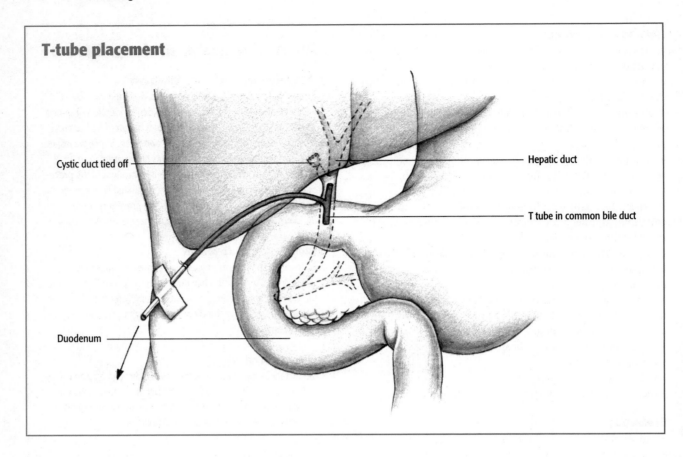

Cystic duct tied off

Hepatic duct

T tube in common bile duct

Duodenum

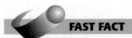 **FAST FACT**

Incidence of gallstone formation increases with the use of oral contraceptives, estrogens, and clofibrate because these drugs increase biliary cholesterol.

Data collection findings
- Belching
- Clay-colored stools
- Dark amber urine
- Ecchymosis
- Episodic colicky pain in the epigastric area, which radiates to the back and shoulder
- Fever
- Flatulence
- Indigestion or chest pain after eating fatty or fried foods
- Jaundice
- Nausea and vomiting
- Pruritus
- Steatorrhea

Diagnostic findings
- Hematologic studies, such as CBC, serum bilirubin levels, aspartate aminotransferase (AST), alanine aminotransferase (ALT), alkaline phosphatase, and serum amylase, reveal elevated enzyme levels if the liver has stasis or cell destruction. Elevated bilirubin levels (as well as alkaline phosphatase) reveal obstructed bile flow through the common bile duct, and elevated serum amylase levels may indicate concurrent pancreatitis. Also, WBC count may be elevated.
- Radiologic studies include GI series, ultrasound, chest X-ray, cholecystogram (rare), and endoscopic retrograde cholangiopancreatography, which show any abnormalities, the extent of the disease, and the client's ability to tolerate the proposed surgery.
- Bilirubin studies show darkened urine (cola-colored) and clay-colored stools if there's an obstruction.

Nursing diagnoses
- Acute pain
- Chronic pain

- Imbalanced nutrition: Less than body requirements
- Risk for infection

Treatment

- Small, frequent meals of a low-fat, low-calorie diet high in carbohydrates, protein, and fiber with restricted intake of gas-forming foods or no foods or fluids, as directed
- Extracorporeal shock wave lithotripsy
- Incentive spirometry
- Laparoscopic cholecystectomy or open cholecystectomy

Drug therapy options

- Analgesic: meperidine (Demerol), morphine (MS Contin)
- Antibiotic: cephalothin (Keflin)
- Anticholinergic: dicyclomine (Bentyl), propantheline (Pro-Banthine)
- Antiemetic: prochlorperazine (Compazine)
- Antipruritic: diphenhydramine (Benadryl)

Patient care goals

- The client will have relief from pain.
- The client will maintain or regain adequate nutritional intake.
- The client will undergo the procedure for removal of gallstones without complications.

Nursing interventions

- Assess abdominal status and pain *to determine baselines and detect changes in the client's condition.*
- Monitor and record vital signs and intake and output, laboratory studies, and urine specific gravity *to assess fluid and electrolyte balance.*
- Weigh the client daily *to detect signs of decreased food intake.*
- Monitor the client's appetite, food intake, and food tolerance; assess the client for pain after eating, abdominal distention, nausea, and vomiting *to help determine his nutritional status and detect passage of stones from the duct or increasing obstruction.*
- Use the guaiac test *to detect occult blood in stools.* Guaiac testing detects occult bleeding caused by decreased prothrombin synthesis if the liver is inflamed.
- Monitor the administration of I.V. fluids *to provide needed fluids and electrolytes.*

For diagnostic testing

- Prepare the client for upper GI studies, including explaining procedures and their rationales, administering a

laxative if ordered, and instituting any dietary restrictions required by testing, such as clear liquids the evening before, *to decrease client anxiety and help reduce contents in the GI tract.*
- If necessary, prepare the client for a cholecystogram, as follows:
– Explain the procedure and its rationale to the client *to help relieve fear and anxiety.*
– Provide a clear-liquid dinner the evening before the cholecystogram *to help reduce contents in the GI tract.*
– Assess the client for allergies to iodine or seafood and contact the physician if the client has an allergy. Administer dye tablets, as ordered (usually, Telepaque, Tablets VI, one every 5 minutes beginning at 6 p.m.); provide a full glass of water with each tablet, monitoring for signs of an allergic reaction. *Telepaque is a dye that collects in the gallbladder to outline it on the X-ray. Ultrasound examinations substitute for or accompany the cholecystogram.*
– Administer enemas, as ordered. One or two enemas may be needed *to clean the colon.*
– Provide nothing by mouth after midnight *to keep the colon free from contents.*
– After the client returns from the examination, resume the client's diet and fluids as ordered, *which promotes return to a normal bowel pattern.*

Preoperative care (traditional surgery)

- Perform usual preoperative preparations, including an explanation of the T tube the client may have after surgery. If the surgery involves exploration of the common bile duct, the client will have a T tube placed in the common duct to promote drainage.

Postoperative care

- Perform routine postoperative care. Check the client's vital signs, fluid and electrolyte levels, Hb level, WBC count, and $Paco_2$ level *to help determine the client's postoperative status.*
- Check the client's skin for relief from jaundice and edema. *Jaundice should gradually fade. Edema shouldn't be present postoperatively.*
- Have the client turn, deep-breathe, cough, and use a respiratory aid every 2 hours; increase walking as tolerated *to help prevent such complications as atelectasis after surgery;* administer pain medications as needed *to relieve pain with breathing caused by the right upper quadrant incision.*
- Observe drainage in the T tube bile collection container, and keep the container below the incisional level; main-

Caring for surgical wounds

Purpose

Proper care of surgical wounds helps prevent infection, protects the skin from maceration and excoriation, allows removal and measurement of wound drainage, and promotes comfort. When a surgical incision is primarily closed, the incision is covered with a sterile dressing for 24 to 48 hours. After 48 hours, the incision can be covered by a dressing or left open to air.

Implementation

- Because many physicians prefer to change the first postoperative dressing, avoid changing it unless ordered. If you have no such order and drainage is seeping through the dressing, reinforce the dressing with fresh sterile gauze. To prevent bacterial growth, don't allow a reinforced dressing to remain in place longer than 24 hours. Replace any dressing that becomes wet from the outside as soon as possible.
- Check the physician's order for wound care instructions
- Explain the procedure to the client.
- Position the client as comfortably as possible, with the wound site exposed.
- Wash your hands.
- Put on a gown, if necessary, and clean gloves.
- When the procedure is complete, document appearance of wound site and color, consistency, amount, and odor of any drainage.

Removing the old dressing

- Hold the skin and pull the tape or dressing toward the wound. Remove the soiled dressing. If needed, loosen gauze with sterile normal saline solution.
- Check the dressing for the amount, type, color, and odor of drainage. Discard the dressing and gloves in a waterproof trash bag.

Caring for the wound or incision

- Establish a sterile field for equipment and supplies. Squeeze the needed amount of ordered ointment onto the sterile field. Put on sterile gloves.
- If you aren't using prepackaged swabs, saturate sterile gauze pads with the prescribed cleaning agent.
- Squeeze excess solution from the pad or swab. Wipe once from the top to the bottom of the incision and then discard the pad or swab. With a second pad, wipe from top to bottom in a vertical path next to the incision and then discard the pad.

- Continue to work outward from the incision in lines running parallel to it. Always wipe from the clean area toward the less-clean area. Use each pad or swab for only one stroke. Use sterile cotton-tipped applicators to clean tight-fitting wire sutures, deep wounds, or wounds with pockets.
- If the client has a surgical drain, clean the drain's surface last. Clean the surrounding skin by wiping in half or full circles from the drain site outward.
- Clean at least 1″ (2.5 cm) beyond the new dressing or 2″ (5 cm) beyond the incision.
- Check for signs of infection, dehiscence, or evisceration. If you observe such signs or the client reports pain, notify the physician.
- Wash the surrounding skin with soap and water, and pat it dry. Apply prescribed topical medication and a skin protectant, if warranted.
- Pack open wounds with sterile moist gauze using the wet-to-damp method. Avoid using cotton-lined gauze pads.

Applying a fresh gauze dressing

- Place a sterile 4″ × 4″ gauze pad at the wound center, and move the pad outward to the edges of the wound site. Extend the gauze at least 1″ beyond the incision in each direction. Use enough sterile dressings to absorb all drainage until the next dressing change.
- Secure the dressing with strips of tape, a T-binder, or Montgomery straps.

Dressing a wound with a drain

- Use a precut sterile 4″ × 4″ gauze pad.
- Place the pad close to the skin around the drain so that the tubing fits into the slit. Press a second pad around the drain from the opposite direction to encircle the tubing.
- Layer as many uncut sterile pads around the tubing as needed to absorb drainage. Secure the dressing with tape, a T-binder, or Montgomery straps.

Pouching a wound

- To create a pouch, first measure the wound, and cut an opening in the collection pouch's facing ⅛″ (0.3 cm) larger than the wound.
- Make sure surrounding skin is clean and dry and then apply a skin protectant.

Caring for surgical wounds (continued)

- Make sure the drainage port at the bottom of the pouch is closed. Then press the contoured pouch opening around the wound, beginning at its lower edge.
- To empty the pouch, put on gloves, insert bottom half of the pouch into a graduated container, and open the drainage port.

- Wipe the bottom of the pouch and the drainage port with a sterile gauze pad; reseal the port. Change the pouch if it leaks or becomes loose.

---

tain the client on I.V. fluids only, as ordered. *The T tube uses gravity. I.V. fluids nourish the client until GI functions return; then food intake provides nourishment.*
- Clamp the T tube, when ordered, to aid fat digestion. If the client experiences no pain, nausea, or vomiting after eating, the physician removes the T tube. (A cholangiogram may be performed to confirm the absence of stones before the T tube is removed.) If the client is discharged with a T tube in place, provide instructions for home care *to ensure adequate care.* Maintain gravity drainage until the surgeon decides healing has occurred and bile is draining into the duodenum. The tube will then be clamped. Instruct the client to take a daily shower to keep the insertion site clean.
- Check the wound site every 4 hours for 24 to 48 hours *to observe for signs of bleeding and infection.* Change the dressing as needed and perform wound care, using aseptic technique. (See *Caring for surgical wounds.*)
- Measure the client's abdominal girth, check stool color, and monitor for flatus. Begin a clear liquid diet, when ordered, after bowel sounds return and the client can pass flatus; advance to a regular diet as tolerated. *The GI tract begins to regain function after the second postoperative day. Passage of flatus represents significant progress. The client's appetite slowly increases. Abdominal girth measurement will detect the development of ileus.*
- Prepare the client for discharge by reviewing home care instructions and activity restrictions *to ensure appropriate care.* Wound care includes washing the area while the client is bathing, noting untoward signs (drainage, warmth, tenderness), and keeping the area free from dressings and pressure from clothing. The client may not lift or carry heavy items for 6 weeks but can perform light household activities and cooking, as desired. The client should return to the physician if pain or food intolerance recurs.

Evaluation
- The client gains relief from jaundice, gallstones, and pain after surgery.
- The client has no postoperative complications.
- The client performs self-care activities and increases nutritional intake to restore nutritional balance.

Cirrhosis

CIRRHOSIS of the liver is a severe, life-threatening condition. Fibrotic, scarred tissues and fatty deposits gradually replace functioning liver cells. About 50% of cirrhosis results from alcoholism. Other causes include HEPATITIS, chemical destruction (from drugs, such as vinyl chloride), and bacterial liver infections. The cirrhotic liver shows patchy areas of regenerated cells that give the liver capsule a hobnailed, irregular appearance.

The pathophysiologic changes of cirrhosis arise from portal vein hypertension, leading to hypoalbuminemia and excessive venous pressures and causing esophageal varices and hemorrhoids, ascites, hyperaldosteronism, and hepatic encephalopathy. (See *Pathophysiologic changes caused by cirrhosis,* page 438.)

Possible causes
- Alcoholism and resulting malnutrition
- Autoimmune disease, such as sarcoidosis or chronic inflammatory bowel disease
- Exposure to hepatitis (types A, B, C, and D viral hepatitis) or toxic substances

Data collection findings
- Weakness
- Nausea
- Vomiting
- Fatigue
- Diarrhea
- Constipation

Pathophysiologic changes caused by cirrhosis

This table outlines and defines the pathophysiologic changes in the client with cirrhosis.

CHANGES	DEFINITION
Portal vein hypertension	The portal vein empties into the liver. Scarring or obstruction in the liver causes backup in the portal vein, producing portal vein hypertension.
Hypoalbuminemia	The contents of the portal vein and blood serum contain albumin and globulin, two serum proteins. Albumin leaks out of the portal vein into the peritoneal cavity because the portal vein is distended by portal vein hypertension. Hypoalbuminemia is loss of albumin from the blood serum.
Esophageal varices	Portal vein hypertension leads to increased pressures in veins, causing esophageal varices and hemorrhoids.
Ascites	Albumin draws fluids with it into the abdominal cavity, causing a fluid accumulation called ascites.
Hyperaldosteronism	Only the liver metabolizes aldosterone. A cirrhotic liver can't perform its normal functions. Therefore, aldosterone builds up (hyperaldosteronism), leading to fluid retention and edema.
Portal-systemic (hepatic) encephalopathy	Buildup of nitrogenous and biliary products in the blood causes a pathologic brain cell condition (encephalopathy). The wastes accumulate because the dysfunctional liver can't metabolize and excrete them.

- Anorexia
- Indigestion
- Gynecomastia
- Muscle cramps
- Jaundice
- Pallor
- Petechiae
- Edema
- Asterixis
- Ascites
- Abdominal pain (possibly because of an enlarged liver)
- Decreased mental function and fine motor skills

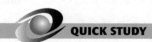 **QUICK STUDY**

To remember the signs of impending hepatic encephalopathy, know your **ABC**s:
>   **A**sterixis – Ask the client to hold his arms straight in front and look for hand tremors.
>   **B**ehavioral changes – Assess the client for personality changes.
>   **C**larity – Assess the client for mental status changes.

Diagnostic findings
- Esophagogastroduodenoscopy reveals bleeding esophageal varices, stomach irritation or ulceration, or duodenal bleeding and irritation.
- Chest X-ray reveals pulmonary condition.
- Liver biopsy confirms the diagnosis.
- EEG determines cerebral functioning.
- Blood studies reveal decreased platelets and HCT and decreased levels of Hb, albumin, serum electrolytes (sodium, potassium, chloride, magnesium), and folate.
- Blood studies reveal elevated levels of globulin, ammonia, total bilirubin, alkaline phosphatase, AST, ALT, and LD and increased thymol turbidity.
- Urine studies show increased levels of bilirubin and urobilinogen.
- Stool studies reveal decreasing urobilinogen levels.

Nursing diagnoses
- Imbalanced nutrition: Less than body requirements
- Ineffective breathing pattern
- Risk for impaired skin integrity
- Risk for injury

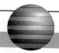

CLINICAL SITUATION

Caring for the client with cirrhosis

A 54-year-old male client, a manufacturer of plastic ornaments, enters the hospital with a tentative medical diagnosis of cirrhosis of the liver. The client has been ill at home for the past 6 weeks after developing viral hepatitis B. For 25 years, he has worked in a plastics factory, handling liquid materials. The client appears pale, weak, and fatigued. He's scheduled for a liver biopsy.

What nursing measures can help prevent hemorrhage after the liver biopsy?

● Apply a snug dressing over the biopsy sight and have the client lie on his right side to assist in splinting the site for 1 to 4 hours, as ordered.

● Check vital signs frequently to ensure the client's safety. For example, check vital signs every 15 minutes for 1 hour, then every 30 minutes for 1 hour, and then every hour for the first 8 to 12 hours. After 8 to 12 hours, begin ambulation, if ordered.

The nurse is monitoring the client for nausea and vomiting. If the vomitus contains blood, the nurse should
prepare for treatment of esophageal varices. What treatment would be anticipated?

Treatment can vary:

● Minor bleeding may warrant nasogastric tube insertion and antacid administration.

● Major bleeding may require I.V. administration of vasopressin to cause splanchnic vasoconstriction.

● Uncontrolled bleeding may necessitate a Sengstaken-Blakemore (S-B) tube. The S-B tube has a triple lumen to the esophageal balloon, gastric balloon, and gastric suction. Periodically, the esophageal balloon must be deflated and reinflated to prevent compression trauma to the esophageal venous circulation. The physician may order ice-water saline lavages to decrease the client's bleeding. The nurse will need to deflate and reinflate the esophageal balloon, as ordered.

Questions for further thought

● Why would vitamin K be ordered for a client with bleeding?
● What are key assessments after the removal of an S-B tube?

Treatment

● Blood transfusions
● Fluid restriction (usually to 1,500 ml per day)
● Gastric intubation and esophageal balloon tamponade for bleeding esophageal varices (Sengstaken-Blakemore method and Minnesota tube method)
● I.V. therapy using colloid volume expanders or crystalloids
● Oxygen therapy (may require ET intubation and mechanical ventilation)
● Paracentesis to reduce abdominal pressure from ascites
● Portal-systemic shunting as a last resort for a client with bleeding esophageal varices and portal hypertension
● Sclerotherapy, if the client continues to experience repeated hemorrhagic episodes despite conservative treatment
● Sodium restriction (usually up to 500 mg per day)
● Surgical intervention, such as peritoneovenous shunt

Drug therapy options
● Antibiotic: neomycin (Neo-fradin)
● Antiemetic: trimethobenzamide (Tigan)
● Beta-adrenergic blocker: propranolol (Inderal)
● Diuretic: furosemide (Lasix), spironolactone (Aldactone)
● Hemostatic: vasopressin (Pitressin)
● Laxative: lactulose (Cephulac)
● Vitamin K: phytonadione (AquaMEPHYTON)

Patient care goals
● The client will retain maximum liver functioning.
● The client won't experience uncontrolled bleeding episodes, infections, or respiratory complications.
● The client's skin integrity will remain intact.
● The client will retain mental capacity and functions.

Nursing interventions
● Assess respiratory status frequently *because abdominal distention may interfere with lung expansion.* Position the client to facilitate breathing.
● Check skin, gums, stool, and emesis regularly for bleeding *to recognize early signs of bleeding and prevent hemorrhage.*
● Apply pressure to injection sites *to prevent bleeding.*
● Warn the client against taking aspirin, straining during defecation, and blowing his nose or sneezing too vigor-

ously *to avoid bleeding.* Also, suggest using an electric razor and soft toothbrush.

● Observe the client closely for signs of behavioral or personality changes — especially increased stupor, lethargy, hallucinations, and neuromuscular dysfunction — *which may indicate increased ammonia levels.*

● Wake the client periodically *to determine LOC.*

● Watch for asterixis, *a sign of developing hepatic encephalopathy.*

 SPOT CHECK

What is the underlying cause of hepatic encephalopathy?
Answer: Elevated blood ammonia levels.

● Monitor ammonia levels *to determine the effectiveness of lactulose therapy.*

● Weigh the client and measure abdominal girth daily, inspect the ankles and sacrum for dependent edema, and accurately record intake and output *to assess fluid retention.*

● Carefully evaluate the client before, during, and after paracentesis *because drastic loss of fluid may induce shock.*

● Avoid using soap when bathing the client; instead, use lubricating lotion or moisturizing agents *to prevent skin breakdown associated with edema and pruritus.*

● Handle the client gently and turn and reposition him often *to keep the skin intact.*

● Encourage rest and good nutrition *to help the client conserve energy and to decrease metabolic demands on the liver.*

● Review dietary instructions *to ensure nutritional needs are met,* including following a diet of modified protein (70 to 100 g daily), carbohydrate intake to spare protein, and modified fat as desired; total intake should range from 2,000 to 3,000 calories daily. Dietary needs result from the liver's inability to use nutrients properly.

Evaluation

● The client exhibits no evidence of respiratory distress.

● The client doesn't exhibit altered LOC or confusion.

● The client's skin exhibits no evidence of redness, breakdown, or infection.

● The client remains free from coagulation complications and is aware of how to help prevent bleeding episodes.

● The client verbalizes understanding of dietary restrictions, the need to avoid exposure to infections, abstaining

from alcohol, and medication regimen. (See *Caring for the client with cirrhosis,* page 439.)

Colorectal cancer

Colorectal cancer is a malignant tumor of the colon or rectum. It may be primary or metastatic. It begins when unregulated cell growth and uncontrolled cell division develop into a neoplasm. Adenocarcinomas then infiltrate and cause obstruction, ulcerations, and hemorrhage.

Possible causes

● Aging
● Chronic constipation
● Chronic ulcerative colitis
● Diverticulosis
● Familial polyposis
● Low-fiber, high-carbohydrate diet
● Diet high in animal fat

Data collection findings

● Abdominal cramping
● Abdominal distention
● Anorexia
● Change in bowel habits and shape of stools
● Diarrhea and constipation
● Fecal oozing
● Melena
● Pallor
● Palpable mass
● Rectal bleeding
● Vomiting
● Weakness
● Weight loss

Diagnostic findings

● Barium enema is used to locate a mass.
● Biopsy is positive for cancer cells.
● Carcinoembryonic antigen (CEA) is positive.
● Colonoscopy or sigmoidoscopy is used to identify and locate a mass.
● Digital rectal examination is used to detect a mass.
● Fecal occult blood test is positive.
● Lower GI series shows the location of a mass.
● Hematology shows decreased Hb level and HCT.

Nursing diagnoses

● Anxiety
● Imbalanced nutrition: Less than body requirements
● Risk for deficient fluid volume

Treatment
- Radiation therapy
- Surgery, depending on tumor location

Drug therapy options
- Antiemetic: prochlorperazine (Compazine), ondansetron (Zofran)
- Antineoplastic: doxorubicin (Adriamycin), 5-fluorouracil (Adrucil)
- Folic acid derivative: leucovorin (citrovorum factor)
- Immunomodulator: levamisole (Ergamisol)

Patient care goals
- The client will verbalize decreased anxiety.
- The client will maintain adequate fluid balance.
- The client will receive adequate nutritional intake.

Nursing interventions
- Assess GI status *to determine baseline and detect changes in the client's condition.*
- Monitor and record vital signs and intake and output, laboratory studies, and daily weight *to assess fluid and electrolyte status.*
- Monitor and record the color, consistency, amount, and frequency of stools *to detect early changes and bleeding.*
- Monitor for bleeding, infection, and electrolyte imbalance *to detect early changes and prevent complications.*
- Maintain the client's diet *to meet metabolic needs and promote healing.*
- Keep the client in semi-Fowler's position *to promote emptying of the GI tract.*
- Instruct the client about the need for TPN *to improve nutritional status when the client can't consume adequate calories through the GI tract.*
- Administer postoperative care if indicated (monitor vital signs and intake and output; make sure the NG tube is kept patent; monitor the dressing for drainage; assess the wound for infection; assist with turning, coughing, deep breathing, and incentive spirometry; medicate for pain as necessary or guide the client with use of client-controlled analgesia) *to prevent complications and promote healing.* (See *Performing nasogastric tube care.*)
- Encourage the client to express feelings about changes in his body image and a fear of dying, and support coping mechanisms *to increase the potential for further adaptive behavior.*
- Provide skin and mouth care *to maintain tissue integrity.*
- Provide rest periods *to promote healing and conserve energy.*

NURSING PROCEDURE

Performing nasogastric tube care

Purpose
Providing effective nasogastric (NG) tube care requires meticulous monitoring of the client and the equipment. Monitoring the client involves checking drainage from the NG tube and assessing GI function. Monitoring the equipment involves verifying correct tube placement and irrigating the tube to ensure patency and to prevent mucosal damage.

Implementation
- Explain the procedure to the client and provide privacy.
- Wash your hands and put on gloves.
- Inject 10 cc of air and auscultate the epigastric area with a stethoscope. Aspirate stomach contents *to check correct positioning in the stomach and to prevent the client from aspirating the irrigant.*
- Measure the amount of irrigant in the bulb syringe or in the 60-ml catheter-tip syringe (usually 10 to 20 ml) *to maintain an accurate intake and output record.*
- When suctioning with a Salem sump tube or a Levin tube, unclamp and disconnect the tube from the suction equipment while holding it over a linen-saver pad or an emesis basin *to collect any drainage.*
- Slowly instill the irrigant into the NG tube. When irrigating a Salem sump tube, you may instill small amounts of solution into the vent lumen without interrupting suction; however, you should instill greater amounts into the larger, primary lumen.
- Gently aspirate the solution with the bulb syringe or a 60-ml catheter-tip syringe or connect the tube to the suction equipment as ordered. *Gentle aspiration prevents excessive pressure on the suture line and the delicate gastric mucosa.* Report any bleeding.
- Reconnect the tube to suction after completing irrigation.
- Document tube placement confirmation (usually every 4 to 8 hours). Keep a precise record of fluid intake and output, including the instilled irrigant in fluid input. Track the irrigation schedule and note the actual time of each irrigation. Describe drainage color, consistency, odor, and amount. Also, note tape change times and the condition of the nares.

- Provide postchemotherapeutic and postradiation nursing care *to promote healing and prevent complications.*
- Administer antiemetics and antidiarrheals, as prescribed, *to prevent further fluid loss.*

- Review key teaching topics with the client *to ensure adequate knowledge about his condition and treatment,* including:
  - performing ostomy self-care if indicated
  - monitoring changes in bowel elimination
  - self-monitoring for infection
  - alternating rest periods with activity
  - contacting the United Ostomy Association and the American Cancer Society.

Evaluation

- The client verbalizes knowledge about the disease and treatment, expresses feelings of anxiety, and describes coping skills to help manage increased anxiety.
- The client has a balanced intake and output and normal vital signs.
- The client maintains adequate nutritional intake through diet or TPN and understands dietary instructions for discharge.

Crohn's disease

CROHN'S DISEASE is a chronic inflammatory disease of the small intestine, usually affecting the terminal ileum. It also sometimes affects the large intestine, usually in the ascending colon. It's slowly progressive with exacerbations and remissions.

Possible causes

- Emotional upsets
- Fried foods
- Milk and milk products
- Unknown

Data collection findings

- Abdominal cramps and spasms after meals
- Chronic diarrhea with blood
- Fever
- Flatulence
- Nausea
- Pain in lower right quadrant
- Weight loss

Diagnostic findings

- Abdominal X-ray shows congested, thickened, fibrosed, and narrowed intestinal wall.
- Barium enema shows lesions in the terminal ileum.
- Fecal fat test shows increased fat.

- Fecal occult blood test is positive.
- Proctosigmoidoscopy shows ulceration.
- Upper GI series shows a classic string sign: segments of stricture separated by normal bowel.
- CBC usually shows a decreased Hb level and HCT and may show elevated WBC count.
- Low albumin and protein levels reflect poor absorption of protein.
- ESR is elevated due to inflammation.

Nursing diagnoses

- Anxiety
- Diarrhea
- Imbalanced nutrition: Less than body requirements

Treatment

- Colectomy with ileostomy in many clients with extensive disease of the large intestine and rectum
- Small, frequent meals of a diet high in protein, calories, and carbohydrates and low in fat, fiber, and residue with bland foods and restricted intake of milk and gas-forming foods or no food or fluids
- TPN to rest the bowel

Drug therapy options

- Analgesic: meperidine (Demerol), morphine (MS Contin)
- Antianemic: ferrous sulfate (Feosol), ferrous gluconate (Fergon)
- Antibiotic: sulfasalazine (Azulfidine), metronidazole (Flagyl)
- Anticholinergic: propantheline (Pro-Banthine), dicyclomine (Bentyl)
- Antidiarrheal: diphenoxylate with atropine (Lomotil)
- Antiemetic: prochlorperazine (Compazine)
- Anti-inflammatory: olsalazine (Dipentum)
- Corticosteroid: prednisone (Deltasone)
- Immunosuppressant: mercaptopurine (Purinethol), azathioprine (Imuran)
- Potassium supplement: potassium chloride (K-Lor) administered with food, potassium gluconate (Kaon)

Patient care goals

- The client will verbalize decreased anxiety.
- The client will regain normal bowel function.
- The client will receive adequate nutritional intake.

SPOT CHECK

Why is TPN commonly administered to a client with Crohn's disease?

Answer: To allow the bowel to rest and to treat the client for malnutrition.

Nursing interventions

- Assess GI status (note excessive abdominal distention) and fluid balance *to determine baseline and detect changes in the client's condition.*
- Monitor and record vital signs and intake and output, laboratory studies, daily weight, urine specific gravity, and fecal occult blood *to detect bleeding and dehydration.*
- Monitor the number, amount, and character of stools *to detect deterioration in GI status.*
- Instruct the client about the need for TPN administration *to rest the bowel and promote nutritional status.*
- Administer medications, as prescribed, *to maintain or improve the client's condition.*
- Maintain the client's diet, including withholding food and fluids as necessary, *to minimize GI discomfort.*
- Minimize stress and encourage verbalization of feelings *to allay the client's anxiety.*
- Provide skin and perianal care *to prevent skin breakdown.*
- If surgery is necessary, provide postoperative care (monitor vital signs; monitor dressings for drainage; monitor ileostomy drainage and perform ileostomy care as needed; assess incision for signs of infection; assist with turning, coughing, and deep breathing; get the client out of bed on the 1st postoperative day if stable) *to promote healing and prevent complications.*
- Review key teaching topics with the client *to ensure adequate knowledge about his condition and treatment*, including:
  – performing ileostomy self-care
  – avoiding laxatives and aspirin
  – performing perianal care daily
  – reducing stress
  – recognizing the signs and symptoms of rectal hemorrhage and intestinal obstruction.

Evaluation

- The client verbalizes knowledge about the disease and treatment, expresses feelings of anxiety, and relates coping skills to help manage increased anxiety.

- The client is free from diarrhea and abdominal cramps.
- The client maintains adequate nutritional intake and verbalizes understanding of dietary instructions for discharge.

Diverticular disease

Diverticular disease has two clinical forms: DIVERTICULOSIS and DIVERTICULITIS. Diverticulosis occurs when the intestinal mucosa protrudes through the muscular wall. The common sites for diverticula are in the descending and sigmoid colon, but they may develop anywhere from the proximal end of the pharynx to the anus.

Diverticulitis is an inflammation of the diverticula that may lead to infection, hemorrhage, or obstruction.

Possible causes

- Age (most common in people over age 40)
- Chronic constipation
- Congenital weakening of the intestinal wall
- Low intake of roughage and fiber
- Straining during defecation
- Stress

FAST FACT

The incidence of diverticular disease increases with age, secondary to structural changes in the muscle layers of the colon. Symptoms may be less pronounced and blood in the stool may go undetected due to the poor vision of elderly clients.

Data collection findings

- Anorexia
- Bloody stools
- Change in bowel habits
- Constipation and diarrhea
- Fever
- Flatulence
- Left lower quadrant pain or midabdominal pain that radiates to the back
- Nausea
- Rectal bleeding

Diagnostic findings

- Barium enema (contraindicated in clients with acute diverticulitis) shows inflammation, narrow lumen of the bowel, and diverticula.

Gastrointestinal tubes

TYPE	SITE AND PURPOSE	NURSING CONSIDERATIONS
Salem sump	Nasogastric (NG) Suctioning or feeding	• Make sure that blue tubing is free from secretions • Clamp tube for ambulation and note its tolerance • Irrigate tube with 20 to 30 ml of normal saline solution.
Levin tube	NG Suctioning or feeding	• Be sure to connect tube to low suction to prevent gastric irritation • Irrigate tube with 20 to 30 ml of normal saline solution
Nutriflex	NG Feeding	• Use 50-ml syringe with 20 ml of water to irrigate (small syringe may cause tube to rupture from excessive pressure) • Use infusion pump, which can exert only up to 40 psi (tube bursting pressure is 80 psi)
Gastrostomy	Stomach Suctioning or feeding	• Know that tube uses gravity drainage • As required, clamp tube and open for residuals
Sengstaken-Blakemore	Esophagus and stomach Compressing esophageal varices	• Inflate (never irrigate) esophageal balloon with air and irrigate stomach tube with 20 to 30 ml normal saline solution as required
Jejunostomy	Jejunum Feeding	• Know that feedings may be intermittent or continuous with an infusion pump
Dobhoff	Jejunum Feeding	• Know that tube has mercury tip for X-ray visualization and assists in passage • Know that tube has same cautions as Nutriflex tube
Cantor	Small to large intestine Suctioning	• Know that mercury is inserted into balloon before insertion to aid passage • Connect tube to suction • Irrigate tube with 20 to 30 ml of normal saline solution
Miller-Abbott	Small to large intestine Suctioning	• Know that mercury is instilled into properly marked opening after tube reaches stomach, to aid passage • Irrigate tube with 20 to 30 ml normal saline solution

• Hematologic study shows increased WBC count and ESR.
• Sigmoidoscopy (contraindicated in clients with acute diverticulitis) shows a thickened wall in the diverticula.
• CT scan shows abscesses or thickening of the bowel.

Nursing diagnoses
• Acute pain
• Chronic pain
• Constipation
• Diarrhea
• Imbalanced nutrition: Less than body requirements

Treatment
• Generally, no treatment for asymptomatic diverticulosis
• Colon resection (for diverticulitis refractory to medical treatment)
• Bland diet, stool softeners, and occasional doses of mineral oil for diverticulosis with pain, mild GI distress, constipation, or difficult defecation

- Bland diet (for diverticulosis after pain subsides) or liquid diet (for mild diverticulitis or diverticulosis before pain subsides); low-fiber diet indicated following the liquid diet; when the client is asymptomatic, low-fat, high-fiber diet recommended
- Temporary colostomy possible for perforation, peritonitis, obstruction, or fistula that accompanies diverticulitis

Drug therapy options
- Analgesic: meperidine (Demerol)
- Antibiotic: gentamicin (Garamycin), tobramycin (Nebcin), clindamycin (Cleocin) (for mild diverticulitis)
- Anticholinergic: propantheline (Pro-Banthine)
- Stool softener: docusate (Colace) for diverticulosis or mild diverticulitis
- Bulk laxative

Patient care goals
- The client's diarrhea or constipation will be controlled.
- The client will verbalize pain relief.
- The client will maintain or regain adequate nutrition.

Nursing interventions
- Assess abdominal distention and bowel sounds *to determine baseline and to detect changes in the client's condition.*
- Monitor and record vital signs, intake and output, and laboratory studies *to assess fluid status.*
- Monitor stools for occult blood *to detect bleeding.*
- Maintain the client's diet *to improve his nutritional status and promote healing.*
- Maintain the position, patency, and low suction of the NG tube *to prevent nausea and vomiting.* (See *Gastrointestinal tubes.*)
- Keep the client in semi-Fowler's position *to promote comfort and GI emptying.*
- Prepare the client for surgery (administer cleansing enemas, osmotic purgative, and antibiotics), if necessary, *to avoid wound contamination from bowel contents during surgery.*
- Provide postoperative care (watch for signs of infection; perform meticulous wound care; watch for signs of postoperative bleeding; assist with turning, coughing, and deep breathing; teach ostomy self-care) *to promote healing and prevent complications.*
- Instruct the client about the need for TPN *to improve nutritional status when the client can't receive nutrition through the GI tract.*
- Administer medications as prescribed *to maintain or improve the client's condition.*

- Review key teaching topics with the client *to ensure adequate knowledge about his condition and treatment,* including:
  – decreasing constipation
  – following dietary recommendations and restrictions
  – avoiding corn, nuts, and fruits and vegetables with seeds
  – monitoring stools for bleeding.

Evaluation
- The client exhibits improved stool consistency and decreased incidence of constipation or diarrhea.
- The client verbalizes adequate pain relief or pain control and can demonstrate pain-relief measures.
- The client maintains adequate nutrition.

Esophageal cancer
Esophageal cancer attacks the esophagus, the muscular tube that runs from the back of the throat to the stomach. Cells in the lining of the esophagus start to multiply rapidly and form a tumor that may spread to other parts of the body.

Nearly always fatal, esophageal cancer usually develops in men over age 60. This disease occurs worldwide, but incidence varies geographically. It's most common in Japan, China, the Middle East, and parts of South Africa.

Possible causes
- Excessive use of alcohol
- Nutritional deficiency
- Smoking

Data collection findings
- Dysphagia
- Weight loss

Diagnostic findings
- Endoscopic examination of the esophagus, punch and brush biopsies, and an exfoliative cytologic test confirm esophageal tumors.
- X-rays of the esophagus, with barium swallow and motility studies, reveal structural and filling defects and reduced peristalsis.

Nursing diagnoses
- Impaired swallowing
- Imbalanced nutrition: Less than body requirements
- Risk for aspiration

NURSING PROCEDURE

Delivering a gastric feeding

Purpose

Gastric tube feedings involve delivery of a liquid feeding formula directly to the stomach (known as *gastric gavage*). Tube feedings may also be delivered to the duodenum or jejunum. Gastric gavage is typically indicated for a client who can't eat normally due to dysphagia, oral or esophageal obstruction, or injury. Gastric feedings also may be given to an unconscious or intubated client or to a client recovering from GI tract surgery who can't ingest food orally.

Implementation

- Explain the procedure to the client.
- Place the client in semi Fowlers or high-Fowler's position (if possible).
- If the client has a nasal or oral tube, cover his chest with a towel or linen-saver pad *to protect him and the bed linens from spills.*
- Assess the client's abdomen for bowel sounds and distention.
- Check placement of the feeding tube *to ensure that it hasn't slipped out since the last feeding.* Never give a tube feeding until you're certain the tube is properly positioned in the client's stomach.
- *To check tube patency and position,* remove the cap or plug from the feeding tube and use a bulb or piston syringe to inject 5 to 10 cc of air through the tube. At the same time, auscultate the client's stomach with the stethoscope. Listen for a whooshing sound to confirm tube positioning in the stomach. Also, aspirate stomach contents to confirm tube patency and placement.
- *To assess gastric emptying,* aspirate and measure residual gastric contents. Hold feedings if residual volume is greater then the amount specified in the physician's order (usually 50 to 100 ml). Reinstill any aspirate obtained.
- Connect the gavage bag tubing to the feeding tube.
- If you're using a bulb or piston syringe, remove the bulb or plunger and attach the syringe to the pinched-off feeding tube to prevent excess air from entering the client's stomach, which causes distention. If you're using an infusion controller, thread the tube from the formula container through the controller, according to the manufacturer's directions. Blue food dye can be added to the feeding to quickly identify aspiration. Purge the tubing of air, and attach it to the feeding tube.

- Open the flow regulator clamp on the gavage bag tubing, and adjust the flow rate as appropriate. When using a bulb syringe, fill the syringe with formula and release the feeding tube *to allow formula to flow through it.* The height at which you hold the syringe determines the flow rate. When the syringe is three-quarters empty, pour more formula into it.
- *To prevent air from entering the tube and the client's stomach,* never allow the syringe to empty completely. If you're using an infusion controller, set the flow rate according to the manufacturer's directions. Always administer a tube feeding slowly — typically 200 to 350 ml over 15 to 30 minutes, depending on the client's tolerance and the physician's order — to prevent sudden stomach distention, which can cause nausea, vomiting, cramps, and diarrhea.
- After administering the appropriate amount of formula, flush the tubing by adding about 60 ml of water to the gavage bag or bulb syringe, or manually flush it using a barrel syringe. This maintains the tube's patency by removing excess formula, which could occlude the tube.
- If you're administering a continuous feeding, flush the feeding tube every 4 hours to help prevent tube occlusion. Monitor gastric emptying every 4 hours.
- To discontinue gastric feeding (depending on the equipment you're using), close the regulator clamp on the gavage bag tubing, disconnect the syringe from the feeding tube, or turn off the infusion controller.
- Cover the end of the feeding tube with its plug or cap *to prevent leakage and contamination.*
- Leave the client in semi-Fowler's or high Fowler's position for at least 30 minutes.
- On the intake and output sheet, record the date, volume of formula, and volume of water. In your notes, document abdominal assessment findings (including tube exit site, if appropriate); amount of residual gastric contents; verification of tube placement; amount, type, and time of feeding; and tube patency. Discuss the client's tolerance of the feeding, including nausea, vomiting, cramping, diarrhea, and distention.

Treatment

- Endoscopic laser treatment and bipolar electrocoagulation to help restore swallowing by vaporizing cancerous tissue
- Esophageal dilation
- Gastrostomy or jejunostomy to help provide adequate nutrition
- Radiation therapy

● Radical surgery to excise the tumor and resect either the esophagus or the stomach and the esophagus

Drug therapy options
● Analgesic: morphine (MS Contin), fentanyl (Duragesic-25)
● Antineoplastic: porfimer (Photofrin)

Patient care goals
● The client will have improved swallowing abilities related to diet modification.
● The client will maintain weight within an acceptable range.
● The client won't aspirate.

Nursing interventions
● Before surgery, answer the client's questions and let him know what to expect after surgery (gastrostomy tubes, closed chest drainage, NG suctioning) *to allay his anxiety.*
● After surgery, monitor vital signs and watch for unexpected changes *to detect early signs of complications and avoid treatment delay.* If surgery included an esophageal anastomosis, keep the client flat on his back *to avoid tension on the suture line.*
● Promote adequate nutrition, and assess the client's nutritional and hydration status *to determine the need for supplementary parenteral feedings.*
● Place the client in Fowler's position for meals and allow plenty of time to eat *to avoid aspiration of food.*
● Provide high-calorie, high-protein, pureed food as needed *to meet increased metabolic demands and to prevent aspiration.*
● If the client has a gastrostomy tube, give food slowly, using gravity to adjust the flow rate *to prevent abdominal discomfort.* The prescribed amount usually ranges from 200 to 500 ml. Offer him something to chew before each feeding *to promote gastric secretions and a semblance of normal eating.* (See *Delivering a gastric feeding.*)
● Instruct the family in gastrostomy tube care (checking tube patency before each feeding, providing skin care around the tube, and keeping the client upright during and after feedings) *to avoid complications.*
● Provide emotional support for the client and his family *to help them cope with the terminal illness.*

Evaluation
● The client reports improved swallowing abilities.
● The client maintains an adequate weight.

● The client doesn't display signs or symptoms of aspiration.

Gastric cancer
Gastric cancer involves a malignant stomach tumor. It may be primary or metastatic. Its precise cause is unknown, but it's commonly associated with gastritis, gastric atrophy, and other conditions. About one-half of gastric cancers occur in the pyloric area of the stomach.

Possible causes
● Achlorhydria
● Chronic gastritis
● Peptic ulcer
● High intake of salted and smoked foods
● Low intake of vegetables and fruits
● Pernicious anemia

Data collection findings
● Indigestion
● Pain after eating that isn't relieved by antacids
● Fatigue
● Malaise
● Anorexia
● Nausea and vomiting
● Epigastric fullness and pain
● Weakness
● Hematemesis
● Melena
● Regurgitation
● Syncope
● Weight loss
● Shortness of breath

Diagnostic findings
● Blood chemistry shows increased levels of AST, LD, and amylase.
● CEA test is positive.
● Fecal occult blood test is positive.
● Gastric analysis shows positive cancer cells and achlorhydria.
● Gastroscopy biopsy is positive for cancer cells.
● Upper GI series reveals a gastric mass.
● Hematology shows decreased Hb level and HCT.
● Gastric hydrochloric acid level is decreased.

SPOT CHECK

The nurse is reviewing the diagnostic data of a client suspected of having gastric cancer. What laboratory finding is the nurse most likely to find?

A. Elevated Hb level and HCT
B. Negative fecal occult blood test
C. Subnormal gastric hydrochloric acid level
D. Negative CEA test

Answer: C. One manifestation of gastric cancer is achlorhydria, an absence of free hydrochloric acid in the stomach. In gastric cancer, subnormal Hb level and HCT is most likely; fecal occult blood test is most likely to be positive. The CEA test would most likely be positive in gastric cancer.

Nursing diagnoses
- Acute pain
- Risk for deficient fluid volume
- Fear

Treatment
- Gastric surgery: gastroduodenostomy, gastrojejunostomy, partial gastric resection, total gastrectomy
- TPN
- High-calorie diet
- Radiation therapy

Drug therapy options
- Analgesic: meperidine (Demerol), morphine (MS Contin)
- Antiemetic: prochlorperazine (Compazine)
- Antineoplastic: carmustine (BiCNU), 5-fluorouracil (Adrucil)
- Vitamin supplement: folic acid (Folvite), cyanocobalamin (vitamin B_{12}) for clients who have undergone total gastrectomy

Patient care goals
- The client will express feelings of increased comfort and pain relief.
- The client will maintain adequate fluid status.
- The client will have decreased fear over illness.

Nursing interventions
- Assess GI status postoperatively *to monitor the client for dumping syndrome (weakness, nausea, flatulence, and palpitations 30 minutes after a meal).*
- Monitor and record vital signs, intake and output, laboratory studies, and daily weight *to determine baseline and detect early changes in the client's condition.*
- Monitor the consistency, amount, and frequency of stools *to detect GI compromise.*
- Monitor the color of stools *to detect bleeding and to prevent hemorrhage.*
- Maintain the client's diet *to promote nutritional balance.*
- Maintain the position, patency, and low suction of the NG tube (without irrigating or repositioning the NG tube because it may put pressure on the suture line) *to prevent complications, nausea, and vomiting.*
- Instruct the client on the need for TPN administration for 1 week or longer if gastric surgery is extensive *to meet metabolic needs and to promote wound healing.*
- Administer medications, as prescribed, *to maintain or improve the client's condition.*
- Support client coping mechanisms *to increase the potential for adaptive behavior.*
- Provide skin and mouth care *to prevent skin breakdown and damage to the oral mucosa and to improve nutritional intake.*
- Provide rest periods *to conserve energy.*

Evaluation
- The client reports adequate pain control.
- The client doesn't display signs of dehydration.
- The client expresses less fear over his illness.

Gastritis
GASTRITIS is an inflammation of the gastric mucosa (the stomach lining). It may be acute or chronic. Acute gastritis produces mucosal reddening, edema, hemorrhage, and erosion. Chronic gastritis is common among elderly people and people with pernicious anemia. In chronic atrophic gastritis, all stomach mucosal layers are inflamed.

Possible causes
Acute gastritis
- Chronic ingestion of irritating foods, spicy foods, or alcohol
- Drugs, such as aspirin and other NSAIDs (in large doses), cytotoxic agents, caffeine, corticosteroids, antimetabolites, phenylbutazone, and indomethacin
- Ingestion of poisons, especially dichlorodiphenyltrichloroethane (DDT), ammonia, mercury, carbon tetrachloride, and corrosive substances

- Endotoxins released from infecting bacteria, such as staphylococci, *Escherichia coli*, and salmonella

Chronic gastritis
- Alcohol ingestion
- Cigarette smoke
- Environmental irritants
- Peptic ulcer disease

Data collection findings
- Abdominal cramping
- Epigastric discomfort
- Hematemesis
- Indigestion

Diagnostic findings
- Fecal occult blood test can detect occult blood in vomitus and stools if the client has gastric bleeding.
- Blood studies show low Hb level and HCT when significant bleeding has occurred.
- Upper GI endoscopy with biopsy confirms the diagnosis when performed within 24 hours of bleeding.
- Upper GI series may be performed to exclude serious lesions.

Nursing diagnoses
- Risk for deficient fluid volume
- Imbalanced nutrition: Less than body requirements
- Acute pain

Treatment
- Angiography with vasopressin infused in normal saline solution (when gastritis causes massive bleeding)
- Blood transfusion
- I.V. fluid therapy
- NG lavage to control bleeding
- Oxygen therapy, if necessary
- Partial or total gastrectomy (rare)
- Vagotomy and pyloroplasty (limited success when conservative treatments have failed)

Drug therapy options
- Antibiotics: according to sensitivity of the infecting organism (if the cause is bacterial)
- Antidote: according to the ingested poison (if the cause is poisoning)
- H_2-receptor antagonist: cimetidine (Tagamet), ranitidine (Zantac), famotidine (Pepcid), nizatidine (Axid) to block gastric secretions

Patient care goals
- The client will maintain normal fluid volume.
- The client will maintain weight.
- The client will express feelings of increased comfort and pain relief.

Nursing interventions
- If the client is vomiting, give antiemetics and I.V. fluids *to prevent dehydration and electrolyte imbalance.*
- Monitor fluid intake and output and electrolyte levels *to detect early signs of dehydration and electrolyte loss.*
- Provide a bland diet *to prevent recurrence.* Monitor the client for recurrent symptoms as food is reintroduced.
- Offer smaller, more frequent meals *to reduce irritating gastric secretions.* Eliminate foods that cause gastric upset *to prevent gastric irritation.*
- If surgery is necessary, prepare the client preoperatively and provide appropriate postoperative care *to decrease preoperative anxiety and prevent intraoperative and postoperative complications.*
- Administer antacids and other prescribed medications *to promote gastric healing.*
- Urge the client to seek immediate attention for recurring symptoms, such as hematemesis, nausea, and vomiting, *to prevent complications such as GI hemorrhage.*
- Urge the client to take prophylactic medications as prescribed *to prevent recurring symptoms.*
- Provide emotional support to the client *to help him manage his symptoms.*

Evaluation
- The client doesn't display signs of dehydration.
- The client maintains his weight.
- The client reports adequate pain control.

Gastroenteritis

GASTROENTERITIS is irritation and inflammation of the digestive tract characterized by diarrhea, nausea, vomiting, and abdominal cramping. It occurs in all age-groups and is usually self-limiting in adults.

In the United States, gastroenteritis ranks second to the common cold as a cause of lost work time and fifth as the cause of death among young children. It can also be life-threatening in elderly and debilitated persons. It's a major cause of morbidity and mortality in developing nations.

This disorder is also called *intestinal flu, traveler's diarrhea, viral enteritis,* and *food poisoning.*

Possible causes

- Amoebae, especially *Entamoeba histolytica*
- Bacteria (responsible for acute food poisoning), such as *Staphylococcus aureus*, salmonella, shigella, *Clostridium botulinum*, *Escherichia coli*, *C. perfringens*
- Drug reactions (especially antibiotics)
- Enzyme deficiencies
- Food allergens
- Ingestion of toxins, such as plants or toadstools (mushrooms)
- Parasites, such as ascaris, Enterobius, *Trichinella spiralis*
- Viruses (may be responsible for traveler's diarrhea), such as adenovirus, echovirus, or coxsackievirus

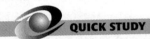 **QUICK STUDY**

Fight the **WAR** against gastroenteritis by remembering these tips:
Wash your hands before handling all foods.
Always cook food thoroughly.
Refrigerate perishable foods promptly.

Data collection findings

- Abdominal discomfort
- Diarrhea
- Nausea

Diagnostic findings

- Stool culture identifies the causative bacterium, parasite, or amoeba.
- Blood culture identifies causative organism.

Nursing diagnoses

- Diarrhea
- Risk for deficient fluid volume
- Acute pain

Treatment

- Increased fluid intake
- I.V. fluid and electrolyte replacement
- Nutritional support

Drug therapy options

- Antibiotic: according to the sensitivity of the causative organism
- Antidiarrheal: camphorated opium tincture (Paregoric), diphenoxylate with atropine (Lomotil), loperamide (Imodium)

- Antiemetic: prochlorperazine (Compazine), trimethobenzamide (Tigan) (should be avoided in clients with viral or bacterial gastroenteritis)

Patient care goals

- The client will maintain adequate fluid volume.
- The client will express feeling of comfort and pain relief.

Nursing interventions

- Administer medications and correlate dosages, routes, and times appropriately with the client's meals and activities; for example, give antiemetics 30 to 60 minutes before meals *to prevent onset of symptoms.*
- If the client is unable to tolerate food, replace lost fluids and electrolytes with clear liquids and sport drinks *to prevent dehydration.*
- Vary the client's diet *to make it more enjoyable and allow some choice of foods.*
- Instruct the client to avoid milk and milk products, *which may exacerbate the condition.*
- Record strict intake and output. Watch for signs of dehydration, such as dry skin and mucous membranes, fever, and sunken eyes, *to prevent complications of dehydration.*
- Wash your hands thoroughly after giving care *to avoid the spread of infection.*
- Instruct the client to perform warm sitz baths three times per day *to relieve anal irritation.*

Evaluation

- The client doesn't display signs of dehydration.
- The client reports adequate pain control.

Gastroesophageal reflux disease

GASTROESOPHAGEAL REFLUX DISEASE (GERD) refers to the backflow, or reflux, of gastric and duodenal contents past the lower esophageal sphincter and into the esophagus. Reflux may cause symptoms or pathologic changes. Persistent reflux may cause reflux esophagitis (inflammation of the esophageal mucosa). The prognosis varies with the underlying cause.

Possible causes

- Any action that decreases lower esophageal sphincter pressure, such as smoking cigarettes and ingesting food, alcohol, anticholinergics (atropine, belladonna, propantheline), and other drugs (morphine, diazepam, meperidine)
- Any condition or position that increases intra-abdominal pressure

- Hiatal hernia (especially in children)
- Long-term NG intubation (more than 5 days)
- Pressure within the stomach that exceeds lower esophageal sphincter pressure
- Pyloric surgery (alteration or removal of the pylorus), which allows reflux of bile or pancreatic juice

Data collection findings
- Heartburn (burning sensation in the upper abdomen)
- Dysphagia

Atypical symptoms
- Asthma
- Atypical chest pain
- Chronic cough
- Laryngitis
- Sore throat

Diagnostic findings
- Barium swallow fluoroscopy indicates reflux.
- Esophageal pH probe reveals reflux.
- Esophagoscopy shows reflux.
- Acid perfusion (Bernstein) test shows that reflux is the cause of symptoms.
- Endoscopy allows visualization and confirmation of pathologic changes in the mucosa.
- Biopsy allows visualization and confirmation of pathologic changes in the mucosa.

Nursing diagnoses
- Risk for aspiration
- Chronic pain
- Deficient knowledge (diet)

Treatment
- Oxygen therapy
- Positional therapy to help relieve symptoms by decreasing intra-abdominal pressure
- Dietary modifications (see *Dietary factors affecting LES pressure*)
- Surgery, which reduces reflux by creating an artificial closure at the gastroesophageal junction (in extreme, chronic cases)

Drug therapy options
- Antacid: aluminum hydroxide (AlternaGEL) administered 1 hour and 3 hours after meals and at bedtime
- GI prokinetic: cisapride (Propulsid)
- GI stimulant: metoclopramide (Reglan), bethanechol (Urecholine)

Dietary factors affecting LES pressure

Various dietary and lifestyle elements can increase or decrease lower esophageal sphincter (LES) pressure. Take these into account as you plan the patient's treatment program.

Increase LES pressure
- Protein
- Carbohydrate
- Nonfat milk
- Low-dose ethanol

Decrease LES pressure
- Fat
- Whole milk
- Orange juice
- Tomatoes
- Antiflatulent (simethicone)
- Chocolate
- High-dose ethanol
- Cigarette smoking
- Lying on right or left side
- Sitting

- H_2-receptor antagonist: cimetidine (Tagamet), ranitidine (Zantac), famotidine (Pepcid), nizatidine (Axid)

Patient care goals
- The client won't show signs of aspiration.
- The client will express feelings of comfort and pain relief.
- The client will have improved knowledge regarding dietary guidelines for GERD.

Nursing interventions
- Develop a diet that takes food preferences into account while helping to minimize reflux symptoms *to ensure compliance.*
- Have the client sleep in reverse Trendelenburg's position (with the head of the bed elevated 6″ to 12″ [15 to 30 cm]) *to reduce intra-abdominal pressure.*

After surgery using a thoracic approach
- Carefully watch and record chest tube drainage and respiratory status *to detect early signs of respiratory distress.*

- If needed, give chest physiotherapy and oxygen *to mobilize secretions and prevent hypoxemia.*
- Place the client with an NG tube in semi-Fowler's position *to help prevent reflux.*
- Offer reassurance and emotional support *to help the client cope with pain and discomfort.*

Evaluation
- The client doesn't display signs of aspiration.
- The client reports adequate pain control.
- The client relates appropriate dietary guidelines.

Hepatitis

HEPATITIS is an inflammation of liver tissue that causes hypertrophy and proliferation of Kupffer's cells and bile stasis. Hepatitis is typically caused by one of five viruses: hepatitis A, B, C, D, or E. Hepatitis may also be drug- or toxin-induced or secondary to infection.

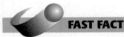
FAST FACT

All health care workers and others at risk should be vaccinated with hepatitis B vaccine. Boosters are given 1 month and 6 months after the initial dose. Antibody response can be checked 1 to 3 months after completing the course of vaccination.

Possible causes
Hepatitis A
- Contaminated food
- Milk
- Water
- Feces

Hepatitis B
- Parenteral (needle sticks)
- Blood
- Sexual contact
- Secretions

Hepatitis C
- Blood or serum (blood transfusion, exposure to contaminated blood)
- Sexual contact

Hepatitis D
- Similar to causes of type B virus

Hepatitis E
- Fecal-oral route

Toxin- and drug-induced hepatitis
- Hepatotoxins, such as alcohol, medications, and industrial toxins

Hepatitis secondary to other infections
- Epstein-Barr
- Herpes simplex
- Varicella zoster
- Cytomegalovirus

Data collection findings
Assessment findings are consistent for the different types of hepatitis, but signs and symptoms progress over several stages: the preicteric phase (usually 1 to 5 days), the icteric phase (usually 1 to 2 weeks), and the posticteric or recovery phase (usually 2 to 12 weeks but sometimes longer in clients with hepatitis B, C, or E). (See *Recognizing fulminant hepatitis.*)

Preicteric phase
- Anorexia
- Aversion to the taste of cigarettes
- Constipation and diarrhea
- Fatigue
- Fever
- Headache
- Hepatomegaly
- Malaise
- Nasal discharge
- Nausea and vomiting
- Pharyngitis
- Pruritus
- Right upper quadrant pain
- Splenomegaly
- Weight loss

Icteric phase
- Clay-colored stools
- Dark urine
- Fatigue
- Hepatomegaly
- Jaundice
- Pruritus
- Splenomegaly
- Weight loss

Posticteric phase
- Decreased hepatomegaly
- Decreased jaundice
- Fatigue
- Improved appetite

Diagnostic findings

● Blood chemistry shows increased ALT, AST, alkaline phosphatase, LD, and bilirubin levels; increased ESR; positive antibody to hepatitis A; positive immunoglobulin anti-delta antigens (in type D); positive hepatitis B surface antigen; and positive hepatitis E antigen.
● Hematology shows increased PT and fibrin-split products.
● Stool specimen reveals hepatitis A virus (in hepatitis A cases).
● Urine chemistry shows increased urobilinogen.

Nursing diagnoses

● Deficient knowledge (client)
● Fatigue
● Imbalanced nutrition: Less than body requirements
● Risk for deficient fluid volume

Treatment

● High-calorie, moderate-protein, high-carbohydrate, low-fat diet in small, frequent meals
● Rest

Drug therapy options

● Antiemetic: prochlorperazine (Compazine)
● Vitamins and minerals: vitamin K (AquaMEPHYTON), ascorbic acid (vitamin C), vitamin B-complex (Mega-B)
● Alpha-interferon and ribavirin (Rebetron) for hepatitis B and C (has demonstrated efficacy in the treatment of hepatitis C)

Patient care goals

● The client will regain adequate nutritional and fluid intake.
● The client will exhibit a decreased level of fatigue.
● The client will learn about the disease and how to prevent infection and transmission.

Nursing interventions

● Assess GI status and watch for bleeding and fulminant hepatitis *to detect early complications.*
● Maintain the client's diet *to meet metabolic needs.*
● Monitor and record vital signs, intake and output, and laboratory studies *to detect early signs of deficient fluid volume.*
● Administer medications, as prescribed, *to maintain or improve the client's condition.*
● Maintain standard precautions. *Hand washing prevents the spread of pathogens to others.*
● Provide rest periods *to conserve the client's energy and reduce his metabolic demands.*

Recognizing fulminant hepatitis

Fulminant hepatitis is a rare but severe form of hepatitis that rapidly causes massive liver necrosis. It usually occurs in clients with hepatitis B, D, or E. Mortality is extremely high (more than 80% of clients lapse into deep coma), but those who survive may recover completely.

Assessment

In a client with viral hepatitis, suspect fulminant hepatitis if you detect:
● confusion
● somnolence
● ascites
● edema
● rapidly rising bilirubin level
● markedly prolonged prothrombin time.

As the disease progresses quickly to the terminal phase, the client may experience cerebral edema, brain stem compression, GI bleeding, sepsis, respiratory failure, cardiovascular collapse, and renal failure.

Emergency actions

If you suspect fulminant hepatitis, you should:
● notify the physician immediately
● provide supportive care, such as maintaining fluid volume, supporting ventilation through mechanical means, controlling bleeding, and correcting hypoglycemia
● restrict protein intake
● expect to administer oral lactulose or neomycin and, possibly, massive doses of glucocorticoids
● prepare the client for a liver transplant if necessary and if the client meets the criteria.

● Encourage small, frequent meals *to improve the client's nutritional status.*
● Change the client's position every 2 hours *to reduce the risk of skin breakdown.*
● Monitor for signs of bleeding *to prevent hemorrhage.*
● Review key teaching topics with the client *to ensure adequate knowledge about his condition and treatment,* including:
– avoiding exposure to people with infections
– avoiding alcohol
– maintaining good personal hygiene
– refraining from donating blood
– increasing fluid intake to 3,000 ml per day (approximately twelve 8-oz glasses)

– abstaining from sexual intercourse until serum liver studies are within normal limits

– avoiding over-the-counter medications, such as acetaminophen, until discussing their use with a health care professional.

Evaluation

● The client has balanced intake and output, adequate nutritional intake, and normal vital signs.
● The client verbalizes decreased fatigue, energy-saving measures, and the need for rest.
● The client demonstrates understanding about the disease process, the need for follow-up care, the necessity for good personal hygiene, and practices to avoid disease infection and transmission.

Hiatal hernia

A HIATAL HERNIA, also known as an *esophageal hernia*, is a protrusion of the stomach through the diaphragm into the thoracic cavity. Hiatal hernia is the most common problem of the diaphragm affecting the alimentary canal.

Possible causes

● Aging
● Congenital weakness
● Increased abdominal pressure
● Obesity
● Pregnancy
● Trauma
● Unknown

Data collection findings

● Cough
● Dysphagia
● Dyspnea
● Feeling of fullness
● Pyrosis
● Regurgitation
● Sternal pain after eating
● Tachycardia
● Vomiting

Diagnostic findings

● Barium swallow reveals protrusion of the hernia.
● Chest X-ray shows protrusion of abdominal organs into the thorax.
● Esophagoscopy shows incompetent cardiac sphincter.
● Gastric analysis reveals increased pH.

Nursing diagnoses

● Acute pain
● Anxiety
● Chronic pain
● Imbalanced nutrition: Less than body requirements

Treatment

● Antireflux surgical repair, if complications develop
● Bland diet with decreased intake of caffeine and spicy foods
● Weight loss, if necessary

Drug therapy options

● Anticholinergic: propantheline (Pro-Banthine)
● H_2-receptor antagonist: cimetidine (Tagamet), famotidine (Pepcid), ranitidine (Zantac), nizatidine (Axid)

Patient care goals

● The client will have a decreased level of anxiety.
● The client will have improved nutritional status.
● The client will experience pain relief.

Nursing interventions

● Assess respiratory status *to detect early signs of respiratory distress.*
● Monitor and record vital signs, intake and output, and daily weight *to determine baseline and detect early signs of nutritional deficit.*
● Administer oxygen *to help relieve respiratory distress.*
● Avoid flexion at the waist in positioning the client *to promote comfort.*
● Maintain the client's diet *to maintain and improve nutritional status.*
● Maintain position, patency, and low suction of NG tube *to prevent nausea and vomiting.*
● Keep the client in semi-Fowler's position *to promote comfort.*
● Monitor the administraton of medications, as prescribed, *to improve GI function.*
● Review key teaching topics with the client *to ensure adequate knowledge about his condition and treatment,* including:
– eating small, frequent meals
– avoiding carbonated beverages and alcohol
– remaining upright for 2 hours after eating
– avoiding constrictive clothing
– avoiding lifting, bending, straining, and coughing
– sleeping with upper body elevated to reduce gastric reflux.

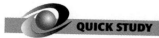

Evaluation

- The client expresses feelings, verbalizes decreased anxiety, and discusses coping skills to handle anxiety.
- The client regains and maintains adequate nutritional intake.
- The client acknowledges changes in his eating habits and interventions that can help promote comfort before, during, and after eating.

Intestinal obstruction

An INTESTINAL OBSTRUCTION occurs when the intestinal lumen becomes blocked, causing gas, fluid, and digested substances to accumulate near the obstruction and increasing peristalsis in the area of the obstruction. Water and electrolytes are then secreted into the blocked bowel, causing inflammation and inhibiting absorption.

Possible causes

- Adhesions
- Diverticulitis
- Fecal impaction
- Hernia
- Inflammation (Crohn's disease)
- Mesenteric thrombosis
- Paralytic ileus
- Tumors
- Volvulus

Data collection findings

- Nausea
- Cramping pain
- Abdominal distention
- Diminished or absent bowel sounds
- Constipation
- Fever
- Vomiting fecal material
- Weight loss

Diagnostic findings

- Abdominal X-ray shows an increased amount of gas in the bowel.
- Barium enema stops at obstruction.
- Blood chemistry shows decreased sodium and potassium levels.
- Hematologic study shows an increased WBC count.

Nursing diagnoses

- Ineffective tissue perfusion (GI)
- Acute pain
- Imbalanced nutrition: Less than body requirements

Treatment

- Bowel resection with or without anastomosis, if other treatment fails
- GI decompression using NG tube, Miller-Abbott tube, or Cantor tube
- Withholding food and fluids

Drug therapy options

- Analgesic: meperidine (Demerol)
- Antibiotic: gentamicin (Garamycin)

Patient care goals

- The client will have adequate perfusion of GI system.
- The client will express feelings of comfort and pain relief.
- The client will maintain adequate caloric intake.

Nursing interventions

- Assess GI status. Assess and record bowel sounds once per shift *to determine GI status.*
- Monitor and record vital signs, intake and output, and laboratory studies *to detect early signs of fluid volume deficit.*

- Withhold food and fluids *to prevent nausea and vomiting.*
- Monitor and record the frequency, color, and amount of stools *to assess and determine nutritional status.*
- Measure and record the client's abdominal girth *to determine the presence of distention.*
- Monitor the administration of I.V. fluids *to maintain hydration.*
- Maintain the position, patency, and low intermittent suction of the NG and Miller-Abbott tubes *to prevent nausea and vomiting and to resolve the obstruction, if possible.*
- Keep the client in semi-Fowler's position *to promote comfort.*
- Administer postoperative care if indicated (monitor vital signs and intake and output; make sure the NG tube is kept patent; monitor the dressing for drainage; assess the wound for infection; assist with turning, coughing, and deep breathing; medicate for pain as necessary or guide the client with use of postoperative client-controlled analgesia) *to promote healing and detect early postoperative complications.*
- Administer medications as prescribed *to maintain or improve the client's condition.*

Evaluation
- The client doesn't display signs of ischemic bowel.
- The client reports adequate pain control.
- The client maintains an adequate weight.

Irritable bowel syndrome
IRRITABLE BOWEL SYNDROME is marked by chronic symptoms of abdominal pain, alternating constipation and diarrhea, and abdominal distention. This disorder is extremely common; a substantial portion of clients, however, never seek medical attention.

This disorder may also be referred to as *spastic colon* or *spastic colitis.*

Possible causes
- Diverticular disease
- Irritants (caffeine, alcohol)
- Stress

Data collection findings
- Abdominal bloating
- Constipation, diarrhea, or both
- Dyspepsia
- Faintness
- Heartburn
- Lower abdominal pain

- Passage of mucus
- Pasty, pencil-like stools
- Weakness

Diagnostic findings
- Barium enema may reveal colonic spasm and tubular appearance of the descending colon. It also rules out certain other disorders, such as diverticula, tumors, and polyps.
- Sigmoidoscopy may disclose spastic contractions.
- Stool examination for occult blood, parasites, and pathogenic bacteria is negative.

Nursing diagnoses
- Chronic pain
- Diarrhea
- Constipation

Treatment
- Elimination diet to determine if symptoms result from food intolerance (in this type of diet, certain foods, such as citrus fruits, coffee, corn, dairy products, tea, and wheat, are sequentially eliminated; then each food is gradually reintroduced to identify which foods, if any, trigger the client's symptoms)
- Diet containing 15 to 20 g daily of bulky foods, such as wheat bran, oatmeal, oat bran, rye cereals, prunes, dried apricots, and figs (if the client has constipation and abdominal pain)
- Increasing fluid intake to at least eight 8-oz glasses per day
- Stress management
- Heat application

Drug therapy options
- Sedative: diazepam (Valium)
- Antiflatulent: simethicone (Mylicon)
- Antispasmodic: propantheline (Pro-Banthine)
- Antidiarrheal: diphenoxylate with atropine (Lomotil)

FAST FACT

The client with irritable bowel syndrome needs to ingest 15 to 20 g of bulk per day.

Patient care goals
- The client will express feelings of comfort and pain relief.
- The client's bowel function will return to normal.

Nursing interventions

- Help the client deal with stress, and warn against dependence on sedatives or antispasmodics *because stress may be the underlying cause of irritable bowel syndrome.*
- Encourage regular checkups. For clients over age 40, emphasize the need for a yearly flexible sigmoidoscopy and rectal examination. *Irritable bowel syndrome is associated with a higher-than-normal incidence of diverticulitis and colon cancer.*

Evaluation

- The client reports adequate pain control.
- The client reports a decreased incidence of diarrhea and constipation.

Pancreatitis

PANCREATITIS is the inflammation of the pancreas. In acute pancreatitis, pancreatic enzymes are activated in the pancreas rather than the duodenum, resulting in tissue damage and autodigestion of the pancreas.

In chronic pancreatitis, chronic inflammation results in fibrosis and calcification of the pancreas, obstruction of the ducts, and destruction of the secreting acinar cells.

Possible causes

- Alcoholism
- Bacterial or viral infection
- Biliary tract disease
- Blunt trauma to the pancreas or abdomen
- Drugs: steroids, thiazide diuretics, oral contraceptives
- Duodenal ulcer
- Hyperlipidemia
- Hyperparathyroidism

Data collection findings

- Abrupt onset of pain in the epigastric area that radiates to the shoulder, substernal area, back, and flank
- Abdominal tenderness and distention
- Aching, burning, stabbing, pressing pain
- Knee-chest position, fetal position, or leaning forward for comfort
- Decreased or absent bowel sounds
- Nausea and vomiting
- Tachycardia
- Dyspnea
- Fever
- Hypotension
- Jaundice
- Steatorrhea
- Weight loss

Diagnostic findings

- Arteriography reveals fibrous tissue and calcification of the pancreas.
- Blood chemistry shows increased amylase, lipase, LD, glucose, AST, and lipid levels and decreased calcium and potassium levels. (See *Caring for the client with pancreatitis,* page 458.)
- CT scan shows an enlarged pancreas.
- Cullen's sign is positive.
- Endoscopic retrograde cholangiopancreatography reveals biliary obstruction.
- Fecal fat test is positive.
- Glucose tolerance test shows decreased tolerance.
- Grey-Turner's sign is positive.
- Hematology shows increased WBC count and decreased Hb level and HCT.
- Ultrasonography reveals cysts, bile duct inflammation, and dilation.
- Urine chemistry shows increased amylase.

Nursing diagnoses

- Acute pain
- Ineffective breathing pattern
- Deficient fluid volume

Treatment

- Bland, low-fat, high-protein diet of small, frequent meals with restricted intake of caffeine, alcohol, and gas-forming foods (nothing by mouth as the disease progresses)
- Bed rest
- I.V. fluids (vigorous replacement of fluids and electrolytes)
- Dialysis
- Sequential compression device to prevent blood clot formation
- Surgical intervention to treat the underlying cause, if appropriate
- Transfusion therapy with packed RBCs

Drug therapy options

- Analgesic: meperidine (Demerol) (morphine is contraindicated)
- Anticholinergic: propantheline (Pro-Banthine), dicyclomine (Bentyl)
- Antidiabetic: insulin (possible infusion to stabilize blood glucose levels)
- Antiemetic: prochlorperazine (Compazine)
- Calcium supplement: calcium gluconate (Kalcinate)
- Corticosteroid: hydrocortisone (Solu-Cortef)
- Digestant: pancrelipase (Pancrease)

Caring for the client with pancreatitis

The client is a 34-year-old male with a history of alcohol abuse. He presents with a complaint of severe abdominal pain that radiates to his back. He has also had several incidents of nausea and vomiting.

Which diagnostic tests should be ordered in order to confirm a diagnosis of pancreatitis?

A. Amylase, lipase, chest X-ray

B. Amylase, lipase, abdominal X-ray

C. Amylase, lipase, computer tomography (CT) scan

D. Complete blood count, urine analysis, electrolytes, electrocardiogram

Answer: C. Elevated serum amylase and lipase are the diagnostic hallmarks that confirm acute pancreatitis. Characteristically, serum amylase reaches peak levels 24 hours after the onset of pancreatitis and then returns to normal within 48 to 72 hours, despite continued symptoms. Serum lipase levels remain elevated longer than amylase levels.

A CT scan reveals an increased pancreatic diameter. Abdominal and chest X-rays rule out other diseases that cause similar symptoms and detect pleural effusions.

True or false?

During acute pancreatitis, the client should be placed on a clear liquid diet.

Answer: False. In acute pancreatitis, the client can't eat or drink. Nasogastric suctioning is usually required to decrease gastric distention and suppress pancreatic secretions.

Questions for further thought

● Which nursing diagnoses would be appropriate for the client with pancreatitis?

● What complications of pancreatitis can occur?

● H_2-receptor antagonist: cimetidine (Tagamet), ranitidine (Zantac), famotidine (Pepcid), nizatidine (Axid)
● Mucosal barrier fortifier: sucralfate (Carafate)
● Potassium supplement: I.V. potassium chloride
● Tranquilizer: lorazepam (Ativan), alprazolam (Xanax)

Patient care goals
● The client will express feelings of comfort and pain relief.
● The client will maintain adequate ventilation.
● The client will maintain a normal fluid volume.

Nursing interventions
● Assess abdominal, cardiac, and respiratory status (as the disease progresses, watch for respiratory failure, tachycardia, and worsening GI status) *to determine baseline and detect early changes and signs of complications.*
● Assess fluid balance *to detect fluid volume deficit or excess.*
● Assist with monitoring and recording vital signs, intake and output, laboratory studies, CVP, daily weight, and urine specific gravity *to detect signs of fluid volume deficit.*

● Monitor urine and stool for color, character, and amount *to detect bleeding.*
● Maintain the client's diet; withhold food and fluids as necessary *to rest the pancreas and to prevent nausea and vomiting.*
● Perform bedside glucose monitoring *to assess for hyperglycemia.*
● Administer oxygen and maintain ET tube and mechanical ventilation if necessary *to improve oxygenation* and provide suctioning as needed *to stabilize secretions.*
● Monitor the administration of I.V. fluids *to treat or prevent hypovolemic shock and restore electrolyte balance.*
● Maintain position, patency, and low suction of NG tube *to prevent nausea and vomiting.*
● Keep the client in semi-Fowler's position (if his blood pressure allows) *to promote comfort and lung expansion.*
● Maintain the safety and the patency of the central venous line for administration of TPN. *In severe cases, reintroduction of food may be associated with pancreatic abscess. TPN is necessary to meet the client's metabolic needs.*
● Keep the client in bed and turn him every 2 hours, or utilize a specialty rotation bed *to prevent pressure ulcers.*

- Administer medications as prescribed *to improve or maintain the client's condition.*
- Provide skin, nares, and mouth care *to prevent tissue damage.*
- Provide a quiet, restful environment *to conserve energy and decrease metabolic demands.*

Evaluation
- The client reports adequate pain relief.
- The client's breathing pattern remains normal and unlabored.
- The client doesn't display signs of dehydration.

Peptic ulcer

PEPTIC ULCERS are breaks in the continuity of esophageal, gastric, or duodenal mucosa. They can occur in any part of the GI tract that comes in contact with gastric substances, hydrochloric acid, and pepsin. The ulcers may be found in the esophagus, stomach, duodenum, or (after gastroenterostomy) jejunum.

Possible causes
- Alcohol abuse
- Drugs: salicylates, steroids, NSAIDs, reserpine
- Gastritis
- *Helicobacter pylori*
- Smoking
- Stress
- Zollinger-Ellison syndrome

Data collection findings
- Anorexia
- Diarrhea or constipation (secondary to antacid use)
- Dizziness
- Fainting
- Hematemesis
- Left epigastric pain 1 to 2 hours after eating
- Melena
- Nausea and vomiting
- Relief from pain after administration of antacids
- Weight loss

Diagnostic findings
- Acid-base studies may indicate metabolic alkalosis caused by overuse of antacids.
- Barium swallow shows ulceration of the gastric mucosa.
- Fecal occult blood test is positive.

- Gastric analysis is normal.
- Gastric sampling may be positive for *H. pylori.*
- Hematologic study shows decreased Hb level and HCT (if bleeding is present).
- Serum gastrin level is normal or increased.
- Upper GI endoscopy shows location of the ulcer.

Nursing diagnoses
- Acute pain
- Anxiety
- Chronic pain
- Risk for deficient fluid volume

Treatment
- Endoscopic laser to control bleeding
- If GI hemorrhage, gastric surgery that may include gastroduodenostomy, gastrojejunostomy, partial gastric resection, and total gastrectomy
- Low-fiber diet in small, frequent meals
- Photocoagulation to control bleeding
- Saline lavage by NG tube until return is clear (if bleeding is present)
- Transfusion therapy with packed RBCs (if bleeding is present and Hb level and HCT are low)

Drug therapy options
- Antacid: magnesium and aluminum hydroxide (Maalox), aluminum hydroxide gel (AlternaGEL)
- Antibiotic, if *H. pylori* is present
- Anticholinergic: propantheline (Pro-Banthine), dicyclomine (Bentyl)
- H_2-receptor antagonist: cimetidine (Tagamet), famotidine (Pepcid), nizatidine (Axid), ranitidine (Zantac)
- Mucosal barrier fortifier: sucralfate (Carafate)
- Pituitary hormone: vasopressin (Pitressin) to manage bleeding
- Prostaglandin: misoprostol (Cytotec) to protect the stomach lining
- Proton pump inhibitor: lansoprazole (Prevacid), omeprazole (Prilosec)

Patient care goals
- The client will display decreased anxiety.
- The client will regain and maintain adequate fluid balance and nutritional intake.
- The client will experience pain relief through healing.

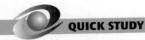

Nursing interventions

● Assess GI status to monitor *for signs of bleeding.*
● Assess cardiovascular status *to detect early signs of GI hemorrhage.*
● Monitor and record vital signs, intake and output, laboratory studies, fecal occult blood, and gastric pH *to detect signs of bleeding.*
● Monitor the consistency, color, amount, and frequency of stools *to detect early signs of GI bleeding.*
● Maintain the client's diet with small, frequent feedings *to meet metabolic needs and promote healing.*
● Maintain the position, patency, and low suction of the NG tube if gastric decompression is ordered *to prevent nausea and vomiting.*
● Administer medications, as prescribed, *to maintain or improve the client's condition.*
● Provide nose and mouth care *to maintain tissue integrity.*
● Provide postoperative care if necessary (don't reposition the NG tube, irrigate it gently if ordered, medicate for pain as needed and ordered, monitor the dressings for drainage, assess bowel sounds, get the client out of bed as tolerated) *to detect early complications and promote healing.*
● Review key teaching topics with the client *to ensure adequate knowledge about his condition and treatment,* including:
– reducing stress
– relaxation techniques
– following dietary recommendations and restrictions such as avoiding caffeine, alcohol, and spicy or fried foods
– following postoperative care and restrictions.

Evaluation

● The client verbalizes decreased anxiety and is able to describe positive outlets for stress and learn stress management techniques.
● The client has a balanced intake and output and normal vital signs.
● The client maintains adequate nutritional intake to restore nutritional balance.

Peritonitis

PERITONITIS results from a localized or generalized inflammation of the peritoneal cavity. It occurs when irritants in the peritoneal area cause inflammatory edema, vascular congestion, and hypermotility of the bowel.

Possible causes

● Bacterial invasion
● Chemical invasion

Data collection findings

● Abdominal resonance and tympany on percussion
● Abdominal rigidity and distention
● Anorexia
● Constant, diffuse, and intense abdominal pain
● Decreased or absent bowel sounds
● Decreased peristalsis
● Decreased urine output
● Fever
● Malaise
● Nausea
● Rebound tenderness
● Shallow respirations
● Weak, rapid pulse

Diagnostic findings

● Abdominal X-ray shows free air in the abdomen under the diaphragm.
● Hematologic study shows increased WBC count and HCT.
● Peritoneal aspiration is positive for blood, pus, bile, bacteria, or amylase.

Nursing diagnoses

● Decreased cardiac output
● Acute pain
● Deficient fluid volume

Treatment

● Withholding food or fluid
● Surgical intervention when the client's condition is stabilized (chosen to treat the cause; for example, if the client has a perforated appendix, an appendectomy is indicated; drains will also be placed for drainage of infected material)

Drug therapy options

● Analgesic: meperidine (Demerol)
● Antibiotic: gentamicin (Garamycin), clindamycin (Cleocin), cephalothin (Keflin), ampicillin and sulbactam (Unasyn)

Patient care goals

- The client will remain hemodynamically stable.
- The client will express feelings of comfort and pain relief.
- The client will maintain normal fluid volume.

Nursing interventions

- Assess abdominal and respiratory status and fluid balance *to detect and assess signs of fluid volume deficit.*
- Assist with monitoring and recording vital signs, intake and output, laboratory studies, CVP, daily weight, and urine specific gravity *to detect signs of fluid volume deficit.*
- Measure and record the client's abdominal girth *to assess for abdominal distention.*
- Withhold food and fluids *to prevent nausea and vomiting.*
- Monitor the administration of I.V. fluids *to maintain hydration and electrolyte balance.*
- Provide routine postoperative care (monitor vital signs and intake and output, including drainage from drains; assist with turning, incentive spirometry, coughing, and deep breathing; and get the client out of bed on the 1st postoperative day if his condition allows) *to promote healing and to prevent and detect early complications.*
- Maintain the position, the patency, and low suction of the NG tube *to prevent nausea and vomiting.*
- Keep the client in semi-Fowler's position *to promote comfort and prevent pulmonary complications.*
- Maintain the safety and the patency of the central venous line for administration of TPN *to meet the client's metabolic needs.*
- Administer medications, as prescribed, *to treat infection and control pain.*

Evaluation

- The client has stable vital signs.
- The client reports adequate pain control.
- The client doesn't display signs of dehydration.

Ulcerative colitis

ULCERATIVE COLITIS is a major health problem and a potentially debilitating disease. It's a type of inflammatory bowel disease that produces lesions primarily confined to the large bowel, with ulcerations of the large bowel's mucosa and submucosa. Healing of lesions causes scarring and strictures, leading to bowel obstruction, and ulcers may perforate, causing hemorrhage and peritonitis. Ulcerative colitis usually develops in people between ages 18 and 35 and occurs more commonly in women than in men.

Possible causes

- Genetics
- Idiopathic cause
- Allergies
- Autoimmune disease
- Emotional stress
- Viral and bacterial infections

Data collection findings

- Abdominal cramping, distention, and tenderness
- Anorexia
- Bloody, purulent, mucoid, watery stools (15 to 20 per day)
- Dehydration
- Fever
- Hyperactive bowel sounds
- Nausea and vomiting
- Weakness
- Weight loss

Total parenteral nutrition

Total parenteral nutrition (TPN) is administered to meet a client's total nutritional needs when oral feedings, tube feedings, and standard I.V. feedings are contraindicated. It's used for clients with various GI problems or other conditions that necessitate nutritional support such as some oncology clients.

Key facts

- In most cases, TPN is administered through a central vein such as the subclavian. The fluid is highly concentrated to provide rapid dilution and thus decrease the risks of peripheral inflammation and thrombosis.
- TPN is administered at a constant rate, using filtered tubing and an infusion pump.
- The infusion should never be stopped abruptly. Dextrose 10% in water is given if the infusion must be stopped. During TPN administration, the pancreas secretes increased insulin; abrupt cessation can lead to hypoglycemia.
- Maintain strict asepsis. An occlusive dressing is used on the site. The dressing, tubing, and filter are changed every 48 hours.
- Monitor blood glucose levels or check urine for glucose every 6 hours. Note that the client might need insulin.
- Observe the client for headache, nausea, vomiting, and fever. These indicate an allergy to the protein.
- Closely monitor intake and output.
- Weigh the client daily. Expect a weight gain of ½ lb per day.
- Never use a filter when infusing fat emulsions. Monitor for nausea and fever, which are common adverse reactions.

Comparing ulcerative colitis and regional enteritis

Use this table to compare ulcerative colitis and regional enteritis. Clinical symptoms usually don't aid differentiation.

	ULCERATIVE COLITIS	REGIONAL ENTERITIS (CROHN'S DISEASE)
Site of inflammation	Colon and rectum	Small intestine (primarily terminal ileum), although the disease may occur in any part of the small or large intestine
Type of lesion	Continuous ulcerated lesions involving mucosal and submucosal layers (may create abscesses)	Skip lesions (inflamed areas skip around in the tract); lesions involve all intestinal layers (mucosa, submucosa, muscle, and serous layers); may abscess or perforate, scar, or form fistulas
Common patterns	Frequent diarrhea (30 to 40 bowel movements per day) – profuse, mucus-filled, watery, bloody, and debilitating; dehydration and weight loss; electrolyte imbalances (common); fever common in acute attacks	Watery, mucus-filled diarrhea, less bloody than in ulcerative colitis; cramping, distention, and low-grade fever
Treatments	*Medical:* Diet high in protein, calories, and vitamins; anticholinergic drugs and anti-inflammatory, antibacterial, or antibiotic drugs; emotional support	*Medical:* Same as for ulcerative colitis
	Surgical: Ileostomy with colectomy and removal of the rectum	*Surgical:* Bowel resection (possibly repeated resections)

Diagnostic findings
- Barium enema shows ulcerations.
- Blood chemistry shows decreased potassium level and increased osmolality.
- Hematology shows decreased Hb level and HCT.
- Intestinal biopsy helps to differentiate between ulcerative colitis and regional enteritis. (See *Comparing ulcerative colitis and regional enteritis.*)
- Sigmoidoscopy shows ulceration and hyperemia.
- Stool specimen is positive for blood and mucus.
- Urine chemistry displays increased urine specific gravity.

Nursing diagnoses
- Deficient knowledge (client)
- Diarrhea
- Disturbed body image
- Imbalanced nutrition: Less than body requirements
- Risk for deficient fluid volume

Treatment
- Colectomy or pouch ileostomy
- High-protein, high-calorie, low-residue diet, with bland foods in small, frequent meals and restricted intake of milk and gas-forming foods or no food or fluids
- TPN if necessary to rest the GI tract (see *Total parenteral nutrition,* page 461)
- Transfusion therapy with packed RBCs

Drug therapy options
- Analgesic: meperidine (Demerol)
- Antianemic: ferrous gluconate (Fergon), ferrous sulfate (Feosol)
- Antibiotic: sulfasalazine (Azulfidine)
- Anticholinergic: dicyclomine (Bentyl), propantheline (Pro-Banthine)
- Antidiarrheal: diphenoxylate with atropine (Lomotil), loperamide (Imodium)
- Antiemetic: prochlorperazine (Compazine)
- Anti-inflammatory: olsalazine (Dipentum)

Low-residue diet

A low-residue diet is prescribed to avoid irritation of the mucosal lining. A regular diet containing normal amounts of protein and gradually incorporating fiber should be instituted when the client can tolerate it.

FOODS	ALLOWED	NOT ALLOWED
Breads and cereals	Refined breads without seeds	High-fiber cereals (All Bran, Grape Nuts); whole-grain breads
Fruit	Canned fruits without skins or seeds; ripe banana; strained fruit juice	Raw fruits
Fats	All	None
Meats, fish, poultry	Roasted, baked, or broiled	Fried or highly spiced
Dairy	Milk, eggs, cheese	Fried eggs
Soups	Bouillon, broth, strained cream soups	All others
Vegetables	Canned or cooked strained vegetables; tomato juice	Raw or whole cooked vegetables
Miscellaneous	Salt, gravy, jelly, syrups, chocolate, puddings, and plain cakes	Nuts, olives, pickles, jam, alcohol, rich pastries

- Corticosteroid: hydrocortisone (Solu-Cortef)
- Immunosuppressant: azathioprine (Imuran), cyclophosphamide (Cytoxan)
- Potassium supplement: potassium chloride (K-Lor), potassium gluconate (Kaon)
- Sedative: lorazepam (Ativan)

Patient care goals

- The client will understand the disease and possible complications of ulcerative colitis.
- The client will follow the treatment regimen.
- The client will maintain adequate fluid balance and nutritional intake.
- The client will express feelings about the disease and treatment and will participate in care.

Nursing interventions

- Assess GI status and fluid balance *to determine deficient fluid volume.*
- Monitor and record vital signs, intake and output, laboratory studies, daily weight, urine specific gravity, calorie count, and fecal occult blood *to determine deficient fluid volume.*

- Monitor the number, amount, and character of stools *to determine status of nutrient absorption.*
- Maintain the client's diet; withhold food and fluids as necessary *to prevent nausea and vomiting.*
- Monitor the administration of I.V. fluids and maintain the safety and patency of central venous line for administration of TPN *to maintain hydration and improve nutritional status.*
- Maintain the position, patency, and low suction of the NG tube *to prevent nausea and vomiting.*
- Keep the client in semi-Fowler's position *to promote comfort.*
- Administer medications, as prescribed, *to maintain or improve the client's condition.*
- Provide skin, mouth, nares, and perianal care *to promote comfort and prevent skin breakdown.*
- Review key teaching topics with the client *to ensure adequate knowledge about his condition and treatment,* including:
  – monitoring weight
  – reducing stress and performing relaxation techniques
  – recognizing the early signs and symptoms of rectal hemorrhage and intestinal obstruction

– following a low-residue, high protein diet during an acute exacerbation (see *Low-residue diet*, page 463)
– contacting the United Ostomy Association and the National Foundation of Ileitis and Colitis.

Evaluation

- The client can explain the treatment regimen and possible complications.
- The client has a balanced intake and output and normal vital signs.
- The client maintains adequate nutritional intake to restore nutritional balance.
- The client recovers from surgery and can perform self-care.

GENITOURINARY SYSTEM

The genitourinary system serves as the body's water treatment plant, filtering waste products from the body and expelling them as urine through the kidneys and other parts of the urinary system. The genitourinary system also encompasses the female and male reproductive systems, including external and internal genitalia.

Urinary structure and function

The key structures of the urinary system include the kidneys, ureter, bladder, urethra, and prostate gland. The urinary system processes and filters waste products by continuously exchanging water and solutes, such as hydrogen, potassium, chloride, bicarbonate, sulfate, and phosphate, across cell membranes.

Kidneys

The kidneys are two bean-shaped organs that produce urine and maintain fluid and acid-base balance. To help maintain acid-base balance, the kidneys secrete hydrogen ions, reabsorb sodium and bicarbonates, acidify phosphate salts, and produce ammonia.

The kidneys have four main components:

- cortex, which makes up the outer layer of the kidney and contains the glomeruli, the proximal tubules of the nephron, and the distal tubules of the nephron
- medulla, which makes up the inner layer of the kidney and contains the loops of Henle and the collecting tubules
- renal pelvis, which collects urine from the calices
- nephron, which makes up the functional unit of the kidney and contains Bowman's capsule and the glomerulus as well as the renal tubule (which consists of the proximal convoluted tubule and collecting segments).

Urine production

Urine is produced through a complex process in the kidneys.

- Blood from the renal artery is filtered across the glomerular capillary membrane in the Bowman's capsule. Filtration requires adequate intravascular volume and adequate cardiac output.
- ADH and aldosterone control the reabsorption of water and electrolytes. The composition of the filtrate is similar to blood plasma without proteins.
- Formed filtrate moves through the tubules of the nephron, which reabsorb and secrete electrolytes, water, glucose, amino acids, ammonia, and bicarbonate.
- What remains in the filtrate is excreted as urine.

Blood pressure control

The kidneys are involved in regulating blood pressure by removing water from the body in the form of urine. The renin-angiotensin system is activated by decreased blood pressure and can be altered by renal disease.

Ureter

The ureter, which transports urine from the kidney to the bladder, is a tubule that extends from the renal pelvis to the bladder floor.

Bladder

The bladder, a muscular, distensible sac, can contain up to 1 L of urine.

Urethra

The urethra, extending from the bladder to the urinary meatus, transports urine from the bladder to the exterior of the body.

Prostate gland

The prostate gland surrounds the male urethra. It contains ducts that secrete the alkaline portion of seminal fluid.

Female external genitalia

The external female genitalia include the mons pubis, labia majora, labia minora, clitoris, vestibule, urethral meatus, paraurethral glands, and breasts.

Mons pubis

The mons pubis provides an adipose cushion over the anterior symphysis pubis and protects the pelvic bones and contributes to the rounded contour of the female body.

Labia majora

The labia majora are two folds that converge at the mons pubis and extend to the posterior commissure. The labia majora consist of connective tissue, elastic fibers, veins, and sebaceous glands. They protect components of the vulval cleft.

Labia minora

The labia minora are located within the labia majora. The labia minora:
- consist of connective tissue, sebaceous and sweat glands, nonstriated muscle fibers, nerve endings, and blood vessels
- unite to form the fourchette and vaginal vestibule
- serve to lubricate the vulva, which adds to sexual enjoyment and fights bacteria.

Clitoris

The clitoris — located in the anterior portion of the vulva above the urethral opening — is made up of erectile tissue, nerves, and blood vessels and, homologous to the penis, provides sexual pleasure. The clitoris consists of:
- glans
- body
- two crura.

Vestibule

The vaginal vestibule extends from the clitoris to the posterior fourchette and consists of:
- vaginal orifice
- hymen — a thin, vascularized mucous membrane at the vaginal orifice
- fossa navicularis — a depressed area between the hymen and fourchette
- Bartholin's glands — two bean-shaped glands on either side of the vagina that secrete mucus during sexual stimulation
- perineal body — the area between the vagina and the anus that's the site of episiotomy during childbirth.

Urethral meatus

The urethral meatus is located ¼″ to 1″ (0.5 to 2.5 cm) below the clitoris.

Paraurethral glands

The paraurethral glands, also called *Skene's glands,* are located immediately inside the urethral meatus.

Breasts

The breasts consist of glandular, fibrous, and adipose tissue. The breasts:
- are stimulated by secretions from the hypothalamus, anterior pituitary, and ovaries
- provide nourishment to the infant and transfer maternal antibodies during breast-feeding
- enhance sexual pleasure.

Female internal genitalia

The internal female genitalia include the vagina, uterus, fallopian tubes, and ovaries.

Vagina

The vagina is a vascularized musculomembranous tube that extends from the external genitals to the uterus.

Uterus

The uterus is a hollow, pear-shaped, muscular organ that's divided by a slight constriction (isthmus) into an upper portion (body or corpus) and a lower portion (cervix). The uterus:
- consists of a body or corpus with three layers (perimetrium, myometrium, and endometrium)
- receives support from broad, round, uterosacral ligaments
- provides an environment for fetal growth and development.

Fallopian tubes

The fallopian tubes are about 4¼″ (11 cm) long and consist of four layers (peritoneal, subserous, muscular, mucous) divided into four portions (interstitial, isthmus, ampulla, fimbria). The fallopian tubes:
- transport ova from the ovary to the uterus
- provide a nourishing environment for zygotes
- serve as the site of fertilization.

Ovaries

The ovaries are two almond-shaped glandular structures that rest below and behind the fallopian tubes on either side of the uterus. The ovaries produce sex hormones (estrogen, progesterone, androgen) and serve as the site of ovulation.

Male external genitalia

The male external genitalia include the penis and scrotum.

Penis

The penis consists of the body (shaft) and glans and has three layers of erectile tissue — two corpora cavernosa and one corpus spongiosum. The penis deposits spermatozoa in the female reproductive tract and provides sexual pleasure.

Scrotum

The scrotum is a pouchlike structure composed of skin, fascial connective tissue, and smooth muscle fibers that houses the testes and serves to protect spermatozoa from high body temperature.

Male internal genitalia

The internal male genitalia serve to produce and transport semen and seminal fluid. They include the testes, epididymides, vas deferens, urethra, seminal vesicles, prostate gland, and bulbourethral glands.

Testes

The testes are two oval-shaped glandular organs inside the scrotum that function to produce spermatozoa and testosterone.

Epididymides

The epididymides serve as the initial section of the testes' excretory duct system that store spermatozoa as they mature and become motile.

Vas deferens

The vas deferens connect the epididymal lumen and the prostatic urethra and serve as conduits for spermatozoa. The vas deferens:
- consist of ejaculatory ducts
- are located between the seminal vesicles and the urethra
- serve as passageways for semen and seminal fluid.

Urethra

The urethra extends from the bladder through the penis to the external urethral opening and serves as the excretory duct for urine and semen.

Seminal vesicles

The seminal vesicles are two pouchlike structures between the bladder and the rectum that secrete a viscous fluid that aids in spermatozoa motility and metabolism.

Prostate gland

The prostate gland is located just below the bladder and is considered homologous to Skene's glands in females. The prostate gland:
- produces an alkaline fluid that enhances spermatozoa motility
- lubricates the urethra during sexual activity.

Bulbourethral glands

The bulbourethral glands, also called *Cowper's glands,* are two pea-sized glands opening into the posterior portion of the urethra. They secrete a thick alkaline fluid that neutralizes acidic secretions in the female reproductive tract, thus prolonging spermatozoa survival.

GENITOURINARY DISORDERS

The major disorders that affect the genitourinary system include ACUTE POSTSTREPTOCOCCAL GLOMERULONEPHRITIS (APSGN), acute renal failure, BENIGN PROSTATIC HYPERPLASIA (BPH), bladder cancer, breast cancer, cervical cancer, chlamydia, chronic glomerulonephritis, chronic renal failure, cystitis, gonorrhea, herpes simplex virus, neurogenic bladder, ovarian cancer, prostate cancer, renal calculi, syphilis, and testicular cancer.

Acute poststreptococcal glomerulonephritis

Also called *acute glomerulonephritis,* APSGN is a relatively common bilateral inflammation of the glomeruli, the kidney's blood vessels. It follows a streptococcal infection of the respiratory tract or, less commonly, a skin infection such as impetigo.

Possible causes

- Trapped antigen-antibody complexes (produced as an immunologic mechanism in response to streptococci) in the glomerular capillary membranes, inducing inflammatory damage and impeding glomerular function
- Untreated pharyngitis (inflammation of the pharynx)

Data collection findings

- Oliguria
- Hematuria
- Fatigue
- Azotemia
- Edema
- Proteinuria

Diagnostic findings

- Blood tests show elevated serum creatinine levels.
- 24-hour urine sample shows low creatinine clearance and impaired glomerular filtration.
- Elevated antistreptolysin-O titers (in 80% of clients), elevated streptozyme and anti-DNase B titers, and low serum complement levels verify recent streptococcal infection.
- Renal biopsy may confirm the diagnosis in a client with APSGN or may be used to assess renal tissue status.
- Renal ultrasonography may show a normal or slightly enlarged kidney.
- Throat culture may also show group A beta-hemolytic streptococci.
- Urinalysis typically reveals proteinuria and hematuria. RBCs, WBCs, and mixed cell casts are common findings in urinary sediment.
- Kidney-ureter-bladder X-rays show bilateral kidney enlargement.

Nursing diagnoses

- Impaired urinary elimination
- Excess fluid volume
- Fatigue

Treatment

- Bed rest
- Fluid restriction
- High-calorie, low-sodium, low-potassium, low-protein diet
- Dialysis (occasionally necessary)

Drug therapy options

- Diuretic: metolazone (Zaroxolyn) and furosemide (Lasix) to reduce extracellular fluid overload
- Antihypertensive: hydralazine (Apresoline)

Patient care goals

- The client will maintain urine specific gravity within the designated limits.
- The client will maintain fluid balance.
- The client will have increased energy.

Nursing interventions

- Check vital signs and electrolyte values. Monitor fluid intake and output and daily weight. Assess renal function daily through serum creatinine and BUN levels and urine creatinine clearance. Watch for signs of acute renal failure (oliguria, azotemia, acidosis). *These measures detect early signs of complications and guide the treatment plan.*

- Consult the dietitian to provide education regarding a diet high in calories and low in protein, sodium, potassium, and fluids.
- Provide good nutrition, use good hygienic technique, and prevent contact with infected people *to protect the debilitated client against secondary infection.*
- Bed rest is necessary during the acute phase. Encourage the client to gradually resume normal activities as symptoms subside *to prevent fatigue.*
- Provide emotional support for the client and family. If the client is on dialysis, explain the procedure fully. *These measures may help ease his anxiety.*

Evaluation

- The client has normal urine specific gravity.
- The client doesn't display signs of fluid overload.
- The client reports feeling of increased energy.

Acute renal failure

ACUTE RENAL FAILURE is a sudden interruption of renal function resulting from obstruction, poor circulation, or kidney disease. With treatment, this condition is usually reversible; if untreated, it may progress to end-stage renal disease (ESRD) or death.

Acute renal failure is classified as:

- prerenal — results from conditions that diminish blood flow to the kidneys
- intrarenal — results from damage to the kidneys, usually from acute tubular necrosis
- postrenal — results from bilateral obstruction of urine flow.

Acute renal failure has four phases: onset, oliguric-anuric, diuretic, and convalescent. The convalescent period can last up to 12 months.

Possible causes

- Acute glomerulonephritis
- Acute tubular necrosis
- Anaphylaxis
- BPH
- Blood transfusion reaction
- Burns
- Cardiopulmonary bypass
- Collagen diseases
- Congenital deformity
- Dehydration
- Diabetes mellitus
- Heart failure
- Cardiogenic shock
- Endocarditis

Types of dialysis

Dialysis is the process of diffusion, osmosis, and ultrafiltration used to reestablish fluid and electrolyte balance and to remove toxic substances and metabolic wastes:

● *Diffusion* is the passage of ions from an area of high concentration across a semipermeable membrane to an area of lower concentration.

● *Osmosis* is the passage of water molecules across a semipermeable membrane from a less concentrated solution to a more concentrated one.

● *Ultrafiltration* uses positive pressure to cause fluid to pass across a semipermeable membrane from an area of lesser concentration to one of greater concentration. It's faster than osmosis.

Peritoneal dialysis

In peritoneal dialysis, a commercially prepared sterile dialysate (an electrolyte solution) flows by gravity through a catheter inserted through the abdominal wall into the peritoneal cavity. The peritoneum acts as a semipermeable membrane for osmosis and diffusion. After the solution has remained in the peritoneal cavity for the prescribed time, the dialysate is removed. The physician will order this process repeated until the client's fluid and electrolyte levels fall within acceptable limits.

Hemodialysis

In hemodialysis, the client's blood is passed through a dialyzer where, through the processes of diffusion and ultrafiltration, body fluids and electrolytes are exchanged with the dialysate. In this way, excess fluid, electrolytes, and nitrogenous wastes are removed from the body. Access to the client's bloodstream is essential in hemodialysis. This is achieved by external arteriovenous shunt (for acute situations), subclavian or femoral catheters (for acute situations), or internal arteriovenous fistula or graft (used for chronic dialysis).

Continuous ambulatory peritoneal dialysis

Continuous ambulatory peritoneal dialysis (CAPD) is a variation of peritoneal dialysis. CAPD involves infusing 500 to 1,000 ml of a personalized dialysate through a peritoneal catheter, clamping the catheter with the empty bag still attached, rolling up the bag, and placing it in a waistband, with the client then going about his usual activities. Every 4 hours, the client drains the fluid from his peritoneal cavity into the empty bag, removes the bag and drainage from the catheter, aseptically attaches a new bag of dialysate, and repeats the infusion. CAPD proves much less confining to those who can assume the responsibility of maintaining the proper techniques. Major complications of CAPD include peritonitis, fluid and electrolyte imbalances, dehydration, catheter sepsis, abdominal pain and tenderness, organ trauma, and hemorrhage.

Continuous cyclic peritoneal dialysis uses a machine to deliver and drain the peritoneal fluid. Cycling time lasts from 6 to 8 hours, so the client can usually be dialyzed while sleeping at night. The machine has an alarm to protect the client from malfunction.

● Malignant hypertension
● Hemorrhage
● Infections, such as pyelonephritis and septicemia
● Nephrotoxins, such as antibiotics, X-ray dyes, pesticides, and anesthetics
● Thrombi or emboli

Data collection findings
● Anorexia
● Nausea
● Vomiting
● Costovertebral pain
● Headache
● Diarrhea or constipation
● Irritability
● Restlessness
● Lethargy
● Drowsiness
● Stupor
● Coma

● Pallor
● Ecchymosis
● Stomatitis
● Thick tenacious sputum
● Urine output less than 400 ml per day for 1 to 2 weeks, followed by diuresis (3 to 5 L per day) for 2 to 3 weeks
● Weight gain

Diagnostic findings
● ABG analysis shows metabolic acidosis.
● Blood chemistry shows increased potassium, phosphorus, magnesium, BUN, creatinine, and uric acid levels and decreased calcium, carbon dioxide, and sodium levels.
● Creatinine clearance is low.
● Excretory urography shows decreased renal perfusion and function.
● Glomerular filtration rate is 20 to 40 ml/minute (renal insufficiency); 10 to 20 ml/minute (renal failure); or less than 10 ml/minute (ESRD).

- Hematology shows decreased Hb level, HCT, and erythrocytes; and increased PT and PTT.
- Urine chemistry shows albuminuria; proteinuria; increased sodium levels; casts, RBCs, and WBCs; and urine specific gravity greater than 1.025, and then fixed at less than 1.01.

Nursing diagnoses
- Ineffective tissue perfusion (renal)
- Excess fluid volume
- Risk for infection
- Risk for deficient fluid volume

Treatment
- Continuous arteriovenous hemofiltration
- Low-protein, increased-carbohydrate, moderate-fat, and moderate-calorie diet with potassium, sodium, and phosphorus intake regulated according to serum levels
- Peritoneal dialysis or hemodialysis (see *Types of dialysis*)
- Fluid intake restricted to the amount needed to replace fluid loss
- Transfusion therapy with packed RBCs administered over 1 to 3 hours as tolerated

Drug therapy options
- Alkalinizing agent: sodium bicarbonate
- Antacid: aluminum hydroxide (AlternaGEL)
- Antibiotic: cefazolin (Ancef)
- Anticonvulsant: phenytoin (Dilantin)
- Antiemetic: prochlorperazine (Compazine)
- Antipyretic: acetaminophen (Tylenol)
- Beta-adrenergic blocker: dopamine (Intropin) initially to improve renal perfusion
- Cation exchange resin: sodium polystyrene sulfonate (Kayexalate)
- Diuretic: furosemide (Lasix), metolazone (Zaroxolyn)

Patient care goals
- The client will have normal fluid and electrolyte levels.
- The client will experience no preventable complications.
- The client will understand the means by which she and her family members will implement health teaching after discharge.

Nursing interventions
Oliguric-anuric phase
During the oliguric-anuric phase, the client's urine output falls below 400 ml per day, with resultant electrolyte imbalance, metabolic acidosis, and retention of nitrogenous

NURSING PROCEDURE

Inserting an indwelling urinary catheter

Purpose
A urinary catheter, inserted through the urethra into the urinary bladder, is used to empty the bladder before surgery, treat incontinence or urine retention, obtain a sterile urine specimen, determine the amount of residual urine, or monitor urine output continuously in a seriously ill client.

Implementation
- Explain the procedure to the client; provide privacy; and arrange for good lighting.
- Place the female client in the dorsal recumbent position with knees flexed and feet positioned about 2 feet (61 cm) apart. Place the male client in the supine position.
- Place a waterproof pad under the client; clean the genital area with soap and water and then dry it.
- Open the supplies, put on sterile gloves, and set up sterile supplies.
- Spread the labia or position the penis with your nondominant hand. Identify the meatus (in an uncircumcised male, retract the foreskin). Using cotton balls held by forceps, clean the area with antiseptic (use each cotton ball only once).
- Using the dominant hand, insert the catheter into the meatus until urine flows; for a female, insert the indwelling catheter 3″ to 4″ (7.5 to 10 cm); for a male, 7″ to 9″ (17.5 to 23.5 cm). Don't use force when advancing the catheter. If you meet resistance, rotate the catheter slightly (for a male, exert slight upward tension on the penis).
- Inflate the balloon with sterile water; then tug gently on the catheter to check placement
- Attach the catheter to the drainage system (if not connected already). Position the collection bag on the bed frame. Secure the catheter to the patient's thigh, allowing sufficient slack for leg movement.
- Document the date and time of the catheter insertion, the amount of urine initially obtained, urine characteristics, the size of the catheter, and the client response to the procedure.

wastes from nonfunctioning nephrons. This phase may last up to 14 days. Follow these interventions:
- Maintain the client on complete bed rest; organize care *to provide long rest periods. Activity increases the rate of metabolism, which increases production of nitrogenous waste products.*

Key nursing measures during dialysis

Before dialysis
- Explain the procedure to the client.
- Weight the client and measure his vital signs.

Peritoneal dialysis
- Ask the client to urinate before you insert the catheter into the peritoneum to prevent bladder puncture.
- Warm the bottles of dialysate in warm water or by using a heating pad on a low setting.
- Permit 2 L of dialysate to flow unrestricted into the peritoneal cavity (this should take about 10 minutes).
- Allow fluid to remain in the cavity for the time ordered by the physician (about 20 to 30 minutes).
- Reverse the bottles; allow fluid to drain from the peritoneal cavity unrestricted (about 20 to 30 minutes). Facilitate drainage by changing the client's position or massaging the abdomen.
- Keep accurate intake and output records related to the amount of dialysis fluid entering the peritoneal cavity and the amount in the drainage. *Important:* Remove all the dialysis fluid.

Hemodialysis
- Observe carefully for breaks or kinks in membranes to prevent hemorrhage.
- Monitor the chemical composition of the dialysate solution, the fluid rate and pressure, and blood clotting time (anticoagulants are administered throughout hemodialysis).
- Provide shunt care:
  – Keep the area clean, dry, and sterile.
  – Observe the internal fistula for patency. If it's working, you can feel a thrill on palpation or hear a bruit with a stethoscope; if the shunt is discolored, patency is questionable.
  – Immediately report clotting to the physician.
  – Avoid trauma to the extremity with the shunt (no blood pressure measurement, intramuscular or intravenous medications, or blood drawn).
  – Have clamps available to prevent exsanguination if the external shunt disconnects.
- Provide comfort measures for the client.

After dialysis
- Monitor the client's pulse rate and blood pressure every 15 minutes until the client becomes stable and then every 4 hours.
- Monitor the client's weight daily.
- Monitor the client's temperature every 4 hours.

- Implement interventions to prevent infection and the complications of immobility. *Because she's on bed rest, the client becomes susceptible to the hazards of immobility. Infection is a serious risk and the leading cause of death in clients with acute renal failure.*
- Observe the client for metabolic acidosis *to identify complications of renal failure.*
- Observe fluid and electrolyte balance hourly. Insert an indwelling urinary catheter, and measure output and specific gravity hourly. *These actions allow the nurse to monitor the kidneys, which have the major role in regulating fluid and electrolyte balance. High potassium levels can occur.* (See *Inserting an indwelling urinary catheter,* page 469.)
- Provide only enough fluid intake to replace urine output *to avoid edema caused by excessive fluid intake.*
- Monitor the client's diet *to provide high carbohydrates, adequate fats, and low protein.* (Protein should be of high biologic value, or complete protein, such as from beef, eggs, milk, and chicken.) Offer carbohydrate supplements (hard candy, jelly beans, Kool-Aid, tapioca, honey, and jelly). If the client receives adequate calories from fat and carbohydrate metabolism, the body doesn't break down protein for energy. Protein is thus available for growth and repair. There's an accompanying decrease in nonprotein waste products, which result from protein metabolism.
- Reduce the client's potassium intake *to help prevent elevated potassium levels. Protein catabolism causes potassium release from cells into the serum.*
- Assist with observation of arrhythmias and cardiac arrest *to identify complications of high serum potassium.*
- Provide frequent oral hygiene *to avoid tissue irritation and, sometimes, ulcer formation caused by urea and other acid waste products excreted through the skin and mucous membranes.*
- Provide the client with hard candy and chewing gum *to stimulate saliva flow and decrease thirst.*
- Maintain skin care with cool water *to relieve pruritus and remove uremic frost (white crystals formed on the skin from the excretion of urea).*
- Administer stool softeners *to prevent colon irritation from high levels of urea and organic acids.*
- Provide emotional reassurance to the client and family members *to help decrease anxiety levels caused by the fact that the client has an acute illness with an unknown prognosis.*
- Explain treatments and progress to the client *to help reduce anxiety.*

● Assist with providing hemodialysis or peritoneal dialysis, as ordered, *which reduces nonprotein nitrogen waste levels in the blood and improves the fluid and electrolyte balance until the kidneys regain function.* (See *Key nursing measures during dialysis.*)

Early diuretic phase

During the early diuretic phase, which lasts about 10 days, the client excretes a large volume (usually over 3,000 ml per day) of very dilute urine; the glomeruli are beginning to function effectively, but the tubules aren't, and the client still experiences electrolyte imbalance, retention of nitrogenous waste products, and metabolic acidosis. Follow these interventions:

● Assess fluid and electrolyte balance *to identify continued fluid and electrolyte imbalance when the renal tubules aren't functioning.*

● Assess the emotional status of the client and family members *to provide support because the prognosis is still uncertain.*

● Continue interventions used during the oliguric phase, except for:

– increasing fluid intake dramatically to keep up with output *to prevent dehydration that may be experienced during the polyuric phase*

– administering potassium or other electrolyte replacements, if needed, *to prevent imbalances caused by loss of electrolytes and fluid.*

Late diuretic phase

In the late diuretic phase, the client is still excreting more fluid than normal; urine specific gravity is increasing because the tubules are beginning to function effectively; and fluid, electrolyte, and acid-base balances are returning to normal. Follow these interventions:

● Continue implementations of the early diuretic phase. Allow the client to engage in nonstrenuous activity for brief periods, and increase the activity level gradually; don't let her become fatigued, *which may increase the rate of metabolism and overwork the kidneys.*

● Teach the client to prevent infection and to avoid the factors that caused renal failure *to help prevent a recurrence.*

Evaluation

● The client regains fluid and electrolyte balance.
● The client understands the rationale behind activity restrictions.

Benign prostatic hyperplasia

Benign prostatic hyperplasia (BPH) affects about one-half of all men over age 50. In BPH, the prostate gland enlarges, compresses the urethra, and causes urinary obstruction. If hyperplasia becomes severe and causes obstruction, infection, or impaired renal function, surgical intervention becomes necessary. Surgeons most commonly use transurethral resection.

Possible causes

● Hormonal
● Unknown

Data collection findings

● Decreased force and amount of urination
● Dribbling
● Hesitancy
● Nocturia
● Urgency, frequency, and burning on urination

Diagnostic findings

● BUN level (normally 8 to 20 mg/dl) is elevated, indicating dehydration or renal damage.
● Creatinine level (normally 0.8 to 1.5 mg/dl) is elevated, indicating renal damage.
● Excretory urography, an X-ray of the kidney and pelvis using a contrast material injected I.V., shows urethral obstruction and hydronephrosis. A check for hypersensitivity to the dye may be necessary.
● Cystoscopy, which permits visualization of the bladder and urethra through a lighted tube, shows an enlarged prostate gland, obstructed urine flow, and urinary stasis. (See *Nursing interventions for cystoscopy,* page 472.)
● Rectal examination discloses an enlarged prostate gland.
● Urinary flow rate determination shows a small volume, prolonged flow pattern, and low peak flow.
● Urine chemistry shows bacteria, hematuria, alkaline pH, and increased urine specific gravity.

Nursing diagnoses

● Acute pain
● Urinary retention
● Impaired urinary elimination
● Sexual dysfunction

Treatment

● Forced fluids
● Transurethral resection of the prostate or prostatectomy

Nursing interventions for cystoscopy

Before cystoscopy
● Force fluids for several hours to maintain a constant flow of urine and prevent bacterial stasis.
● Provide sedation 1 hour before the cystoscopy with either diazepam (Valium) or meperidine (Demerol), as ordered, to reduce stress and anxiety in the client.

After cystoscopy
● Evaluate the client's ability to void after the procedure. Urine may be pink-tinged from the trauma of cystoscopy.
● Check for complaints of pain, spasms, and urinary frequency. Warm sitz baths, analgesics, or antispasmodics may be needed to promote comfort.
● Force fluids to keep the urinary tract flushed and provide internal irrigation.
● Observe the client for complications, such as an elevated temperature, chills, flushing, and hypotension, which may signal hemorrhage or infection.

Drug therapy options
● Alpha-adrenergic antagonist: prazosin (Minipress), terazosin (Hytrin)
● Alpha-adrenergic blocker: phenoxybenzamine (Dibenzyline)
● Analgesic: oxycodone hydrochloride with acetaminophen (Tylox)
● Antianxiety: oxazepam (Serax)
● Antibiotic: co-trimoxazole (Bactrim)
● Urinary antiseptic: phenazopyridine (Pyridium)

Patient care goals
● The client will have normal urine output and unobstructed flow.
● The client will be free from postoperative complications.
● The client will discuss concerns related to temporary sexual dysfunction.

Nursing interventions
Preoperative care
● Gradually drain urine through a urethral catheter *to relieve the obstruction.* With severe obstruction, the bladder may contain more than 1,000 ml of urine; *gradual decompression is necessary to prevent shock and hemorrhage.*
● Prepare the client for the transurethral resection. Tell him to expect a catheter in the bladder. Explain that he'll feel like voiding and that urine will drain through the tube *to ensure that the client doesn't attempt to void around the tube. That would strain the bladder and contribute to spasms.*
● Reassure the client that he'll probably be able to resume sexual activity after he's healed *to help alleviate the client's fears about sexual dysfunctioning.* Impotence rarely occurs except after a radical prostatectomy for prostate cancer.

Postoperative care
● Inspect the client's urine, and observe him for signs of shock *to monitor response to surgery and to identify signs of complications.* Dark red blood in the urine is normal for the first few days after surgery; bright red blood and clots indicate an active hemorrhage. Tissue sloughing and straining can cause delayed hemorrhaging 6 to 10 days postoperatively.
● Maintain catheter patency. Keep accurate intake and output records, and account for irrigating fluid *to monitor the client's status.* Assess him for water intoxication *to identify signs of complications.* The client is likely to have a three-way indwelling urinary catheter in place with continuous irrigation for the first 24 hours. The catheter maintains flow and prevents and eliminates clots. The venous sinusoids of the bladder may absorb the irrigating fluid.
● Force fluids *to keep urine diluted.*
● Irrigate catheter as needed to prevent voiding around the catheter and *to decrease strain and reduce the discomfort of bladder spasms. Irrigation removes clots. The catheter has a 30-ml balloon, and applied traction prevents bleeding. Both the large balloon and traction contribute to spasms, which usually decrease within 24 to 48 hours.*
● Administer anticholinergic drugs (for example, belladonna and opium suppositories) as ordered *to decrease bladder spasms.*
● Remove the catheter 2 to 3 days after surgery, as ordered, and periodically check for voiding *to assess urinary status and to check for occasional dribbling.* The catheter typically is removed by the time the client is discharged, usually 3 days after surgery.
● Teach perineal (Kegel) exercises, with the client tightly squeezing the perineal muscles 5 to 10 times each hour. *Perineal exercises increase sphincter tone.* Full bladder capacity may not return for 2 months.
● Help the client walk *to prevent a thromboembolism and to reduce bladder spasms.*
● Before discharge, provide the following instructions *to protect the client from injury and hemorrhage, which can occur if he sustains trauma before healing is complete:*

– Don't strain at stool.
– Use a stool softener.
– Don't drive a car for 3 weeks.
– Do no heavy lifting for 6 weeks.
– Resume sexual activity when healing is complete.
Without complications, the client is usually discharged on day 4.

 SPOT CHECK

When is surgical intervention necessary for a client with BPH?
Answer: Surgical intervention is performed if prostatic enlargement causes obstruction, infection, or impaired renal function.

Evaluation
● The client shows no evidence of hemorrhage or infection.
● The client has an unobstructed urine flow.
● Follow-up care reveals that the client isn't experiencing sexual dysfunction.

Bladder cancer
Bladder cancer is a malignant tumor that invades the mucosal lining of the bladder. It may metastasize to the ureters, prostate gland, vagina, rectum, and periaortic lymph nodes.

Possible causes
● Chronic bladder irritation
● Cigarette smoking
● Drugs (cyclophosphamide [Cytoxan])
● Excessive intake of coffee, phenacetin, sodium, saccharin, or sodium cyclamate
● Exposure to industrial chemicals
● Radiation

Data collection findings
● Frequency of urination
● Urgency of urination
● Dysuria
● Painless hematuria
● Anuria
● Chills
● Fever
● Flank or pelvic pain
● Peripheral edema

Diagnostic findings
● Cystoscopy reveals a mass.
● Cytologic examination is positive for malignant cells.
● Excretory urography shows a mass or an obstruction.
● Hematology shows decreased RBC count, Hb level, and HCT.
● Kidney-ureter-bladder X-ray shows mass or obstruction.
● Urine chemistry shows hematuria.

Nursing diagnoses
● Impaired urinary elimination
● Acute pain
● Anxiety

Treatment
● Transfusion therapy with packed RBCs
● Surgery, depending on the location and progress of the tumor

Drug therapy options
● Analgesic: meperidine (Demerol), morphine (MS Contin)
● Antispasmodic: phenazopyridine (Pyridium)
● Sedative: oxazepam (Serax)

Patient care goals
● The client will maintain adequate intake and output.
● The client will express feelings of comfort and pain relief.
● The client will exhibit adequate coping mechanisms.

Nursing interventions
● Assess renal status *to determine baseline and detect early changes.*
● Monitor and record vital signs and intake and output. *Accurate intake and output are essential for correct fluid replacement therapy.*
● Provide postoperative care *to promote healing and prevent complications.* (Closely monitor urine output. Observe for hematuria [reddish tint to gross bloodiness] or infection [cloudy, foul smelling, with sediment]. Maintain continuous bladder irrigation, if indicated. Assist with turning, coughing and deep breathing.)
● Maintain the client's diet *to improve nutrition and to meet metabolic demands.*
● Force fluids *to prevent dehydration.*
● Monitor the administration of I.V. fluids *to maintain hydration.*
● Administer medications, as prescribed, *to maintain or improve the client's condition.*

- Encourage the client to express his fear of dying *to encourage adequate coping mechanisms.*
- Provide postchemotherapeutic care (watch for myelosuppression, chemical cystitis, and skin rash) and postradiation nursing care *to prevent complications associated with treatment.*

SPOT CHECK

Following a diagnosis of bladder cancer, a client receives local radiation therapy and experiences a dry skin reaction. In recommending care of the skin, the nurse should instruct the client to avoid:

A. lubrication.
B. cleansers.
C. cold packs.
D. cotton garments.

Answer: C. Cold packs over the area of a dry reaction to radiation therapy are contraindicated because they reduce capillary circulation to the site and hamper healing. Lubrication, cleansers, and cotton garments aren't unconditionally contraindicated.

Evaluation

- The client has an appropriate fluid balance.
- The client reports adequate pain control.
- The client demonstrates appropriate coping mechanisms.

Breast cancer

Breast cancer is the most common cancer in women in the United States; however, since 1986, breast cancer has been second to lung cancer as the leading cause of death due to cancer in women. Current statistical data indicate that one in every eight women in the United States develops breast cancer in her lifetime. While breast cancer can also develop in men, its incidence is very low.

Most primary breast cancers are adenocarcinomas and occur in the upper outer quadrant of the breast. The most common sites of metastasis from breast cancer are the:

- liver
- bone
- lungs.

Possible causes
Primary risk factors
- Female gender
- Age older than 50 years
- Country of origin

- Personal or family history of breast cancer
- Breast cancer gene
- Benign breast disease

Secondary risk factors
- Postmenopausal obesity
- Early menarche (before age 12)
- Nulliparity or parity (first, full-term pregnancy) after age 35
- Late menopause (after age 55)
- Use of oral contraceptives before age 20 and for more than 6 years
- Exposure to ionizing radiation, especially during young adulthood

Other potential risk factors
- Prolonged postmenopausal estrogen replacement therapy
- Diet high in animal fat
- Moderate alcohol consumption

Data collection findings
- Asymmetry of breasts
- Dimpling or puckering of the skin
- Enlargement of axillary or supraclavicular lymph nodes
- Lump or thickening in the breast
- Nipple retraction or inversion
- Peau d'orange skin changes
- Redness, ulceration, edema, or dilated veins in the breast
- Scaly skin around the nipple
- Spontaneous, persistent, and unilateral nipple discharge that's serosanguineous, bloody, or watery in character

Diagnostic findings
- Sonogram or ultrasound is used to differentiate between a solid or cystic lesion.
- MRI (or magnetic resonance mammography) of the breast can be used to distinguish between a benign or malignant lesion.
- Fine-needle aspiration (FNA) is used when a known lesion is solid or to determine if a lump is cystic. If cystic, a lump should resolve after the FNA is completed.
- Biopsy, such as stereotactic needle-guided biopsy, wire-localized biopsy, or excisional biopsy, reveals a malignant lesion.
- Estrogen-progesterone receptor analysis (biomarker) identifies hormone-dependent tumors that may respond to hormonal therapy. Receptor-positive tumors occur more

commonly in postmenopausal women and generally confer an improved overall prognosis.

● Radiographic scans of the bone, brain, liver, and other organs can reveal distant metastases.

Nursing diagnoses
● Disturbed body image
● Fear
● Acute pain

Treatment
● Surgery, such as lumpectomy, skin-sparing mastectomy, partial mastectomy, total mastectomy, or modified radical mastectomy
● Radiation therapy

FAST FACT

Breast reconstruction surgery can be performed immediately after mastectomy, or it may be delayed if adjuvant chemotherapy or radiation therapy is necessary.

Drug therapy options
● Analgesic: fentanyl (Duragesic), morphine (MS Contin), NSAIDs
● Antiemetic: granisetron (Kytril), ondansetron (Zofran), prochlorperazine (Compazine), trimethobenzamide (Tigan)
● Chemotherapeutic drug: cyclophosphamide (Cytoxan), doxorubicin (Adriamycin), and methotrexate (Folex)
● Hormonal therapy: tamoxifen (Nolvadex), letrozole (Femara), toremifine (Fareston)
● Transfusion therapy, if needed

Patient care goals
● The client will maintain a positive body image and positive self-concept.
● The client will demonstrate a decreased level of fear.
● The client will receive adequate pain relief.

Nursing interventions
● Assess the client's feelings about her illness, and determine what she knows about breast cancer and her expectations *to identify her needs and to aid in developing a plan of care.*
● Provide routine postoperative care *to prevent complications.*
● Perform comfort measures *to promote relaxation and relieve anxiety.*

● Administer analgesics as ordered, and monitor their effectiveness *to promote the client's comfort.*
● Watch for treatment-related complications, such as nausea, vomiting, anorexia, leukopenia, thrombocytopenia, GI ulceration, and bleeding, *to ensure that measures are taken to prevent further complications.*
● Monitor the client's weight and nutritional intake *to detect evidence of malnutrition.* Encourage a high-protein diet. Dietary supplements may be necessary to meet increased metabolic demands.
● Assess the client's and family member's ability to cope, especially if the cancer is terminal. Counseling may be necessary *to help them cope with the fear of death and dying.*
● In the immediate postoperative phase, teach arm exercises, as ordered, *to facilitate drainage, prevent contractures, and relieve muscle spasms.* Such factors as wound healing, grafts, temperature elevation, and increased drainage may delay exercises. Consult with the surgeon to determine when to undertake a full regimen.
● Before discharge, encourage the client to view her incision *to help her adjust to an altered body image.* Explain that after healing has occurred, the incision can be massaged with cocoa butter or cold cream to soften the incision.
● Take precautions to prevent lymphedema and infection *to prevent long-term problems.* Permit no invasive procedures on the affected arm, and give the client these instructions:
– Don't permit blood pressure checks on the affected arm.
– Wear gloves when gardening.
– Avoid all burns, including sunburn.
– Wear a thimble when sewing.
– Immediately provide care for even minor cuts and scratches.
– Whenever possible, keep the arm elevated.
– Don't wear constrictive clothing.
– Avoid undue pressure such as from a shoulder purse.
● Before discharge, review these instructions with the client and family members *to ensure adequate knowledge about her condition and treatment,* including:
– treatment options
– management of adverse reactions to treatment
– importance of immediately reporting signs of infection to the physician
– breast self-examination
– availability of community support services
– contacting the American Cancer Society.

CLINICAL SITUATION

Caring for the client with breast cancer

A 62-year-old female arrives at the surgery unit at 6 a.m. on the day of her scheduled right modified radical mastectomy. One week ago, she had a biopsy that showed a 1" (2.5 cm) adenocarcinoma in the upper outer quadrant of her right breast. Since that time, she's had a full workup to check for metastasis. All tests have been negative. Her husband, who seems attentive and concerned about her condition, accompanies her to the hospital. The client had her preoperative teaching 3 days ago at the preadmission testing unit. She'll stay 3 to 4 days if she remains free from complications.

After surgery, what are appropriate nursing actions?
● Observe the client's vital signs *to establish her condition.*
● Inspect the dressing for bleeding and report any bleeding to the physician immediately. Be sure to check under the client. *Gravity may cause the blood to flow beneath the client, thereby obscuring it.*
● Ensure proper functioning of the Hemovac unit, *which removes excess fluid. Show the client how to empty the drain because the drain may remain in place after discharge.*

● Identify the type and severity of the client's pain. Initially, the operation causes trauma pain. Later, pain may result from nerve irritation and muscle spasm. The client may also feel a phantom breast.
● Elevate the affected arm in an abducted position; observe for edema. Transient or long-term edema can occur after removal of the lymph nodes. *Arm elevation in the abducted position facilitates drainage, increases venous return, and prevents lymphedema and shoulder contracture.*
● Encourage ambulation. Have the client deep-breathe every 2 hours. Relieve pain with analgesics.
● Spend time with the client, encourage her to express feelings and concerns, and provide generous emotional support. After breast removal, the client will grieve. *The nurse's presence can be a source of comfort during this difficult time.*

Questions for further thought
● How can the nurse help the husband to reassure the client of continued love and nurturing?
● What actions by the client indicate she's beginning to accept the change to her body?

Evaluation
● The client expresses feelings about her body image changes and expresses positive feelings about herself.
● The client verbalizes a decreased level of fear and can discuss her feelings, the diagnosis, and treatment options.
● The client verbalizes relief from pain and has normal vital signs.
● The client discusses self-care activities to promote full recovery. (See *Caring for the client with breast cancer.*)

Cervical cancer
Cervical cancer is second to breast cancer as the most common malignancy in women throughout the world. Preinvasive cancers range from minimal cervical dysplasia, in which the lower third of the epithelium contains abnormal cells, to carcinoma in situ, in which the full thickness of epithelium contains abnormally proliferating cells.

In many underdeveloped countries, invasive cervical cancer is the leading cause of death in women of reproductive age, largely due to the absence of effective screen-

ing programs for the early detection and treatment of preinvasive disease. The average age of diagnosis is 50 years. Cervical cancer is largely a preventable disease. The American Cancer Society recommends that all women who are sexually active or who are age 18 or older have a Papanicolaou (Pap) test performed every year.

Most cervical cancers are squamous; the rest are adenocarcinomas. The incidence of adenocarcinomas and adenocarcinomas in situ more than doubled between the early 1970s and the mid-1980s, especially in women younger than age 35.

Possible causes
● Unknown

Sexual risk factors
● High number of sexual partners
● Partners with multiple sexual partners
● Early age at first sexual intercourse, particularly before age 16
● Multiple pregnancies

• History of sexually transmitted diseases (STDs), especially herpes simplex virus II (HSV-2) or human papillomavirus (HPV)

SPOT CHECK

Name two STDs that put a client at risk for cervical cancer.
Answer: Two STDs that put a client at risk for cervical cancer are HPV and HSV-2.

Other risk factors

• Race (the incidence of cervical cancer is highest in Native American, African-American, and Hispanic-American women; double or more than double that for white women)
• Long-term cigarette smoking or exposure to passive cigarette smoke
• Diets low in beta-carotene, alpha-tocopherol, ascorbic acid, folate, or retinol
• Rural or socioeconomic factors that limit access to health care

Data collection findings

• Abnormal bleeding (amount may vary from scant spotting to frank bleeding)
• Prolonged menstrual period or intermittent
• Bleeding following sexual intercourse
• Difficulty voiding, urgency, hematuria, rectal tenesmus, or rectal bleeding (direct invasion of the bladder or rectum)
• Lower extremity edema (lymphatic involvement)
• Odor or pain in the lower back, leg, or groin (extensive tumor involvement)
• Serosanguineous discharge (uncommon)

Diagnostic findings

• A Pap test is used for screening purposes.
• Colposcopy is used to determine the source of abnormal cells found through the Pap test.
• Cone biopsy is performed if endocervical curettage is positive.
• Reflex HPV typing can distinguish between cells or lesions requiring aggressive treatment (intermediate or high-risk HPV), such as colposcopy, and those that can be managed conservatively (negative or low-risk HPV) through repeated Pap tests in 3 to 6 months.
• For invasive cervical cancer, the initial workup and clinical staging includes chest radiography, excretory urography or CT scan, cystoscopy, proctosigmoidoscopy, and

HIV testing (especially for younger at-risk women) for clinical staging and evaluation of metastasis.
• CT scan can reveal enlarged lymph nodes, which can then be assessed histologically and cytologically with either surgical excision or FNA.
• MRI can be used to detect early parametrial and nodal disease.
• Barium enema, bone scans, cystography, and lymphangiography can be used to detect metastasis.

Nursing diagnoses

• Acute pain
• Fear
• Risk for infection

Treatment

• Varies depending on the stage and extent of the cancer

Preinvasive

• Laser therapy, cryosurgery, cervical conization
• Total excisional biopsy
• Hysterectomy (rare)

Invasive

• Radiation therapy (internal, external, or both)
• Radical hysterectomy
• Pelvic exoneration (rare)

Patient care goals

• The client will have a decreased level of fear.
• The client will be free from signs of infection.
• The client will receive adequate pain relief.

Nursing interventions

• Encourage the client to use relaxation techniques *to promote comfort during diagnostic procedures.*
• When assisting with a biopsy, drape and prepare the client as for a routine pelvic examination. Have a container of formaldehyde ready *to preserve the specimen during transfer to the pathology laboratory.* Assist the physician as needed and provide support for the client throughout the procedure *to allay the client's anxiety.*
• If assisting with laser therapy, drape and prepare the client as for a routine pelvic examination. Assist the physician as needed and provide support to the client *to alleviate the client's anxiety.*
• Watch for complications related to therapy *to ensure that measures can be instituted to prevent or alleviate complications.*

● Administer pain medication, as needed, and note its effectiveness. If pain relief isn't achieved, an alternative dose or medication may be required.

● Review key teaching topics with the client and family members *to ensure adequate knowledge about her condition and treatment,* including:

– treatment options

– postexcisional biopsy care (expecting discharge or spotting for about 1 week; avoiding douching, using tampons, or engaging in sexual intercourse during this time; reporting signs of infection)

– follow-up Pap tests and pelvic examinations.

Postoperative care
After abdominal hysterectomy

● Check abdominal and perineal dressings for excessive bleeding every 15 minutes for 2 hours and then every 4 hours for at least 8 hours. A moderate amount of sanguineous drainage on the perineal pad is normal. *The risk of hemorrhage after an abdominal hysterectomy is greatest during the first 24 hours because of the abundant blood supply to the pelvis.*

● Insert an indwelling urinary catheter or encourage the client to void *to maintain urine output.*

● Allow no food or fluids for 24 to 48 hours, as ordered, until peristalsis returns and bowel sounds are normal. When the client is able to eat, allow no gas-forming foods *because flatus causes intense discomfort.*

● Encourage ambulation *to promote peristalsis.*

● Encourage ambulation and exercises *to promote circulation.* Have the client walk the day after surgery, if ordered. Avoid high Fowler's position, which may result in pelvic congestion. Don't use the knee gatch (resulting in flexed knees) on the bed. Use antiembolic stockings and pneumatic compression stockings as appropriate *to promote venous return.*

● Review key teaching topics with the client and family members *to ensure adequate knowledge about the condition and treatment,* including:

– avoiding sexual intercourse and douching until instructed otherwise by the physician

– avoiding heavy lifting and other strenuous activities for about 2 months, as instructed by the physician

– notifying the physician of bleeding or abnormal vaginal discharge

– understanding the importance of continued follow-up care at frequent intervals, which allows for an assessment of the client's psychological adjustment (while most clients successfully resolve their feelings of loss and fear associated with hysterectomy and a diagnosis of cancer,

some will have unusual difficulty coping and may need referral for psychological counseling).

Evaluation

● The client verbalizes a decreased level of fear and can discuss her feelings, the diagnosis, and treatment options.

● The client has normal vital signs, an incision site without signs of redness, or drainage, and exhibits no signs of complication from surgery.

● The client verbalizes relief from pain.

Chlamydia

CHLAMYDIA refers to a group of infections linked to one organism: *Chlamydia trachomatis.* Chlamydial infections are the most common STDs in the United States. Chlamydia infection causes urethritis in men and urethritis and cervicitis in women. Untreated, chlamydial infections can lead to such complications as acute epididymitis, salpingitis, pelvic inflammatory disease (PID) and, eventually, sterility.

Possible causes

● Exposure to *C. trachomatis* through sexual contact

Data collection findings
In women

● Pelvic pain
● Dyspareunia
● Mucopurulent discharge
● Cervical erosion

In men

● Urinary frequency
● Dysuria
● Pruritus
● Erythema
● Tenderness of the meatus
● Urethral discharge

Diagnostic findings

● A swab from the site of infection (urethra, cervix, or rectum) establishes a diagnosis of urethritis, cervicitis, salpingitis, endometritis, or proctitis.

● A culture of aspirated material establishes a diagnosis of epididymitis.

● Antigen detection methods, ELISA and the direct fluorescent antibody test, are the diagnostic tests of choice for identifying chlamydial infection, although tissue cell cultures are more sensitive and specific.

Nursing diagnoses
- Deficient knowledge (disease transmission)
- Acute pain
- Ineffective sexuality patterns

Treatment
- The only treatment available for chlamydial infection is drug therapy.

Drug therapy options
- Antibiotic: doxycycline (Vibramycin), azithromycin (Zithromax) a single 1-gram dose for pregnant women with chlamydial infections

Patient care goals
- The client will relate appropriate information concerning disease transmission and treatment.
- The client will express feelings of comfort and pain relief.
- The client will voice feelings about changes in sexual practice.

Nursing interventions
- Practice standard precautions when caring for a client with a chlamydial infection *to prevent the spread of infection.*
- Make sure that the client fully understands the dosage requirements of all prescribed medications for this infection *to ensure compliance with the treatment regimen.*
- If required in your state, report all cases of chlamydial infection to the appropriate local public health authorities, who will then conduct follow-up notification of the client's sexual contacts. *These measures help ensure that an infected sexual contact will receive medical care to treat the infection.*
- Suggest that the client and his sexual partners receive HIV testing. *The unsafe sex practices that lead to chlamydial infection also place the client at risk for contracting HIV.*
- Check neonates of infected mothers for signs of chlamydial infection *to ensure prompt recognition and treatment of infection.* Obtain appropriate specimens for diagnostic testing *to confirm diagnosis of chlamydial infection.*

Evaluation
- The client relates appropriate knowledge regarding the disease.
- The client reports adequate pain control.
- The client reports responsible sexual behavior.

Chronic glomerulonephritis

A slowly progressive disease, CHRONIC GLOMERULONEPHRITIS is characterized by inflammation of the glomeruli, which results in sclerosis, scarring and, eventually, renal failure. By the time it produces symptoms, chronic glomerulonephritis is usually irreversible.

Possible causes
- Renal disorders
- Systemic disorders (SLE, Goodpasture's syndrome, and diabetes mellitus)

Data collection findings
- Hematuria
- Edema
- Hypertension
- Uremic symptoms (in the late stages of the disease)

Diagnostic findings
- Kidney biopsy identifies the underlying disease and provides the data needed to guide therapy.
- Blood studies reveal rising BUN and serum creatinine levels, which indicate advanced renal insufficiency.
- Urinalysis reveals proteinuria, hematuria, cylindruria, and RBC casts.
- X-ray or ultrasonography shows smaller kidneys.

Nursing diagnoses
- Impaired urinary elimination
- Excess fluid volume
- Fatigue

Treatment
- Dialysis
- Low-sodium, high-calorie with adequate protein diet
- Kidney transplant

Drug therapy options
- Antibiotic for symptomatic urinary tract infections
- Antihypertensive: metoprolol (Lopressor)
- Diuretic: furosemide (Lasix)

Patient care goals
- The client will maintain fluid balance.
- The client will experience increased energy and decreased fatigue.

Nursing interventions
- Understand that client care is primarily supportive, focusing on continual observation and sound client teach-

ing. *Supportive measures encourage the client to cope with chronic disease.*
- Accurately monitor vital signs, intake and output, and daily weight *to evaluate fluid retention.*
- Observe for signs of fluid, electrolyte, and acid-base imbalances *to ensure early treatment and prevent complications.*
- Consult the dietitian *to plan low-sodium, high-calorie meals with adequate protein.*
- Administer medications and provide good skin care *to combat pruritus and edema.*
- Provide good oral hygiene *to prevent the breakdown of the oral mucosa.*

Evaluation
- The client doesn't display signs of fluid overload.
- The client reports increased energy.

Chronic renal failure

CHRONIC RENAL FAILURE is progressive, irreversible destruction of the kidneys, leading to loss of renal function. It may result from a rapidly progressing disease of sudden onset that destroys the nephrons and causes irreversible kidney damage.

FAST FACT

ESRD is more common among African Americans and Native Americans. Increased incidence among African Americans results from hypertension; Native Americans, diabetes.

Possible causes
- Congenital abnormalities
- Dehydration
- Diabetes mellitus
- Exacerbations of nephritis
- Hypertension
- Nephrotoxins
- Recurrent urinary tract infection
- SLE
- Urinary tract obstructions

Data collection findings
- Anorexia
- Nausea and vomiting
- Azotemia
- Bone pain
- Brittle nails and hair
- Decreased urine output
- Ecchymosis
- Heart failure
- Irritability (early metabolic acidosis)
- Apathy
- Drowsiness
- Coma (late metabolic acidosis)
- Lethargy
- Muscle twitching
- Weakness
- Paresthesia
- Pruritus
- Uremic frost
- Stomatitis
- Seizures
- Susceptibility to infection
- Weight gain

Diagnostic findings
- ABG analysis shows metabolic acidosis.
- Blood chemistry shows increased BUN, creatinine, phosphorus, and lipid levels and decreased calcium, carbon dioxide, and albumin levels.
- Hematology shows decreased Hb level, HCT, and platelet count.
- Urine chemistry shows proteinuria, glycosuria, erythrocytes, leukocytes, or casts, depending on the cause.
- Urine specific gravity is fixed.

Nursing diagnoses
- Excess fluid volume
- Ineffective tissue perfusion (renal)
- Powerlessness

Treatment
- Limited fluids
- Low-protein, low-sodium, low-potassium, low-phosphorus, high-calorie, and high-carbohydrate diet
- Peritoneal dialysis and hemodialysis (for more information on dialysis, see *Types of dialysis*, page 468, and *Key nursing measures during dialysis*, page 470)
- Transfusion therapy with packed RBCs and platelets

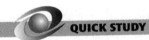

QUICK STUDY

To remember contraindications for peritoneal dialysis, think **SHE**:
Severe obstructive pulmonary diseases
History of multiple abdominal surgical procedures
Excessive obesity, large abdominal wall, and fat deposits

Drug therapy options
- Alkalinizing agent: sodium bicarbonate
- Antacid: aluminum hydroxide gel (AlternaGEL)
- Antianemic: epoetin alfa (recombinant human erythropoietin, Epogen), ferrous sulfate (Feosol), iron dextran (InFeD)
- Antiarrhythmic: procainamide (Pronestyl)
- Antibiotic: cefazolin (Ancef)
- Antiemetic: prochlorperazine (Compazine)
- Antipyretic: acetaminophen (Tylenol)
- Beta-adrenergic blocker: dopamine (Intropin)
- Calcium supplement: calcium carbonate (Os-Cal)
- Cation exchange resin: sodium polystyrene sulfonate (Kayexalate)
- Cardiac glycoside: digoxin (Lanoxin)
- Diuretic: furosemide (Lasix)
- Stool softener: docusate (Colace)
- Vitamin: ascorbic acid (vitamin C), pyridoxine (vitamin B_6)

Patient care goals
- The client will understand how dialysis works and why it's needed.
- The client and family members will be able to cope with the prognosis and the need for lifelong dialysis.

Nursing interventions
- Assess renal, respiratory, and cardiovascular status and fluid balance. *An increase in hemodynamic status and vital signs may indicate fluid overload caused by lack of kidney function.*
- Assess the dialysis access site for bruits and thrills *to ensure patency and detect complications.*
- Monitor and record vital signs, intake and output, electrocardiogram values, daily weight, laboratory studies, and stools for occult blood *to assess baseline and to detect early changes in the client's condition.*
- Monitor for ecchymosis and GI bleeding *because the blood clotting mechanism may be affected.*
- Maintain standard precautions *to prevent the spread of infection.*
- Maintain the client's diet *to promote nutritional status.* Allow him to select foods from the diet prescribed *to encourage him to eat.*
- Restrict fluids *to prevent fluid overload.*
- Administer medications, as prescribed, and observe for adverse effects of medications *to improve or maintain the client's condition and monitor his increased sensitivity to medications.*

CLINICAL SITUATION

Caring for the client with chronic renal failure

A 57-year-old steelworker has had several urinary tract infections. Recently, he has been experiencing muscle weakness, and he tires more easily than usual, being exhausted at the end of a workday. After a thorough physical examination and a diagnostic testing, the client receives a medical diagnosis of chronic renal failure.

The nurse formulates the following nursing diagnoses:
- Excess fluid volume related to impaired excretory function
- Impaired physical mobility related to fatigue and anemia
- Powerlessness related to dependence on dialysis.

The nurse formulates a fourth nursing diagnosis: *Risk for situational low self-esteem.*

Provide at least three reasons why this nursing diagnosis is appropriate with this medical condition. Possible reasons that the client's self-esteem may be affected by this medical condition include:
- lifestyle changes
- dependency on dialysis
- chronic fatigue
- body-image changes
- role maintenance
- occupational problems.

Questions for further thought
- What medications excreted by the kidney need to be avoided?
- What type of diet is appropriate for the client with chronic renal failure and why?
- When should the nurse instruct the client to take his diuretics and why?

- Encourage the client to express his feelings about the chronicity of his illness *to encourage the use of coping mechanisms.*
- Provide tepid baths *to promote comfort and reduce skin irritation.*
- Maintain a cool and quiet environment *to reduce metabolic demands.*
- Provide mouth care using plain water *to promote comfort and enhance the ability to eat.* The client's breath will have an ammonia odor, resembling that of urine, which

may limit the ability to eat. His gums may bleed and stomatitis or ulcers may form.

● Avoid giving the client I.M. injections *to prevent bleeding from the injection site.*

● The client and family members may become depressed by the problems of continuing therapy and the poor prognosis. Encourage them to express their feelings and provide emotional support *to aid communication to provide an outlet for the client's and family members' feelings and to identify the need for further support measures.*

● Review key teaching topics with the client and family members *to ensure adequate knowledge about the condition and treatment,* including:

– required care techniques and what symptoms to report to the physician

– importance of getting sufficient rest

– importance of completing skin and mouth care daily

– ways to avoid infection.

Evaluation

● The client can explain the principles of dialysis and his participation in the procedure.

● The client and family members are learning to cope with their situation. (See *Caring for the client with chronic renal failure,* page 481.)

Cystitis

CYSTITIS, an inflammation of the urinary bladder, usually results from pathologic microorganisms. Most commonly, it's related to a superficial infection that doesn't extend to the bladder mucosa.

Possible causes

● Diabetes mellitus

● Incorrect aseptic technique during catheterization

● Incorrect perineal care

● Kidney infection

● Obstruction of the urethra

● Pregnancy

● Radiation

● Sexual intercourse

● Stagnation of urine in the bladder

Data collection findings

● Low-grade fever

● Urinary burning, frequency, and urgency

● Suprapubic or flank tenderness

● Pus or blood in the urine (present with advanced infection)

● Presence of predisposing factors or disease

Diagnostic findings

● Cystoscopy shows obstruction or deformity.

● Urine chemistry shows hematuria, pyuria, and increased protein, leukocytes, and urine specific gravity.

● Urine culture and sensitivity positively identifies organisms (*Escherichia coli, Proteus vulgaris,* or *Streptococcus faecalis*).

Nursing diagnoses

● Acute pain

● Impaired urinary elimination

● Risk for infection

Treatment

● Increased intake of fluids and vitamin C

Drug therapy options

● Antibiotic: co-trimoxazole (Bactrim)

● Antipyretic: acetaminophen (Tylenol)

● Urinary antiseptic: phenazopyridine (Pyridium)

Patient care goals

● The client will be free from cystitis.

● The client will understand how to prevent cystitis.

● The client will have decreased discomfort.

Nursing interventions

● Assess renal status *to determine baseline and to detect changes.*

● Monitor and record vital signs, intake and output, and laboratory studies *to assess the client's status and to detect early complications.*

● Maintain the client's diet *to promote nutrition.*

● Force fluids (cranberry or orange juice) to 3 qt (3 L) per day *because dilute urine lessens irritation of the bladder mucosa and lowering urine pH with orange juice and cranberry juice consumption helps diminish bacterial growth.*

● Administer medications, as prescribed, *to maintain or improve the client's condition.*

● Perform sitz baths and perineal care *to relieve perineal or suprapubic discomfort.* (See *Performing a sitz bath.*)

● Encourage voiding every 2 to 3 hours *to decrease bladder irritation and prevent urine stasis.*

● Review key teaching topics with the client *to ensure adequate knowledge about his condition and treatment,* including:

– avoiding coffee, tea, alcohol, and cola

NURSING PROCEDURE

Performing a sitz bath

Purpose

Also known as a hip bath, a sitz bath involves immersion of the pelvic area in warm or hot water. It's used to relieve discomfort, especially after perineal or rectal surgery or childbirth. The bath promotes wound healing by cleaning the perineum and anus, increasing circulation, and reducing inflammation. It also helps relax local muscles.

Implementation

● Explain the procedure to the patient.
● Wash your hands thoroughly and put on gloves, if necessary.
● Assist the patient to the bath area, provide privacy, and make sure the area is warm and free from drafts. Help the patient undress as needed.
● Remove and dispose of any soiled dressings. If a dressing adheres to a wound, allow it to soak off in the tub.
● If you're using the sitz bath kit, open the clamp on the irrigation tubing *to allow a stream of water to flow continuously over the wound site.* Refill the bag with water of the correct temperature as needed and encourage the patient to regulate the flow himself. Place the patient's overbed table in front of him *to provide support and comfort.*
● If you're using a tub, check the water temperature frequently with the bath thermometer. If the temperature drops significantly, add warm water. *For maximum safety,* first help the patient stand up slowly to prevent dizziness and loss of balance. Then, with the patient holding the safety rail for support, run warm water into the tub. Check the water temperature. When the water reaches the correct temperature, help the patient sit down again to resume the bath.
● When the prescribed bath time has elapsed — usually 15 to 20 minutes — tell the patient to use the safety rail for balance, and help him to a standing position slowly *to prevent dizziness and to allow him to regain his equilibrium.*
● Document the date, time, duration, and temperature of the bath; wound condition before and after treatment, including color, odor, and amount of drainage; any complications; and the patient's response to treatment.

– increasing fluid intake to 3 L per day using orange juice and cranberry juice
– voiding every 2 to 3 hours and after intercourse

– performing perineal care correctly; wiping the perineal area from front to back after voiding and defecation
– avoiding bubble baths, vaginal deodorants, and tub baths
– recognizing that urine may be orange while taking phenazopyridine
– seeking early treatment if cystitis symptoms are noticed.

FAST FACT

Encourage the client to void every 2 to 3 hours to empty the bladder completely. This enhances bacteria removal and reduces urinary stasis.

Evaluation

● The client remains free from cystitis.
● The client can explain how to prevent recurrence.
● The client reports no pain or bladder spasms.

Gonorrhea

A common STD, GONORRHEA is an infection of the genitourinary tract (especially the urethra and cervix) and, occasionally, the rectum, pharynx, and eyes. Untreated gonorrhea can spread through the blood to the joints, tendons, meninges, and endocardium; in females, it can also lead to chronic PID and sterility.

After adequate treatment, the prognosis in males and females is excellent, although reinfection is common. Gonorrhea is especially prevalent among young people and people with multiple partners, particularly those between ages 19 and 25.

Possible causes

● Exposure to *Neisseria gonorrhoeae* through sexual contact

Data collection findings

● Dysuria
● Purulent urethral or cervical discharge
● Redness and swelling
● Itching, burning, and pain

Diagnostic findings

● A culture from the site of infection (urethra, cervix, rectum, or pharynx), grown on a Thayer-Martin or Transgrow medium, usually establishes the diagnosis by isolating the organism.

- A Gram stain showing gram-negative diplococci supports the diagnosis and may be sufficient to confirm gonorrhea in males.

Nursing diagnoses
- Risk for infection
- Acute pain
- Ineffective sexuality patterns

Treatment
- Moist heat to affected joints if gonococcal arthritis is present

Drug therapy options
- Antibiotic: ceftriaxone (Rocephin), doxycycline (Vibramycin), erythromycin (E-Mycin)
- Prophylactic antibiotic: 1% silver nitrate or erythromycin (EryPed) eye drops to prevent infection in neonates

Patient care goals
- The client will remain free from signs and symptoms of infection.
- The client will express feelings of comfort and pain relief.
- The client will voice concerns over alterations in sexual practice.

Nursing interventions
- Before treatment, establish whether the client has any drug sensitivities. Watch closely for adverse effects during therapy *to prevent severe adverse reactions.*
- Warn the client that until cultures prove negative, he's still infectious and can transmit gonococcal infection; *this helps prevent the spread of infection to others.*
- Practice standard precautions *to prevent the spread of infection.*
- In the client with gonococcal arthritis, apply moist heat *to ease pain in affected joints.*
- Urge the client to inform his sexual contacts of his infection *so that they can seek treatment, even if cultures are negative.* Advise him to avoid sexual intercourse until treatment is complete *to prevent the spread of infection.*
- Routinely instill two drops of 1% silver nitrate or erythromycin in the eyes of all neonates immediately after birth. Check neonates of infected mothers for signs of infection. Take specimens for culture from the infant's eyes, pharynx, and rectum. *These measures ensure prompt recognition and treatment of infection in the neonate.*
- Report all cases of gonorrhea in children to child abuse authorities.

Evaluation
- The client doesn't display signs of infection.
- The client reports adequate pain control.
- The client reports safe sexual practice.

Herpes simplex virus

A recurrent viral infection, HERPES SIMPLEX VIRUS is caused by two types of *Herpesvirus hominis,* a widespread infectious agent. HSV-1, which is transmitted by oral and respiratory secretions, affects the skin and mucous membranes and commonly produces cold sores and fever blisters. HSV-2 primarily affects the genital area and is transmitted by sexual contact. Cross-infection may result from orogenital sex.

Possible causes
- Exposure to HSV-2 herpes through sexual contact
- Contact with HSV-1 herpes through oral or respiratory secretions

Data collection findings
- Blisters on any part of the mouth accompanied by erythema and edema
- Fever
- Swelling of the lymph nodes under the jaw
- Appetite loss
- Increased salivation
- Conjunctivitis (herpetic keratoconjunctivitis, or herpes of the eye)

Genital herpes
- Fluid-filled blisters
- Painful urination
- Fever
- Swollen lymph nodes

Diagnostic findings
- Confirmation requires isolation of the virus from local lesions and a histologic biopsy.
- Blood studies reveal a rise in antibodies and moderate leukocytosis.

Nursing diagnoses
- Acute pain
- Impaired oral mucous membrane
- Impaired social interaction

Treatment
- Symptomatic and supportive treatment

Drug therapy options

- Analgesic-antipyretic agent: acetaminophen (Tylenol) to reduce fever and relieve pain
- Drying agent: calamine lotion to relieve pain of genital lesions
- Antiviral agent: idoxuridine (Herplex Liquifilm), trifluridine (Viroptic), vidarabine (Vira-A), 5% acyclovir (Zovirax) ointment (possible relief to clients with genital herpes or to immunosuppressed clients with *H. hominis* skin infections; I.V. acyclovir to treat more severe infections)

Patient care goals

- The client will express feelings of comfort and pain relief.
- The client will exhibit improved or healed lesions or wounds.
- The client will resume effective communication patterns.

Nursing interventions

- Observe standard precautions. For clients with extensive cutaneous, oral, or genital lesions, institute contact precautions *to prevent the spread of infection.*
- Administer pain medications and prescribed antiviral agents as ordered *to relieve pain and to treat infection.*
- Provide supportive care, as indicated, such as oral hygiene, nutritional supplementation, and antipyretics for fever. *These measures enhance the client's well-being.*
- Abstain from direct client care if you have herpetic whitlow (an *H. hominis* finger infection that commonly affects health care workers) *to prevent the spread of infection.*

Evaluation

- The client reports adequate pain control.
- The client displays healing lesions.
- The client reports improved social interaction.

Neurogenic bladder

NEUROGENIC BLADDER refers to all types of bladder dysfunction caused by an interruption of normal bladder innervation. Subsequent complications include incontinence, residual urine retention, urinary infection, stone formation, and renal failure. A neurogenic bladder may be described as spastic (resulting from an upper motor neuron lesion) or flaccid (resulting from a lower motor neuron lesion).

This disorder is also known as neuromuscular dysfunction of the lower urinary tract, neurologic bladder dysfunction, and neuropathic bladder.

Possible causes

- Acute infectious diseases such as Guillain-Barré syndrome
- Cerebral disorder (stroke, brain tumor [meningioma and glioma], Parkinson's disease, multiple sclerosis, dementia)
- Chronic alcoholism
- Collagen diseases such as SLE
- Disorders of peripheral innervation
- Distant effects of cancer such as primary oat cell carcinoma of the lung
- Heavy metal toxicity
- Herpes zoster
- Metabolic disturbances (hypothyroidism, porphyria, or uremia)
- Sacral agenesis
- Spinal cord disease or trauma
- Vascular diseases such as atherosclerosis

Data collection findings

- Altered micturition
- Flaccid neurogenic bladder (overflow incontinence, diminished anal sphincter tone, greatly distended bladder with an accompanying feeling of bladder fullness)
- Hydroureteronephrosis (distention of the ureter and the renal pelvis and calices)
- Incontinence
- Spastic neurogenic bladder (involuntary or frequent scanty urination without a feeling of bladder fullness, possible spontaneous spasms of the arms and legs, increased anal sphincter tone)
- Vesicoureteral reflux (passage of urine from the bladder back into a ureter)

Diagnostic findings

- Voiding cystourethrography evaluates bladder neck function, vesicoureteral reflux, and continence.
- Urodynamic studies help evaluate how urine is stored in the bladder, how well the bladder empties, and the rate of movement of urine out of the bladder during voiding.
- Retrograde urethrography reveals the presence of strictures and diverticula.

Nursing diagnoses

- Impaired urinary elimination
- Disturbed body image
- Impaired skin integrity

Treatment
- Credé's maneuver (application of manual pressure over the lower abdomen) to evacuate the bladder)
- Valsalva's maneuver to promote complete emptying of the bladder
- Indwelling urinary catheter insertion, including teaching the client self-catheterization techniques
- Surgical repair if the client has structural impairment
- Surgical insertion of an artificial urinary sphincter

Drug therapy options
- Urinary tract stimulant: bethanechol (Urecholine)
- Antimuscarinic agent: propantheline (Pro-Banthine), flavoxate (Urispas), dicyclomine (Antispas)

Patient care goals
- The client will demonstrate skill in managing the urinary elimination problem.
- The client will maintain a positive self-image.
- The client will maintain intact skin integrity.

Nursing interventions
- Use strict aseptic technique during insertion of an indwelling urinary catheter (a temporary measure to drain the incontinent client's bladder). Don't interrupt the closed drainage system for any reason *to prevent infection.*
- Obtain urine specimens with a syringe and small-bore needle inserted through the aspirating port of the catheter itself (below the junction of the balloon instillation site). Irrigate in the same manner, if necessary, *to prevent infection.*
- Clean the catheter insertion site with soap and water at least twice per day *to prevent infection.*
- Don't allow the catheter to become encrusted; *this is a medium for bacteria growth.*
- Use a sterile applicator to apply antibiotic ointment around the meatus after catheter care, if prescribed. Keep the drainage bag below the tubing, and don't raise the bag above the level of the bladder *to prevent urine reflux and infection.*
- Clamp the tubing or empty the catheter bag before transferring the client to a wheelchair or stretcher *to prevent accidental urine reflux.*
- Watch for signs of infection (fever, cloudy or foul-smelling urine) *to ensure early treatment intervention and prevent complications.*
- Try to keep the client as mobile as possible. Perform passive range-of-motion exercises, if necessary. *These measures prevent complications of immobility.*

- If a urinary diversion procedure is to be performed, arrange for consultation with an enterostomal therapist and coordinate the care *to help the client cope with his change in body image.*

Evaluation
- The client demonstrates the ability to control his urinary problem.
- The client demonstrates a positive self-image.
- The client's skin integrity is intact.

Ovarian cancer

Ovarian cancer attacks the ovaries, which are the organs in women that produce the hormones estrogen and progesterone. After cancers of the lung, breast, and colon, primary ovarian cancer ranks as the most common cause of cancer deaths among women in the United States. In women with previously treated breast cancer, metastatic ovarian cancer is more common than cancer at any other site.

The prognosis varies with the histologic type and stage of the disease but is generally poor because ovarian tumors produce few early signs and are usually advanced at diagnosis. About 40% of women with ovarian cancer survive for 5 years.

Possible causes
- Unknown

Risk factors
- Early menarche
- Late menopause
- Celibacy
- Exposure to asbestos, talc, and industrial pollutants
- Familial tendency and history of breast or uterine cancer
- High-fat diet
- Upper socioeconomic levels and age between 20 and 54 (highest incidence)
- Infertility

Data collection findings
- Abdominal discomfort, dyspepsia, and other mild GI disturbances
- Pelvic discomfort
- Abdominal distention
- Constipation
- Urinary frequency
- Weight loss

Diagnostic findings

● Diagnosis requires clinical evaluation, a complete client history, surgical exploration, and histologic studies. Preoperative evaluation includes a complete physical examination, including pelvic examination with a Pap test (positive in only a small number of women with ovarian cancer) and the following special tests:

– Abdominal ultrasonography, CT scan, or X-ray may delineate tumor size.

– Chest X-ray may reveal distant metastasis and pleural effusions.

– Barium enema (especially in clients with GI symptoms) may reveal obstruction and size of tumor.

– Lymphangiography may show lymph node involvement.

– Mammography may rule out primary breast cancer.

– Liver scan in clients with ascites may rule out liver metastasis.

– Blood tests such as ovarian carcinoma antigen, CEA, and human chorionic gonadotropin reveal the presence of cancer.

● Despite extensive testing, accurate diagnosis and staging are impossible without exploratory laparotomy, including lymph node evaluation and tumor resection.

Nursing diagnoses

● Acute pain
● Fear
● Imbalanced nutrition: Less than body requirements

Treatment

Conservative treatment (for girls or young women with a unilateral encapsulated tumor who wish to maintain fertility)

● Resection of the involved ovary
● Biopsies of the omentum and the uninvolved ovary
● Peritoneal washings for cytologic examination of pelvic fluid
● Careful follow-up, including periodic chest X-rays to rule out lung metastasis

Aggressive treatment (for ovarian cancer)

● Total abdominal hysterectomy and bilateral salpingo-oophorectomy with tumor resection, omentectomy, and appendectomy
● Lymph node biopsies with lymphadenectomy, tissue biopsies, and peritoneal washings

Drug therapy options

● Antineoplastic: cisplatin (Platinol), paclitaxel (Taxol), topotecan (Hycamtin)

● Analgesic: morphine (MS Contin), fentanyl (Duragesic-25)
● Antipyretic: aspirin, acetaminophen (Tylenol)
● Immunotherapy: bacille Calmette-Guérin vaccine

Patient care goals

● The client will express feelings of comfort and pain relief.
● The client will express feelings about her illness.
● The client will maintain an appropriate weight.

Nursing interventions

Before surgery

● Thoroughly explain all preoperative tests, the expected course of treatment, and surgical and postoperative procedures *to allay the client's anxiety.*

● In premenopausal women, explain that bilateral oophorectomy artificially induces early menopause, so they may experience hot flashes, headaches, palpitations, insomnia, depression, and excessive perspiration *to help her cope with changes in her body image that occur as a result of surgery.*

After surgery

● Monitor vital signs frequently *to detect early signs of postoperative complications such as fluid volume deficit.*

● Monitor fluid intake and output *to detect fluid volume excess or deficit* while maintaining good catheter care *to prevent infection.*

● Check the dressing regularly for excessive drainage or bleeding, and watch for signs of infection. *These measures detect early signs of complications and prevent treatment delay.*

● Provide abdominal support *to promote comfort,* and watch for abdominal distention, *which may indicate the presence of ascites.*

● Encourage coughing and deep breathing *to mobilize secretions and prevent postoperative pneumonia.*

● Reposition the client often *to prevent skin breakdown,* and encourage her to walk shortly after surgery *to prevent complications of immobility.*

● Monitor and treat adverse effects of radiation and chemotherapy *to prevent complications.*

● Enlist the help of a social worker, chaplain, and other members of the health care team *to provide additional supportive care.*

Evaluation

● The client reports adequate pain control.

- The client demonstrates appropriate coping mechanisms.
- The client has an appropriate weight.

Prostate cancer

Prostate cancer is a malignant tumor of the prostate gland, which can obstruct urine flow when encroaching on the bladder neck. It commonly metastasizes to bone, lymph nodes, brain, and lungs. Next to skin cancer, prostate cancer is the most common type of cancer in men in the United States.

Possible causes

- Family history
- Age
- Race
- Vasectomy
- Increased dietary fat
- No known etiology

Data collection findings

- Decreased size and force of urine stream
- Difficulty and frequency of urination
- Hematuria
- Urine retention

Diagnostic findings

- Digital rectal examination reveals palpable firm nodule in gland or diffuse induration in posterior lobe.
- Serum acid phosphatase level is increased.
- Radioimmunoassay for acid phosphatase is increased.
- Prostatic-specific antigen is increased.
- Transurethral ultrasound studies show mass or obstruction.
- Prostate biopsy has cytology positive for cancer cells.
- Excretory urogram shows mass or obstruction.

Nursing diagnoses

- Acute pain
- Impaired urinary elimination
- Sexual dysfunction

Treatment

- High-protein diet with restrictions on caffeine and spicy foods
- Radiation implant
- Radical prostatectomy (for localized tumors without metastasis), cryosurgery, or transurethral resection of the prostate (to relieve obstruction in metastatic disease)

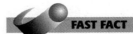 **FAST FACT**

Because many prostate cancers grow slowly, many elderly men never need treatment. Active treatment can be started later if the cancer begins to grow more quickly or causes other problems.

Drug therapy options

- Analgesic: meperidine (Demerol), morphine (MS Contin), oxycodone with acetaminophen (Tylox)
- Antiemetic: granisetron (Kytril), ondansetron (Zofran)
- Antineoplastic: cisplatin (Platinol), doxorubicin (Adriamycin)
- Corticosteroid: prednisone (Deltasone)
- Immunosuppressant: cyclophosphamide (Cytoxan)
- Luteinizing hormone-releasing hormone agonist: goserelin acetate (Zoladex), leuprolide (Lupron)
- NSAID: ibuprofen (Motrin), indomethacin (Indocin), sulindac (Clinoril)
- Oral flutamide (Eulexin) to block circulating testosterone
- Stool softener: docusate (Colace)

Patient care goals

- The client will verbalize adequate pain relief.
- The client will discuss concerns related to sexual dysfunction.
- The client will have normal urine output and unobstructed flow.

Nursing interventions

- Assess renal and fluid status *to determine baseline and detect early changes.*
- Monitor and record vital signs, fluid intake and output, and laboratory studies. *Accurate intake and output are essential for correct fluid replacement therapy.*
- Monitor for signs of infection *to assess for complications.*
- Assess pain and note the effectiveness of analgesia *to promote comfort.*
- Administer medications, as prescribed, *to maintain or improve the client's condition.*
- Maintain the client's diet *to maintain nutritional level and meet increased metabolic demands.*
- Maintain patency of the urinary catheter and note drainage *to ensure effective urine drainage.*
- Encourage the client to express his feelings about the changes in his body image and fear of sexual dysfunction *to encourage coping and adaptation.*

● Encourage ambulation *to prevent complications of immobility.*
● Provide postoperative, postchemotherapeutic, and postradiation nursing care *to prevent complications.*
● Review key teaching topics with the client and family members *to ensure adequate knowledge about the condition and treatment,* including:
– managing changes in sexual activity
– avoiding prolonged sitting, standing, and walking
– avoiding the strain of exercise and lifting
– urinating frequently
– avoiding coffee and cola beverages
– decreasing fluid intake during evening hours
– performing perineal exercises
– completing catheter care, as directed
– self-monitoring for bloody urine, pain, burning, frequency, decreased urine output, and loss of bladder control
– contacting the American Cancer Society and other community agencies and resources for additional information or support.

Evaluation

● The client verbalizes relief from pain and has normal vital signs.
● The client indicates he isn't experiencing sexual dysfunction when seen for follow-up care.
● The client's urine flow isn't obstructed.

Renal calculi

RENAL CALCULI, also known as *kidney stones,* result from the precipitation of salts in the urine. These include salts of:
● phosphate
● oxalate
● carbonate
● uric acid
● urate
● cystine.

Under normal circumstances, calculi are dissolved and excreted in the urine. However, larger calculi can cause great pain and may become lodged in the ureter.

Possible causes

● Chemotherapy
● Dehydration
● Diet high in calcium, vitamin D, milk, protein, oxalate, alkali
● Genetics
● Gout
● Hypercalcemia
● Hyperparathyroidism
● Idiopathic origin
● Immobility
● Leukemia
● Polycythemia vera
● Urinary stasis
● Urinary tract infection
● Urinary tract obstruction

Data collection findings

● Costovertebral tenderness
● Nausea and vomiting
● Pallor
● Diaphoresis
● Renal colic
● Urinary frequency and urgency

Diagnostic findings

● 24-hour urine collection shows increased uric acid, oxalate, calcium, phosphorus, and creatinine levels.
● Blood chemistry shows increased calcium, phosphorus, creatinine, BUN, uric acid, protein, and alkaline phosphatase levels.
● Cystoscopy allows visualization of stones.
● Excretory urography reveals stones.
● Kidney-ureter-bladder X-ray reveals stones.
● Urine chemistry shows pyuria, proteinuria, hematuria, presence of WBCs, and increased urine specific gravity.

Nursing diagnoses

● Acute pain
● Impaired urinary elimination
● Risk for infection

Treatment

For calcium stones

● Acid-ash with limited intake of calcium and milk products

For oxalate stones

● Alkaline-ash with limited intake of foods high in oxalate (cola, tea)

For uric acid stones

● Alkaline-ash with limited intake of foods high in purine (see *Diet considerations for the client with renal calculi,* page 490)

Diet considerations for the client with renal calculi

Use this table as a guide for what foods to consider and avoid when planning a diet for the client with renal calculi.

FOODS THAT ACIDIFY URINE	FOODS THAT ALKALINIZE URINE	FOODS TO AVOID WITH CALCIUM CALCULI	FOODS TO AVOID WITH OXALATE CALCULI
Fish (halibut)	Dried apricots	Cheddar cheese	Rhubarb
Bacon	Dried figs	Cheese food	Asparagus
Veal	Molasses	Cheese spread	Dandelion greens
Lamb	Beet greens	Whole milk	Spinach
Chicken	Green olives	Evaporated milk	Cranberries
Roast beef	Dandelion greens	Skim milk	Beets and beet greens
Pork	Navy beans	Powdered dry skim milk	Cashew nuts
Cranberries	Milk		Chocolate
Prunes	Milk products		Cocoa
Plums	Citrus fruit and juice		Okra
			Potatoes
			Tomatoes
			Corn
			Swiss chard

Other treatments

- Extracorporeal shock wave lithotripsy to shatter calculi
- Increased fluid intake to 3 qt (3 L) per day
- Moist heat to flank; hot baths
- Percutaneous nephrostolithotomy
- Surgery if other measures to remove the stone aren't effective (type of surgery depends on the location of the stone)

Drug therapy options

- Acidifier: ammonium chloride, methenamine mandelate (Mandelamine)
- Alkalinizing agent: potassium acetate, sodium bicarbonate
- Analgesic: meperidine (Demerol) or morphine (MS Contin)
- Antibiotic: cefazolin (Ancef), cefoxitin (Mefoxin)
- Antiemetic: prochlorperazine (Compazine)
- Antigout agent: sulfinpyrazone (Anturane)

Patient care goals

- The client will eliminate calculi.
- The client will experience pain relief.
- The client won't experience complications.
- The client will understand how to prevent calculi.

Nursing interventions

- Assess the client's renal status *to determine baseline and to detect complications.*
- Assess pain and the effectiveness of analgesia. *Assessment allows for modification of the plan of care as needed.*
- Monitor and record vital signs, intake and output, daily weight, urine specific gravity, laboratory studies, and urine pH *to assess renal status.*
- Monitor the client's urine for evidence of renal calculi. Strain all urine and save all solid material *for analysis of spontaneous passage of calculi.*
- Force fluids to 3,000 ml/day *to moisten mucous membranes and to dilute chemicals within the body.*

 SPOT CHECK

When providing care for a client with renal calculi, the nurse carefully records urine output. What other nursing action must be conducted each time the client voids?
Answer: The urine should be strained for calculi each time the client voids.

- Maintain the client's diet *to promote adequate nutrition.*
- Administer medications, as prescribed, *to maintain and improve the client's condition.*

- Apply warm soaks to the client's flank *to promote comfort.*
- If surgery was performed, check dressings regularly for bloody drainage and report excessive amounts of bloody drainage to the physician; use sterile technique to change the dressing; maintain nephrostomy tube or indwelling urinary catheter if indicated; and monitor incision for signs of infection *to promote healing and detect complications.*
- Review key teaching topics with the client *to ensure adequate knowledge about his condition and treatment,* including:
  – increasing fluid intake, especially during hot weather, illness, and exercise
  – voiding whenever the urge is felt
  – testing urine pH
  – increasing fluids at night and voiding frequently.

Evaluation
- The client excretes calculi without complications.
- The client verbalizes pain relief.
- The client can explain how to prevent renal calculi.

Syphilis

A chronic, infectious STD, SYPHILIS begins in the mucous membranes and quickly becomes systemic, spreading to nearby lymph nodes and the bloodstream. This disease, when untreated, is characterized by progressive stages: primary, secondary, latent, and late (formerly called *tertiary*).

In the United States, incidence of syphilis is highest among urban populations, especially in persons ages 15 to 39, drug users, and those infected with HIV.

Possible causes
- Exposure to the spirochete *Treponema pallidum* through sexual contact
- Transmission from an infected mother to her fetus

Data collection findings
Primary syphilis
- Chancres on the genitalia, anus, fingers, lips, tongue, nipples, tonsils, or eyelids

Secondary syphilis
- Symmetrical mucocutaneous lesions
- General lymphadenopathy
- Headache

- Malaise
- Anorexia
- Weight loss
- Nausea
- Vomiting
- Sore throat
- Slight fever

Diagnostic findings
- Dark-field examination identifies *T. pallidum* from a lesion. This method is most effective when moist lesions are present, as in primary, secondary, and prenatal syphilis.
- Fluorescent treponemal antibody-absorption test identifies antigens of *T. pallidum* in tissue, ocular fluid, CSF, tracheobronchial secretions, and exudates from lesions. This is the most sensitive test available for detecting syphilis at all stages. When reactive, it remains so permanently.
- Venereal Disease Research Laboratory (VDRL) slide test and rapid plasma reagin test detect nonspecific antibodies. Both tests, if positive, become reactive within 1 to 2 weeks after the primary lesion appears or 4 to 5 weeks after the infection begins.
- CSF examination identifies neurosyphilis when the total protein level is above 40 mg/100 ml, VDRL slide test is reactive, and CSF cell count exceeds five mononuclear cells per microliter.

Nursing diagnoses
- Ineffective sexuality patterns
- Impaired skin integrity
- Deficient knowledge (STD)

Treatment
- Antibiotic therapy is the only treatment for syphilis.

Drug therapy options
- Antibiotic: penicillin G benzathine (Permapen); if allergic to penicillin, erythromycin (Erythrocin) or tetracycline (Panmycin P)

Patient care goals
- The client will relate appropriate information regarding his illness and safe sexual practice.
- The client will exhibit healing lesions or wounds.

Nursing interventions
- Follow standard precautions when assessing the client, collecting specimens, and treating lesions *to prevent the spread of infection.*

● Check for a history of drug sensitivity before administering the first dose of penicillin *to prevent anaphylaxis.*

● In secondary syphilis, keep the lesions clean and dry. If they're draining, dispose of contaminated materials properly *to prevent the spread of infection.*

● In late syphilis, provide supportive care *to relieve the client's symptoms during prolonged treatment.*

● In cardiovascular syphilis, check for signs of decreased cardiac output (decreased urine output, hypoxia, and decreased sensorium) and pulmonary congestion *to prevent shock and respiratory distress.*

● In neurosyphilis, regularly check level of consciousness, mood, and coherence. Watch for signs of ataxia. *These measures detect neurologic complications early and prevent treatment delay.*

● Urge clients to seek VDRL testing after 3, 6, 12, and 24 months *to detect possible relapse.* Clients treated for latent or late syphilis should receive blood tests at 6-month intervals for 2 years *to detect possible relapse.*

● Be sure to report all cases of syphilis to local public health authorities. Urge the client to inform his sexual partners of his infection *so that they can also receive treatment.*

● Refer the client and his sexual partners for HIV testing. *High-risk behaviors that caused the client to contract syphilis also place the client at risk for HIV.*

Evaluation
● The client relates appropriate information regarding his illness and safe sexual practice.
● The client has improved skin integrity.

Testicular cancer

Testicular cancer affects the testes or testicles, the two oval-shaped glandular organs inside the scrotum that produce spermatozoa and testosterone. Malignant testicular tumors primarily affect young to middle-aged men. Testicular tumors in children are rare.

Most testicular tumors originate in gonadal cells. About 40% are seminomas (uniform, undifferentiated cells resembling primitive gonadal cells). The rest are nonseminomas (tumor cells showing various degrees of differentiation).

The prognosis varies with the cell type and disease stage. When treated with surgery and radiation, almost all clients with localized disease survive beyond 5 years.

Possible causes
Contributing factors include:
● age (incidence peaks between ages 20 and 40)
● higher incidence in men with cryptorchidism and in men whose mothers used diethylstilbestrol during pregnancy.

Data collection findings
● Firm, painless, smooth testicular mass, varying in size and sometimes producing a sense of testicular heaviness

Advanced stages
● Abdominal mass
● Cough
● Fatigue
● Hemoptysis
● Lethargy
● Pallor
● Shortness of breath
● Ureteral obstruction
● Weight loss

Diagnostic findings
● Regular self-examinations and testicular palpation during a routine physical examination may disclose testicular tumors.
● Transillumination can be used to distinguish between a tumor (which doesn't transilluminate) and a hydrocele or spermatocele (which does transilluminate).
● CT scan can be used to detect metastasis.
● Scrotal ultrasonography can be used to differentiate between a cyst and a solid mass.
● Chest X-ray may show pulmonary metastasis.
● Excretory urography may reveal ureteral deviation resulting from para-aortic node involvement.
● Serum alpha-fetoprotein and beta-human chorionic gonadotropin levels — indicators of testicular tumor activity — provide a baseline for measuring the client's response to therapy and determining the prognosis.
● Surgical excision and biopsy of the tumor and testis permits histologic verification of the tumor cell type.
● Inguinal exploration (examination of the groin) is used to determine the extent of nodal involvement.

 SPOT CHECK

True or False? The incidence of testicular cancer peaks between ages 50 and 75.
Answer: False. Incidence peaks between ages 20 and 40.

Nursing diagnoses
- Disturbed body image
- Fear
- Sexual dysfunction

Treatment
- Radiation therapy
- Surgery: orchiectomy (testicle removal; most surgeons remove the testicle but not the scrotum to allow for a prosthetic implant)
- Retroperitoneal lymph node dissection (dissection of lymph nodes posterior to the peritoneum)
- Bone marrow transplantation (follows chemotherapy and radiation therapy in clients with unresponsive tumors)
- High-calorie diet provided in small, frequent feedings
- I.V. fluid therapy

Drug therapy options
- Antineoplastic: bleomycin (Blenoxane), carboplatin (Paraplatin), cisplatin (Platinol), dactinomycin (Cosmegen), etoposide (VePesid), ifosfamide (IFEX), plicamycin (Mithracin), vinblastine (Velban)
- Analgesic: fentanyl (Duragesic-25), morphine (MS Contin)
- Antiemetic: granisetron (Kytril), ondansetron (Zofran)
- Diuretic: furosemide (Lasix), mannitol (Osmitrol)
- Hormone replacement therapy (after bilateral orchiectomy)

Patient care goals
- The client will maintain a positive body image and positive self-concept.
- The client will demonstrate a decreased level of fear.
- The client will discuss concerns related to sexual dysfunction.

Nursing interventions
- Develop a treatment plan that addresses the client's psychological and physical needs *to enhance his sense of well-being.*

Before orchiectomy
- Reassure the client that sterility and impotence need not follow unilateral orchiectomy, that synthetic hormones can restore hormonal balance, and that most surgeons don't remove the scrotum. In many cases, a testicular prosthesis can correct anatomic disfigurement. *These interventions can help allay the client's anxiety.*

- If bilateral orchiectomy is planned, facilitate the proper referral or discussions about sperm-banking options, as appropriate, *to promote client and family understanding of the available options.*

After orchiectomy
- For the first day after surgery, apply an ice pack to the scrotum *to reduce swelling* and provide analgesics *to promote comfort.*
- Check for excessive bleeding, swelling, and signs of infection *to detect early signs of complications and to prevent treatment delay.*
- Provide a scrotal athletic supporter *to minimize pain during ambulation.*

During chemotherapy
- Give antiemetics, as needed, *to treat or prevent nausea and vomiting.*
- Encourage small, frequent meals *to maintain oral intake despite anorexia.*
- Establish a mouth care regimen to prevent breakdown of the oral mucosa and check for stomatitis *to detect early signs and to avoid treatment delay.*
- Watch for signs of myelosuppression so precautions can be taken *to avoid infection.*
- Encourage increased fluid intake and provide I.V. fluids, a potassium supplement, and diuretics *to prevent renal damage.*
- Review key teaching topics with the client and family members *to ensure adequate knowledge about the condition and treatment,* including:
  - understanding the disease process and treatment options
  - preventing and reporting infection
  - managing adverse reactions to chemotherapy and radiation.

Evaluation
- The client verbalizes feelings about his body image change and expresses positive feelings about himself.
- The client verbalizes a decreased level of fear and can discuss his feelings, the diagnosis, and treatment options.
- The client indicates he isn't experiencing sexual dysfunction when seen for follow-up care.

Appendices Part IV

A NANDA Taxonomy II codes

The North American Nursing Diagnosis Association (NANDA) endorsed its first nursing diagnosis taxonomic structure, NANDA Taxonomy I, in 1986. This taxonomy has been revised several times, most recently in 2000. The new Taxonomy II has a code structure that's compliant with recommendations from the National Library of Medicine concerning health care terminology codes. The taxonomy that appears here represents the currently accepted classification system for nursing diagnosis.

NURSING DIAGNOSIS	TAXONOMY II CODE	NURSING DIAGNOSIS	TAXONOMY II CODE
Imbalanced nutrition: More than body requirements	00001	Urinary retention	00023
Imbalanced nutrition: Less than body requirements	00002	Ineffective tissue perfusion (specify type: renal, cerebral, cardiopulmonary, gastrointestinal, peripheral)	00024
Risk for imbalanced nutrition: More than body requirements	00003	Risk for imbalanced fluid volume	00025
Risk for infection	00004	Excess fluid volume	00026
Risk for imbalanced body temperature	00005	Deficient fluid volume	00027
Hypothermia	00006	Risk for deficient fluid volume	00028
Hyperthermia	00007	Decreased cardiac output	00029
Ineffective thermoregulation	00008	Impaired gas exchange	00030
Autonomic dysreflexia	00009	Ineffective airway clearance	00031
Risk for autonomic dysreflexia	00010	Ineffective breathing pattern	00032
Constipation	00011	Impaired spontaneous ventilation	00033
Perceived constipation	00012	Dysfunctional ventilatory weaning response	00034
Diarrhea	00013	Risk for injury	00035
Bowel incontinence	00014	Risk for suffocation	00036
Risk for constipation	00015	Risk for poisoning	00037
Impaired urinary elimination	00016	Risk for trauma	00038
Stress urinary incontinence	00017	Risk for aspiration	00039
Reflex urinary incontinence	00018	Risk for disuse syndrome	00040
Urge urinary incontinence	00019	Latex allergy response	00041
Functional urinary incontinence	00020	Risk for latex allergy response	00042
Total urinary incontinence	00021	Ineffective protection	00043
Risk for urge urinary incontinence	00022	Impaired tissue integrity	00044

NURSING DIAGNOSIS	TAXONOMY II CODE	NURSING DIAGNOSIS	TAXONOMY II CODE
Impaired oral mucous membrane	00045	Ineffective community therapeutic regimen management	00081
Impaired skin integrity	00046	Effective therapeutic regimen management	00082
Risk for impaired skin integrity	00047	Decisional conflict (specify)	00083
Impaired dentition	00048	Health-seeking behaviors (specify)	00084
Decreased intracranial adaptive capacity	00049	Impaired physical mobility	00085
Disturbed energy field	00050	Risk for peripheral neurovascular dysfunction	00086
Impaired verbal communication	00051	Risk for perioperative-positioning injury	00087
Impaired social interaction	00052	Impaired walking	00088
Social isolation	00053	Impaired wheelchair mobility	00089
Risk for loneliness	00054	Impaired transfer ability	00090
Ineffective role performance	00055	Impaired bed mobility	00091
Impaired parenting	00056	Activity intolerance	00092
Risk for impaired parenting	00057	Fatigue	00093
Risk for impaired parent/infant/child attachment	00058	Risk for activity intolerance	00094
Sexual dysfunction	00059	Disturbed sleep pattern	00095
Interrupted family processes	00060	Sleep deprivation	00096
Caregiver role strain	00061	Deficient diversional activity	00097
Risk for caregiver role strain	00062	Impaired home maintenance	00098
Dysfunctional family processes: Alcoholism	00063	Ineffective health maintenance	00099
Parental role conflict	00064	Delayed surgical recovery	00100
Ineffective sexuality patterns	00065	Adult failure to thrive	00101
Spiritual distress	00066	Feeding self-care deficit	00102
Risk for spiritual distress	00067	Impaired swallowing	00103
Readiness for enhanced spiritual well-being	00068	Ineffective breast-feeding	00104
Ineffective coping	00069	Interrupted breast-feeding	00105
Impaired adjustment	00070	Effective breast-feeding	00106
Defensive coping	00071	Ineffective infant feeding pattern	00107
Ineffective denial	00072	Bathing or hygiene self-care deficit	00108
Disabled family coping	00073	Dressing or grooming self-care deficit	00109
Compromised family coping	00074	Toileting self-care deficit	00110
Readiness for enhanced family coping	00075	Delayed growth and development	00111
Readiness for enhanced community coping	00076	Risk for delayed development	00112
Ineffective community coping	00077	Risk for disproportionate growth	00113
Ineffective therapeutic regimen management	00078	Relocation stress syndrome	00114
Noncompliance (specify)	00079	Risk for disorganized infant behavior	00115
Ineffective family therapeutic regimen management	00080	Disorganized infant behavior	00116
		Readiness for enhanced organized infant behavior	00117
		Disturbed body image	00118

NURSING DIAGNOSIS	TAXONOMY II CODE
Chronic low self-esteem	00119
Situational low self-esteem	00120
Disturbed personal identity	00121
Disturbed sensory perception (specify: visual, auditory, kinesthetic, gustatory, tactile, olfactory)	00122
Unilateral neglect	00123
Hopelessness	00124
Powerlessness	00125
Deficient knowledge (specify)	00126
Impaired environmental interpretation syndrome	00127
Acute confusion	00128
Chronic confusion	00129
Disturbed thought processes	00130
Impaired memory	00131
Acute pain	00132
Chronic pain	00133
Nausea	00134
Dysfunctional grieving	00135
Anticipatory grieving	00136
Chronic sorrow	00137
Risk for other-directed violence	00138
Risk for self-mutilation	00139
Risk for self-directed violence	00140
Posttrauma syndrome	00141
Rape-trauma syndrome	00142
Rape-trauma syndrome: Compound reaction	00143
Rape-trauma syndrome: Silent reaction	00144
Risk for posttrauma syndrome	00145
Anxiety	00146
Death anxiety	00147
Fear	00148

NURSING DIAGNOSIS	TAXONOMY II CODE
New Nursing Diagnoses: Effective April 2000	
Risk for relocation stress syndrome	00149
Risk for suicide	00150
Self-mutilation	00151
Risk for powerlessness	00152
Risk for situational low self-esteem	00153
Wandering	00154
Risk for falls	00155

Positioning clients

The chart below lists various positions in which clients may be placed. These positions may be used for client comfort, but proper positioning also maintains functional body alignment and client safety, promotes respiration and circulation, relieves pressure, and aids in administering treatment.

POSITION	IMPLEMENTATION	RATIONALE	INDICATIONS
Elevation of extremity	Use the bed controls to elevate the lower extremities, or use pillows to elevate the upper and lower extremities.	● Promotes circulation and comfort ● Enables examinations and procedures	● Thrombophlebitis ● Post cast application ● Edema ● Post surgery on extremity
Dorsal recumbent (supine)	Place the client on his back with the knees slightly flexed. Place a pillow beneath the head for comfort.	● Immobilizes the spine	● Spinal cord injury ● Urinary catheter insertion ● Vaginal examination
Fowler's	Elevate the head of the bed to 45 degrees, and raise the bed section under the client's knees, flexing the knees slightly.	● Enables examination ● Immobilizes the spine ● Promotes drainage, cardiac output, and ventilation ● Prevents aspiration of food and secretions	● Head injury, cranial surgery, increased intracranial pressure ● Post abdominal surgery ● Dyspnea ● Vomiting ● Post thyroidectomy ● Post eye surgery
High Fowler's	Elevate the head of the bed to 90 degrees, and raise the bed section under the client's knees, flexing the knees slightly.	● Promotes drainage, cardiac output, and ventilation ● Prevents aspiration of food and secretions	● Head injury, cranial surgery, increased intracranial pressure ● Dyspnea, respiratory distress ● Feeding (during and after meals) ● Hiatus hernia
Lateral (side-lying)	Place the client on his side, with weight being mostly supported by the lateral aspect of the lower scapula and the lower ileum. Support with pillows.	● Promotes safety ● Prevents atelectasis, pressure sores, and aspiration of food and secretions	● Post abdominal surgery ● Coma ● Pressure ulcer ● Enema or rectal irrigation

(continued)

POSITION	IMPLEMENTATION	RATIONALE	INDICATIONS
Lithotomy	Place the client on his back (either flat or with the head slightly elevated). Knees should be flexed at right angles and feet placed in stirrups.	• Enables examination of the pelvis	• Perineal or rectal procedure
Prone	Place the client on his stomach with the head turned to one side. Position the arms at the side or above the head. Make sure that the legs are extended.	• Enables examination of the back and spine • Promotes gas exchange	• Immobilization • Adult respiratory distress syndrome • Post lumbar puncture or myelogram
Reverse Trendelenburg's	Elevate the head of the bed and lower the feet.	• Provides counterbalance for traction • Promotes blood flow to the lower extremities	• Cervical traction • Post lower extremity vessel surgery
Semi-Fowler's	Elevate the head of the bed to 30 degrees, and raise the bed section under the client's knees, flexing the knee slightly.	• Promotes drainage, cardiac output, and ventilation • Prevents aspiration of food and secretions	• Head injury, cranial surgery, increased intracranial pressure • Post abdominal surgery • Dyspnea • Vomiting • Post thyroidectomy • Post eye surgery
Sims'	Position the client on his side with a small pillow beneath the head. Flex one knee toward the abdomen, with the other knee only slightly flexed. Place one arm behind the body and the other in a comfortable position. Support with pillows.	• Enables examination of the back and rectum • Prevents pressure sores and atelectasis	• Coma • Rectal injuries
Trendelenburg's	Position the client supine with the feet elevated 30 to 40 degrees higher than the head.	• Promotes postural drainage and venous return	• Shock • Cystic fibrosis

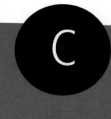

Recommended childhood immunization schedule
United States, January – December 2001

Vaccines[1] are listed under routinely recommended ages. Bars indicate range of recommended ages for immunization. Any doses not given at the recommended age should be given as a "catch-up" immunization at any subsequent visit when indicated and feasible. Ovals indicate vaccines to be given if previously recommended doses were missed or given earlier than the recommended minimum age.

VACCINE	BIRTH	1 MONTH	2 MONTHS	4 MONTHS	6 MONTHS	12 MONTHS	15 MONTHS	18 MONTHS	24 MONTHS	4 to 6 YEARS	11 to 12 YEARS	14 to 18 YEARS
AGE												
Hepatitis B[2]	Hep B #1	Hep B #1										
		Hep B #2	Hep B #2	Hep B #2	Hep B #3	Hep B #3	Hep B #3	Hep B #3			Hep B[2]	
Diptheria, tetanus, pertussis[3]		DTaP	DTaP	DTaP			DTaP[3]	DTaP[3]		DTaP	Td	Td
Haemophilus influenzae type b[4]		Hib	Hib	Hib		Hib	Hib					
Inactivated polio[5]		IPV	IPV		IPV[5]	IPV[5]	IPV[5]			IPV[5]		
Pneumococcal conjugate[6]		PCV	PCV	PCV	PCV	PCV						
Measles, mumps, rubella[7]						MMR	MMR			MMR[7]	MMR[7]	
Varicella[8]						Var	Var	Var			Var	
Hepatitis A[9]									Hep A — in selected areas[9]	Hep A — in selected areas[9]	Hep A — in selected areas[9]	Hep A — in selected areas[9]

Var — Range of recommended ages for immunization   Var — "Catch-up" immunization

Approved by the Advisory Committee on Immunization Practices (ACIP), the American Academy of Pediatrics (AAP), and the American Academy of Family Physicians (AAFP).

1. This schedule indicates the recommended ages for routine administration of currently licensed childhood vaccines, as of 11/1/00, for children and adolescents through 18 years of age. Additional vaccines may be licensed and recommended during the year. Licensed combination vaccines may be used whenever any components of the combination are indicated and its other components aren't contraindicated. Providers should consult the manufacturers' package inserts for detailed recommendations.

2. *Infants born to hepatitis B surface antigen (HBsAg)–negative mothers* should receive the first dose of hepatitis B (Hep B) vaccine by age 2 months. The second dose should be at least 1 month after the first dose. The third dose should be administered at least 4 months after the first dose and at least 2 months after the second dose, but not before 6 months of age for infants.

Infants born to HBsAg-positive mothers should receive hepatitis B vaccine and 0.5 ml hepatitis B immune globulin (HBIG) within 12 hours of birth at separate sites. The second dose is recommended at 1 to 2 months of age, and the third dose at 6 months of age.

*Infants born to mothers whose HBSAg status is un-*known should receive hepatitis B vaccine within 12 hours of birth. Maternal blood should be drawn at the time of delivery to determine the mother's HBsAg status; if the HBsAg test is positive, the infant should receive HBIG as soon as possible (no later than 1 week of age).

All children and adolescents who haven't been immunized against hepatitis B should begin the series during any visit. Special efforts should be made to immunize children who were born or whose parents were born in areas of the world with moderate or high endemicity of hepatitis B virus infection.

3. The fourth dose of diphtheria and tetanus toxoids and acellular pertussis vaccine (DTaP) may be administered as early as 12 months of age, provided 6 months have elapsed since the third dose and the child is unlikely to return at 15 to 18 months of age. Tetanus and diphtheria toxoids (Td) is recommended at 11 to 12 years of age if at least 5 years have elapsed since the last dose of DTP, DTaP, or DT. Subsequent routine Td boosters are recommended every 10 years.

4. Three *Haemophilus influenzae* type b (Hib) conjugate vaccines are licensed for infant use. If PRP-OMP (Pedvaxhib or ComVax) is administered at 2 and 4 months of age, a dose at 6 months isn't required. Because clinical studies in infants have demonstrated that using some combination products may induce a lower immune response to the Hib vaccine component, DTaP/Hib combination products shouldn't be used for primary immunization in infants at 2, 4, or 6 months of age, unless FDA-approved for these ages.

5. An all–poliovirus inactivated vaccine (IPV) schedule is recommended for routine childhood polio vaccination in the United States. All children should receive four doses of IPV at 2 months, 4 months, 6 to 18 months, and 4 to 6 years of age. Poliovirus vaccine live oral (OPV) should be used only in selected circumstances. (See *MMWR*, May 19, 2000, 49[RR-5]:1-22.)

6. The heptavalent conjugate pneumococcal vaccine (PCV) is recommended for all children 2 to 23 months of age. It's also recommended for certain children 24 to 59 months of age. (See *MMWR*, Oct. 6, 2000, 49[RR-9]:1-35).

7. The second dose of measles-mumps-rubella (MMR) vaccine is recommended routinely at 4 to 6 years of age but may be administered during any visit, provided at least 4 weeks have elapsed since receipt of the first dose and that both doses are administered beginning at or after 12 months of age. Those who haven't previously received the second dose should complete the schedule by 11 to 12 years of age.

8. Varicella (Var) vaccine is recommended at any visit on or after the first birthday for susceptible children — for example, those who lack a reliable history of chickenpox (as judged by a health care provider) and who haven't been immunized. Susceptible persons 13 years of age or older should receive two doses, given at least 4 weeks apart.

9. Hepatitis A (Hep A) is shaded to indicate its recommended use in selected states or regions and for certain high-risk groups; consult your local public health authority. (See *MMWR*, Oct. 1, 1999, 48[RR-12]:1-37.)

Common drug prototypes

The following chart is a general review of some of the more common drug classes. Each drug class is presented with a prototype drug, actions, indications, and nursing considerations. This chart should be used only for a review; a drug handbook should be used for more in-depth information about the medications and drug classes.

CLASSIFICATION	PROTOTYPE	ACTIONS	INDICATIONS	NURSING CONSIDERATIONS
Alpha-adrenergic blocker	Minipress	Inhibits alpha-adrenergic receptors causing arterial and venous dilation, which reduces peripheral vascular resistance	• Mild to moderate hypertension	• Monitor for adverse effects, such as dizziness, first-dose syncope, palpitations, and nausea. • Monitor pulse rate and blood pressure frequently. • Advise the client to arise slowly and to avoid abrupt position changes.
Aminoglycoside	Gentamicin	Inhibits protein synthesis by binding directly to the 30S ribosomal subunit; usually bactericidal	• Serious infections caused by susceptible organisms • Endocarditis prophylaxis for GI and genitourinary procedures or surgery	• Monitor for adverse effects, such as seizures, ototoxicity, nephrotoxicity, apnea, anaphylaxis, leukopenia, thrombocytopenia, and agranulocytosis. • Obtain peak gentamicin level 1 hour after I.M. injection or 30 minutes after I.V. infusion; check trough levels prior to next dose.
Angiotensin-converting enzyme inhibitor	Vasotec	Prevents the conversion of angiotensin I to angiotensin II; decreases vasoconstriction, reducing peripheral arterial resistance; causes inhibition of angiotensin II and decreases adrenocortical secretion of aldosterone;	• Hypertension • Management of symptomatic heart failure	• Monitor for adverse effects, such as hypotension, dry cough, and angioedema. • Monitor serum potassium levels and complete blood count with differential.

(continued)

CLASSIFICATION	PROTOTYPE	ACTIONS	INDICATIONS	NURSING CONSIDERATIONS
Angiotensin-converting enzyme inhibitor *(continued)*		results in decreased sodium and water retention and extracellular fluid volume		
Antiarrhythmic (atrial)	Quinaglute	Causes direct and indirect effects on cardiac tissue; decreases automaticity, conduction velocity, and membrane responsiveness; prolongs effective refractory period; reduces vagal tone reduced by anticholinergic action	• Atrial fibrillation and flutter • Atrial tachycardia; premature atrial and ventricular contractions • Paroxysmal supra ventricular tachycardia	• Monitor for adverse effects, such as vertigo, headache, arrhythmias, hypotension, heart failure, tinnitus, diarrhea, nausea, vomiting, hematologic disorders, hepatotoxicity, respiratory arrest, angioedema, fever, and cinchonism. • Monitor pulse and blood pressure frequently. • Anticoagulation may be performed prior to treatment.
Antiarrhythmic (ventricular)	Lidocaine	Decreases depolarization, automaticity, and excitability in the ventricles during the diastole phase by direct action on the tissues (especially the Purkinje network)	• Ventricular arrhythmias	• Monitor for adverse effects, such as confusion, tremor, restlessness, seizures, hypotension, new arrhythmias, cardiac arrest, tinnitus, blurred vision, respiratory depression, and anaphylaxis. • Monitor serum lidocaine levels for toxicity. • Monitor electrolytes, blood urea nitrogen, and creatinine levels.
Anticholinergic	Atropine	Antagonizes actions of acetylcholine and other cholinergic agonists at muscarinic and nicotinic receptors within the parasympathetic nervous system and smooth muscles that lack cholinergic innervation	• Symptomatic bradycardia • Given preoperatively to diminish secretions and block cardiac vagal reflexes • Adjunct treatment for peptic ulcer disease; treatment for functional GI disorders	• Monitor for adverse effects, such as headache, restlessness, insomnia, urine retention, urinary hesitancy, dizziness, blurred vision, dry mouth, constipation, anaphylaxis, and uticara. • Recommend monitoring the client's vital signs, urine output, and vision and for signs of impending toxicity. • Constipation may be relieved by stool softeners or bulk laxatives.

CLASSIFICATION	PROTOTYPE	ACTIONS	INDICATIONS	NURSING CONSIDERATIONS
Anticoagulant	Heparin	Accelerates formation of antithrombin III–thrombin complex and deactivates thrombin; prevents conversion of fibrinogen to fibrin	• Treatment for deep vein thrombosis (DVT), myocardial infarction (MI), pulmonary embolism, and consumption coagulopathy • Prevention of DVT and pulmonary embolism	• Monitor for adverse effects, such as hemorrhage, prolonged clotting time, thrombocytopenia, and hypersensitivity reactions. • Regularly inspect the client for bleeding gums, bruises, petechiae, epistaxis, tarry stools, hematuria, and hematemesis. • Effects can be neutralized by protamine sulfate. • Monitor partial thromboplastin time regularly.
	Coumadin	Inhibits vitamin K-dependent activation of clotting factors II, VII, IX, and X formed in the liver	• Prevention of pulmonary embolism caused by DVT, MI, rheumatic fever, prosthetic heart valves, or chronic atrial fibrillation	• Monitor for adverse effects, such as hemorrhage, prolonged clotting time, rash, fever, diarrhea, and hepatitis. • Regularly inspect the client for bleeding gums, bruises, petechiae, epistaxis, tarry stools, hematuria, and hematemesis. • Monitor prothrombin time regularly. • Effects can be neutralized by vitamin K.
Anticonvulsant	Dilantin	Stabilizes neuronal membranes and limits seizure activity by either increasing efflux or decreasing influx of sodium ions across cell membranes in the motor cortex during generation of nerve impulses	• Control of tonic-clonic and complex partial seizures • Status epilepticus • Prevention of and treatment for seizures during neurosurgery	• Monitor for adverse effects, such as ataxia, slurred speech, mental confusion, nystagmus, blurred vision, gingival hyperplasia, nausea, vomiting, hematologic disorders, hepatitis, Stevens-Johnson syndrome, and hirsutism. • Don't withdraw suddenly; seizures may occur. • Monitor drug levels as ordered; therapeutic levels range from 10 to 20 µg/ml.

CLASSIFICATION	PROTOTYPE	ACTIONS	INDICATIONS	NURSING CONSIDERATIONS
Antidepressant	Prozac	Inhibits central nervous system (CNS) neuronal uptake of serotonin	• Depression • Obsessive-compulsive disorder • Eating disorders	• Monitor for adverse effects, such as nervousness, anxiety, insomnia, headache, drowsiness, tremor, dizziness, nausea, diarrhea, dry mouth, and anorexia. • Use cautiously in the client with high suicide risk.
Antihistamine	Benadryl	Competes with histamine for H_1-receptor sites on the smooth muscle of the bronchi, GI tract, uterus, and large blood vessels, binding to the cellular receptors and preventing access and subsequent activity of histamine; doesn't directly alter histamine or prevent its release; antagonizes the action of histamine that causes increased capillary permeability and resultant edema and suppresses flare and pruritus associated with the endogenous release of histamine	• Rhinitis • Allergy symptoms • Motion sickness • Parkinson's disease	• Monitor for adverse effects, such as drowsiness, sedation, seizures, nausea, dry mouth, thrombocytopenia, agranulocytosis, thickening of secretions, and anaphylactic shock. • Use with extreme caution in clients with prostatic hyperplasia, asthma, chronic obstructive pulmonary disease, hyperthyroidism, cardiovascular disease, and hypertension.
Antilipemic	Lipitor	Inhibits 3-hydroxy-3-methylglutaryl-coenzyme A reductase, an early (and rate-limiting) step in cholesterol biosynthesis	• Treatment for various dyslipidemias	• Monitor for adverse effects, such as headache and muscle aches. • Monitor lipid profile and liver enzymes periodically.
Antiparkinsonian	Sinemet	Converts to dopamine in the CNS; increases dopamine levels in the brain; carbidopa inhibits peripheral decarboxylation of levodopa without affecting its metabolism within the CNS, leaving more to be decarboxylated to dopamine in the brain	• Parkinson's disease	• Monitor for adverse effects, such as involuntary grimacing, head movements, myoclonic jerks, ataxia, suicidal tendencies, hypotension, dry mouth, nausea, vomiting, hematologic disorders, hepatotoxicity, and choreiform, dystonic, dyskinetic movements.

CLASSIFICATION	PROTOTYPE	ACTIONS	INDICATIONS	NURSING CONSIDERATIONS
Antiparkinsonian (*continued*)				• Clients on long-term therapy should be tested for acromegaly and diabetes.
Antitubercular	Laniazid	Appears to inhibit cell wall biosynthesis by interfering with lipid and deoxyribonucleic acid (DNA) synthesis	• Tuberculosis	• Monitor for adverse effects, such as peripheral neuropathy, seizures, hematologic disorders, hepatitis, and hypersensitivity reactions. • Always give with other antituberculotics to prevent development of resistant organisms.
Antiviral	Acyclovir	Interferes with DNA synthesis and inhibits viral multiplication	• Treatment for herpes simplex viruses Types 1 and 2; varicella	• Monitor for adverse effects, such as malaise, headache, encephalopathy, renal failure, thrombocytopenia, and pain at injection site.
Barbiturate	Phenobarbital	Induces imbalance in central inhibitory and facilitatory mechanisms that influence cerebral cortex and reticular formation; decreases presynaptic and postsynaptic membrane excitability; exact mechanism of action not known, and which cellular and synaptic actions resulting in sedative-hypnotic effects not clear; produces all levels of CNS depression (mild sedation to coma to death); exerts its effect by facilitating the actions of gamma-aminobutyric acid (GABA); exerts a central effect, which depresses respiration and GI motility; no analgesic action, and may increase the reaction to	• Epilepsy • Febrile seizures • Sedation	• Monitor for adverse effects, such as drowsiness, lethargy, hangover, respiratory depression, apnea, Stevens-Johnson syndrome, and angioedema. • Don't withdraw abruptly; seizures may worsen. • Watch for signs of toxicity: coma, asthmatic breathing, cyanosis, clammy skin, and cyanosis.

(continued)

CLASSIFICATION	PROTOTYPE	ACTIONS	INDICATIONS	NURSING CONSIDERATIONS
Barbiturate (*continued*)		painful stimuli at sub-anesthetic doses; reduces nerve transmission and decreases excitability of the nerve cell as its principal anticonvulsant mechanism of action; raises the seizure threshold		
Benzodiazepine	Xanax	Sites and mechanisms of action not known; enhances or facilitates the action of GABA, an inhibitory neurotransmitter in the CNS; acts at the limbic, thalamic, and hypothalamic levels of the CNS; produces anxiolytic, sedative, hypnotic, skeletal muscle relaxant, and anticonvulsant effects; CNS-depressant activities; individual derivatives act more selectively at specific sites, allowing them to be subclassified into five categories based on their predominant clinical use	● Anxiety ● Panic disorders	● Monitor for adverse effects, such as drowsiness, light-headedness, depression, dry mouth, diarrhea, and constipation. ● Drug isn't recommended for long-term use. ● Don't withdraw abruptly; seizures may occur.
Beta-adrenergic blocker	Lopressor	Competes with beta-agonists for available beta-receptor sites	● Hypertension ● Angina pectoris	● Monitor for adverse effects, such as fatigue, dizziness, bradycardia, hypotension, heart failure, and atrioventricular block. ● Drug may be held if apical pulse is less than 60 beats/minute. ● Monitor blood pressure frequently.

CLASSIFICATION	PROTOTYPE	ACTIONS	INDICATIONS	NURSING CONSIDERATIONS
Calcium channel blocker	Verapamil	Inhibits calcium influx across the slow channels of myocardial and vascular smooth muscle cells; reduces intracellular calcium concentrations; dilates coronary arteries, peripheral arteries, and arterioles and slows cardiac conduction	• Vasospasm angina • Hypertension • Supraventricular arrhythmias	• Monitor for adverse effects, such as hypotension, heart failure, constipation, and ventricular asystole or fibrillation. • Monitor blood pressure frequently.
Cardiac glycoside	Digoxin	Inhibits sodium potassium–activated adenosine triphosphate; promotes movement of calcium from extracellular to intracellular cytoplasm and strengthens myocardial contraction; acts on the CNS to enhance vagal tone, slowing contraction through the sinoatrial and atrioventricular nodes and providing an antiarrhythmic effect	• Heart failure • Atrial fibrillation and flutter • Supraventricular tachycardia	• Monitor for adverse effects, such as fatigue, agitation, hallucinations, arrhythmias, anorexia, and nausea. • Drug may be held if apical pulse is less than 60 beats/minute. • Monitor serum potassium and digoxin levels periodically.
Cephalosporin	Cefazolin	Inhibits cell wall synthesis, promoting osmotic instability; usually bactericidal	• Infection caused by susceptible organisms	• Monitor for adverse effects, such as diarrhea, hematologic disorders, rash, and hypersensitivity reactions. • With large doses or prolonged treatment, monitor for superinfections. • Obtain specimen for culture and sensitivity prior to first dose; therapy may begin prior to results.

CLASSIFICATION	PROTOTYPE	ACTIONS	INDICATIONS	NURSING CONSIDERATIONS
Corticosteroid	Prednisone	Decreases inflammation; stabilizes leukocyte lysomal membranes; suppresses immune response; stimulates bone marrow; influences protein, fat, and carbohydrate metabolism	● Severe inflammation, immunosuppression	● Monitor for adverse effects, such as euphoria, insomnia, seizures, heart failure, arrhythmias, thromboembolism, peptic ulcers, pancreatitis, and acute adrenal insufficiency. ● Monitor the client's weight, blood pressure, and serum electrolytes. ● May mask signs of infection. ● Dose must be gradually reduced after long-term therapy.
Diuretic, loop	Lasix	Inhibits sodium and chloride reabsorption in the ascending loop of Henle, thus increasing renal excretion of sodium, chloride, and water; like thiazide diuretic, increases excretion of potassium; produces greater maximum diuresis and electrolyte loss than a thiazide diuretic	● Acute pulmonary edema ● Edema ● Hypertension	● Monitor for adverse effects, such as pancreatitis, hematologic disorders, and electrolyte imbalances (especially hypokalemia). ● Monitor weight and blood pressure frequently. ● Signs of hypokalemia may include leg cramps and muscle aches.
Diuretic, thiazide	Hydrochloro-thiazide	Interferes with sodium transport across tubules of the cortical diluting segment of the nephron; increases renal excretion of sodium, chloride, water, potassium, and calcium; increases bicarbonate, magnesium, phosphate, bromide, and iodide excretion; decreases excretion of ammonia, causing increased serum ammonia levels	● Edema ● Hypertension	● Monitor for adverse effects, such as pancreatitis, hematologic disorders, and electrolyte imbalances (especially hypokalemia). ● Monitor weight and blood pressure frequently. ● Signs of hypokalemia may include leg cramps and muscle aches.

CLASSIFICATION	PROTOTYPE	ACTIONS	INDICATIONS	NURSING CONSIDERATIONS
Hematinic	Ferrous sulfate	Provides elemental iron	• Iron deficiency	• Monitor for adverse effects, such as nausea, constipation, and black, tarry stools. • Use cautiously for long-term treatment.
Histamine-2 receptor antagonist	Pepcid	Inhibits histamine's action at H_2 receptors in gastric parietal cells; reduces gastric acid output and concentration regardless of the stimulatory agent (histamine, food, insulin, caffeine, betazole, pentagastrin) or basal conditions	• Gastroesophageal reflux disease • Zollinger-Ellison syndrome • Duodenal ulcer • Gastric ulcer • Heartburn	• Monitor for adverse effects such as headache. • Monitor for signs of GI bleeding such as blood in the stools.
Hypoglycemic agent (sulfonylurea)	Micronase	Stimulates insulin release from the pancreatic beta cells and reduces glucose output by the liver; extrapancreatic effect increases peripheral sensitivity to insulin and causes a mild diuretic effect	• Diabetes mellitus type 2	• Monitor for adverse effects, such as hypoglycemia, angioedema, and hematologic disorders. • During times of stress, clients may need insulin. Monitor for signs of hypoglycemia.
Hypoglycemic agent	Insulin	Increases glucose transport across muscle and fat cell membranes to reduce blood glucose levels; promotes conversion of glucose to its storage form glycogen; triggers amino acid uptake and conversion to protein in muscle cells and inhibits protein degradation; stimulates triglyceride formation and inhibits release of free fatty acids from adipose tissue; stimulates lipoprotein lipase activity, which converts circulating lipoproteins to fatty acids	• Diabetes mellitus type 1 • Adjunct treatment in diabetes mellitus type 2 • Diabetic ketoacidosis	• Monitor for adverse effects, such as hypoglycemia and hypersensitivity reactions.

CLASSIFICATION	PROTOTYPE	ACTIONS	INDICATIONS	NURSING CONSIDERATIONS
Nitrate	Nitroglycerin	Relaxes vascular smooth muscle relaxation; causes generalized vasodilation	• Acute or chronic anginal attacks	• Monitor for adverse effects, such as headache, dizziness, orthostatic hypotension, tachycardia, flushing, palpitations, and hypersensitivity reactions. • Monitor vital signs closely. • Treat headaches with acetaminophen or aspirin.
Nonsteroidal anti-inflammatory drug (NSAID)	Motrin	Interferes with the prostaglandins involved in pain; appears to sensitize pain receptors to mechanical stimulation or to other chemical mediators (such as bradykinin and histamine); inhibits synthesis of prostaglandins peripherally and possibly centrally; inhibits prostaglandin synthesis and release during inflammation; antipyretic effect due to suppression of prostaglandin synthesis in the CNS	• Rheumatoid arthritis • Osteoarthritis • Juvenile arthritis • Mild to moderate pain • Fever	• Monitor for adverse effects, such as bronchospasm, Stevens-Johnson syndrome, hematologic disorders, and aseptic meningitis. • It may take 1 to 2 weeks for full anti-inflammatory effects. • NSAIDs may mask the signs and symptoms of infection.
Opioid	Morphine	Acts on opiate receptors in the CNS	• Pain	• Monitor for adverse effects, such as sedation, euphoria, seizures, dizziness, nightmares, bradycardia, shock, cardiac arrest, nausea, constipation, vomiting, thrombocytopenia, and respiratory depression. • Keep narcotic antagonist (naloxone) and resuscitation equipment available.

CLASSIFICATION	PROTOTYPE	ACTIONS	INDICATIONS	NURSING CONSIDERATIONS
Proton pump inhibitor	Prilosec	Inhibits activity of acid (proton) pump and binds to hydrogen-potassium adenosine-triphosphatase, located at secretory surface of the gastric parietal cells, to block formation of gastric acid	• Gastroesophageal reflux disease • Zollinger-Ellison syndrome • Duodenal ulcer • Gastric ulcer • *Helicobacter pylori* infection	• Monitor for adverse effects, such as headache, dizziness, and nausea. • Administer 30 minutes before meals.
Sulfonamide	Bactrim	Bacteriostatic; mechanism of action correlating directly with the structural similarities it shares with para-aminobenzoic acid; inhibits biosynthesis of folic acid; susceptible bacteria being those that synthesize folic acid	• Infections of the urinary tract, respiratory tract, and ear caused by susceptible organisms • Chronic bacterial prostatitis • Prevention of recurrent urinary tract infection in women and of "traveler's diarrhea"	• Monitor for adverse effects, such as seizures, nausea, vomiting, diarrhea, hematologic disorders, Stevens-Johnson syndrome, toxic nephrosis, and hypersensitivity reactions. • Reduced dosages are needed in clients with renal and hepatic impairment. • With large doses or prolonged treatment, monitor for superinfections. • Obtain specimen for culture and sensitivity prior to first dose; therapy may begin prior to results.
Tetracycline	Tetracycline	Bacteriostatic but may be bactericidal against certain organisms; binds reversibly to 30S and 50S ribosomal subunits; inhibits bacterial protein synthesis; bacterial resistance to tetracyclines usually mediated by plasmids (R-factor resistance), which decrease bacterial cell wall permeability	• Infections due to susceptible organism • Gonorrhea	• Monitor for adverse effects, such as nausea, vomiting, diarrhea, hematologic disorders, Stevens-Johnson syndrome, intracranial hypertension, rash, photosensitivity, and hypersensitivity reactions. • With large doses or prolonged treatment, monitor for superinfections. • Obtain specimen for culture and sensitivity prior to first dose; therapy may begin prior to results.

CLASSIFICATION	PROTOTYPE	ACTIONS	INDICATIONS	NURSING CONSIDERATIONS
Thrombolytic	Streptokinase	Lyses clots by converting plasminogen to plasmin; in contrast, anticoagulants act by preventing thrombi from developing	• Venous thrombosis; pulmonary embolism; arterial thrombosis and embolism • Lysis of a clot during an MI	• Monitor for adverse effects, such as arrhythmias, bleeding, pulmonary edema, and hypersensitivity reaction. • Monitor vital signs and for bleeding frequently.
Thyroid hormone	Synthroid	Stimulates metabolism of all body tissues by accelerating rate of cellular oxidation	• Cretinism • Myxedema coma • Thyroid hormone replacement	• Monitor for adverse effects, such as nervousness, insomnia, tremor, tachycardia, palpitations, angina, arrhythmias, and cardiac arrest. • Use with extreme caution in elderly clients and those with cardiovascular disorders.

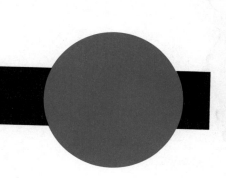

515

Posttest

Instructions

This posttest has been designed to evaluate your nursing ability, skill, and knowledge as you prepare to take the NCLEX-PN. This posttest can also be used for review by nurses returning to active practice after an absence and by those moving to a different clinical area of practice.

The posttest is based on the question-and-response format used on the NCLEX-PN. The questions on the posttests focus primarily on practical application of nursing principles rather than on simple recall of facts.

The posttest contains 85 questions, written in the same format used in the computerized examination. There are four possible answers for each question, labeled A, B, C, and D. (These letters don't appear in the computerized NCLEX-PN but are provided here so that you can later identify the correct answers and the rationales.) Read each question and all possible answers carefully; then select the best answer. Take no more than 85 minutes to complete the posttest.

Like the NCLEX-PN, the *Springhouse Review* posttest doesn't contain deliberately misleading questions. Each question has only one correct answer. Before selecting your answer, read the entire question carefully to make sure you understand it. Then choose the best answer. Be aware that for some questions, all four answer choices might represent appropriate nursing behavior. However, the question will ask which behavior is *most important* or should be done *first*.

If you don't know the answer to a particular question, try to eliminate one, or preferably two, of the possible answers and then choose the best answer from the remaining choices. Remember that on the computerized examination, you will *not* be able to go back to a question or go on to the next question without selecting an answer choice.

Remember to:
- read each question carefully
- choose the best answer from the four possible choices
- select only one answer for each question
- answer each question on the test.

Before beginning the posttest, select a quiet room where you'll be undisturbed and set a timer for 85 minutes. After you've completed the posttest or the 85-minute time limit expires, check your responses against the answers and rationales on pages 525 to 535. Carefully study the rationales for any questions you answered incorrectly. This will give you an additional opportunity to recall important nursing information.

1. A client with cervical cancer is receiving internal radiation treatment. The intensity of radiation is estimated by using the principle of the inverse square rule. If the nurse is 4′ from the radiation source, the exposure would be:
- ☐ **A.** ½ of the exposure at 1′.
- ☐ **B.** ¼ of the exposure at 1′.
- ☐ **C.** ⅛ of the exposure at 1′.
- ☐ **D.** ¹⁄₁₆ of the exposure at 1′.

2. A client in a nursing home has Alzheimer's disease. She's very forgetful and frequently asks what time it is. How should the nurse respond the next time the client asks the time?
- ☐ **A.** Ask the client what time it was the last time she asked.
- ☐ **B.** Ask the client why she can't remember the time.
- ☐ **C.** Tell the client the correct time.
- ☐ **D.** Tell the client this is the last time she'll be told.

3. The nurse is administering the prescribed morning dose of NPH insulin to a client with diabetes. Within 30 minutes after administering NPH insulin, the nurse should assign highest priority to which of the following interventions?

- ☐ **A.** Testing the client's urine for glucose
- ☐ **B.** Observing the client for a skin reaction
- ☐ **C.** Checking the injection site for drug absorption
- ☐ **D.** Instructing the client to eat breakfast

4. While on the examining table, a client who is 19 weeks pregnant tells the nurse that she's experiencing quickening. Which action should the nurse take?

- ☐ **A.** Inform the charge nurse of the client's symptom.
- ☐ **B.** Turn the client onto her left side.
- ☐ **C.** Tell the client that quickening is normal.
- ☐ **D.** Remind the client that she soon may have bloody show.

5. A client is recovering from abdominal surgery. Which finding indicates that the client is ready for removal of the nasogastric (NG) tube?

- ☐ **A.** The client no longer complains of feeling nauseated.
- ☐ **B.** The client burps after taking a sip of clear fluids.
- ☐ **C.** Drainage from the client's stomach has diminished in volume.
- ☐ **D.** The client has been passing flatus.

6. A 2-month-old infant who has been vomiting formula and passing watery green stools is admitted to the pediatric unit. The physician diagnoses infectious diarrhea and dehydration. An I.V. infusion is started in a scalp vein, and all oral intake is withheld. Which action should the nurse assigned to care for the child take first?

- ☐ **A.** Obtain a stool specimen.
- ☐ **B.** Measure the infant's axillary temperature.
- ☐ **C.** Place the infant on isolation precautions.
- ☐ **D.** Test urine specific gravity.

7. A client is receiving digoxin (Lanoxin). Which of the following adverse effects should the nurse observe for during digoxin therapy?

- ☐ **A.** Blurred vision
- ☐ **B.** Hand tremors
- ☐ **C.** Urine retention
- ☐ **D.** Hearing loss

8. For a client with osteoporosis, the nurse should provide which dietary instruction?

- ☐ **A.** "Decrease your intake of red meat."
- ☐ **B.** "Decrease your intake of popcorn, nuts, and seeds."
- ☐ **C.** "Eat more fruits to increase your potassium intake."
- ☐ **D.** "Eat more dairy products to increase your calcium intake."

9. A client undergoes an abdominal-perineal resection and a permanent colostomy in the descending colon. Postoperatively, a nasogastric tube is attached to low intermittent suction and a urethral catheter is attached to straight drainage. Two hours after surgery, the nurse notes that the perineal dressing is saturated with serosanguineous drainage. The nurse's next action should be based on the conclusion that the drainage resulted from:

- ☐ **A.** abrupt movement by the client.
- ☐ **B.** slippage of the suture holding the stoma in place.
- ☐ **C.** a properly functioning Penrose drain.
- ☐ **D.** a displaced urinary catheter.

10. A client with benign prostatic hyperplasia undergoes transurethral prostatic resection. Postoperatively, an indwelling catheter is in place. During the immediate postoperative period, the nurse should expect which assessment finding?

- ☐ **A.** Discomfort when urinating
- ☐ **B.** Distended bladder
- ☐ **C.** Neurogenic bladder
- ☐ **D.** Bloody urinary drainage

11. The physician prescribes ferrous gluconate (Fergon) in liquid form for a client with iron deficiency anemia. How should the nurse administer this preparation?

- ☐ **A.** Undiluted, with a dropper onto the tongue
- ☐ **B.** Undiluted, from a teaspoon
- ☐ **C.** Diluted with milk, in a glass
- ☐ **D.** Diluted with water, through a straw

12. The physician orders 1,000 ml of 5% dextrose in water every 8 hours for a client. The I.V. setup delivers 20 gtt/ml. About how many drops should be administered per minute?

- ☐ **A.** 27
- ☐ **B.** 35
- ☐ **C.** 42
- ☐ **D.** 50

13. A client is admitted to an alcohol treatment clinic. During the first meeting with the nurse, the client says, "Why am I meeting with you? You can't make me stop drinking." Which response by the nurse would be most therapeutic?
- ☐ **A.** "What makes you think I want to make you stop drinking?"
- ☐ **B.** "That's true. Quitting is truly your decision."
- ☐ **C.** "It's your life. I hope you'll give the program a fair try."
- ☐ **D.** "Your family really cares about you, and I think you care, too."

14. Which action by the nurse may help prevent a urinary tract infection in a client who is in labor?
- ☐ **A.** Providing the client with ice chips
- ☐ **B.** Encouraging the client to void frequently
- ☐ **C.** Testing the client's urine for glycosuria
- ☐ **D.** Providing frequent perineal care

15. A 4-year-old girl is scheduled for a bone marrow aspiration. Which nursing action would help prepare her for this procedure?
- ☐ **A.** Using a doll to show her what will happen during the procedure.
- ☐ **B.** Telling her a story about a little girl who had the procedure.
- ☐ **C.** Discussing the procedure with her parents and letting them explain it to her.
- ☐ **D.** Asking her parents whether she knows anyone who has had this procedure.

16. A client with rectal cancer is scheduled for an abdominal-perineal resection. Before surgery, the nurse tells the client that this procedure will cause a change in the client's:
- ☐ **A.** urine output.
- ☐ **B.** eating habits.
- ☐ **C.** physical activity.
- ☐ **D.** body image.

17. The physician prescribes an I.M. injection of iron dextran (DexFerrum) for a client with anemia. Which nursing action applies to administering this medication?
- ☐ **A.** Asking whether the client drinks alcoholic beverages
- ☐ **B.** Finding out whether the client is allergic to fish oil
- ☐ **C.** Giving the medication by the Z-track method
- ☐ **D.** Using a 1″ 25G needle to inject the medication

18. A client with rectal cancer is scheduled for an abdominal-perineal resection. The client is placed on a low-residue diet initially; then he's switched to a liquid diet for 24 hours before surgery. The nurse teaches the client that the low-residue and liquid diets are needed to:
- ☐ **A.** eliminate stress in the diseased bowel.
- ☐ **B.** empty the bowel of fecal material.
- ☐ **C.** reduce bowel motility.
- ☐ **D.** decrease pain in the diseased bowel.

19. A client is to take ferrous sulfate (Feosol). Which adverse effect can this preparation cause?
- ☐ **A.** Tinnitus
- ☐ **B.** Ataxia
- ☐ **C.** Blurred vision
- ☐ **D.** Black stools

20. A depressed client talks, walks, and moves at a slow pace. Which measure should the nurse include in the care plan?
- ☐ **A.** Try to slow the pace of care activities.
- ☐ **B.** Encourage the client to move at a faster pace.
- ☐ **C.** Remind the client that this behavior isn't appropriate.
- ☐ **D.** Provide the client with a more stimulating environment.

21. The nurse teaches a client with anemia to eat iron-rich foods. The client shows an understanding of the dietary instructions by selecting which snack?
- ☐ **A.** 1 cup of popcorn
- ☐ **B.** ½ cup of raisins
- ☐ **C.** ½ cup of blueberries
- ☐ **D.** 1 cup of hot chocolate

22. A multigravida client has her urine tested for protein. The purpose of this test is to help determine whether the client has:
- ☐ **A.** pregnancy-induced hypertension.
- ☐ **B.** ketoacidosis.
- ☐ **C.** placenta previa.
- ☐ **D.** gestational diabetes.

23. After learning that their child has acute lymphocytic leukemia, the child's parents become angry and hostile toward the staff. How should the nurse respond to the parents?

☐ **A.** Tell them that their behavior isn't helping their child.

☐ **B.** Give them a chance to talk, and help them cope with their feelings.

☐ **C.** Limit their visiting time with their child.

☐ **D.** Tell them that everything possible is being done to restore their child's health.

24. A client with iron deficiency anemia reports episodes of feeling dizzy and faint. To manage these episodes, the nurse should include which intervention in the care plan?

☐ **A.** Have the client lie down until the episode is over.

☐ **B.** Instruct the client to do breathing exercises when an episode occurs.

☐ **C.** Advise the client to drink highly sweetened beverages when an episode occurs.

☐ **D.** Teach the client to rise slowly from a lying or sitting position to a standing position.

25. After a client has a sigmoidoscopy, the nurse should observe for which potential complication of this procedure?

☐ **A.** Muscle atony of the colon

☐ **B.** Fissure of the anal sphincter

☐ **C.** Perforation of the intestinal wall

☐ **D.** Intestinal hyperactivity

26. A client with iron deficiency anemia is most likely to make which of the following statements?

☐ **A.** "My skin feels warm."

☐ **B.** "I get short of breath."

☐ **C.** "My tongue is swollen."

☐ **D.** "I've lost my sense of smell."

27. The nurse teaches a client how to prepare for a barium enema. Which statement by the client indicates a correct understanding of the teaching?

☐ **A.** "I'll cleanse my bowel with laxatives and enemas before the test."

☐ **B.** "I'll receive a muscle relaxant during the test."

☐ **C.** "I'll drink a contrast medium during the test."

☐ **D.** "I'll stop eating red meat 3 days before the test."

28. A client receives instructions on breast-feeding. Which statement indicates that she understands the instructions?

☐ **A.** "I should pull my baby's mouth from my nipple gently to detach him from my breast."

☐ **B.** "I should use cold compresses to relieve breast discomfort between feedings."

☐ **C.** "I should clean my nipples with soap and water gently after each feeding."

☐ **D.** "I should alternate breasts with each feeding."

29. Which of the following behavior modification techniques is useful in the treatment of phobias?

☐ **A.** Aversion therapy

☐ **B.** Imitation or modeling

☐ **C.** Positive reinforcement

☐ **D.** Systemic desensitization

30. A client is found sitting in a car with the motor running in an enclosed garage. When brought to the emergency department by the rescue squad, the client is unresponsive and hypotensive, he has a respiratory rate of 6 breaths/minute, and his skin appears bright red. Which nursing diagnosis takes highest priority for this client?

☐ **A.** Ineffective coping related to depression

☐ **B.** Ineffective tissue perfusion (peripheral) related to decreased cardiac output

☐ **C.** Ineffective tissue perfusion (cerebral) related to depressed neurological functioning

☐ **D.** Ineffective breathing pattern related to depressed respirations

31. An 18-month-old infant falls down a flight of stairs and is admitted to the hospital with a fractured right femur. The infant is placed in Bryant's traction. Which of the following observations by the nurse necessitates intervention?

☐ **A.** The weights are hanging freely over the foot of the crib.

☐ **B.** The infant's buttocks are resting on the crib mattress.

☐ **C.** The ropes are resting in the pulley grooves.

☐ **D.** The infant's legs are flexed at a 90-degree angle to the body.

32. Which goal of nursing care takes priority for a female client with cystitis?

☐ **A.** Increasing urine alkalinity

☐ **B.** Maintaining a balanced fluid intake and output

☐ **C.** Providing instructions on perineal hygiene

☐ **D.** Screening urine for sedimentation

33. The nurse teaches a client about a high-fiber diet. The client shows an understanding of the instructions by selecting which food from a sample menu?
- ☐ **A.** Cheese
- ☐ **B.** White bread
- ☐ **C.** Grapefruit
- ☐ **D.** Broccoli

34. A client had abdominal surgery 2 days ago. Which observation indicates that peristaltic activity has returned?
- ☐ **A.** The client is belching.
- ☐ **B.** The client is hungry.
- ☐ **C.** The client is passing flatus.
- ☐ **D.** The client is thirsty.

35. A client complains of irritability and poor concentration. These symptoms indicate which level of anxiety?
- ☐ **A.** Mild
- ☐ **B.** Moderate
- ☐ **C.** Severe
- ☐ **D.** Panic

36. An elderly client with emphysema is scheduled for discharge. During discharge preparation, the nurse reminds the client to stop smoking. The client replies angrily, "Who are you to tell me what to do? I'm older than you." Which response by the nurse would be most appropriate?
- ☐ **A.** "I'm giving you this information in your best interest."
- ☐ **B.** "You have the right to make your own decisions."
- ☐ **C.** "I'm sorry. I don't mean to be disrespectful."
- ☐ **D.** "If you don't want to take my advice, do whatever you wish."

37. The nurse is assessing a 2-year-old child for signs of increased intracranial pressure. Which of the following signs might this include?
- ☐ **A.** Increasing irritability
- ☐ **B.** Tachycardia
- ☐ **C.** Narrowing pulse pressure
- ☐ **D.** Pinpoint pupils

38. The physician prescribes promethazine hydrochloride (Phenergan) for a client who is being prepared for surgery. What's the purpose of administering this drug to the client?
- ☐ **A.** To provide sedation
- ☐ **B.** To inhibit oral secretions
- ☐ **C.** To prevent bleeding problems
- ☐ **D.** To enhance wound healing

39. After being admitted for diagnostic tests to rule out a cardiac problem, a client complains of nervousness, irritability, and an upset stomach. To best assist the client, the nurse should understand that:
- ☐ **A.** the client's symptoms are an inappropriate reaction to the diagnostic tests.
- ☐ **B.** a client may invent symptoms to gain the nurse's attention.
- ☐ **C.** the client's symptoms may indicate increased anxiety.
- ☐ **D.** an exaggerated reaction to unpleasant situations is common.

40. A client is receiving a transfusion of whole blood. Which assessment finding indicates that a hemolytic reaction is occurring?
- ☐ **A.** Lower back pain
- ☐ **B.** Positive Homans' sign
- ☐ **C.** Hyperreflexia
- ☐ **D.** Hematemesis

41. A child is scheduled for surgery. Which statement by the child indicates the need for more preoperative teaching?
- ☐ **A.** "I'll wake up in another room and then come back to my room."
- ☐ **B.** "I'll see Mom and Dad after the operation."
- ☐ **C.** "I'll have my favorite ice cream after I wake up."
- ☐ **D.** "I'll feel sleepy for a while after the operation."

42. A 74-year-old client has vascular disease. Which nursing intervention would be most appropriate for this client?
- ☐ **A.** Encourage him to avoid caffeine and nicotine.
- ☐ **B.** Advise him to wear knee-length stockings.
- ☐ **C.** Instruct him to soak both feet in cool water.
- ☐ **D.** Caution him not to exercise daily.

43. A client undergoes a left-sided mastectomy with removal of the axillary lymph nodes. During discharge preparation, the nurse should provide which instruction?
- ☐ **A.** "Wear an elastic bandage on your left arm at all times."
- ☐ **B.** "Don't let anyone draw blood from your left arm or take your blood pressure on that arm."
- ☐ **C.** "Avoid sleeping on your left side or putting pressure on your left arm."
- ☐ **D.** "Keep your left arm elevated or in a sling most of the day."

44. After a tonsillectomy and an adenoidectomy, a child returns to the pediatric unit. Until he's fully awake, the child should be maintained in which position?
- ☐ **A.** Side-lying
- ☐ **B.** Supine
- ☐ **C.** Knee-to-chest
- ☐ **D.** Lithotomy

45. Which of the following interventions would the nurse recommend to a client having severe heartburn during her pregnancy?
- ☐ **A.** Eat several small meals daily.
- ☐ **B.** Eat crackers on waking every morning.
- ☐ **C.** Drink a preparation of salt and vinegar.
- ☐ **D.** Drink orange juice frequently during the day.

46. A 40-week pregnant client is scheduled for a cesarean delivery because of cephalopelvic disproportion. Which of the following interventions should be included in her preoperative care plan?
- ☐ **A.** The client may be out of bed as tolerated and side-lying while in bed.
- ☐ **B.** The client may have clear fluids as desired because of planned spinal anesthesia.
- ☐ **C.** Vital signs should be taken every half hour until surgery.
- ☐ **D.** Pain medication should be given as directed.

47. A client's daughter tells the nurse, "Since I found out that my mother needs heart surgery, I've had trouble eating and sleeping." Which response by the nurse is best?
- ☐ **A.** "You must keep up your strength."
- ☐ **B.** "Your mother's condition is upsetting you."
- ☐ **C.** "Don't be concerned. These operations are common now."
- ☐ **D.** "I have the opposite reaction when I'm troubled."

48. Which response pattern best describes Babinski's reflex?
- ☐ **A.** Flexion of the forearm when the biceps tendon is tapped
- ☐ **B.** Extension of the leg when the patellar tendon is struck
- ☐ **C.** Tremor of the foot following brisk, forcible dorsiflexion
- ☐ **D.** Dorsiflexion of the great toe when the sole is scratched

49. Which assessment finding would indicate that a client's abdominal ascites are decreasing?
- ☐ **A.** The amount of ankle edema remains the same.
- ☐ **B.** Abdominal skin becomes shinier.
- ☐ **C.** Urine output per void increases.
- ☐ **D.** Pulse rate increases over time.

50. An 18-month-old infant is being placed in Bryant's traction after a fall down a flight of stairs. What position would the infant be in for this type of traction?
- ☐ **A.** Flat in bed with the affected leg extended wrapped in an elastic bandage with traction applied
- ☐ **B.** Flat in bed with a padded sling under the knee on the affected leg with traction applied
- ☐ **C.** Both legs at a 90-degree angle with the buttocks off the bed with traction applied
- ☐ **D.** Affected leg at a 90-degree angle with a skeletal pin inserted in the distal end of the femur with traction applied

51. A client is recovering from abdominal surgery. During the immediate postoperative period, which action should the nurse take to help prevent hypostatic pneumonia?
- ☐ **A.** Splint the incisional area while the client breathes deeply.
- ☐ **B.** Have the client use an incentive spirometer four times daily.
- ☐ **C.** Encourage the client to exhale through pursed lips.
- ☐ **D.** Support the client in an orthopneic position.

52. Which action by the nurse helps prevent thrombophlebitis in the calves of a postoperative client?
- ☐ **A.** Obtaining an order for the use of elastic stockings
- ☐ **B.** Keeping the knee gatch of the bed in a slightly elevated position
- ☐ **C.** Elevating the client's legs higher than the heart
- ☐ **D.** Encouraging the client to dorsiflex the feet three times daily

53. Nursing actions important in the secondary prevention of violence and abuse include:
- ☐ **A.** helping participants discuss the problem and developing alternatives for dealing with the tension that could lead to violence.
- ☐ **B.** identifying "red flag" behaviors, including isolation and depression.
- ☐ **C.** emphasizing safety as a top priority.
- ☐ **D.** teaching clients the importance of respect and care for family members.

54. The mother of a child who has been hospitalized for status asthmaticus stands outside the child's room crying. Which comment by the nurse would be most therapeutic?
- ☐ **A.** "This must be upsetting for you."
- ☐ **B.** "Talking to the doctor will help."
- ☐ **C.** "Most mothers feel this way."
- ☐ **D.** "Come talk with other parents in the waiting room."

55. A client with type 1 diabetes mellitus is taking NPH insulin. Which dietary instruction should the nurse provide?
- ☐ **A.** "When you skip a meal, reduce your insulin dosage."
- ☐ **B.** "Substitute 1 oz of fat for 2 oz of protein."
- ☐ **C.** "Eat your meals and snacks on schedule."
- ☐ **D.** "Use artificial sweeteners instead of complex sugars."

56. The physician prescribes ibuprofen (Motrin) for a client with osteoarthritis. The nurse should instruct the client to take this drug with any of the following except:
- ☐ **A.** food.
- ☐ **B.** an antacid.
- ☐ **C.** milk.
- ☐ **D.** aspirin.

57. A neonate is 8 hours old. Which assessment finding indicates that the neonate is in satisfactory condition?
- ☐ **A.** Axillary temperature of 94.6° F (34.8° C)
- ☐ **B.** Apical pulse rate of 124 beats/minute
- ☐ **C.** Slight yellowish tinge to the sclera
- ☐ **D.** Respiratory grunting on expiration

58. Based on multiple referrals, the nurse determines that childhood injuries are increasing in the community in which she practices. The first step the nurse would take in developing an educational program is:
- ☐ **A.** assessing for a decrease in referrals following a pediatric safety class.
- ☐ **B.** assessing the strengths and needs of the community while identifying barriers to learning.
- ☐ **C.** choosing a health promotion or health belief model as a framework.
- ☐ **D.** developing and implementing a specific plan to decrease childhood injuries.

59. Which of the following treatments is the definitive one for a ruptured aneurysm?

- ☐ **A.** Antihypertensive medication administration
- ☐ **B.** Aortogram
- ☐ **C.** Beta-adrenergic blocker administration
- ☐ **D.** Surgical intervention

60. Which of the following recurring conditions most commonly occurs in clients with cardiomyopathy?
- ☐ **A.** Heart failure
- ☐ **B.** Diabetes mellitus
- ☐ **C.** Myocardial infarction
- ☐ **D.** Pericardial effusion

61. Which of the following symptoms of hypertension is most common?
- ☐ **A.** Blurred vision
- ☐ **B.** Epistaxis
- ☐ **C.** Headache
- ☐ **D.** Peripheral edema

62. A 36-year-old client complains of fatigue, weight loss, and a low-grade fever. He also has pain in his fingers, elbows, and ankles. Which of the following conditions is suspected?
- ☐ **A.** Anemia
- ☐ **B.** Leukemia
- ☐ **C.** Rheumatic arthritis
- ☐ **D.** Systemic lupus erythematosus

63. When examining a nursery school–age child, the nurse finds multiple contusions over the body. Child abuse is suspected. Which of the following statements regarding this type of injury is true?
- ☐ **A.** Contusions confined to one body area are typically suspicious.
- ☐ **B.** All lesions, including location, shape, and color, should be documented.
- ☐ **C.** Natural injuries usually have straight linear lines, while injuries from abuse have multiple curved lines.
- ☐ **D.** The depth, location, and amount of bleeding that initially occurs are constant, but the sequence of color change is variable.

64. Although a client's physiologic response to a health crisis is important to the health outcome, which of the following nursing interventions also must be addressed?

- ☐ **A.** Teach the family how to care for the client.
- ☐ **B.** Help the client effectively cope with the crisis.
- ☐ **C.** Maintain I.V. access, medications, and diet.
- ☐ **D.** Teach the client basic information about the illness.

65. A client was infected with tuberculosis bacillus (TB) 10 years ago but never developed the disease. He's now being treated for cancer. The client begins to develop signs of TB. This is known as which of the following types of infection?
- ☐ **A.** Active infection
- ☐ **B.** Primary infection
- ☐ **C.** Superinfection
- ☐ **D.** Tertiary infection

66. A client has active tuberculosis. Which of the following symptoms will he exhibit?
- ☐ **A.** Chest and lower back pain
- ☐ **B.** Chills, fever, night sweats, and hemoptysis
- ☐ **C.** Fever of more than 104° F (40° C) and nausea
- ☐ **D.** Headache and photophobia

67. Which of the following measures best determines that a chest tube is no longer needed for a client who had a pneumothorax?
- ☐ **A.** The drainage from the chest tube is minimal.
- ☐ **B.** Arterial blood gas levels are obtained to ensure proper oxygenation.
- ☐ **C.** The tube is removed and the client is assessed to see whether he's breathing adequately.
- ☐ **D.** No fluctuation in the water seal chamber occurs when no suction is applied.

68. Which of the following nursing interventions should be used to prevent footdrop and contractures in a client recovering from a subdural hematoma?
- ☐ **A.** High-topped sneakers
- ☐ **B.** Low-dose heparin therapy
- ☐ **C.** Physical therapy consultation
- ☐ **D.** Sequential compression device

69. The treatment for osteoarthritis commonly includes salicylates. Salicylates can be dangerous in older people because they can cause which of the following adverse effects?
- ☐ **A.** Hearing loss
- ☐ **B.** Increased pain in joints
- ☐ **C.** Decreased calcium absorption
- ☐ **D.** Increased bone demineralization

70. Clients with osteoarthritis may be on bed rest for prolonged periods. Which of the following nursing interventions would be appropriate for these clients?
- ☐ **A.** Encourage coughing and deep breathing, and limit fluid intake.
- ☐ **B.** Provide only passive range of motion, and decrease stimulation.
- ☐ **C.** Have the client lie as still as possible, and give adequate pain medicine.
- ☐ **D.** Turn the client every 2 hours, and encourage coughing and deep breathing.

71. A client describes a foul odor from his cast. Which of the following responses or interventions would be the most appropriate?
- ☐ **A.** Assess further because this may be a sign of infection.
- ☐ **B.** Teach him proper cast care, including hygiene measures.
- ☐ **C.** This is normal, especially when a cast is in place for a few weeks.
- ☐ **D.** Assess further because this may be a sign of neurovascular compromise.

72. Which of the following substances is most likely to cause gastritis?
- ☐ **A.** Milk
- ☐ **B.** Bicarbonate of soda, or baking soda
- ☐ **C.** Enteric-coated aspirin
- ☐ **D.** Nonsteroidal anti-inflammatory drugs (NSAIDs)

73. Which of the following tasks should be included in the immediate postoperative management of a client who has undergone gastric resection?
- ☐ **A.** Monitoring gastric pH to detect complications
- ☐ **B.** Assessing for bowel sounds
- ☐ **C.** Providing nutritional support
- ☐ **D.** Monitoring for symptoms of hemorrhage

74. Which of the following treatments should be included in the immediate management of acute gastritis?
- ☐ **A.** Reducing work stress
- ☐ **B.** Completing gastric resection
- ☐ **C.** Treating the underlying cause
- ☐ **D.** Administering enteral tube feedings

75. Which of the following nursing interventions should be taken for a client who complains of nausea and vomits 1 hour after taking his morning glyburide (DiaBeta)?
- [ ] **A.** Give glyburide again.
- [ ] **B.** Give subcutaneous insulin, and monitor blood glucose.
- [ ] **C.** Monitor blood glucose closely, and look for signs of hypoglycemia.
- [ ] **D.** Monitor blood glucose, and assess for symptoms of hyperglycemia.

76. Which of the following chronic complications is associated with diabetes mellitus?
- [ ] **A.** Dizziness, dyspnea on exertion, and angina
- [ ] **B.** Retinopathy, neuropathy, and coronary artery disease
- [ ] **C.** Leg ulcers, cerebral ischemic events, and pulmonary infarcts
- [ ] **D.** Fatigue, nausea, vomiting, muscle weakness, and cardiac arrhythmias

77. Rotating injection sites when administering insulin prevents which of the following complications?
- [ ] **A.** Insulin edema
- [ ] **B.** Insulin lipodystrophy
- [ ] **C.** Insulin resistance
- [ ] **D.** Systemic allergic reactions

78. What tests should be ordered if hypothyroidism is suspected?
- [ ] **A.** Liver function tests
- [ ] **B.** Hemoglobin A_{1C}
- [ ] **C.** T_4 and thyroid-stimulating hormone
- [ ] **D.** 24-hour urine free cortisol measurement

79. A client with hypothyroidism may present with which of the following symptoms?
- [ ] **A.** Polyuria, polydipsia, and weight loss
- [ ] **B.** Heat intolerance, nervousness, weight loss, and hair loss
- [ ] **C.** Coarsening of facial features and extremity enlargement
- [ ] **D.** Tiredness, cold intolerance, weight gain, and constipation

80. Which of the following statements best explains why it's important to empty the bowel before treatment with intracavitary radiation for cancer of the cervix?

- [ ] **A.** Feces in the bowel increase the risk of ileus.
- [ ] **B.** An empty bowel allows the applicator to be positioned with little or no discomfort.
- [ ] **C.** Bowel movements increase the risk of inadvertent contamination of the vagina and urethra.
- [ ] **D.** Pressure changes in the pelvis associated with bowel movements can alter the position of the applicator and the radiation source.

81. A nurse enters the room of a client who had a left modified mastectomy 8 hours earlier. Which of the following observations indicates that the nursing assistant assigned to the client needs further instruction and guidance?
- [ ] **A.** The client is squeezing a ball in her left hand.
- [ ] **B.** The client is wearing a robe with elastic cuffs.
- [ ] **C.** The client's affected arm is elevated on a pillow.
- [ ] **D.** A blood pressure cuff is on the client's right arm.

82. For which of the following symptoms should a client at risk for evisceration be monitored after an abdominal hysterectomy?
- [ ] **A.** Tachycardia accompanied by a weak, thready pulse
- [ ] **B.** Hypotension with a decreased level of consciousness
- [ ] **C.** Shallow, rapid respirations and increasing vaginal drainage
- [ ] **D.** Low-grade fever with increasing serosanguineous incisional drainage

83. Which of the following findings indicates that oxycodone (Percodan) given to a client with breast cancer metastasized to the bone is exerting the desired effect?
- [ ] **A.** Bone density is increased.
- [ ] **B.** Pain is rated at 0 to 2 on a 10-point scale.
- [ ] **C.** Alpha-fetoprotein level is decreased.
- [ ] **D.** Serum calcium level is within normal range.

84. Which of the following adverse reactions may be caused by the use of isotretinoin (Accutane)?
- [ ] **A.** Birth defects
- [ ] **B.** Nausea and vomiting
- [ ] **C.** Vaginal yeast infection
- [ ] **D.** Gram-negative folliculitis

85. A client complains of small, red, pruritic dots between his fingers and toes. Which of the following conditions is the most likely diagnosis?

☐ **A.** Contusion
☐ **B.** Herpes zoster
☐ **C.** Scabies
☐ **D.** Varicella

Answers and rationales

In the posttest answers below, the question number appears in boldface type, followed by the letter of the correct answer. Rationales for correct answers and, where appropriate, for incorrect options follow. To help you evaluate your knowledge base and application of nursing behaviors, each rationale is classified as follows:

- nursing process step
- client needs category
- client needs subcategory
- cognitive level.

1. CORRECT ANSWER: D
The exposure to radiation at 4′ from the source is determined by squaring ¼, which yields ⅟₁₆. The other options are incorrect.
Nursing process step: Implementation
Client needs category: Safe, effective care environment
Client needs subcategory: Safety and infection control
Cognitive level: Comprehension

2. CORRECT ANSWER: C
Alzheimer's disease typically affects the memory, so the nurse should tell the client the time whenever she asks. Asking the client what time it was the last time she asked is demeaning. Asking the client why she can't remember the time would upset her. Telling the client that this is the last time she'll be told is threatening and nontherapeutic.
Nursing process step: Implementation
Client needs category: Psychosocial integrity
Client needs subcategory: Psychosocial adaptation
Cognitive level: Application

3. CORRECT ANSWER: D
NPH insulin starts to act within 2 hours after administration. Eating breakfast 30 minutes after administration ensures that the blood glucose level will be elevated. Hypoglycemia could result if the client didn't eat after NPH administration. The urine glucose level doesn't reliably reflect the blood glucose level. Insulin injection doesn't cause a skin reaction. Drug absorption rarely is a problem with insulin.
Nursing process step: Planning
Client needs category: Safe, effective care environment
Client needs subcategory: Safety and infection control
Cognitive level: Analysis

4. CORRECT ANSWER: C
Quickening, the pregnant woman's first awareness of fetal movement, normally is felt after 16 to 20 weeks. Informing the charge nurse of the client's symptom, turning the client onto her left side, and reminding the client that she soon may have bloody show are inappropriate nursing actions for a client who is experiencing quickening.
Nursing process step: Implementation
Client needs category: Health promotion and maintenance
Client needs subcategory: Growth and development through the life span
Cognitive level: Comprehension

5. CORRECT ANSWER: D
Anesthesia and surgery impede intestinal peristalsis, leading to gas accumulation in the intestine and distention. An NG tube is inserted to prevent distention. The tube can be removed when the bowel resumes normal function, as indicated by passing flatus.
Nursing process step: Data collection
Client needs category: Physiological integrity
Client needs subcategory: Physiological adaptation
Cognitive level: Comprehension

6. CORRECT ANSWER: C
Infectious diarrhea is highly contagious, and all persons on the pediatric unit should be protected from exposure. Obtaining a stool specimen and measuring the infant's axillary temperature are appropriate measures to take after isolating the infant. Testing urine specific gravity also may be required but isn't done first.
Nursing process step: Planning
Client needs category: Safe, effective care environment
Client needs subcategory: Safety and infection control
Cognitive level: Application

7. CORRECT ANSWER: A
Adverse effects of digoxin include nausea, vomiting, anorexia, and visual disturbances, such as blurred or yellow vision.
Nursing process step: Evaluation
Client needs category: Physiological integrity
Client needs subcategory: Pharmacological therapies
Cognitive level: Knowledge

8. CORRECT ANSWER: D
Osteoporosis causes a severe, general reduction in skeletal bone mass. To offset this reduction, the nurse should advise the client to increase calcium intake by consuming more dairy products, which provide about 75% of the calcium in the average diet. None of the other options would prevent osteoporosis from worsening.
Nursing process step: Implementation
Client needs category: Physiological integrity
Client needs subcategory: Basic care and comfort
Cognitive level: Comprehension

9. CORRECT ANSWER: C
The wound site is the probable source of serosanguineous drainage. After an abdominal-perineal resection, a Penrose drain is typically used to drain the wound site, and serosanguineous drainage on the perineal dressing is normal.
Nursing process step: Evaluation
Client needs category: Physiological integrity
Client needs subcategory: Physiological adaptation
Cognitive level: Analysis

10. CORRECT ANSWER: D
During a transurethral prostatic resection, the surgeon removes prostate tissue through the urethra with a resectoscope, cutting away slices of the prostate bit by bit. Bloody urinary drainage is expected during the immediate postoperative period. During this time, the client has a catheter attached to an irrigation system that continuously drains urine, so discomfort on urination and a distended bladder shouldn't occur. A neurogenic bladder develops secondary to central or peripheral nervous system lesions.
Nursing process step: Planning
Client needs category: Physiological integrity
Client needs subcategory: Physiological adaptation
Cognitive level: Comprehension

11. CORRECT ANSWER: D
Ferrous gluconate should be well diluted and administered through a straw or placed on the back of the client's tongue with a dropper to prevent staining and to mask the taste. This preparation shouldn't be administered undiluted. Although it may be mixed with water, it isn't compatible with milk.
Nursing process step: Implementation
Client needs category: Physiological integrity
Client needs subcategory: Pharmacological therapies
Cognitive level: Application

12. CORRECT ANSWER: C
The I.V. should deliver about 42 drops/minute, as indicated by the following formula:

$$\frac{\text{Volume of infusion in ml} \times \text{Drip factor (gtt/ml)}}{\text{Time of infusion in minutes}} = \text{Drops/minute}$$

Therefore:
$$1{,}000 \times 20/480 = 20{,}000/480 =$$
$$41.6, \text{ or } 42 \text{ drops/minute.}$$
Nursing process step: Implementation
Client needs category: Physiological integrity
Client needs subcategory: Pharmacological therapies
Cognitive level: Comprehension

13. CORRECT ANSWER: B
This response places the responsibility for recovery squarely on the client. Option A sounds like a dare. Options C and D suggest that others also are responsible for the client's recovery.
Nursing process step: Implementation
Client needs category: Psychosocial integrity
Client needs subcategory: Psychosocial adaptation
Cognitive level: Application

14. CORRECT ANSWER: D
Keeping the perineal area clean reduces the risk of an infection that ascends the urinary tract. The nurse encourages the client to void frequently to provide more space for the descending fetus. Providing the client with ice chips and testing the client's urine for glycosuria don't prevent infection.
Nursing process step: Planning
Client needs category: Physiological integrity
Client needs subcategory: Basic care and comfort
Cognitive level: Comprehension

15. CORRECT ANSWER: A

Typically, a 4-year-old child is at the preoperational level of cognitive development and has trouble understanding anything beyond her own experience. Using a doll provides a near-life experience, giving the child both an understanding of the procedure and a sense of control. The other options require abstract thinking, which is beyond the cognitive developmental level of a 4 year old.
Nursing process step: Implementation
Client needs category: Safe, effective care environment
Client needs subcategory: Coordinated care
Cognitive level: Application

16. CORRECT ANSWER: D

Because an abdominal-perineal resection commonly necessitates a colostomy and prevents defecation through the rectum, it causes a permanent change in body image to which the client must adapt. Although the client may have a catheter postoperatively and may need to restrict the diet and activity level, these changes are only temporary.
Nursing process step: Planning
Client needs category: Psychosocial integrity
Client needs subcategory: Coping and adaptation
Cognitive level: Application

17. CORRECT ANSWER: C

The nurse should administer iron dextran using the Z-track method to prevent drug leakage along the needle track and brown staining of subcutaneous tissue. Asking whether the client drinks alcoholic beverages and finding out whether the client is allergic to fish oil are unrelated to iron dextran administration. Iron dextran must be injected deep into the muscle mass, so the nurse should use a 2″ or 3″ 19G or 20G needle — not a 1″ 25G needle.
Nursing process step: Implementation
Client needs category: Physiological integrity
Client needs subcategory: Pharmacological therapies
Cognitive level: Application

18. CORRECT ANSWER: B

Low-residue and liquid diets rid the bowel of bacteria and reduce feces formation. They don't eliminate stress in the bowel, reduce bowel motility, or decrease pain.
Nursing process step: Implementation
Client needs category: Physiological integrity
Client needs subcategory: Reduction of risk potential
Cognitive level: Comprehension

19. CORRECT ANSWER: D

Ferrous sulfate may cause black or dark green stools.
Nursing process step: Data collection
Client needs category: Physiological integrity
Client needs subcategory: Pharmacological therapies
Cognitive level: Knowledge

20. CORRECT ANSWER: A

Slowing the pace of care activities will help the client feel more in touch. A depressed client can't move at a faster pace and lacks the energy to change behavior. A highly stimulating environment isn't helpful to a depressed client and may make the client even more conscious of the depression.
Nursing process step: Planning
Client needs category: Psychosocial integrity
Client needs subcategory: Coping and adaptation
Cognitive level: Analysis

21. CORRECT ANSWER: B

Iron-rich foods include raisins and other dried fruits, liver, meat, dark green vegetables, and egg yolks.
Nursing process step: Evaluation
Client needs category: Health promotion and maintenance
Client needs subcategory: Prevention and early detection of disease
Cognitive level: Comprehension

22. CORRECT ANSWER: A

Proteinuria (protein in the urine) is a cardinal sign of pregnancy-induced hypertension. It doesn't occur in ketoacidosis, placenta previa, or gestational diabetes.
Nursing process step: Data collection
Client needs category: Health promotion and maintenance
Client needs subcategory: Growth and development through the life span
Cognitive level: Analysis

23. CORRECT ANSWER: B

Parents of a child with a catastrophic illness typically feel guilty about the child's illness and wonder whether something they did (or failed to do) might have caused it. To cope with their guilt feelings, they may become angry at those around them — particularly health care providers. The nurse should let them talk and help them cope with their feelings. Telling them that their behavior isn't helping their child and limiting their visiting time with their child serve only to chastise the parents, not help them.

Telling them that everything possible is being done to restore their child's health doesn't respond to their needs.
Nursing process step: Planning
Client needs category: Psychosocial integrity
Client needs subcategory: Coping and adaptation
Cognitive level: Application

24. CORRECT ANSWER: A
A client with iron deficiency anemia may become dizzy and faint from lack of hemoglobin, which in turn reduces oxygen to the brain. Lying down improves circulation, reduces oxygen demands, and promotes safety. Instructing the client to do breathing exercises when an episode occurs and advising the client to drink highly sweetened beverages when an episode occurs wouldn't alleviate the symptoms. Teaching the client to rise slowly from a lying or sitting position to a standing position would be appropriate to alleviate dizziness from hypotension but wouldn't aid in preventing symptoms of iron deficiency anemia.
Nursing process step: Planning
Client needs category: Physiological integrity
Client needs subcategory: Reduction of risk potential
Cognitive level: Application

25. CORRECT ANSWER: C
In sigmoidoscopy, an endoscope is inserted into the rectum. Improper insertion may cause perforation of the intestinal wall. The other options aren't potential complications of sigmoidoscopy.
Nursing process step: Data collection
Client needs category: Physiological integrity
Client needs subcategory: Physiological adaptation
Cognitive level: Application

26. CORRECT ANSWER: B
Iron deficiency anemia is characterized by decreased hemoglobin in the blood, which reduces the amount of oxygen transported to body tissues. Therefore, the client may complain of shortness of breath. Other signs and symptoms of iron deficiency anemia include chills, pallor, faintness, and appetite loss.
Nursing process step: Data collection
Client needs category: Physiological integrity
Client needs subcategory: Physiological adaptation
Cognitive level: Comprehension

27. CORRECT ANSWER: A
Barium sulfate is administered rectally. To ensure that it adheres to the lower portion of the intestine, the area must be properly cleaned, using laxatives and enemas. A muscle relaxant isn't administered during the test. Barium sulfate isn't administered orally. The client is put on a liquid diet the night before the procedure and receives nothing by mouth the morning of the procedure.
Nursing process step: Evaluation
Client needs category: Safe, effective care environment
Client needs subcategory: Safety and infection control
Cognitive level: Application

28. CORRECT ANSWER: D
Alternating breasts with each breast-feeding session promotes emptying of milk from the breasts. Pulling the infant from the breast before suction is broken may cause nipple trauma. Warm compresses are more effective in relieving breast discomfort than cold compresses. Soap and water may dry the nipples.
Nursing process step: Evaluation
Client needs category: Health promotion and maintenance
Client needs subcategory: Growth and development through the life span
Cognitive level: Application

29. CORRECT ANSWER: D
Systemic desensitization is a common behavior modification technique successfully used to help treat phobias. Aversion therapy and positive reinforcement aren't behavior modification techniques used in the treatment of phobias. Imitation and modeling are social learning techniques, not behavior modification techniques.
Nursing process step: Implementation
Client needs category: Psychosocial integrity
Client needs subcategory: Psychosocial adaptation
Cognitive level: Application

30. CORRECT ANSWER: D
Respiratory problems, such as ineffective breathing pattern, always take highest priority. Ineffective coping and ineffective tissue perfusion have lower priority.
Nursing process step: Evaluation
Client needs category: Physiological integrity
Client needs subcategory: Physiological adaptation
Cognitive level: Analysis

31. CORRECT ANSWER: B
Proper countertraction occurs when the child's buttocks are raised approximately 2″ (5.1 cm) above the mattress. Options A and C describe proper traction. Option D describes correct alignment for a child in Bryant's traction.

Nursing process step: Evaluation
Client needs category: Safe, effective care environment
Client needs subcategory: Safety and infection control
Cognitive level: Analysis

32. CORRECT ANSWER: C
The nurse should teach a client with cystitis to wipe from front to back after using the toilet to avoid bacterial contamination caused by close proximity of the urethra and rectum. An acidic, not alkaline, urine helps to discourage bacterial growth.
Nursing process step: Planning
Client needs category: Physiological integrity
Client needs subcategory: Physiological adaptation
Cognitive level: Analysis

33. CORRECT ANSWER: D
One cup of cooked broccoli contains a moderate amount of total dietary fiber. Cheese, white bread, and grapefruit contain smaller amounts of fiber.
Nursing process step: Evaluation
Client needs category: Health promotion and maintenance
Client needs subcategory: Prevention and early detection of disease
Cognitive level: Application

34. CORRECT ANSWER: C
The return of peristaltic activity is signaled by movement in the bowel, which causes expulsion of bowel contents (usually gas). Belching, hunger, and thirst don't indicate movement in the entire bowel.
Nursing process step: Data collection
Client needs category: Physiological integrity
Client needs subcategory: Physiological adaptation
Cognitive level: Comprehension

35. CORRECT ANSWER: B
Irritability and poor concentration are associated with a moderate anxiety level. Mild anxiety doesn't cause irritability and poor concentration. Severe anxiety and panic cause more marked symptoms. For instance, a client with panic-level anxiety typically is out of touch with reality.
Nursing process step: Data collection
Client needs category: Psychosocial integrity
Client needs subcategory: Coping and adaptation
Cognitive level: Comprehension

36. CORRECT ANSWER: C
When a client becomes angry and resents advice from a younger health care provider to give up a lifelong habit,

the nurse should apologize and assure the client that no disrespect was intended. The other options would antagonize the client rather than reduce anger.
Nursing process step: Implementation
Client needs category: Psychosocial integrity
Client needs subcategory: Coping and adaptation
Cognitive level: Analysis

37. CORRECT ANSWER: A
In a 2-year-old child, increasing irritability suggests increased intracranial pressure (ICP). The other options describe findings opposite those expected in a child with increased ICP.
Nursing process step: Data collection
Client needs category: Physiological integrity
Client needs subcategory: Reduction of risk potential
Cognitive level: Comprehension

38. CORRECT ANSWER: A
Promethazine hydrochloride, an antihistamine, has prominent sedative effects. It doesn't inhibit oral secretions, prevent bleeding problems, or enhance wound healing.
Nursing process step: Planning
Client needs category: Safe, effective care environment
Client needs subcategory: Safety and infection control
Cognitive level: Comprehension

39. CORRECT ANSWER: C
Fear of the unknown may cause anxiety, which may manifest in such symptoms as irritability, nervousness, and upset stomach as well as pain. The client's anxiety isn't inappropriate. Anxiety causes real symptoms, not imaginary ones. No evidence suggests that the client's anxiety is an exaggerated reaction.
Nursing process step: Evaluation
Client needs category: Psychosocial integrity
Client needs subcategory: Coping and adaptation
Cognitive level: Analysis

40. CORRECT ANSWER: A
A hemolytic reaction to a blood transfusion usually results from blood group incompatibility. Signs and symptoms include back pain, reduced blood pressure, decreased urine output, tightness in the chest, dyspnea, and shock.
Nursing process step: Data collection
Client needs category: Physiological integrity
Client needs subcategory: Physiological adaptation
Cognitive level: Comprehension

41. CORRECT ANSWER: C

After awakening, the child will receive sips of water and a clear liquid diet, including ice popsicles. Milk products rarely are given immediately. The child will probably go to the postanesthesia care unit immediately after surgery and will be allowed to see his parents. The child will feel drowsy from the effects of general anesthesia.

Nursing process step: Evaluation
Client needs category: Physiological integrity
Client needs subcategory: Physiological adaptation
Cognitive level: Analysis

42. CORRECT ANSWER: A

The client should be taught to avoid caffeine and nicotine because they constrict blood vessels and would further impair the circulation. Wearing knee-length stockings would impair circulation. Clients with peripheral vascular disease should keep the extremities warm and dry. The client should exercise daily, not avoid exercise.

Nursing process step: Implementation
Client needs category: Physiological integrity
Client needs subcategory: Reduction of risk potential
Cognitive level: Analysis

43. CORRECT ANSWER: B

Because the client's axillary lymph nodes were removed, the risk of lymphedema is high. Therefore, the client must avoid any actions that carry a risk of constriction, such as using a tourniquet or a blood pressure cuff. Wearing an elastic bandage may decrease circulation and cause edema, leading to skin breakdown (option A). The client's position and movement need not be restricted (options C and D).

Nursing process step: Implementation
Client needs category: Physiological integrity
Client needs subcategory: Reduction of risk potential
Cognitive level: Application

44. CORRECT ANSWER: A

The side-lying position should be used to help prevent aspiration. The other options don't provide this advantage.

Nursing process step: Implementation
Client needs category: Physiological integrity
Client needs subcategory: Reduction of risk potential
Cognitive level: Comprehension

45. CORRECT ANSWER: A

Eating small, frequent meals places less pressure on the esophageal sphincter, reducing the likelihood of the regurgitation of stomach contents into the lower esophagus. None of the other interventions reduces heartburn.

Nursing process step: Planning
Client needs category: Physiological integrity
Client needs subcategory: Basic care and comfort
Cognitive level: Application

46. CORRECT ANSWER: A

The weight of the pregnant uterus compresses the abdominal aorta and may cause a decrease in blood pressure, so the recommended positions include walking, side-lying, and sitting for short periods. Even though spinal anesthesia is anticipated, fluids are restricted in case general anesthesia is required. Vital signs and pain medication are more important after the procedure.

Nursing process step: Implementation
Client needs category: Physiological integrity
Client needs subcategory: Basic care and comfort
Cognitive level: Analysis

47. CORRECT ANSWER: B

This response shows respect for the daughter's feelings and encourages her to express these feelings further. Giving advice is inappropriate and doesn't acknowledge the daughter's feelings (option A). Telling the daughter not to worry denies her the right to her feelings (option C). The nurse's response should focus on the daughter's feelings, not the nurse's (option D).

Nursing process step: Implementation
Client needs category: Psychosocial integrity
Client needs subcategory: Coping and adaptation
Cognitive level: Analysis

48. CORRECT ANSWER: D

Babinski's reflex is characterized by dorsiflexion of the great toe and fanning of the other toes when the sole is stimulated. This reflex usually is absent in adults and in children over age 24 months; its presence may indicate damage to pyramidal tracts. Flexion of the forearm when the biceps tendon is tapped describes the biceps reflex. Extension of the leg when the patellar tendon is struck describes the patellar reflex. Tremor of the foot following brisk, forcible dorsiflexion occurs with ankle clonus.

Nursing process step: Evaluation
Client needs category: Physiological integrity
Client needs subcategory: Physiological adaptation
Cognitive level: Comprehension

49. CORRECT ANSWER: C
Increased urine output means ascitic fluid is being absorbed into the circulation and then excreted. As this fluid is absorbed, ankle edema should decrease, not remain the same, and abdominal skin should become less shiny, not shinier. With decreasing ascites, lower fluid volume would cause the pulse rate to slow, not to increase.
Nursing process step: Data collection
Client needs category: Physiological integrity
Client needs subcategory: Physiological adaptation
Cognitive level: Comprehension

50. CORRECT ANSWER: C
Bryant's traction may be used in infants and children weighing 25 to 30 lb (11 to 13.5 kg) to reduce a fractured femur. It's also used to reduce congenital hip dislocation. Flat in bed with an elastic wrap is Buck's extension; flat in bed with a pad under the knee is Russell traction; traction with a pin or wire is skeletal traction.
Nursing process step: Data collection
Client needs category: Safe, effective care environment
Client needs subcategory: Coordinated care
Cognitive level: Knowledge

51. CORRECT ANSWER: A
During the immediate postoperative period, breathing deeply is essential to prevent hypostatic pneumonia and other complications. However, many clients are afraid to breathe deeply because this may cause incisional pain; therefore, the nurse must support the incisional area. The other options don't enhance expansion and air exchange in the lungs and therefore don't help prevent hypostatic pneumonia.
Nursing process step: Implementation
Client needs category: Physiological integrity
Client needs subcategory: Reduction of risk potential
Cognitive level: Application

52. CORRECT ANSWER: A
Thrombophlebitis refers to clot formation in a vein, caused by such conditions as venous stasis. It may result from lying in bed, which causes pooling of blood. Elastic stockings compress superficial blood vessels, promoting circulation. The other options are less effective than elastic stockings in preventing thrombophlebitis.
Nursing process step: Implementation
Client needs category: Physiological integrity
Client needs subcategory: Reduction of risk potential
Cognitive level: Application

53. CORRECT ANSWER: A
Nursing measures in the secondary prevention of violence and abuse are intended to reduce further incidence of violence and abuse once those behaviors have occurred. Nursing interventions in these situations are aimed at helping the participants, notably the victim, discuss the problem, develop alternative actions, and move to a safe haven, if needed.
Nursing process step: Data collection
Client needs category: Safe, effective care environment
Client needs subcategory: Coordinated care
Cognitive level: Analysis

54. CORRECT ANSWER: A
Because this comment reflects the mother's feelings, it encourages her to express her feelings further, thereby reducing her anxiety. The nurse should avoid giving false reassurance (option B). Option C belittles the mother's feelings by implying that they aren't unique. Although sharing feelings in a group session may be helpful, this client's mother is too upset to talk with other parents, who aren't necessarily experiencing similar emotions (option D).
Nursing process step: Implementation
Client needs category: Psychosocial integrity
Client needs subcategory: Coping and adaptation
Cognitive level: Application

55. CORRECT ANSWER: C
An intermediate-acting insulin, NPH insulin starts to act within 2 hours and peaks in 8 to 10 hours. To ensure adequate blood glucose control, the client must eat meals or snacks at scheduled times. The client shouldn't skip a meal. One ounce of fat isn't an equal exchange for 2 oz of protein. The client should use artificial sweeteners instead of simple sugars, not complex sugars.
Nursing process step: Implementation
Client needs category: Health promotion and maintenance
Client needs subcategory: Prevention and early detection of disease
Cognitive level: Application

56. CORRECT ANSWER: D
Concomitant use of aspirin and ibuprofen isn't recommended. To reduce the risk of adverse GI effects, the client can take ibuprofen with food, an antacid, or milk.
Nursing process step: Implementation
Client needs subcategory: Physiological integrity
Client needs subcategory: Pharmacological therapies
Cognitive level: Application

57. CORRECT ANSWER: B

For neonates, normal apical pulse rates range from 120 to 160 beats/minute. The axillary temperature should measure 97.7° F (36.5° C) to 98.6° F (37° C). The sclera should be white, not yellowish. Respiratory grunting may be a sign of respiratory obstruction or distress.

Nursing process step: Evaluation
Client needs category: Health promotion and maintenance
Client needs subcategory: Growth and development through the life span
Cognitive level: Analysis

58. CORRECT ANSWER: B

Following the identification of a learning need, the first step is to assess the strengths and needs of the community while identifying barriers to learning.

Nursing process step: Planning
Client needs category: Safe, effective care environment
Client needs subcategory: Coordinated care
Cognitive level: Analysis

59. CORRECT ANSWER: D

When the vessel ruptures, surgery is the only intervention that can repair it. Administration of antihypertensive medications and beta-adrenergic blockers can help control hypertension, reducing the risk of rupture. An aortogram is a diagnostic tool used to detect an aneurysm.

Nursing process step: Implementation
Client needs category: Physiological integrity
Client needs subcategory: Basic care and comfort
Cognitive level: Application

60. CORRECT ANSWER: A

Because the structure and function of the heart muscle are affected, heart failure most commonly occurs in clients with cardiomyopathy. Diabetes mellitus is unrelated to cardiomyopathy. Myocardial infarction results from atherosclerosis. Pericardial effusion is most predominant in clients with pericarditis.

Nursing process step: Evaluation
Client needs category: Physiological integrity
Client needs subcategory: Physiological adaptation
Cognitive level: Comprehension

61. CORRECT ANSWER: C

An occipital headache is typical of hypertension secondary to continued increased pressure on the cerebral vasculature. Epistaxis (nosebleed) occurs far less frequently than a headache but can also be a diagnostic sign of hypertension. Blurred vision can result from hypertension due to the arteriolar changes in the eye. Peripheral edema can also occur from an increase in sodium and water retention but is usually a latent sign.

Nursing process step: Evaluation
Client needs category: Health promotion and maintenance
Client needs subcategory: Prevention and early detection of disease
Cognitive level: Comprehension

62. CORRECT ANSWER: C

Fatigue, weight loss, and a low-grade fever are all early signs of many immune system diseases, including anemia, leukemia, and systemic lupus erythematosus (SLE). However, only rheumatic arthritis is associated with pain in the fingers, elbows, wrists, ankles, and knees.

Nursing process step: Data collection
Client needs category: Health promotion and maintenance
Client needs subcategory: Prevention and early detection of disease
Cognitive level: Application

63. CORRECT ANSWER: B

An accurate, precise examination must be properly documented as a legal document. Injuries from normal falls aren't usually linear in nature. The bleeding can cause variations, but the color change is consistent. Contusions that result from falls are typically confined to a single body area and are considered a reasonable finding in a child who is still learning to walk.

Nursing process step: Data collection
Client needs category: Health promotion and maintenance
Client needs subcategory: Prevention and early detection of disease
Cognitive level: Application

64. CORRECT ANSWER: B

Although all of these interventions are important in the care of the client, if the individual can't cope with the emotional, spiritual, and psychological aspects of his crisis, the other components of care may be ineffective as well.

Nursing process step: Implementation
Client needs category: Psychosocial integrity
Client needs subcategory: Coping and adaptation
Cognitive level: Application

65. CORRECT ANSWER: A
Some people carry dormant TB infections that may develop into active disease. In addition, primary sites of infection containing TB bacilli may remain latent for years and then activate when the client's resistance is lowered, such as when a client is being treated for cancer.
Nursing process step: Data collection
Client needs category: Physiological integrity
Client needs subcategory: Physiological adaptation
Cognitive level: Application

66. CORRECT ANSWER: B
Typical signs and symptoms are chills, fever, night sweats, and hemoptysis. Clients with tuberculosis (TB) typically have low-grade fevers, not higher than 102° F (38.9° C). Chest pain may be present from coughing but isn't common. Nausea, headache, and photophobia aren't common TB symptoms.
Nursing process step: Data collection
Client needs category: Physiological integrity
Client needs subcategory: Physiological adaptation
Cognitive level: Application

67. CORRECT ANSWER: D
The chest tube isn't removed until it's determined that the client's lung has adequately reexpanded and will stay that way. One indication of reexpansion is the cessation of fluctuation in the water seal chamber when suction isn't applied. After the lung stays expanded, the chest tube is removed. Drainage should be minimal before the chest tube is removed. An arterial blood gas test may be done to ensure proper oxygenation but isn't necessary if clinical assessment criteria are met.
Nursing process step: Implementation
Client needs category: Physiological integrity
Client needs subcategory: Physiological adaptation
Cognitive level: Application

68. CORRECT ANSWER: A
High-topped sneakers are used to prevent footdrop and contractures in neurologic clients. Low-dose heparin therapy and sequential compression boots prevent deep vein thrombosis. Although a consultation with a physical thera-

pist is important to prevent footdrop, a nurse may use high-topped sneakers independently.
Nursing process step: Implementation
Client needs category: Physiological integrity
Client needs subcategory: Reduction of risk potential
Cognitive level: Application

69. CORRECT ANSWER: A
Many elderly people already have diminished hearing, and salicylate use can lead to further or total hearing loss. Salicylates can cause fluid retention and edema, which is worrisome in older clients, especially those with heart failure. Salicylates don't increase pain in joints, decrease calcium absorption, or increase bone demineralization.
Nursing process step: Data collection
Client needs category: Physiological integrity
Client needs subcategory: Pharmacological therapies
Cognitive level: Comprehension

70. CORRECT ANSWER: D
A bedridden client needs to be turned every 2 hours, have adequate nutrition, and cough and deep-breathe. Adequate pain medication, active and passive range of motion, and hydration are also appropriate nursing measures. The client shouldn't lie as still as possible, to prevent contractures, or limit his fluid intake.
Nursing process step: Implementation
Client needs category: Safe, effective care environment
Client needs subcategory: Coordinated care
Cognitive level: Application

71. CORRECT ANSWER: A
A foul odor from a cast may be a sign of infection. The nurse needs to assess for fever, malaise and, possibly, an elevation in white blood cells. Odor from a cast is never normal and doesn't indicate neurovascular compromise. Signs of neurovascular compromise include decreased pulses, coolness, and paresthesia.
Nursing process step: Data collection
Client needs category: Health promotion and maintenance
Client needs subcategory: Prevention and early detection of disease
Cognitive level: Analysis

72. CORRECT ANSWER: D

NSAIDs are a common cause of gastritis because they inhibit prostaglandin synthesis. Milk, once thought to help reduce gastritis, has little effect on the stomach mucosa. Bicarbonate of soda, or baking soda, may be used to neutralize stomach acid but it should be used cautiously because it may lead to metabolic acidosis. Aspirin with enteric coating shouldn't contribute significantly to gastritis because the coating limits the aspirin's effect on the gastric mucosa.

Nursing process step: Data collection
Client needs category: Physiological integrity
Client needs subcategory: Reduction of risk potential
Cognitive level: Knowledge

73. CORRECT ANSWER: D

The client should be monitored closely for signs and symptoms of hemorrhage, such as bright red blood in the nasogastric tube suction, tachycardia, or a drop in blood pressure. Gastric pH may be monitored to evaluate the need for histamine-2 receptor antagonists. Bowel sounds may not return for up to 72 hours postoperatively. Nutritional needs should be addressed soon after surgery.

Nursing process step: Data collection
Client needs category: Physiological integrity
Client needs subcategory: Reduction of risk potential
Cognitive level: Comprehension

74. CORRECT ANSWER: C

Discovering and treating the cause of gastritis is the most beneficial approach. Reducing or eliminating oral intake until symptoms are gone and reducing the amount of stress are important in the recovery phase. A gastric resection is only an option when serious erosion has occurred.

Nursing process step: Data collection
Client needs category: Safe, effective care environment
Client needs subcategory: Safety and infection control
Cognitive level: Comprehension

75. CORRECT ANSWER: C

When a client who has taken an oral antidiabetic agent vomits, the nurse should monitor glucose level and assess him frequently for signs of hypoglycemia. Most of the medication has probably been absorbed. Therefore, repeating the dose would further lower glucose levels later in the day. Giving insulin also will lower glucose levels, causing hypoglycemia. The client wouldn't have hyperglycemia if the glyburide was absorbed.

Nursing process step: Data collection
Client needs category: Physiological integrity
Client needs subcategory: Pharmacological therapies
Cognitive level: Analysis

76. CORRECT ANSWER: B

Retinopathy, neuropathy, and coronary artery disease are all chronic complications of diabetes mellitus. Dizziness, dyspnea on exertion, and angina are symptoms of aortic valve stenosis. Leg ulcers, cerebral ischemic events, and pulmonary infarcts are complications of sickle cell anemia. Hyperparathyroidism causes fatigue, nausea, vomiting, muscle weakness, and cardiac arrhythmias.

Nursing process step: Evaluation
Client needs category: Physiological integrity
Client needs subcategory: Reduction of risk potential
Cognitive level: Knowledge

77. CORRECT ANSWER: B

Insulin lipodystrophy produces fatty masses at the injection sites, causing unpredictable absorption of insulin injected into these sites. Insulin edema is generalized retention of fluid, sometimes seen after normal blood glucose levels are established in a client with prolonged hyperglycemia. Insulin resistance occurs mostly in overweight clients and is due to insulin binding with antibodies, decreasing the amount of absorption. Systemic allergic reactions range from hives to anaphylaxis; rotating injection sites won't prevent these.

Nursing process step: Planning
Client needs category: Health promotion and maintenance
Client needs subcategory: Prevention and early detection of disease
Cognitive level: Comprehension

78. CORRECT ANSWER: C

Levels of thyroid-stimulating hormone and T_4 should be measured if hypothyroidism is suspected. Liver function tests are used to determine liver disease. Hemoglobin A_{1C} measurement is used to assess hyperglycemia. As part of the screening process for Cushing's syndrome, a 24-hour urinary free cortisol measurement is completed.

Nursing process step: Planning
Client needs category: Physiological integrity
Client needs subcategory: Physiological adaptation
Cognitive level: Knowledge

79. CORRECT ANSWER: D
Tiredness, cold intolerance, weight gain, and constipation are symptoms of hypothyroidism, secondary to a decrease in cellular metabolism. Polyuria, polydipsia, and weight loss are symptoms of type 1 diabetes mellitus. Hyperthyroidism has symptoms of heat intolerance, nervousness, weight loss, and hair loss. Coarsening of facial features and extremity enlargement are symptoms of acromegaly.
Nursing process step: Data collection
Client needs category: Physiological integrity
Client needs subcategory: Physiological adaptation
Cognitive level: Application

80. CORRECT ANSWER: D
A position change of the radioactive implant could deliver more radiation to healthy tissue and less to the malignant lesion. This increases the risk of injury to healthy tissue and decreases the effectiveness of treatment on the cancer. Feces in the bowel increase the likelihood of a bowel movement, which can change the position of the applicator and radiation source. Feces in the bowel don't increase the risk of ileus or inadvertent contamination of the vagina and urethra from a bowel movement. All applicators are inserted under anesthesia in the operating room.
Nursing process step: Planning
Client needs category: Physiological integrity
Client needs subcategory: Reduction of risk potential
Cognitive level: Comprehension

81. CORRECT ANSWER: B
Elastic cuffs can contribute to the development of lymphedema and should be avoided. Blood pressure measurements in the affected arm also should be avoided. Simple exercises, such as squeezing a ball, help promote circulation and should be started as soon as possible after surgery. Elevation of the affected arm promotes venous and lymphatic return from the extremity.
Nursing process step: Evaluation
Client needs category: Safe, effective care environment
Client needs subcategory: Coordinated care
Cognitive level: Analysis

82. CORRECT ANSWER: D
Signs of impending evisceration are low-grade fever and increasing serosanguineous drainage. Tachycardia; weak, thready pulse; shallow, rapid respirations; vaginal drainage; hypotension; and decreased level of consciousness after abdominal hysterectomy are all unrelated to impending evisceration, although they may be associated with other serious problems such as shock.

Nursing process step: Planning
Client needs category: Physiological integrity
Client needs subcategory: Reduction of risk potential
Cognitive level: Comprehension

83. CORRECT ANSWER: B
Oxycodone is an opioid analgesic used for alleviating severe pain, especially in terminal illness. If a client's pain has decreased to 0 to 2 on a 10-point scale (0 is no pain and 10 is the worst pain), the medication is working as desired. The drug doesn't directly affect bone density, alpha-fetoprotein level, or serum calcium level.
Nursing process step: Evaluation
Client needs category: Physiological integrity
Client needs subcategory: Pharmacological therapies
Cognitive level: Analysis

84. CORRECT ANSWER: A
Even small amounts of Accutane are associated with severe birth defects. Most female clients are also prescribed oral contraceptives. Clindamycin phosphate (Cleocin T Gel), another medicine used in the treatment of acne, can cause diarrhea and gram-negative folliculitis. Tetracycline is associated with yeast infections.
Nursing process step: Evaluation
Client needs category: Health promotion and maintenance
Client needs subcategory: Growth and development through the life span
Cognitive level: Knowledge

85. CORRECT ANSWER: C
Scabies are seen as linear burrows between the fingers and toes caused by a mite. Contusions don't have small, pruritic dots. The varicella zoster virus causes herpes zoster, characterized by papulovesicular lesions that erupt along a dermatome, usually with hyperesthesia, pain, and tenderness. The papulovesicular lesions of varicella are distributed over the trunk, face, and scalp and don't follow a dermatome.
Nursing process step: Data collection
Client needs category: Physiological integrity
Client needs subcategory: Physiological adaptation
Cognitive level: Knowledge

Glossary

ABDOMINAL AORTIC ANEURYSM An aneurysm that affects part of the abdominal aorta.

ABRUPTIO PLACENTAE The premature separation of a normally positioned placenta in a pregnancy of at least 20 weeks' gestation, either before or during labor but before delivery. It can result in hemorrhage and death of the mother, the fetus, or both.

ABUSE A wrong or improper action taken toward another that mistreats and injures.

ACNE VULGARIS A form of acne common during puberty and adolescence, characterized by comedones, cysts, papules, and pustules on the face, back, and chest.

ACQUIRED IMMUNODEFICIENCY SYNDROME (AIDS) A disorder of the immune system caused by infection with human immunodeficiency virus and characterized by inability to mount a successful defense against infection, such as by organisms that usually aren't pathogenic (opportunistic infections).

ACROCYANOSIS The bluish discoloration of a neonate's extremities.

ACROMEGALY A metabolic disorder occurring in a middle-aged person that results from excess secretion of somatotropin and is characterized by progressive enlargement of the head, hands, and feet.

ACTIVITY THEORY The social theory that a client is satisfied with becoming older and living a middle-age lifestyle.

ACUTE HEAD INJURY A head injury caused by an incident that leads to brain injury or bleeding within the brain.

ACUTE LYMPHOCYTIC LEUKEMIA (ALL) A common type of leukemia in children that's marked by extreme proliferation of immature lymphocytes (blast cells).

ACUTE POSTSTREPTOCOCCAL GLOMERULONEPHRITIS An inflammatory kidney disease involving the glomeruli and characterized by the sudden onset of facial edema, hematuria, proteinuria, and decreased urine output. It occurs as a late complication of pharyngitis caused by streptococcal infection (beta-hemolytic streptococci).

ACUTE RENAL FAILURE The inability of a kidney to excrete metabolites at normal plasma levels under conditions of normal loading or the inability to retain electrolytes under conditions of normal intake; marked by uremia and usually by oliguria or anuria, with hyperkalemia and pulmonary edema.

ACUTE RESPIRATORY FAILURE Failure of the cardiac and pulmonary systems to adequately exchange oxygen and carbon dioxide in the lungs.

ADDISON'S DISEASE Also known as adrenal hypofunction, failure of the adrenal gland to secrete sufficient mineralocorticoids, glucocorticoids, and androgens.

ADDISONIAN CRISIS Also known as adrenal crisis, critical deficiency of mineralocorticoids and glucocorticoids generally occurring in clients who have chronic adrenal insufficiency and follows acute stress, sepsis, trauma, surgery, or omission of steroid therapy. Medical emergency that necessitates immediate, vigorous treatment.

ADRENERGIC FIBERS The nerve fibers in the sympathetic nervous system that release norepinephrine.

ADULT RESPIRATORY DISTRESS SYNDROME (ARDS) A fulminant pulmonary interstitial and alveolar edema, hemorrhage, and acute hypoxemia, which usually develops a few days after the initiating trauma.

ADVANCE DIRECTIVE Document used as a guideline to determine life-sustaining medical care for clients with advanced disease or disability who are no longer able to indicate their wishes.

AFFECT A feeling, an emotion, or a mood.

AFFECTIVE INAPPROPRIATENESS An inappropriate emotional response to a situation; for example, laughing when sad or crying when happy.

AGRANULOCYTOSIS An abnormal condition of the blood characterized by a severe reduction in the number of granulocytes, resulting in fever, sore throat, and bleeding ulcers of the rectum, mouth, and vagina. It may arise as an adverse reaction to neuroleptic drugs or other medications.

ALOPECIA The absence or loss of hair.

AMBIVALENCE The simultaneous existence of two opposing feelings, needs, or wishes.

AMENORRHEA The absence or cessation of menstruation.

AMYOTROPHIC LATERAL SCLEROSIS (ALS) An incurable disease affecting the spinal cord and the medulla and cortex of the brain, characterized by progressive degeneration of motor neurons, and leading to weakness and wasting of muscles, increased reflexes, and severe muscle spasms.

ANAPHYLAXIS A type of distributive shock that's dramatic and widespread, resulting in a systemic reaction to a previously encountered antigen.

ANEMIA A reduction either in the volume of red blood cells or in hemoglobin concentration that diminishes the blood's capacity to carry oxygen, therefore reducing the amount of oxygen available to tissue.

ANESTHESIA The loss of the ability to feel pain sensation caused by the administration of a drug, which may be general, regional, or local.

ANGINA Severe, spasmodic, crushing, or constricting pain accompanied by a choking feeling.

ANHEDONIA The inability to experience pleasure from acts that normally give it.

ANKYLOSING SPONDYLITIS Spinal arthritis that resembles rheumatoid arthritis, sometimes progressing to fusion of the involved vertebrae.

ANKYLOSIS The fixation or immobility of a joint, usually from cartilage destruction.

ANTICIPATORY GUIDANCE The initiation of interventions before an event occurs to prevent potential problems.

ANTICIPATORY PLANNING The act of preparing for potential situations and outcomes.

ANXIETY An emotional state characterized by fear and dread without a clearly identifiable source.

APPENDICITIS A disorder that causes inflammation of the vermiform appendix.

AORTIC INSUFFICIENCY A defective functioning of the aortic valve with incomplete closure resulting in aortic regurgitation.

AORTIC STENOSIS A narrowing or fusion of the aortic valve that interferes with left ventricular outflow.

APGAR SCORE The physical assessment of heart rate, respiratory effort, muscle tone, reflexes, and color of a neonate at 1 and 5 minutes to test his adjustment to extrauterine life. A score of 0 to 3 reveals severe distress, a score of 4 to 7 reveals moderate distress, and a score of 7 to 10 reveals no distress.

AQUEOUS HUMOR Clear, watery liquid produced by the ciliary processes that fills and circulates in the posterior and anterior chambers of the eye, eventually being reabsorbed into the venous system.

ARRHYTHMIAS A variation from the normal rhythm of the heartbeat encompassing abnormal regular and irregular rhythms as well as loss of rhythm.

ARTERIAL OCCLUSIVE DISEASE An obstruction or narrowing of the lumen of the aorta and its major branches, which interrupts blood flow, usually to the legs and feet. The disease may affect the carotid, vertebral, innominate, subclavian, mesenteric, and celiac arteries.

ASPHYXIA A condition characterized by impairment or cessation of oxygen and carbon dioxide exchange in the body, resulting in a critically insufficient blood oxygen level and a significantly increased carbon dioxide level.

ASSAULT The threat of imminent harmful or offensive bodily contact.

ASSOCIATIVE LOOSENESS The illogical connection of thoughts, so that verbalization is nonsensical or confusing to the listener.

ASTHMA A respiratory disorder characterized by recurrent attacks of paroxysmal dyspnea, bronchospasm, wheezing on expiration, and coughing; triggers may include pollutants, vigorous exercise, emotional stress, and infection.

ATAXIA Poorly coordinated muscle movement.

ATELECTASIS The collapse of lung tissue or incomplete expansion of a lung, caused by the absence of air in a portion of the lung or in the entire lung.

ATONY A lack of normal muscle tone or strength.

ATOPIC DERMATITIS A skin inflammation occurring in individuals with a genetic predisposition to allergies, characterized by intense itching, maculopapular lesions, and excoriation.

ATRESIA The complete closure of a tube or body opening.

ATRIAL SEPTAL DEFECT A defect stemming from a patent foramen ovale or the failure of a septum to develop completely between the atria.

ATTENTION DEFICIT HYPERACTIVITY DISORDER (ADHD) Previously called attention deficit disorder, this disorder includes hyperactivity, impulsiveness, and inattention, which can result in intrusive and disruptive behavior.

ATTITUDINAL ISOLATION A type of isolation that results from societal rejection.

AUSCULTATION The method of listening for sounds from within the body by applying the ear directly to a bare surface or by using an instrument such as a stethoscope.

AUTISTIC WITHDRAWAL Retreat from the external environment through hallucinations, delusions, verbal abuse, refusal to speak, catatonia, or excitation.

AUTOLOGOUS BLOOD TRANSFUSION The process of reinfusing the client with his own blood.

BATTERY Bodily contact with another person without the person's permission or consent.

B CELLS Also known as lymphocytes, any of the mononuclear, nonphagocytic leukocytes found in the blood, lymph, and lymphoid tissues, that are responsible for the body's humoral immunity.

BEHAVIORAL ISOLATION Isolation that results from social withdrawal because of unacceptable social behavior, such as confusion, incontinence, or erratic behavior.

BELL'S PALSY Unilateral facial paralysis of sudden onset, resulting from trauma to the facial nerve, from compression of the nerve by a tumor, or from an unknown cause.

BENIGN PROSTATIC HYPERPLASIA (BPH) An age-related disorder characterized by the enlargement of the prostate resulting from proliferation of glandular and stromal elements; it may cause urethral compression and obstruction.

BINGE-PURGE CYCLE Uncontrolled ingestion of large amounts of food followed by vomiting.

BIPOLAR DISORDER Also known as manic-depression, a severe disturbance in affect, manifested by episodes of extreme sadness alternating with episodes of euphoria.

BLOOD TYPE The specific ABO blood group; consists of four major blood types: O, A, B, and AB. This classification depends on the presence or absence of two major antigens, A and B. Type O occurs when neither is present, and type AB occurs when both are present.

BORDERLINE PERSONALITY DISORDER A condition that results in a pattern of instability in a person's mood, interpersonal relationships, self-esteem, self-identity, behavior, and cognition. Impulsiveness is its most prominent characteristic.

BRACHYTHERAPY Radiation therapy whereby sealed radionuclide sources are placed within or near malignant tumors.

BRAIN TUMOR A neoplasm of the brain characterized by uncontrolled and progressive cell multiplication. Brain tumors are usually invasive but don't cross the cerebrospinal axis.

BREACH OF CONFIDENTIALITY Neglect or failure to keep privileged information private.

BREACH OF DUTY A failure to provide the expected reasonable standard of care under the circumstances.

BRONCHIECTASIS A chronic condition of the bronchial tree marked by irreversible dilation and destruction of the bronchial walls, resulting in a paroxysmal, mucus-producing cough.

BRONCHIOLITIS An infection of the lower respiratory tract that produces inflammation and obstruction of the lungs by thick mucus and edema.

CARDIAC TAMPONADE Compression of the heart resulting from increased intrapericardial pressure secondary to accumulating fluid or blood in the pericardial sac (resulting from cardiac rupture or a penetrating wound).

CARDIOGENIC SHOCK A condition that occurs when the heart fails to pump adequately, thereby reducing cardiac output and compromising tissue perfusion, as in acute myocardial infarction, heart failure, or severe cardiomyopathy.

CARDIOMYOPATHY Primarily a noninflammatory disease of the myocardium.

CARPAL TUNNEL SYNDROME A painful disorder of the wrist and hand resulting from rapid, repetitive use of the fingers or from steady wrist-shaking vibrations, resulting in compression of the median nerve inside the carpal tunnel.

CATATONIC SCHIZOPHRENIA A state of pronounced psychomotor disturbance in which the individual remains immobile with extreme muscle rigidity or, less commonly, exhibits uncontrolled excessive movement.

CELLULITIS A diffuse, commonly infectious inflammation of the skin and underlying tissue, characterized by pain, redness, edema, and heat.

CEPHALOCAUDAL Pertaining to the long axis of the body, in a direction from head to tail, as in the development of an organism. (For example, an infant gains control of his head before his trunk and extremities.)

CEPHALOPELVIC DISPROPORTION (CPD) The incompatibility of the fetal head with the diameter of the maternal pelvis.

CEREBRAL ANEURYSM A saclike dilation of the wall of a cerebral artery, typically resulting from weakness of the wall.

CEREBRAL PALSY A permanent disorder of motor function resulting from nonprogressive brain damage.

CERTIFIED NURSE-MIDWIFE An advanced practice nurse who provides care to low-risk perinatal and gynecologic clients.

CHEILOPLASTY Plastic surgery performed to correct a deformity of the lips.

CHEMICAL CARCINOGENESIS The development of cancer caused by chemical substances, such as hydrocarbons and asbestos.

CHLAMYDIA A genus of bacteria of the Chlamydiaceae family, occurring as gram-negative organisms, which are common animal pathogens and cause various diseases in humans.

CHLOASMA Irregular facial pigmentation — usually on the cheeks, forehead, and nose — that occurs during pregnancy.

CHOLECYSTITIS Inflammation of the gallbladder that may be either acute (usually caused by gallstone) or chronic.

CHOLELITHIASIS Presence or formation of gallstones in the gallbladder.

CHRONIC BRONCHITIS A persistent respiratory disease marked by increased production of mucus by the glands of the trachea and bronchi. It's characterized by a cough with expectoration for at least 3 months of the year for more than 2 consecutive years.

CHRONIC GLOMERULONEPHRITIS An inflammation of the glomerulus of the kidney characterized by decreased urine production, blood and protein in the urine, and edema. It may follow acute glomerulonephritis or occur secondary to a systemic disease and may lead to renal failure.

CHRONIC OBSTRUCTIVE PULMONARY DISEASE (COPD) A disorder that's marked by reduced inspiratory and expiratory capacity of the lungs. COPD is progressive and irreversible and causes such symptoms as dyspnea on exertion, difficulty inhaling or exhaling deeply and, sometimes, a chronic cough.

CHRONIC RENAL FAILURE The inability of a kidney to perform its essential functions of excreting wastes, concentrating urine, and conserving electrolytes.

CHRONIC VENOUS INSUFFICIENCY A condition resulting from inadequate circulation, resulting in decreased blood flow.

CHYLOTHORAX The presence of effused chyle in the pleural space, most commonly resulting from traumatic injury to the neck or a tumor that invades the thoracic duct.

CIRRHOSIS A liver disease characterized by diffuse interlacing bands of fibrous tissue dividing the hepatic parenchyma into micronodular or macronodular areas.

CLEFT LIP A facial malformation that results from failure of the premaxillary process to merge during gestational weeks 7 and 8. The malformation may be unilateral or bilateral and range from a notch in the vermilion border of the lip to a separation extending to the floor of the nose.

CLEFT PALATE A congenital fissure of the roof of the mouth that results from failure of the palatal process to fuse from the 7th to the 12th week of gestation.

CLUB FOOT A congenital deformity in which the foot is twisted out of shape or position.

COARCTATION OF THE AORTA A narrowing of the aortic arch that's usually distal to the ductus arteriosus beyond the left subclavian artery.

COGNITIVE DEVELOPMENT The acquisition of increasingly complex knowledge, thought processes, reasoning, judgment, memory, and problem-solving skills.

COGNITIVE DISORDERS The result of any condition that alters or destroys brain tissue and, in turn, impairs cerebral functioning.

COLOSTRUM The first breast milk, which is high in antibodies that provide passive immunization to the neonate. Production begins early in pregnancy and continues for 1 to 2 days after delivery of the neonate.

COMPARTMENT SYNDROME Compromised circulation — in many cases to an extremity — due to swelling and inflammation as a result of trauma or burns.

COMPENSATORY DAMAGES Reimbursement awarded to the plaintiff for expenses, rehabilitation, and pain and suffering related to the injury.

COMPULSION A repetitive behavior that's performed to decrease escalating anxiety.

CONFABULATION The fabrication of "stories" to fill in memory gaps or to answer questions. The individual considers the "stories" to be factual.

CONGENITAL Existing at birth.

CONJUNCTIVITIS Inflammation and redness of the conjunctiva of the eye as a result of infection, allergy, or a chemical reaction.

CONSCIOUS SEDATION The state when medication is administered I.V. to reduce the intensity or awareness of pain while maintaining defensive reflexes.

CONTINUITY THEORY The social theory whereby the client adjusts successfully to the aging process by continuing the patterns of living that he has established over his lifetime.

CONTRACT A written or oral agreement between two or more individuals that has several elements to its formation, interpretation, and enforcement.

CONVERSION DISORDER A condition that's characterized by symptoms that suggest a physical disorder but for which evaluation and observation can't determine a physiologic cause.

CORNEAL ABRASION The wearing away of the outer layers of the cornea.

CORONARY ARTERY DISEASE (CAD) A disease characterized by atherosclerosis of the coronary arteries, which may cause angina pectoris, myocardial infarction, and sudden death. Genetically determined and avoidable risk factors contribute to CAD, including hypercholesterolemia, hypertension, smoking, diabetes mellitus, and low levels of high-density lipoproteins.

COR PULMONALE A heart condition in which hypertension of the pulmonary circulation leads to enlargement of the right ventricle.

CROHN'S DISEASE A chronic granulomatous inflammatory disease of unknown etiology involving any part of the GI tract from the mouth to the anus but commonly involving the terminal ileum with scarring and thickening of the bowel wall.

CROUP A condition resulting from inflammation of the larynx that commonly occurs in young children and is characterized by a barking, resonant cough.

CUSHING'S SYNDROME Also known as hypercortisolism, hyperactivity of the adrenal cortex that results in excessive secretion of glucocorticoids, particularly cortisol, and may also result in an increase in mineralocorticoids and sex hormones.

CYSTIC FIBROSIS (CF) A disease that affects the pancreas and causes a generalized dysfunction of the exocrine glands. Thickened and tenacious secretions occlude glandular ducts, causing dysfunction in many organ systems.

CYSTITIS An inflammation of the urinary bladder.

DAMAGES *1.* Refers to physical or psychological injury. *2.* Refers to monetary compensation awarded to the plaintiff for incurring the injury.

DEFAMATION The act of injuring the plaintiff's reputation in the community as the result of a false statement, either spoken (slander) or written (libel).

DEHISCENCE The partial or complete separation of wound edges.

DELUSION A false belief to which an individual adheres despite contradictory evidence.

DELUSIONAL DISORDER A condition in which the client holds firmly to false beliefs, despite contradictory information.

DENIAL The unconscious ego defense mechanism whereby an individual refrains from acknowledging stressful aspects about himself or his environment to ease anxiety.

DEPENDENT PERSONALITY DISORDER A disorder in which the client experiences an extreme need to be taken care of, which leads to submissive, clinging behavior and fear of separation.

DEVELOPMENT The increasingly complex functioning that progresses sequentially (for instance, the attainment of cognitive, psychosocial, motor, and communication skills).

DEVELOPMENTAL DYSPLASIA OF THE HIP The abnormal development of the hip socket that occurs when the head of the femur is cartilaginous and the acetabulum (socket) is shallow; as a result, the head of the femur comes out of the hip socket.

DIABETES INSIPIDUS A metabolic disorder marked by extreme polyuria and polydipsia, resulting from deficient secretion or production of antidiuretic hormone (ADH) or the inability of the renal tubules to respond to ADH.

DIABETES MELLITUS A disorder of carbohydrate metabolism characterized by insufficient insulin to allow glucose to cross the cell membrane.

DISORGANIZED SCHIZOPHRENIA A type of schizophrenia in which the client has a flat or inappropriate affect and incoherent thoughts.

DISPLACEMENT Transferring one's emotions about a person, object, or situation to another less-threatening person, object, or situation.

DISSEMINATED INTRAVASCULAR COAGULATION (DIC) Also called consumption coagulopathy and defibrination syndrome, a complication of diseases and conditions that accelerate clotting, causing small blood vessel occlusion, organ necrosis, depletion of circulating clotting factors and platelets, and activation of the fibrinolytic system, which in turn can lead to severe hemorrhage.

DIVERTICULITIS A disease that causes inflammation of a diverticulum, especially inflammation related to colonic diverticula, which may cause perforation with abscess formation.

DIVERTICULOSIS The presence of diverticula, particularly of colonic diverticula, in the absence of inflammation.

DOWN SYNDROME A chromosomal disorder marked by varying degrees of mental retardation and physical characteristics that include a sloping forehead, low-set ears, and short, broad hands with a single palmar crease.

DRUG DEPENDENCE A physical or psychological need to use a drug to experience its effects or to avoid the discomfort of its absence.

DUAL DIAGNOSIS A diagnosis that reveals an addictive disorder and a psychiatric disorder in a client.

DUCHENNE'S MUSCULAR DYSTROPHY A degenerative disease characterized by weakness and progressive atrophy of skeletal muscles with no evidence of involvement of the nervous system.

DURABLE POWER OF ATTORNEY A legal document in which the client identifies a proxy, or surrogate, decision maker in case the client becomes incapacitated; this document should also be included in the client's medical record.

DUTY Refers to the nurse's legal obligation to provide nursing care to a client.

DYSTOCIA Abnormally difficult labor.

ECLAMPSIA The most serious form of toxemia of pregnancy, marked by hypertension, proteinuria, edema, generalized tonic-clonic seizures, and coma.

ECTOPIC PREGNANCY Implantation of a fertilized ovum outside the uterine cavity.

EFFACEMENT The thinning and shortening (obliteration) of the cervix during labor, which is reported in percentages from 0% to 100%.

ELECTRONIC FETAL MONITORING (EFM) The use of a direct or an indirect device to assess fetal status and uterine activity.

EMPHYSEMA A chronic, irreversible lung disorder marked by the enlargement of air spaces distal to terminal bronchioles due to destruction of the alveolar walls; it results in decreased elastic recoil of the lungs.

EMPYEMA The accumulation of pus in a cavity of the body.

ENABLING Helping a chemically dependent client so that the consequences of drug use can be avoided.

ENCEPHALITIS An inflammatory condition of the brain, usually caused by an arbovirus infection transmitted by the bite of an infected mosquito.

ENDOGENOUS Growing from within the body.

EGO The part of the personality that keeps an individual oriented to reality, enables the individual to solve problems, and mediates between the id and the superego.

EPISTAXIS A nosebleed.

ERYTHROCYTES Also called red blood cells, erythrocytes are one of the elements found in peripheral blood.

EVISCERATION The protrusion of abdominal contents through a surgical incision.

EXPECTED DATE OF DELIVERY (EDD) The due date established by calculations, ultrasound, or amniocentesis.

EXTRACORPOREAL Occurring outside of the body.

FAILURE TO THRIVE A condition in which an infant or a young child not only fails to gain weight but may also lose it as a result of physical and psychosocial causation.

FALSE IMPRISONMENT Unlawful restraint of a person against his will.

FAMILIAL CARCINOGENESIS The development of cancer as a result of autosomal dominant traits, such as breast cancer, retinoblastoma, familial polyposis, xeroderma pigmentosum, and Wilms' tumor.

FELONY A type of crime that entails more serious offenses and warrants lengthy prison sentences.

FETAL STATION The relationship of the fetal presenting part to the maternal ischial spines, which is measured in centimeters.

FISTULA An abnormal opening between two organs.

FLIGHT OF IDEAS A nearly continuous flow of rapid speech that jumps from topic to topic.

FREE-FLOATING ANXIETY Anxiety that occurs without cause and produces acute psychic discomfort.

GASTRITIS An inflammation of the stomach and stomach lining.

GASTROENTERITIS An inflammation of the stomach lining and intestines that accompanies numerous GI disorders and is characterized by anorexia, weakness, abdominal pain, nausea, and diarrhea.

GASTROESOPHAGEAL REFLUX DISEASE (GERD) A backflow of stomach and duodenum contents into the esophagus that may result from an incompetent lower esophageal sphincter.

GENERALIZED ANXIETY DISORDER A disorder in which the client worries excessively and experiences tremendous anxiety almost daily.

GESTATIONAL DIABETES MELLITUS Elevated blood sugar levels in an individual as a result of the stress of pregnancy.

GIGANTISM Abnormal stature or overgrowth of the body or any of its parts, caused most frequently by oversecretion of pituitary growth hormone.

GLAUCOMA Visual field loss due to damage to the optic nerve resulting from increased IOP. If untreated, can lead to blindness.

GOITER An enlarged thyroid gland, usually evident as a pronounced swelling in the front of the neck.

GONORRHEA A sexually transmitted disease that commonly infects the genitourinary tract and, occasionally, the pharynx, conjunctiva, or rectum; caused by *Neisseria gonorrhoeae*.

GOUT A group of disorders associated with inborn errors of metabolism that affect purine and pyrimidine use. It causes increased uric acid production or interferes with its excretion and results in hyperuricemia, recurrent acute inflammatory arthritis, deposition of urate crystals in the joints of the extremities, and uric acid urolithiasis.

GRAVIDA   A pregnant woman. Also, the number of pregnancies, including the current one.

GROWTH   A quantitative increase in size resulting from an increase in the number or size of cells, or both.

GUILLAIN-BARRÉ SYNDROME   An acute febrile polyneuritis that occurs after a viral infection and is marked by rapidly ascending paralysis that begins as paresthesia of the feet.

HALLUCINATION   A sensory experience in which no external stimuli exist.

HEAD LICE   *Pediculosis capitis* infestation resulting in lice feeding on human blood and laying their eggs (nits) in body hair on the head. It's commonly due to overcrowded conditions, is common in children, and spreads by the sharing of hats, combs, hairbrushes, or clothing.

HEART FAILURE   The inability of the heart to pump blood at an adequate rate to fill tissue metabolic requirements or the ability to do so only at an elevated filling pressure.

HEMIPARESIS   Muscle weakness in half of the body.

HEMOLYSIS   The destruction of red blood cells and the release of hemoglobin into the fluid medium surrounding them, which may occur after injection of hypotonic saline solutions or after exposure to bacterial toxins, the venom of certain snakes, or certain immune bodies.

HEMOPHILIA   A bleeding disorder characterized by failure of the blood clotting mechanism. It's an inherited condition that occurs almost exclusively in males.

HEMOTHORAX   An accumulation of blood in the pleural cavity, resulting from a traumatic injury or from the rupture of small blood vessels in individuals with inflammatory or malignant lung diseases.

HEPATITIS   A disease that causes inflammation of the liver, usually due to a viral infection but also resulting from exposure to toxic agents.

HERPES SIMPLEX VIRUS (HSV)   An infection caused by herpes virus Type 1 or 2 and characterized by painful, itching lesions consisting of tiny blisters, which commonly appear around the mouth or on the skin and mucous membranes of the genitals.

HERPES ZOSTER   An acute infection characterized by pain resulting from inflammation of the ganglia and dorsal nerve roots as well as the eruption of painful lesions that occur on one side of the body, following the course of a nerve.

HIATAL HERNIA   The herniation of an abdominal organ, usually the stomach, through the esophageal hiatus of the diaphragm.

HIRSCHSPRUNG'S DISEASE   A disease in which a portion of the colon lacks ganglionic cells and the peristaltic waves that are needed to pass feces through that segment of the colon.

HODGKIN'S DISEASE   A type of cancer of the lymphatic system in which Reed-Sternberg cells proliferate in a single lymph node and travel contiguously through the lymphatic system to other lymphatic nodes and organs.

HUMAN IMMUNODEFICIENCY VIRUS (HIV)   A virus of the genus *Lentivirus* separated into two serotypes (HIV-1 and HIV-2) that is the etiologic agent of acquired immunodeficiency syndrome.

HYDATIDIFORM MOLE   A commonly benign neoplasm that occurs at the end of a degenerating pregnancy and arises from enlarged chorionic villi and the proliferation of trophoblastic tissue.

HYDROCEPHALUS   An increase in the amount of cerebrospinal fluid in the ventricles and subarachnoid spaces of the brain.

HYPERCAPNIA   Elevated partial pressure of carbon dioxide in the blood.

HYPEREMESIS GRAVIDARUM   Severe and prolonged vomiting during pregnancy to such a degree that weight loss and fluid and electrolyte imbalance occur.

HYPERPYREXIA   Also known as malignant hyperthermia, a body temperature elevation that may be produced as a reaction to an infection or as a complication of surgery.

HYPERTENSION   A persistent, abnormal elevation in blood pressure, usually defined as systolic pressure exceeding 140 mm Hg or diastolic pressure exceeding 90 mm Hg.

HYPERTHYROIDISM   Increased synthesis of thyroid hormone that can result from overactivity (Graves' disease) or a change in the thyroid gland (toxic nodular goiter).

HYPERVOLEMIA   An abnormal fluid volume increase, usually in the circulatory (blood) system.

HYPOCHONDRIASIS   A mental disorder characterized by a preoccupation with the state of one's physical health.

HYPOTHYROIDISM   A state of low serum thyroid hormone resulting from hypothalamic, pituitary, or thyroid insufficiency that can progress to myxedema coma.

HYPOVOLEMIA   An abnormal fluid volume decrease, usually in the circulatory (blood) system.

HYPOVOLEMIC SHOCK A shock state that results from decreased intravascular volume due to fluid loss, causing circulatory dysfunction and inadequate tissue perfusion.

HYPOXEMIA A deficient blood oxygen level, usually resulting from a ventilation-perfusion imbalance.

HYPOXIA A decreased level of oxygen in inspired air, the arterial blood, or the tissues, although not as severe as anoxia.

ID The part of the personality that houses an individual's needs, drives, and wishes and that has no regard for reality.

IDEAS OF REFERENCE The assumption by a client that the words and actions of another person refer directly to him.

IDENTIFICATION An unconscious ego defense mechanism whereby an individual takes on characteristics of one or more people.

IMMOBILITY The state of being fixed in one position or being rendered incapable of movement. Casts, splints, or surgical fixation are examples of induced immobility.

IMMUNITY A state of protection against a disease, especially one of infectious origin.

IMMUNOGLOBULIN (Ig) One of the five classes (IgA, IgD, IgE, IgG, and IgM) of structurally related glycoproteins that function as antibodies.

INCENTIVE SPIROMETRY The promotion of deep breathing and full expansion of the alveoli by means of a mechanical device that measures the amount of air the client inhales and exhales.

INFECTIVE ENDOCARDITIS Endocarditis caused by infection with microorganisms, especially bacteria and fungi.

INFORMED CONSENT The client's involvement in and agreement with treatment decisions based on careful consideration of all information pertinent to the client's condition.

INSPECTION Observing a client during an examination.

INTENTIONAL TORT A willful act that injures another person or his property.

INTERFERON A class of glycoproteins that are produced after cells are exposed to a virus. Interferon therapy is a potentially valuable treatment for various viral infections because interferons prevent viral replication in noninfected cells.

INTERMITTENT CLAUDICATION Periodic pain and lameness in a limb brought on by activity and relieved by rest; commonly found in arterial peripheral vascular disease.

INTESTINAL OBSTRUCTION A blockage, clogging, or stricture of the lumen in any area of the bowel that prevents the normal passage of intestinal contents.

INTRACRANIAL PRESSURE (ICP) The pressure of the cerebral spinal fluid in the subarachnoid space between the skill and the brain.

INTROJECTION The unconscious ego defense mechanism by which a client incorporates positive or negative aspects of another person or object into his own ego. (This is the mechanism by which anger is turned inward.)

INVASION OF PRIVACY Also known as a breach of confidentiality, the act of revealing personal information about a client to an unauthorized person.

IRON DEFICIENCY ANEMIA Anemia resulting from an iron insufficiency in the serum, decreased iron stores in the bone marrow, and elevated serum iron binding.

IRRITABLE BOWEL SYNDROME A condition characterized by diarrhea and resulting from increased bowel motility.

ISCHEMIA Decreased blood supply to a body part caused by an obstruction or a constriction in a blood vessel.

ISOLATION The unconscious ego defense mechanism that enables an individual to remain unaware of the emotions associated with a thought.

KAPOSI'S SARCOMA A malignant tumor that begins as a soft, brownish or purple nodule, usually on the feet and spreading slowly in the skin, metastasizing to lymph nodes and internal organs.

KERNICTERUS The abnormal toxic accumulation of bilirubin in the brain tissues resulting from hyperbilirubinemia, which may cause brain damage and neonatal death.

LACRIMATION The secretion and discharge of tears.

LANUGO The fine downy hair that appears on the fetal body at about 20 weeks' gestation.

LECITHIN-SPHINGOMYELIN RATIO (L/S RATIO) The ratio of lecithin to sphingomyelin in amniotic fluid; it's useful in predicting fetal lung maturity.

LEGIONNAIRES' DISEASE An acute flulike disease caused by *Legionella pneumophila*. Signs and symptoms include high fever, GI distress, headache, and pneumonia and may involve the liver, kidney, and nervous system.

LEUKEMIA A progressive malignant disease of the blood-forming organs characterized by abnormal numbers or forms of immature circulating white blood cells, with infiltration of the lymph nodes, liver, spleen, and other sites.

LEUKOCYTES Also called white blood cells, leukocytes are a colorless ameboid cell mass.

LEUKOPENIA Abnormally low white blood cell count (below 5,000 µl).

LIABILITY The legal responsibility for failure to act or an action that fails to meet standards of care and causes another person harm.

LIVING WILL A document in which the client instructs family members and health care professionals about medical care that should or shouldn't be provided if he becomes incapacitated.

LOCHIA The postpartum vaginal discharge containing debris from the uterus, such as blood, decidual tissue, mucus, and epithelial cells.

LOOSE EGO BOUNDARY The failure to adequately distinguish between one's thoughts, wishes, and needs and those of others.

LYMPHOMA A type of cancer that occurs in the lymphatic tissue and can be classified as either Hodgkin's disease or malignant lymphoma (also called non-Hodgkin's lymphoma).

MALPRACTICE Negligence by a member of a profession, differing from negligence only in that the standard or duty owed is a professional one, based on special knowledge and skills.

MALIGNANT LYMPHOMA A type of cancer in which tumors occur throughout lymph nodes and lymphatic organs in unpredictable patterns. Malignant lymphoma may be categorized as lymphocytic, histiocytic, or mixed cell type.

MANIPULATION Behaviors directed at getting one's needs met at the expense of another person.

MÉNIÈRE'S DISEASE A chronic inner ear disease characterized by recurrent episodes of vertigo, progressive unilateral nerve deafness, and tinnitus.

MENINGITIS An inflammation of the brain and spinal cord, usually as the result of a bacterial infection.

MENINGOCELE The protrusion of the meninges outside the body through a defect in the vertebral column. The protruding sac is filled with spinal fluid.

METABOLIC ACIDOSIS A state of excess acid accumulation and deficient base bicarbonate.

METABOLIC ALKALOSIS A clinical state marked by decreased amounts of acid or increased amounts of base bicarbonate.

MISDEMEANOR An offense that's considered less serious than a felony and carries with it a lesser penalty, usually a fine or imprisonment for less than 1 year.

MITRAL INSUFFICIENCY A defective functioning of the mitral valve with incomplete closure causing mitral regurgitation.

MITRAL STENOSIS A narrowing of the left atrioventricular orifice.

MITRAL VALVE PROLAPSE (MVP) A prolapse of the mitral valve, often with regurgitation, associated with myxomatous proliferation of the leaflets of the mitral valve.

MULTIPLE SCLEROSIS (MS) A disease in which there are foci of demyelination of various sizes throughout the white matter of the central nervous system, sometimes extending into the gray matter. Typically, the symptoms include weakness, incoordination, paresthesia, speech disturbances, and visual complaints.

MYASTHENIA GRAVIS (MG) A disorder of the neuromuscular function caused by the presence of antibodies to acetylcholine receptors at the neuromuscular junction. Characterized by fatigue and exhaustion of the muscular system, the disorder has a tendency to fluctuate in severity and can affect any muscle of the body.

MYDRIATIC A drug that dilates the pupil.

MYELOMENINGOCELE A meningocele that contains a portion of the spinal cord and spinal nerves in the sac.

MYOCARDIAL INFARCTION (MI) A condition in which gross necrosis of the myocardium occurs as a result of interruption of the blood supply to the area usually caused by atherosclerosis or an embolism of the coronary arteries.

MYOCARDITIS Inflammation of the myocardium, which may arise from a number of conditions, including viral, bacterial, or fungal infection; serum sickness; rheumatic fever; a chemical agent; or a complication of a collagen disease.

NEGLIGENCE An unintentional tort involving four elements: duty, breach of duty, proximate cause, and damages.

NEPHRITIS Inflammation and abnormal function of the kidneys.

NEPHROTIC SYNDROME A clinical classification that includes all kidney diseases characterized by marked proteinuria, hypoalbuminemia, and edema.

NEUROGENIC BLADDER The loss of bladder control from lesions or damage to the nervous system.

NEUROGENIC SHOCK Also known as spinal shock, a form of distributive shock that causes loss of sympathetic (vasomotor) tone.

NEUROLEPTIC MALIGNANT SYNDROME A potentially fatal reaction to neuroleptic (antipsychotic) drugs characterized by fluctuating vital signs, altered consciousness, fever, muscle rigidity, diaphoresis, drooling, and an increased white blood cell count.

NOMINAL DAMAGES Reimbursement awarded to the plaintiff that indicates a defendant's wrongdoing when little, if any, injury occurred.

NYSTAGMUS Rapid, involuntary rolling or vertical movement of the eyeballs.

OBSESSION Ideas or thoughts that a person can't put out of his consciousness.

OBSESSIVE-COMPULSIVE DISORDER (OCD) A disorder characterized by recurrent obsessions (intrusive thoughts, images, and impulses) and compulsions (repetitive behaviors in response to an obsession).

OLIGURIA An abnormally low urine output (less than 500 ml/day) such that metabolic wastes can't be excreted.

OPHTHALMOSCOPE An instrument used to examine the internal structures of the eye.

OSTEOARTHRITIS Also known as degenerative joint disease, characterized by degeneration of cartilage in weight-bearing joints, such as the spine, knees, and hips that occurs when cartilage softens with age, narrowing the joint space. This allows bones to rub together, causing pain and limiting joint movement.

OSTEOMYELITIS An infection of the bone and bone marrow.

OSTEOPOROSIS A metabolic bone disorder in which the rate of bone resorption accelerates while the rate of bone formation slows down, causing a progressive loss of bone mass.

OTITIS MEDIA Inflammation of the middle ear that may be accompanied by infection. Fluid pressing on the tympanic membrane results in pain and leads to possible rupture or perforation.

OTOSCOPE An instrument used to examine the ear canal and tympanic membrane.

OXYTOCIN A posterior pituitary hormone that stimulates uterine contractions and also initiates the let-down reflex of lactation.

PALLIATIVE Relieving symptoms rather than curing a condition.

PALPATION Examining a client by using the hands to feel the shape, texture, consistency, and location of parts of the body.

PANCREATITIS An inflammation, either acute or chronic, of the pancreas.

PANIC DISORDER A disorder in which the client experiences a nonspecific feeling of terror and dread, accompanied by symptoms of physiologic stress.

PARALYTIC ILEUS A temporary paralysis of the intestines, causing abdominal distention and signs of bowel obstruction.

PARAPLEGIA An abnormal condition characterized by loss of sensation and motor function in the lower limbs, which may result in either complete or incomplete paralysis.

PARANOIA An intense, irrational suspicion that can't be changed by giving facts or explaining reality.

PARANOID PERSONALITY DISORDER A disorder characterized by extreme distrust of others.

PARANOID SCHIZOPHRENIA A disorder characterized by delusions unrelated to reality. In many cases, the client displays bizarre behavior, is easily angered, and is at high risk for violence.

PARESTHESIA An abnormal sensation (such as numbness, tingling, or burning) that lacks an objective cause.

PARKINSON'S DISEASE A slowly progressive disease that's characterized by tremor of resting muscles, a slowing of voluntary movements, a festinating gait, peculiar posture, and weakness of the muscles.

PASSIVE IMMUNITY A form of acquired resistance to an infection resulting from transfer of antibodies either naturally through the placenta to a fetus or through the colostrum to an infant, or artificially by inoculation of antiserum.

PATENT DUCTUS ARTERIOSUS (PDA) A defect resulting from the failure of the ductus to close causing shunting of blood to the pulmonary artery.

PATHOLOGIC JAUNDICE A yellowness of the skin caused by hyperbilirubinemia in the neonate that occurs within the first 24 hours after birth.

PATIENT'S BILL OF RIGHTS A document that defines a person's rights while receiving health care. It's designed to protect such basic rights as human dignity, privacy, confidentiality, informed consent, and refusal of treatment. The American Hospital Association, the National League for Nursing, the American Civil Liberties Union, and other organizations and health care facilities have prepared patient's bills of rights, and concepts expressed in these documents may be incorporated into law. Although bills of rights issued by health care facilities and professional organizations don't have the force of law, nurses should regard them as professionally binding.

PEPTIC ULCER An ulceration of the mucous membrane of the esophagus, stomach, or duodenum, caused by the action of the acid gastric juice.

PERCUSSION The act of striking the body with the fist or finger (for example, directly striking the kidney area) or the act of using both hands, by placing either the palm or middle finger on the client and striking with the other fist or finger indirectly (for example, percussing the thorax).

PERICARDITIS   An inflammation of the pericardium, which may be caused by trauma, neoplasm, infection, uremia, myocardial infarction, or collagen disease.

PERINATAL PERIOD   The time from conception through postpartum; also, the time extending from completion of the 20th to 28th week of gestation and ending 28 days after birth.

PERITONITIS   An inflammation of the peritoneum that can be produced by bacteria or irritating substances introduced into the abdominal cavity by a penetrating wound or an organ perforation.

PERNICIOUS ANEMIA   A chronic, progressive, macrocytic anemia caused by a deficiency of intrinsic factor, a substance normally secreted by the stomach. Without intrinsic factor, dietary vitamin B_{12} can't be absorbed by the ileum, inhibiting normal deoxyribonucleic acid (DNA) synthesis and resulting in defective maturation of red blood cells.

PERSONAL LIABILITY   Responsibility for one's acts.

PHYSICAL CARCINOGENESIS   The development of cancer as a result of environmental and other elements, such as ultraviolet radiation, precancerous lesions, acquired disorders (cirrhosis and hepatitis), diet-related foods, and obesity.

PLACENTA PREVIA   Implantation of the placenta so that it adjoins or covers the internal os of the uterine cervix.

PLAINTIFF   A person who files a civil lawsuit initiating a legal action. In criminal actions, the prosecution is the plaintiff acting on behalf of the people in the jurisdiction.

PLASMA   Liquid portion of the blood that's composed of water, proteins (albumin and globulin), glucose, and electrolytes.

PLEURAL EFFUSION   An accumulation of fluid in the interstitial and air spaces of the lung.

PLEURISY   Also known as pleuritis, an inflammation of the pleura characterized by dyspnea and stabbing pain, leading to restriction of breathing.

PNEUMOCYSTIS CARINII PNEUMONIA   Infection with the parasite *P. carinii*, which produces an interstitial plasma cell pneumonia commonly seen in debilitated or immunosuppressed clients.

PNEUMONIA   An acute infection of the lung parenchyma causing impaired gas exchange.

PNEUMOTHORAX   A collection of air in the pleural space that may result from an open chest wound that per-mits the entrance of air or from the rupture of a vesicle on the surface of the lung.

POINT OF MAXIMAL IMPULSE (PMI)   The location at the 4th or 5th left intercostal space, or the midclavicular line, where the heart is usually heard the loudest by using a stethoscope.

POLYCYTHEMIA VERA   A chronic myeloproliferative disorder characterized by increased red blood cell mass, leukocytosis, thrombocytosis, and increased hemoglobin concentration, with normal or increased plasma volume.

POSTTRAUMATIC STRESS DISORDER (PTSD)   A group of symptoms that develop after a traumatic event.

PRESENTATIONAL ISOLATION   Social withdrawal that results from changes in body image, mental or physical functional loss, or self-consciousness.

PRESSURED SPEECH   Frantic speech that's due to a person's attempt to keep up with racing thoughts.

PRIMARY GAIN   The control of anxiety through manifestation of symptoms.

PROJECTION   The unconscious defense mechanism of the ego whereby an individual attributes unacceptable ideas, feelings, and impulses to the external environment or to someone else.

PROXIMATE CAUSE   The causal connection between the breach of duty and the resulting injury.

PROXIMODISTAL   The point from the nearest to the farthest, as in the development of an organism. (For instance, infants gain control of the arm before the hand.)

PSORIASIS   A common, chronic dermatologic condition with polygenic inheritance. Marked by rounded red lesions covered by grayish or silvery white dry scales, psoriasis is caused by an overabundance of epithelial cells. Affected areas include nails, the scalp, genitalia, and the lumbosacral region.

PSYCHOMOTOR AGITATION   The continuous movement or performance of an activity designed to relieve distress.

PSYCHOMOTOR RETARDATION   The slowing of movements to such an extent that the individual appears to perform all physical activity in slow motion. Also, slow and difficult movement that approaches inactivity.

PSYCHOSIS   A condition characterized by major disturbances in ego functioning.

PULMONARY ARTERY STENOSIS   A narrowing or fusing of valve leaflets at the entrance of the pulmonary artery that interferes with right ventricular outflow.

PULMONARY EDEMA   The abnormal accumulation of fluid in the pulmonary tissues and air spaces due to changes in hydrostatic forces in the capillaries or to increased capillary permeability.

PULMONARY EMBOLISM Foreign matter that forms a blockage in a pulmonary artery and can be caused by fat, air, tumor tissue, or a thrombus that usually arises from a peripheral vein.

PULSE OXIMETRY A noninvasive monitoring of the oxygen saturation of arterial blood. A sensor is placed on a finger, a toe, or an earlobe to determine hemoglobin saturation.

PUNITIVE DAMAGES Compensation awarded to the plaintiff in special circumstances, usually to punish the defendant for an especially egregious or outrageous act.

PYLORIC STENOSIS A disorder in which hyperplasia and hypertrophy of the circular muscle at the pylorus cause a narrowing of the pyloric canal preventing the stomach from emptying normally.

QUADRIPLEGIA Paralysis of the arms, legs, and trunk of the body below the level of an associated injury to the spinal cord.

QUICKENING Fetal movement as perceived by the pregnant woman; first noticed between 16 and 20 weeks' gestation.

RADIOLABELED ANTIBODIES Tumor-specific antibodies coupled with radioactive isotopes that can be used to maximize tumor cell kill while sparing healthy tissue.

RATIONALIZATION The unconscious defense mechanism whereby an individual justifies thoughts, wishes, needs, drives, or actions that would otherwise be unacceptable to himself or others.

RAYNAUD'S DISEASE Intermittent bilateral ischemic attacks of the fingers or toes and, sometimes, the ears or nose, characterized by severe pallor and usually accompanied by paresthesia and pain.

REACTION FORMATION An unconscious defense mechanism whereby an individual develops behaviors and attitudes that directly oppose the individual's underlying feelings and attitudes.

REFRAMING Altering one's view of a situation.

REGRESSION An unconscious defense mechanism whereby an individual returns to an earlier, less mature level of functioning.

REGURGITATION Backward flow of fluid or solids from a cavity or tube (for instance, the backward flow of blood through a defective heart valve or stomach contents flowing into the throat and mouth).

RELAPSE A return to using a drug after a period of sobriety has occurred.

RENAL CALCULI Stones formed in the kidneys.

REPRESSION An unconscious defense mechanism whereby an individual keeps unacceptable ideas, impulses, or feelings from conscious awareness.

RESPIRATORY ACIDOSIS An acid-base disturbance caused by reduced alveolar ventilation. This condition is characterized by an excess of carbon dioxide in the blood (hypercapnia) and increased plasma hydrogen-ion concentration.

RESPIRATORY ALKALOSIS An acid-base disturbance characterized by decreased carbon dioxide in the blood (hypocapnia), a decreased hydrogen-ion concentration, and increased pH.

RESPIRATORY SYNCYTIAL VIRUS (RSV) A species of viruses belonging to the genus *Pneumovirus* that causes respiratory disease that can be severe in infants. RSV can lead to pneumonia and bronchiolitis.

RESPONDEAT SUPERIOR The principle that addresses an employer's responsibility for injuries caused by an employee's negligent acts if those acts were performed within the scope of employment and when an employment relationship existed.

RETICULAR ACTIVATING SYSTEM (RAS) A functional system in the brain that controls the overall degree of the central nervous system, including wakefulness, attention, concentration, and introspection.

RETINAL DETACHMENT Separation of the retina from the choroid (the middle vascular coat of the eye between the retina and the sclera), which occurs when the retina develops a hole or tear and the vitreous seeps between the retina and choroid. If untreated, can lead to vision loss.

REYE'S SYNDROME Acute encephalopathy and fatty infiltration of the internal organs following acute viral infections, such as influenza B, chickenpox (varicella), the enteroviruses, and Epstein-Barr virus. It has been associated with administration of aspirin and other salicylates in children.

RHEUMATIC FEVER An inflammatory disease that occurs if a group A beta-hemolytic streptococcal infection is inadequately treated.

RHEUMATIC HEART DISEASE A disease that causes damage to the heart muscle and valves as a result of rheumatic fever.

RHEUMATOID ARTHRITIS A chronic, systemic collagen disease marked by inflammation, stiffness, and pain in the joints and related structures that result in crippling deformities.

SARCOIDOSIS A disease in which granulomatous lesions affect organs and tissues of the body.

SCHIZOPHRENIA A brain disorder characterized by neuro-transmitter imbalances and structural changes within the brain.

SCLERODERMA A relatively rare autoimmune disease characterized by a chronic hardening and thickening of the skin and degeneration of the connective tissue of the skin, lungs, and internal organs.

SCOLIOSIS A lateral curvature of the spine.

SECLUSION An extreme last course of action taken to maintain client safety by placing the person in a room where the nurse can provide protection and intensive monitoring.

SECONDARY GAIN Any benefit that an individual experiences as a result of having a symptom or an illness.

SELF-MUTILATION A self-inflicted action that causes pain or injury without actually attempting to kill oneself.

SEPTIC SHOCK The result of bacterial infection that causes inadequate blood perfusion and circulatory collapse.

SICKLE CELL ANEMIA A chronic and incurable hereditary disorder occurring in people homozygous for hemoglobin S, resulting in erythrocyte fragility.

SITUATION REPETITION When bothersome or problematic behavior is repeated during the course of therapy.

SOMATOFORM DISORDER A disorder characterized by the literal transference of inner conflict onto a body part, commonly resulting in crippling. Clients with somatoform disorders channel anxiety through a body system.

SOUFFLE The soft, blowing sound auscultated as fetal blood flows through the umbilical arteries (funic souffle) or as maternal blood enters the uterine arteries (uterine souffle).

SPINA BIFIDA A congenital cleft of the vertebral column with hernial protrusion of the meninges and sometimes the spinal cord.

SPINAL CORD INJURY A traumatic disruption of the spinal cord, usually accompanied by extensive musculoskeletal involvement.

SPONTANEOUS ABORTION Expulsion of the fetus from the uterus before the 20th week of gestation caused by fetal abnormalities or maternal environment.

STAPHYLORRHAPHY Surgical correction of a midline cleft in the uvula and soft palate.

STATE ANXIETY Anxiety experienced under specific conditions.

STENOSIS The narrowing of the lumen of a tube or body opening.

STEREOTACTIC EXTERNAL-BEAM IRRADIATION A type of radiation that uses a three-dimensional distribution of the radiation beam in the treatment of relatively small intracranial benign lesions, such as arteriovenous malformations, or malignant astrocytomas and brain metastases.

STOMATITIS An inflammation of the oral mucous membrane.

STROKE A condition of sudden onset in which a cerebral blood vessel is occluded by an embolus or a cerebrovascular hemorrhage. Also known as a cerebrovascular accident, or CVA.

SUBLIMATION The process of substituting acceptable activities for impulses that aren't socially acceptable.

SUBSTANCE ABUSE DISORDER A disorder that's characterized by a maladaptive pattern of substance use manifested by recurrent and significant adverse consequences related to the repeated use of substances.

SUDDEN INFANT DEATH SYNDROME (SIDS) The sudden, unexpected, and inexplicable death of an infant who appears healthy. It occurs during sleep, typically in infants between ages 3 weeks and 5 months.

SUPEREGO A part of the personality that's commonly called the conscience or the moral component of the personality.

SYPHILIS An infectious disease, usually transmitted by sexual contact or acquired in utero, that's caused by the spirochete *Treponema pallidum*.

SYSTEMIC LUPUS ERYTHEMATOSUS (SLE) A chronic inflammatory multisystemic disorder of connective tissue characterized principally by involvement of the skin, joints, kidneys, and serosal membranes.

TARDIVE DYSKINESIA A serious, irreversible adverse effect of long-term phenothiazine therapy; symptoms include gait disturbances and involuntary, bizarre movements of the face, tongue, neck, trunk, or pelvis.

T CELLS Also known as lymphocytes, any of the mononuclear, nonphagocytic leukocytes found in the blood, lymph, and lymphoid tissues that are responsible for the body's cellular immunity.

TERATOGEN A substance that causes severely deformed fetal parts. Examples include alcohol, vitamin A, retinoic acid (in excessive doses), rubella virus, and syphilis bacteria.

TETANY Twitching, cramps, and muscle spasms that are caused by hypocalcemia.

TETRALOGY OF FALLOT A congenital anomaly of the heart characterized by pulmonic stenosis, ventricular septal defect, overriding position or dextroposition of the aorta, and compensatory right ventricular hypertrophy.

THORACIC AORTIC ANEURYSM An aneurysm that affects part of the thoracic aorta.

THROMBOCYTE A blood platelet.

THROMBOCYTOPENIA A reduction in the number of blood platelets, usually caused by destruction of erythroid tissue in bone marrow, that may be a result of neoplastic disease or an immune response to a drug.

THROMBOPHLEBITIS Inflammation of a vein that's commonly associated with clot formation.

THYROIDITIS A painful inflammation of the thyroid gland. Acute thyroiditis is caused by infections, such as staphylococcal or streptococcal infections, and its symptoms include abscesses.

TINNITUS Ringing or cracking in one or both ears.

TORT A private wrong or a breach of a legal duty to the rights and interests of another.

TRAIT ANXIETY Anxiety experienced most of the time regardless of the circumstances.

TRANSILLUMINATION The act of observing a body part by shining a light through the part and viewing the quality and quantity of light on the other side.

TRANSPOSITION OF THE GREAT VESSELS A developmental cardiac anomaly characterized by the aorta arising from the right ventricle and the pulmonary artery arising from the left ventricle.

TRICUSPID INSUFFICIENCY The incomplete closure of the tricuspid valve resulting in tricuspid regurgitation.

TRICUSPID VALVULAR ATRESIA A defect characterized by absence of the tricuspid valve and no blood flow between the right atrium and right ventricle, a small right ventricle and large left ventricle, and diminished pulmonary circulation.

TRIGEMINAL NEURALGIA Also called tic douloureux, a painful disorder of one or more branches of the fifth cranial (trigeminal) nerve that produces paroxysmal attacks of excruciating facial pain precipitated by stimulation of a trigger zone.

TUBERCULOSIS (TB) An infectious disease caused by a species of *Mycobacterium* and characterized by the formation of tubercles and caseous necrosis in the tissues. The lung is the major organ affected in TB.

ULCERATIVE COLITIS A chronic, recurrent ulceration in the colon, commonly of the mucosa and submucosa, characterized by cramping abdominal pain, rectal bleeding, and loose discharges of blood, pus, and mucus with scanty fecal particles.

UNDOING An unconscious ego defense mechanism whereby an individual acts to reverse the effects of a previous act.

UNINTENTIONAL TORT An act that fails to meet a duty owed to another person (the plaintiff) and leads to the other person's injury.

URINARY TRACT INFECTION (UTI) A bacterial infection, most commonly caused by *Escherichia coli* or a species of *Klebsiella*, *Proteus*, *Pseudomonas*, or *Enterobacter*, affecting one or more parts of the urinary tract.

VALVULAR HEART DISEASE A disorder characterized by stenosis of a cardiac valve, resulting in obstruction of the flow of blood, or degeneration of the valve, which leads to reflux of blood.

VASCULITIS A disorder in which the blood vessels are inflamed, either from an allergic reaction or as a result of disease.

VENTRICULAR SEPTAL DEFECT A defect that occurs when the ventricular septum fails to complete its formation between the ventricles, resulting in a left-to-right shunt.

VENTRICULOPERITONEAL SHUNT A diversion of cerebrospinal fluid from the cerebral ventricles to the peritoneal cavity using a one-way flow valve and a tubing system.

VERNIX A cheesy substance that covers and protects the fetal body.

VICARIOUS LIABILITY A type of liability in which one is found to have responsibility for the actions of another because a relationship exists between those individuals, such as an employer-employee relationship.

VIRAL CARCINOGENESIS The development of cancer as a result of viral illnesses, such as hepatitis B and hepatocellular carcinoma, herpes virus, herpes simplex type 2, human papillomavirus, and T-cell leukemia or lymphoma.

WITHDRAWAL An adverse physical or psychological reaction to abstinence from a substance to which the individual has become addicted.

Selected references

Introduction to the fundamentals of nursing

Anatomy & Physiology Made Incredibly Easy. Springhouse, Pa.: Springhouse Corp., 2001.

Bickley, L.S., and Szilagyi, P.G. *Bates' Guide to Physical Examination and History Taking,* 8th ed. Philadelphia: Lippincott Williams & Wilkins, 2003.

Craven, R.F., and Hirnle, C.J. *Fundamentals of Nursing: Human Health and Function,* 3rd ed. Philadelphia: Lippincott Williams & Wilkins, 2000.

Dudek, S.G. *Nutrition Essentials for Nursing Practice,* 4th ed. Philadelphia: Lippincott Williams & Wilkins, 2001.

Elkin, M.K., et al. *Nursing Interventions and Clinical Skills,* 2nd ed. St. Louis: Mosby–Year Book, Inc., 2000.

Fuller, J., and Schaller-Ayers, J. *Health Assessment: A Nursing Approach,* 3rd ed. Philadelphia: Lippincott Williams & Wilkins, 2000.

Kee, J.L., and Hayes, E.R. *Pharmacology: A Nursing Process Approach,* 3rd. ed. Philadelphia: W.B. Saunders Co., 2000.

Kelley, M.L., and Fitzsimons, V.M., eds. *Understanding Cultural Diversity: Culture, Curriculum, and Community in Nursing.* Sudbury, Mass.: Jones and Bartlett Pubs., Inc., 2000.

Kozier, B., et al. *Fundamentals of Nursing: Concepts, Process, and Practice,* 6th ed. Upper Saddle River, N.J.: Prentice Hall Health, 2000.

Lippincott Professional Guides: Medical Terms and Abbreviations. Springhouse, Pa.: Lippincott Williams & Wilkins, 2002.

Nursing Procedures, 3rd ed. Springhouse, Pa.: Springhouse Corp., 2000.

Pathophysiology Made Incredibly Easy, 2nd ed. Springhouse, Pa.: Springhouse Corp., 2002.

Perry, A.G. and Potter, P.A. *Clinical Nursing Skills & Techniques,* 5th ed. St. Louis: Mosby–Year Book, Inc., 2002.

Smith-Temple, J., and Johnson, J.Y. *Nurses' Guide to Clinical Procedures,* 4th ed. Philadelphia: Lippincott Williams & Wilkins, 2002.

Townsend, C.E., and Roth, R.A. *Nutrition and Diet Therapy,* 7th ed. Albany, N.Y.: Delmar Pubs., 2000.

Weber, J., and Kelley, J. *Health Assessment in Nursing,* 2nd ed. Philadelphia: Lippincott Williams & Wilkins, 2002.

The nursing process

Ackley, B.J., and Ladwig, G.B. *Nursing Diagnosis Handbook: A Guide to Planning Care,* 5th ed. St. Louis: Mosby–Year Book, Inc., 2002.

Alfaro-LeFevre, R. *Applying Nursing Process: Promoting Collaborative Care,* 5th ed. Philadelphia: Lippincott Williams & Wilkins, 2002.

Carpenito, L.J. *Handbook of Nursing Diagnosis,* 9th ed. Philadelphia: Lippincott Williams & Wilkins, 2002.

Carpenito, L.J. *Nursing Diagnosis: Application to Clinical Practice.* Philadelphia: Lippincott Williams & Wilkins, 2001.

Cox, H., et al. *Clinical Applications of Nursing Diagnosis: Adult, Child, Women's, Psychiatric, Gerontic, and Home Health Considerations,* 4th ed. Philadelphia: F.A. Davis, Co., 2002.

Doenges, M.E., et al. *Application of Nursing Process and Nursing Diagnosis: An Interactive Text for Diagnostic Reasoning,* 3rd ed. Philadelphia: F.A. Davis Co., 2000.

Doenges, M.E., et al. *Nursing Care Plans: Guidelines for Individualizing Patient Care,* 5th ed. Philadelphia: F.A. Davis Co., 2000.

Gordon, M. *Manual of Nursing Diagnosis,* 10th ed. St. Louis: Mosby–Year Book, Inc., 2002.

Johnson, M., et al. *Nursing Outcomes Classification (NOC),* 2nd ed. St. Louis: Mosby–Year Book, Inc., 2000.

Lilley, L.L., and Aucker, R.S. *Pharmacology and the Nursing Process,* 3rd ed. St. Louis: Mosby–Year Book, Inc., 2001.

McCloskey, J.C., and Bulechek, G.M. *Nursing Interventions Classification (NIC),* 3rd ed. St. Louis: Mosby–Year Book, Inc., 2000.

Sparks, S.M., and Taylor, C.M. *Nursing Diagnosis Reference Manual,* 5th ed. Springhouse, Pa.: Springhouse Corp., 2001.

Ulrich, S.P., and Canale, S.W. *Nursing Care Planning Guides: For Adults in Acute, Extended, and Home Care Settings,* 5th ed. Philadelphia: W.B. Saunders Co., 2001.

Wilkinson, J.M. *Nursing Diagnosis Handbook with NIC Interventions and NOC Outcomes,* 7th ed. Upper Saddle River, N.J.: Prentice Hall Health, 2000.

Client needs

Eyles, M. *Mosby's Comprehensive Review of Practical Nursing for NCLEX-PN,* 13th ed. St. Louis: Mosby–Year Book, Inc., 2001.

Healy, P.F. *American Nursing Review: Questions & Answers for NCLEX-PN,* 2nd edition. Springhouse, Pa.: Springhouse Corp., 2001.

Silvestri, L.A. *Saunder's Comprehensive Review for NCLEX-PN.* Philadelphia: W.B. Saunders Co., 2000.

Silvestri, L.A. *Saunder's Q&A Review for NCLEX-PN.* Philadelphia: W.B. Saunders Co., 2000.

Medical-surgical nursing

Abrams, A.C., and Goldsmith, T.L. *Clinical Drug Therapy: Rationales for Nursing Practice,* 6th ed. Philadelphia: Lippincott Williams & Wilkins, 2001.

Assessment Made Incredibly Easy, 2nd ed. Philadelphia: Lippincott Williams & Wilkins, 2002.

Black, J.M., et al. *Medical Surgical Nursing: Clinical Management for Positive Outcomes,* 6th ed. Philadelphia: W.B. Saunders Co., 2001.

Bryant, R.A. *Acute and Chronic Wounds: Nursing Management,* 2nd ed. St. Louis: Mosby–Year Book, Inc., 2000.

Clinical Laboratory Tests: Values and Implications, 3rd ed. Springhouse, Pa.: Springhouse Corp., 2001.

Corrigan, A., et al. *Core Curriculum for Intravenous Nursing, Intravenous Nurses Society,* 2nd ed. Philadelphia: Lippincott Williams & Wilkins, 2000.

Diagnostics: An A-to-Z Nursing Guide to Laboratory Tests & Diagnostic Procedures. Springhouse, Pa.: Springhouse Corp., 2001.

Diseases, 3rd ed. Springhouse, Pa.: Springhouse Corp., 2001.

Fischbach, F.T. *A Manual of Laboratory and Diagnostic Tests,* 6th ed. Philadelphia: Lippincott Williams & Wilkins, 2000.

Fluids and Electrolytes Made Incredibly Easy, 2nd ed. Philadelphia: Lippincott Williams & Wilkins, 2002.

Handbook of Medical-Surgical Nursing, 3rd ed. Springhouse, Pa.: Springhouse Corp., 2001.

Handbook of Pathophysiology. Springhouse, Pa.: Springhouse Corp., 2001.

Hess, C.T. *Wound Care,* 4th ed. Springhouse, Pa.: Springhouse Corp., 2002.

Ignatavicius, D.D., and Workman, M.L. *Medical-Surgical Nursing: Critical Thinking for Collaborative Care,* 4th ed. Philadelphia: W.B. Saunders Co., 2002.

Intravenous Nurses Association. "Infusion Nursing Standards of Practice," *Journal of Intravenous Nursing* 23(6S):S1-S88, November-December 2000.

I.V. Therapy Made Incredibly Easy, 2nd ed. Philadelphia: Lippincott Williams & Wilkins, 2002.

Kee, J.L., and Paulanka, B.J., eds. *Handbook of Fluid, Electrolyte, and Acid-base Imbalances.* Albany, N.Y.: Delmar Pubs., 2000.

Lewis, S.M., et al., eds. *Medical-Surgical Nursing: Assessment and Management of Clinical Problems,* 5th ed. St. Louis: Mosby–Year Book, Inc., 2000.

Luecknotte, A. *Gerontologic Nursing,* 2nd ed. St. Louis: Mosby–Year Book, Inc., 2000.

Maklebust, J., and Sieggreen, M. *Pressure Ulcers: Guidelines for Prevention and Management,* 3rd ed. Springhouse, Pa.: Springhouse Corp., 2001.

Nursing 2003 Drug Handbook. Springhouse, Pa.: Springhouse Corp., 2002.

Nursing I.V. Drug Handbook, 7th ed. Springhouse, Pa.: Springhouse Corp., 2001.

Nursing Procedures, 3rd ed. Springhouse, Pa.: Springhouse Corp., 2000.

Pagana, K.D., and Pagana, T.J. *Mosby's Diagnostic and Laboratory Test Reference,* 5th ed. St. Louis: Mosby–Year Book, Inc., 2001.

Purnell, L.D., and Paulanka, B.J. *Transcultural Health Care: A Culturally Competent Approach.* Philadelphia: F.A. Davis Co., 1998.

Redman, B.K. *The Practice of Patient Education,* 9th ed. St. Louis: Mosby–Year Book, Inc., 2001.

Smeltzer, S.C., and Bare, B.G. *Brunner and Suddarth's Textbook of Medical-Surgical Nursing,* 9th ed. Philadelphia: Lippincott Williams & Wilkins, 2000.

Sussman, C., and Bates-Jensen, B.M. *Wound Care: A Collaborative Practice Manual for Physical Therapists and Nurses,* 2nd ed. Gaithersburg, Md.: Aspen Pubs., Inc., 2001.

Mental health nursing

Boyd, M.A. *Psychiatric Nursing: Contemporary Practice,* 2nd ed. Philadelphia: Lippincott Williams & Wilkins, 2002.

Carson, V.B. *Mental Health Nursing: The Nurse-Patient Journey,* 2nd. ed. Philadelphia: W.B. Saunders Co., 2000.

Copel, L.C. *Psychiatric and Mental Health Care,* 2nd ed. Springhouse, Pa.: Springhouse Corp., 2000.

Fortinash, K.M., and Holoday-Worret, P.A. *Psychiatric Mental Health Nursing,* 2nd ed. St. Louis: Mosby–Year Book, Inc., 2000.

Purnell, L.D., and Paulanka, B.J. *Transcultural Health Care: A Culturally Competent Approach.* Philadelphia: F.A. Davis Co., 1998.

Shives, L.R. and Isaacs, A. *Basic Concepts of Psychiatric-Mental Health Nursing,* 5th ed. Philadelphia: Lippincott Williams & Wilkins, 2002.

Stuart, G.W. *Pocket Guide to Psychiatric Nursing,* 5th ed. St. Louis: Mosby–Year Book, Inc., 2002.

Stuart, G.W., and Laraia, M.T. *Principles and Practice of Psychiatric Nursing,* 7th ed. St. Louis: Mosby–Year Book, Inc., 2001.

Townsend, M.C. *Psychiatric Mental Health Nursing: Concepts of Care,* 3rd ed. Philadelphia: F.A. Davis Co., 2000.

Varcarolis, E.M. *Foundations of Psychiatric Mental Health Nursing: A Clinical Approach,* 4th ed. Philadelphia: W.B. Saunders Co., 2002.

Videbeck, S.D. *Psychiatric Mental Health Nursing.* Philadelphia: Lippincott Williams & Wilkins, 2001.

Maternal-neonatal nursing

Burroughs, A. and Leifer, G. *Maternity Nursing: An Introductory Text,* 8th ed. Philadelphia: W.B. Saunders Co., 2001.

Doenges, M.E., and Moorhouse, M.F. *Maternal/Newborn Plans of Care: Guidelines for Individualizing Care,* 3rd ed. Philadelphia: F.A. Davis Co., 1999.

Kenner, C., et al. *Comprehensive Neonatal Nursing: A Physiologic Perspective,* 2nd ed. Philadelphia: W.B. Saunders Co., 1998.

Lowdermilk, D.L., et al. *Maternity Nursing,* 6th ed. St. Louis: Mosby–Year Book, Inc., 2003.

Mandeville, L.K., and Troiano, N.H. *AWHONN's High Risk and Critical Care Intrapartum Nursing,* 2nd ed. Philadelphia: Lippincott Williams & Wilkins, 1999.

McKinney, E.S, et al. *Maternal-Child Nursing.* Philadelphia: W.B. Saunders Co., 2000.

Melson, K.A., et al. *Maternal-Infant Care Planning,* 3rd ed. Springhouse, Pa.: Springhouse Corp., 1999.

Murray, S., et al. *Foundations of Maternal-Newborn Nursing,* 3rd ed. Philadelphia: W.B. Saunders Co., 2002.

Nursing Procedures, 3rd ed. Springhouse, Pa.: Springhouse Corp., 2000.

Pathophysiology Made Incredibly Easy, 2nd ed. Philadelphia: Lippincott Williams & Wilkins, Corp., 2002.

Pillitteri, A. *Maternal & Child Health Nursing: Care of the Childbearing and Childrearing Family,* 4th ed. Philadelphia: Lippincott Williams & Wilkins, 2002.

Purnell, L.D., and Paulanka, B.J. *Transcultural Health Care: A Culturally Competent Approach.* Philadelphia: F.A. Davis Co., 1998.

Wong, D.L., et al. *Maternal Child Nursing Care,* 2nd ed. St. Louis: Mosby–Year Book, Inc., 2002.

Zastocki, D., and Rovenski-Wagner, C. *Home Care: Patient and Family Instructions,* 2nd edition. Philadelphia: W.B. Saunders Co., 2000.

Pediatric nursing

Baggort, C., et al., eds. *Nursing Care of Children and Adolescents with Cancer,* 3rd ed. Philadelphia: W.B. Saunders Co., 2002.

Handbook of Pediatric Drug Therapy, 2nd ed. Springhouse, Pa.: Springhouse Corp., 2000.

King, C., and Henretig, F.M. *Pocket Atlas of Pediatric Emergency Procedures.* Philadelphia: Lippincott Williams & Wilkins, 2000.

Muscari, M. *Advanced Pediatric Clinical Assessment.* Philadelphia: Lippincott Williams & Wilkins, 2001.

Nursing Procedures, 3rd ed. Springhouse, Pa.: Springhouse Corp., 2000.

Purnell, L.D., and Paulanka, B.J. *Transcultural Health Care: A Culturally Competent Approach.* Philadelphia: F.A. Davis Co., 1998.

Schwartz, M.W., et al. *The 5-minute Pediatric Consult,* 2nd ed. Philadelphia: Lippincott Williams & Wilkins, 2000.

Sussman, C., and Bates-Jensen, B.M. *Wound Care: A Collaborative Practice Manual for Physical Therapists and Nurses,* 2nd ed. Gaithersburg, Md.: Aspen Pubs., Inc., 2001.

Velasco-Whetsell, M., et al. *Pediatric Nursing.* New York: McGraw-Hill Book Co., 2000.

Wong, D.L. *Wong's Essentials of Pediatric Nursing,* 6th ed. St. Louis: Mosby–Year Book, Inc., 2001.

Index

i refers to an illustration; t refers to a table.

---

i refers to an illustration; t refers to a table.

i refers to an illustration; t refers to a table.

Hernia, hiatal, 454-455
Herniated disk, 363-365, 363i
Heroin, abuse of, 142t
Herpes simplex virus, 484-485
Herpes zoster, 376-377
High Fowler's position, xi, xx, 499t
Hip
  developmental dysplasia of, 209-212, 210i
  fracture of, xiv, xxiv, 365-369
Hip bath, 483
Hip-spica cast, care of, 212
Hirschsprung's disease, 215-218, 217t
Histamine-2 receptor antagonist, 511t
Histrionic personality disorder, 127t
Hodgkin's disease, 421, 422
Homans' sign, testing for, 93
Home health care, principles of, 46-47
Homeostasis, maintaining, 60-84
Hormones
  effect of pregnancy on, 154
  thyroid gland, 253
Hot pack, applying, 361
Hot-water bottle, applying, 361
Human immunodeficiency virus infection, 406, 407
  nursing care in, 408
Hydatidiform mole, 160t, 165-166
Hydrocarbon poisoning, 229t
Hydrocephalus, 219
Hydrochlorothiazide, 510t
Hymen, 465
Hyperbilirubinemia, 197
Hypercalcemia, 78, 79, 80
Hypercortisolism, 383
Hyperemesis gravidarum, 160t, 166-167
Hyperglycemia, 258, 259
Hyperkalemia, 77, 78
Hypernatremia, 75, 76
Hyperosmolar hyperglycemic nonketotic syndrome, 386
Hypertension, 287-289, 288i
  portal vein, 438t
  pregnancy-induced, 168-170, 169t
  symptoms of, 522, 532
Hyperthyroidism, 388-389
Hypoalbuminemia, cirrhosis and, 438t
Hypocalcemia, 78, 79
Hypochondriasis, 140
Hypodermis, 372
Hypoglycemia, 258, 259, 386
Hypoglycemic agents, 511t
Hypokalemia, 76, 77
Hyponatremia, 75, 76
Hypoplastic left heart syndrome, 235, 236
Hypothalamus, 300, 381
Hypothermia, neonatal, 195-196
Hypothyroidism, 253-254, 389-390, 524, 534, 535
Hysterectomy
  abdominal, 478, 484
  evisceration following, 524, 535

I

Ibuprofen, xx, xxx, 522, 531
Ice bag, applying, 362
Ilotycin, xvii, xxvii
Immediacy, in therapeutic communication, 24t
Immobility, 82-84

Immune system
  disorders of, 406-431. *See also specific condition.*
  in neonate, 190
  structure and function of, 405-406
Immunization schedule, childhood, 501-502t
Immunoglobulins, 406
Imperforate anus, 216t
Implantation, 151-152
Implant system, as contraceptive method, 149t
Implementation, nursing process and, 14, 14i
Incentive spirometer, 86
Incompetency, 19, 20
Increased intracranial pressure, 312-314
  in children, 221, 520, 529
Indwelling urinary catheter, inserting, 469
Infants
  disorders in, 199-228, 258. *See also specific condition.*
  iron needs in, 232
  nutrition requirements in, 37
  skin turgor in, 81
Infection
  active, 523, 533
  cast and, 523, 533
  chlamydial, 478
  neonatal, 196-197
  puerperal, 188-189
Infection control
  home health care and, 47
  principles of, 47-49
Inflammation, 60-61
Informed consent, 18
Infusion, through secondary I.V. line, 57
Inhalants, abuse of, 142t
Injections, types of, 57
Inspection, 52
Insulin, 381, 511t
  administration of, 260
  NPH, xvii, xix, xxvii, xxix, 7, 525
Insulin lipodystrophy, 524, 534
Integumentary system
  in cystic fibrosis, 263
  disorders of, 372-380. *See also specific condition.*
  effect of aging on, 44
  effect of pregnancy on, 154
  structure and function of, 372
Intentional tort, 18
Intestinal flu, 449
Intestinal obstruction, 455-456
Intra-aortic balloon pump, 66
Intradermal injection, 57
Intramuscular injection, 57
Intrapartum period, 171-182
  complications of, 178-182
  data collection in, 171-173
Intrauterine device, 148t
Intussusception, 216t
Invasion of privacy, 18
Iodine, 38t
Iris, 394
Iron, 38t
Iron deficiency anemia, 230-232, 410-411, 519, 528
Iron dextran, 518, 527
Irritable bowel syndrome, 456-457
Isolation, aging and, 45

Isolation precautions, Centers for Disease Control and Prevention, 47, 48
Isoniazid, xvi, xxvi, 355
Isotretinoin, 524, 535
I.V. administration, 57
  calculation in, xiii, xxii, xvii, xxviii, 517, 526

J

Jaundice, in neonate, 191, 197-198
Jehovah's Witnesses, 50t
Jejunostomy tube, 444t
Joints, 356
  bleeding into, 418
Judaism, 51t
Judicial opinion, 16

K

K pad, applying, 361, 362
Kaposi's sarcoma, 418-420
Kernig's sign, 314
Ketoacidosis, xix, xxix, 386
Kidneys, structure of, 464
Kidney stones, 489
Kübler-Ross, and stages of grieving, 43
Kussmaul's respirations, 73

L

la belle indifference, 139
Labia majora, 465
Labia minora, 465
Labor. *See also* Labor and delivery.
  onset of, 173
  preterm, 161, 181-183
  stages of, 174-175t, 175
Labor and delivery, 171-182
  care plan in, xv, xxiv
  coach's role during, xii, xxi
  complications of, 178-182
  maternal responses to, 177
  nursing care during, 176
  pain relief during, 177
  physiologic changes after, 183
  and urinary tract infection, 518, 526
Labyrinth, 395
Laceration
  during labor and delivery, 180-181
  spinal cord, 323
Lactic acid, and panic attacks, 118
Laminectomy, 364
Landry's syndrome, 310
Laniazid, 507t
Lanoxin, 517, 526
Large intestine, structure of, 432
Laryngeal cancer, 401
Laryngectomy, 401
Laryngopharynx, 395
Laryngotracheobronchitis, acute, 201t
Larynx, 331
Lasix, 510t
Lateral position, 499t
Law
  sources of, 15
  types of, 16
Lead poisoning, 229t
Leg, fractures of, 357-358
Legal competence, 20
Legal principles, 15-22
Legal reporter system, 16

i refers to an illustration; t refers to a table.

---

i refers to an illustration; t refers to a table.

---

i refers to an illustration; t refers to a table.

SPRINGHOUSE REVIEW FOR NCLEX-PN CD-ROM

The *Springhouse Review for NCLEX-PN CD-ROM* is a review-and-test program that gives you unprecedented flexibility in preparing for the NCLEX-PN. This program contains more than 750 NCLEX-style questions. It's designed to pose questions randomly, so you can test yourself repeatedly. You can tailor your test or review to cover any combination of 29 nursing topics, 5 nursing process steps, or 4 client needs categories. The program provides the correct answer and rationales after each question and a performance appraisal at the end of the test. This feature allows you to review any weak areas identified in the performance appraisal.

To operate *Springhouse Review for NCLEX-PN*, we recommend that you have the following computer equipment, at a minimum:

- IBM-compatible personal computer
- Windows®98 or higher
- Pentium 133 MHz or higher (166 MHz recommended)
- 64 MB RAM or more
- 15 MB of free hard-disk space (85 MB of free hard-disk space if Internet Explorer 5.0 must be installed)
- SVGA monitor with High Color (16-bit) — Display area must be set to 800 × 600
- CD-ROM drive
- Mouse
- Internet Explorer 5.0

Installation on Windows®98 or higher

Before installing the *Springhouse Review for NCLEX-PN* program, make sure that your monitor is set up to display High Color (16-bit) or greater and that your display area is set to 800 × 600. If it isn't, consult your monitor's user's manual for instructions about changing the display settings. (The display settings are typically found in the *Start/Settings/Control Panel/Display/Settings* tab.) Set the color palette equal to High Color (16-bit) or True Color (24-bit) and the Display Area to 800 × 600.

To install this program onto the hard drive of your computer, follow these steps:
1. Start Windows®98 or higher.
2. Place the CD in your CD-ROM drive and close the tray. After a few moments, *Springhouse Review for NCLEX-PN* will automatically begin the install process.
3. Follow the on-screen instructions.
Note: If the install program doesn't automatically begin, click the "Start" menu and select "Run." Type **d:\setup.exe** (where **d:** is the letter of your CD-ROM drive) and click *OK*.

For technical support, call toll free 1-800-638-3030, Monday through Friday, 8:30 a.m. to 5 p.m., Eastern Time. You may also write to Lippincott Williams & Wilkins Technical Support, 351 W. Camden Street, Baltimore, Maryland 21201-2436, or e-mail at *techsupp@lww.com*.